Practical Approach to Imaging in Pediatric Oncology

Ishan Kumar • Ashish Verma
Manisha Jana
Editors

Practical Approach to Imaging in Pediatric Oncology

Springer

Editors
Ishan Kumar
Department of Radiodiagnosis and Imaging
Institute of Medical Sciences, Banaras Hindu University
Varanasi, Uttar Pradesh, India

Ashish Verma
Department of Radiodiagnosis and Imaging
Institute of Medical Sciences, Banaras Hindu University
Varanasi, Uttar Pradesh, India

Manisha Jana
Department of Radiodiagnosis and Interventional Radiology
All India Institute of Medical Sciences
New Delhi, India

ISBN 978-981-96-8157-0   ISBN 978-981-96-8158-7 (eBook)
https://doi.org/10.1007/978-981-96-8158-7

This Springer imprint is published by the registered company Springer Nature Singapore Pte Ltd.
The registered company address is: 152 Beach Road, #21-01/04 Gateway East, Singapore 189721, Singapore

This book is dedicated to the ***brave children*** *who, in the face of unimaginable adversity, have battled pediatric cancer with resilience, courage, and hope. Their strength serves as a beacon of inspiration, reminding us all that the human spirit, though small, can shine brighter than the darkest of trials. As the poet A.A. Milne once wrote, "You are braver than you believe, stronger than you seem, and smarter than you think."*

To the ***survivors****—the warriors who, against all odds, have emerged victorious—this work is a tribute to your indomitable will and unyielding hope. To those who have fought and triumphed, and to those whose battles continue, your courage is a light that guides us all.*

This book is also dedicated to the ***parents*** *who, with unshakable faith and love, stand as pillars of strength for their children. You are the unsung warriors, whose sacrifices and sleepless nights speak volumes about the power of parental love. Your courage in the face of adversity is captured in the timeless sentiment, "To the world, you may be one person, but to one person, you are the world." Your sacrifices, your unspoken tears, and your unwavering faith are the quiet force behind every victory.*

This book stands as a testament to you both—the children and the parents—whose journeys define what it means to fight with hope and love.

Foreword

> Gaining knowledge is the first step to wisdom. Sharing it, is the first step to humanity. (Anonymous)

Children getting affected by cancer is a sad reality. Fortunately, advances in healthcare, technology, and collaborations among different streams of science as well as collaborations across the world have improved outcomes and survival in many pediatric cancers. Cancer diagnostics and treatment is one of the most researched and fastest advancing fields of medicine. Thanks to these efforts there is wealth of knowledge in cancer imaging that radiologists and oncologists need to apply in their day-to-day clinical practice. This new book, *Practical Approach to Imaging in Pediatric Oncology*, is a welcome addition to the available resources. It aims to provide thorough information on radiological findings in pediatric oncology, with a particular emphasis on algorithmic reasoning to enhance diagnostic accuracy and management strategies.

This book is edited by the talented team of Dr. Ishan Kumar, Dr. Ashish Verma, and Dr. Manisha Jana. Professors Kumar, Verma, and Jana are well-known radiologists and well-published academicians with years of experience in the field. The proper use of imaging tests requires teamwork and clear communication between radiologists and clinicians. Keeping this in mind, the editors have gathered experts in oncology and radiology from all over India to write chapters in this book. This book offers to benefit oncologists and radiologists from the collective experience and expertise of editors and authors and ultimately, the children we care for.

The editors have done outstanding job of conceptualizing the book with each chapter including essential components like consensus guidelines on management and diagnostic work up for individual tumors or group of malignant conditions, algorithmic approach to interpretation, structured reporting, post-treatment changes on imaging, and future directions. The well-illustrated book is divided into five parts with the first part explaining general concepts, principles, and techniques in oncologic imaging. Other parts cover malignancies in the head and neck region, thoracic and musculoskeletal region, abdominal region, and role of interventional radiology in oncology. Experienced medical surgical oncologists provide clinical perspectives that will be beneficial to radiologists.

In summary, this book provides wholesome comprehensive coverage of oncologic imaging in children, and has the ability to become a bedside or reading room reference book for pediatric oncologic imaging. I congratulate editors and authors on this excellent academic endeavor. To you, the readers, I wish enjoyable reading and learning from this book!

Govind B. Chavhan
The Hospital for Sick Children, Toronto
ON, Canada
University of Toronto, Toronto
ON, Canada

Preface

"Children are not just little adults," a statement which lies at the heart of concept building for most while we differentially learn how to attend to the health needs of little ones over and above what we know about the adult population. "Imaging in pediatric oncology" is one of the lesser trodden paths with paucity of organized literature in a clinically relevant teaching format. The concept and necessity of the book emanated from this very observation. Further, the queries we faced in our everyday practice while interacting with our patients, students, and referring doctors gave a structure to our abstract vision. Being in a university-based tertiary care referral center catering to a huge catchment area of patient population we have been encountering pediatric oncological conditions with diverse array of complex clinical scenarios, both enface and on treatment. This book makes an effort to establish an algorithmic approach one should follow while managing such clinical situations to offer ease of applicability and an organized workflow. The targeted readership would be anyone with specific interest in pediatric oncology whether a medical student, researcher, or a practitioner from any background. Each chapter begins with a short review of classical teaching from referenced database to establish to topic, followed by certain nuances of clinical imaging gathered over the years of practice at our institution as well as those mentioned by other high-volume centers, and researchers across the globe. We end with a structured flowchart to guide daily practice making sure that the foregoing text throughout reflects the buildup toward this final step. The ideal way of reading this text would be to read the concluding part once initially to get an orientation of the whole chapter and then again after going through the entire text to consolidate the concept. We sincerely hope that this text would prove to be a genuine baby step toward alleviating the ailments of babies!

Varanasi, India — Ishan Kumar
Varanasi, India — Ashish Verma
New Delhi, India — Manisha Jana

Contents

Part II Neuro and Head and Neck

Part III Thoracic and Musculoskeletal Systems

Part IV Abdominal

About the Editors

Ishan Kumar is an esteemed Professor in the Department of Radiodiagnosis at the Institute of Medical Sciences, Banaras Hindu University, India. He holds distinguished roles within the radiology community, including serving as a member of the Executive Council of the Indian Society of Pediatric Radiology and as the State Council Member of the Uttar Pradesh Chapter of the Indian Radiological and Imaging Association. His academic contributions are vast, with over 120 peer-reviewed publications and 10 book chapters, alongside his work as Associate Editor for the book Critical Care Imaging. He has also been invited to deliver more than 50 lectures at national and international conferences, sharing his expertise and fostering the growth of pediatric radiology. He is widely recognized for his specialization in Pediatric Radiology, a domain to which he has dedicated much of his career. A devoted educator, he plays an integral role in shaping the future of radiology through his teaching of undergraduate and postgraduate students. His exemplary work has been acknowledged with multiple prestigious awards, including the President Appreciation Award (2023) from the Indian Radiological and Imaging Association and the Hong Kong College of Radiologists Silver Award for Best Oral Presentation (2023).

Ashish Verma, MBBS, DNB, MNAMS, PhD holds the position of professor and ex-head (in-rotation) in the Department of Radiodiagnosis and Imaging at the Institute of Medical Sciences, Banaras Hindu University, Varanasi, India. An author to over 280 research and clinical manuscripts, his personal interest in the field of oncological imaging is seated from the inception of his career. Scientific writing is as much his passion as his hobby, and he serves as a clinical educator not only in his institution but also at various platforms across the globe, with over a hundred invited talks and discussions to his credit. An able clinician, administrator, researcher, and recipient of multiple awards from coveted bodies like the Indian Council of Medical Research and the Radiological Society of North America, interaction with learners is his way of mutual improvisation for which he dedicates a large part of his day. An enthusiastic reader of world history, he ensures that his interest in evolutionary history of culinary traditions, rural and tribal art forms, customs, and traditions, and Indian movies does find some time in his weekly schedule.

Manisha Jana is a Professor in the Department of Radiodiagnosis and Interventional Radiology at the All India Institute of Medical Sciences (AIIMS), New Delhi. She has special interest in Pediatric radiology and is the core faculty of an ongoing Pediatric radiology fellowship program at the institute. She nurtures a love for teaching. With 249 publications in various reputed national and international indexed journals, over 60 book chapters with different reputed publishers, and 5 Radiology textbooks as an editor, she is an ardent academician and teacher par excellence.

Part I

General

1 Pediatric Medical Oncology: A Radiologist's Guide to Treatment Protocols

Priyanka Aggarwal, Nirali Sanghvi, Ishan Kumar, and Vineeta Gupta

1.1 Introduction

Childhood cancer constitutes a small fraction of the global cancer burden. According to WHO, globally an estimated 400,000 children and adolescents (0–19 years) develop cancer each year. In India, annually approximately 45,000 children are diagnosed with malignancy [1, 2]. The causes of these cancers are multifactorial, often involving a combination of genetic predisposition and environmental factors, with only a small percentage attributable to known hereditary syndromes.

Progress in pediatric oncology has become one of the most significant success stories in recent decades, with 5-year survival rates for all pediatric cancers in high-income countries reaching 75–80%. This success stems from a multidisciplinary approach to care, where radiology plays a crucial role at various stages of the disease. In the diagnostic phase, imaging is essential for identifying tumors, assessing their size, location, and extent of involvement in surrounding tissues. Once diagnosed, radiologists assist in staging, guiding biopsies, and other interventional procedures, providing real-time imaging to enhance precision and reduce complications. During treatment, particularly with chemotherapy and radiation therapy, radiologists monitor treatment responses through follow-up imaging, enabling clinicians to adjust regimens as needed. They also play a key role in detecting treatment-related complications, such as infections or secondary malignancies.

In this chapter, we adumbrate the various chemotherapy protocols used in the treatment of common pediatric cancers. Understanding these protocols is vital for radiologists, as it provides context for interpreting imaging findings. Knowledge of specific regimens helps radiologists recognize treatment response patterns, such as tumor necrosis and morphological changes, as well as potential complications. Additionally, being aware of the timing of imaging relative to chemotherapy cycles enhances the radiologist's ability to distinguish between expected therapeutic effects and pathological changes. By linking oncological treatment strategies with radiological assessment, this chapter aims to promote a more cohesive and collaborative approach to pediatric oncology care, ultimately improving patient outcomes.

P. Aggarwal · V. Gupta
Division of Pediatric Hematology and Oncology, Department of Pediatrics, Institute of Medical Sciences, Banaras Hindu University, Varanasi, India
e-mail: tamanna.horizon@bhu.ac.in

N. Sanghvi
Pediatric Hematology-Oncology and BMT, Kokilaben Dhirubhai Ambani Hospital, Mumbai, India

I. Kumar (✉)
Department of Radiodiagnosis and Imaging, Institute of Medical Sciences, Banaras Hindu University, Varanasi, Uttar Pradesh, India

I. Kumar et al. (eds.), *Practical Approach to Imaging in Pediatric Oncology*,
https://doi.org/10.1007/978-981-96-8158-7_1

1.2 Lymphoma

Lymphoma ranks as the third most prevalent cancer in children, following acute leukemia and brain tumors, with an incidence rate of 15 cases per million children annually. This disease is divided into two primary types: Hodgkin lymphoma (HL) and non-Hodgkin lymphoma (NHL). Together, they represent approximately 10% to 12% of cancers diagnosed in the pediatric population, with NHL accounting for about 60% of all lymphomas and generally exhibiting a more aggressive nature compared to the typically indolent HL [3].

1.2.1 Hodgkin Lmphoma

HL is notably the most common malignancy among adolescents aged 15–19 years, but it is rare in children younger than 5 and less common in adults [3]. The classification of HL comprises of classical HL, which makes up 95% of cases, and nodular lymphocyte predominant HL (NLPHL), accounting for 5% of cases. Classical HL is further subdivided into nodular sclerosis, mixed cellularity, lymphocyte-depleted, and lymphocyte-rich forms. In classical HL, the tumor cells are identified as Hodgkin and Reed–Sternberg (HRS) cells, while in NLPHL, they are designated as lymphocyte-predominant (LP) cells [3].

A. **STAGE**

Symptoms

- "A" Symptoms: No "B" symptoms present.
- "B" Symptoms: One or more of the following:
  - Unexplained weight loss over 10% in the last 6 months.
  - Recurrent fever above 38 °C.
  - Severe night sweats.

Bulk Disease (X criteria)

- Mediastinal mass larger than one-third of the chest diameter, or.
- Large extramediastinal lymph node mass > 6 cm.

Extranodal Involvement (E criteria)

- Involvement of an extranodal site next to a known lymph node area.

Treatment In general, chemotherapy, with or without low-dose involved-field radiation therapy, is considered the standard treatment for Hodgkin lymphoma (HL). Patients are typically categorized into low, intermediate, and high-risk groups based on clinical stage, bulk disease presence, and the occurrence of B symptoms (see Tables 1.1 and 1.2). The current treatment strategy also emphasizes a response-based approach, adapting therapy according to the response to initial treatment.

Surgical intervention is usually limited to diagnostic biopsy, except in the case of nodular lymphocyte predominant HL (NLPHL). In Stage IA NLPHL, observation is recommended following complete surgical resection of a single, non-bulky peripheral node [5]. Radiation therapy, ranging from 15 to 25 Gy, is administered with adjustments based on factors such as the patient's age, presence of bulk disease, normal tissue sensitivity, and considerations of both acute and long-term side effects.

Table 1.1 Clinical and staging criteria for Hodgkin lymphoma (Ann Arbor staging system) [4]

Stage	Disease
I	Affects one lymph node region or a single extralymphatic organ (IE)
II	Involves ≥2 lymph node regions on the same side of the diaphragm, OR an extralymphatic organ with nearby lymph node involvement (IIE)
III	Involves lymph nodes on both sides of the diaphragm. This may include: Localized extralymphatic organ involvement, Spleen involvement, or Both.
IV	Widespread involvement of ≥1 extralymphatic organs, possibly with distant lymph node involvement

Table 1.2 Common standard therapy protocols for pediatric classical Hodgkin lymphoma

Stage and presentation	Commonly accepted chemotherapy regimens
IA, IIA (fewer than 4 nodal regions without B symptoms, bulky disease, or extranodal extension)	#OEPA or OPPA for 2 cycles; **OR** ABVD for 2–4 cycles
IA, IIA (with bulk disease, > 3 nodal regions, or extranodal extension), IIB*, IIIA, IVA	#@OEPA for 2 cycles—COPDAC for 2 cycles; **OR** *ABVD for 4–6 cycles
IIB*, IIIB, IVB	#@OEPA for 2 cycles—COPDAC for 4 cycles; **OR** *ABVD for 6–8 cycles

#As per EuroNet-Pediatric Hodgkin Lymphoma Group
*Consider low dose involved field radiotherapy; 15–25 Gy,
@No radiotherapy for patients in at least partial response (PR) and PET negative after two cycles of OEPA
ABVD: Adriamycin, Bleomycin, Vinblastine, Doxorubicin
OEPA: Vincristine, Etoposide, Prednisolone, Doxorubicin)
COPDAC (Cyclophosphamide, Vincristine, Prednisolone, Dacarbazine)

1.2.2 Non-Hodgkin Lymphoma (NHL)

Non-Hodgkin lymphoma (NHL) is a diverse group of lymphoid cancers, representing around 6–8% of all malignancies in <20 years. Approximately 70% of affected children present with advanced-stage disease, frequently involving extranodal sites like the gastrointestinal tract, bone marrow, and central nervous system (CNS). About 25% have anterior mediastinal mass (commonly T-Lymphoblastic Lymphoma or primary mediastinal large B-cell lymphoma) and may exhibit respiratory symptoms or superior vena cava (SVC) syndrome [3]. Gastrointestinal involvement occurs in about 30% of cases, typically manifesting as an abdominal mass or intussusception. Bone marrow involvement is found in 10–30% of patients at diagnosis, while CNS involvement is less common but observed in advanced cases.

Pediatric non-Hodgkin lymphoma (NHL) is primarily characterized by high-grade tumors, accounting for over 95% of cases. It encompasses four principal subtypes: B- and T-lymphoblastic lymphoma (LBL), Burkitt lymphoma (BL), diffuse large B-cell lymphoma (DLBCL), and anaplastic large cell lymphoma (ALCL). Within DLBCL, there are three subcategories; notably, the germinal center B-cell-like subtype is linked to a more favorable prognosis, whereas the activated B-cell-like and primary mediastinal B-cell-like subtypes tend to have worse outcomes [6].

St Jude Staging System for Pediatric Non-Hodgkin Lymphoma

- **Stage I**: Single extranodal tumor or a single nodal area (excluding mediastinum/abdomen).
- **Stage II**: Single tumor with regional lymph node involvement, more than two nodal areas on the same side of the diaphragm, or two tumors on the same side.
- **Stage III**: Tumors on both sides of the diaphragm, more than two nodal areas on both sides, any primary intrathoracic tumor, or extensive intra-abdominal disease.
- **Stage IV**: Any of the above with initial CNS or bone marrow involvement.

Unlike Hodgkin lymphoma (HL), the role of PET scans in initial staging and treatment response for NHL has yet to be clearly defined [7, 8].

Treatment LMB96 is the commonly used treatment protocol for newly diagnosed B lineage NHL (Fig. 1.1) that stratifies patients as follows:

Group A—Stage I (Completely resected)/Stage II (Completely resected abdominal lesion).
Group B—Not eligible for Group A/B.
Group C—CNS involvement (L3 blast in CSF and/or cranial nerve palsy (not due to extracranial tumor) and/or spinal cord compression and/or isolated intracerebral mass and/or parameningeal extension) and/or bone marrow involvement (>25% bone marrow blast).

Current treatment approach for LBL particularly T-LBL has been derived from treatment of T-ALL [9, 10]. Rituximab (anti-CD20 monoclo-

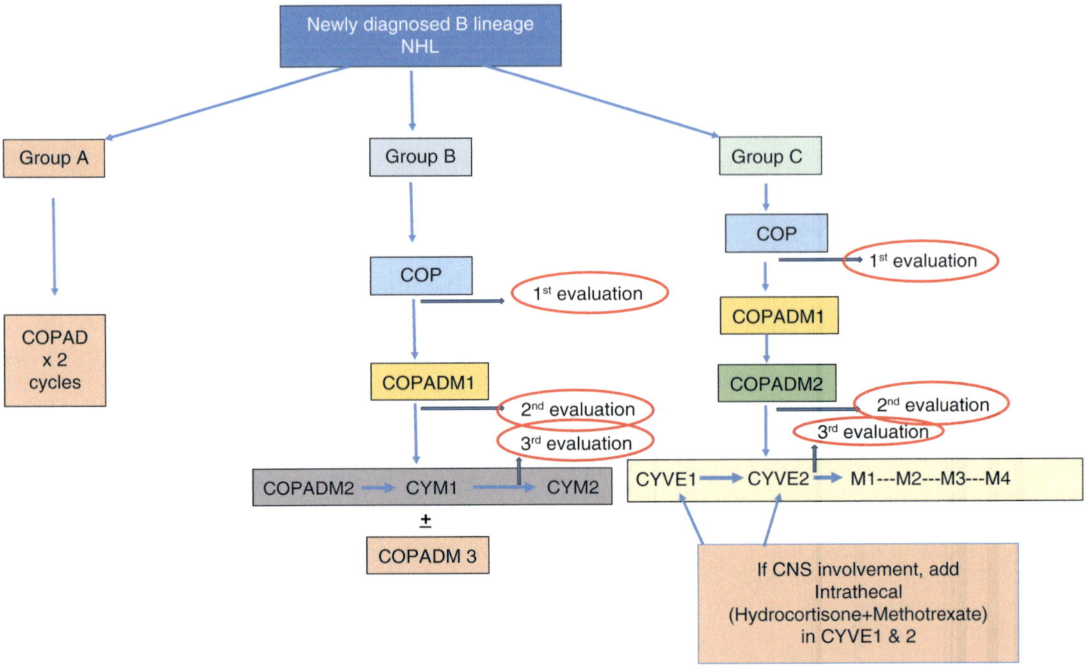

Fig. 1.1 Schema depicting treatment plan in LMB96. first, second, and third evaluation checkpoints are indicated in the treatment schema. *COP* Cyclophosphamide, Vincristine, Prednisolone, *COPADM* Cyclophosphamide, Vincristine, Prednisolone, Doxorubicin, Methotrexate (MTX), *CYM* Cytosine arabinoside, methotrexate, *CYVE* Cytarabine, High dose (HD), Cytosine arabinoside, Etoposide, *M* Maintenance (M1—Cyclophosphamide, Vincristine, Prednisolone, HD-MTX, Doxorubicin, M2-M4—Cytarabine, Etoposide)

Table 1.3 Summary of treatment protocol

Type of NHL	Treatment regimen
Burkitt lymphoma	LMB96 ± rituximab*
Primary mediastinal B cell lymphoma	LMB96 ± rituximab
DLBCL	LMB96 ± rituximab
B and T lymphoblastic lymphoma	Acute lymphoblastic leukemia (ALL) approach
ALCL	ALCL99

nal antibody) is to be added in Stage III tumors with LDH > 2 upper limit of normal (ULN) or stage IV/Burkitt lymphoma. Table 1.3 summarizes the treatment of NHL in a nutshell.

For relapsed ALCL, COG has incorporated newer molecules like anti-CD30, i.e., Brentuximab vedotin [11] and ALK inhibitor, i.e., Crizotinib [12] in the treatment of ALK-negative and ALK-positive ALCL respectively.

1.3 Langerhans Cell Histiocytosis

Langerhans cell histiocytosis (LCH) is a rare disorder without specific age preference, marked by the proliferation of Langerhans cells, a type of dendritic cell involved in immune responses. It affects the bones (80%), skin (33%), pituitary gland (25%), and other organs, including the liver, lungs, spleen, and hematopoietic system (15% each). Less frequently, lymph nodes (5–10%) and the central nervous system (CNS) may be affected (2–4%) [13].

The condition is categorized into two main types: single-system (SS) LCH, which involves a single organ or system, and multisystem (MS) LCH, which affects two or more systems (see Tables 1.4 and 1.5 [14–18]). Patients with SS-LCH, particularly in the skeleton, skin, or lymph nodes, generally have a favorable progno-

Table 1.4 Current clinical classification of LCH

Single System LCH (SS-LCH)	**Bone:** unifocal or multifocal lesions **Skin** **Lymph nodes**: single or multiple (excluding draining nodes) **Lung** **Central nervous system** Other organs (e.g., thyroid, thymus)
Multisystem LCH (MS-LCH)	With or without risk organ involvement Risk organs: Hematopoietic: Anemia (hemoglobin <10 g/dl, infants <9.0 g/dl), leucopenia (WBC < 4000/μL), thrombocytopenia (platelets <100,000/μL) Liver: Hepatomegaly (or hypoproteinemia <5.5 g/dL; hypoalbuminemia <2.5 g/dL Splenomegaly *Currently, sonographic measurements of liver and spleen are not considered for definition of hepatosplenomegaly*

*Bone marrow involvement is defined as presence of CD1a-positive cells on marrow slides

sis and often require minimal treatment. In contrast, MS-LCH can present a wide range of outcomes, from spontaneous resolution to severe progression.

For MS-LCH that does not involve "risk organs," the survival rate exceeds 95% with standard treatments, which include vinblastine and steroids. However, the involvement of risk organs indicates a less favorable prognosis. Notably, the lung is no longer classified as a risk organ [14].

Treatment (see Figs. 1.2 and 1.3): Most patients with localized LCH, especially those with skeletal involvement, typically do not need systemic therapy. A "wait and watch" strategy is often effective for small, asymptomatic lesions due to the likelihood of spontaneous resolution [19, 20]. Surgical options like biopsy, curettage, or resection may be appropriate for solitary bone, lymph node, or skin lesions, but radical surgery is discouraged [13]. An intralesional injection of crystalline methylprednisolone (100–150 mg) can rapidly alleviate symptoms in symptomatic bone lesions [21, 22]. Radiotherapy is generally reserved for specific situations, such as the risk of compressing vital structures (e.g., spinal cord or optic nerve). Treatment approaches for SS-LCH and MS-LCH are outlined in the following schemes [23–25].

Table 1.5 Non-risk organ involvement

Lung	
Confirmed through CECT; biopsy is required if findings are atypical. Histological confirmation is essential for isolated pulmonary LCH	
Skeleton: Two lesions within a single bone are considered one lesion	
Isolated CNS-risk lesion: Isolated lesions in one of the craniofacial bones (i.e., orbit, temporal bone, mastoid, sphenoid, zygomatic, ethmoid, maxilla, paranasal sinuses, or cranial fossa) with or without intracranial soft tissue extension. Lesions in the calvarium (frontal, parietal, and occipital bone) are not "CNS-risk" [5, 6]	
Multifocal bone disease	More than one lesion in different bones.
Central nervous system	
Neurodegenerative CNS-LCH (ND-CNS-LCH)	
Radiological: Detection of typical signal changes on 2 consecutive MRI scans performed within an interval of at least 3 months [17]	
Clinical neurodegeneration Acquired neurological deficits (EDSS, international cooperative ataxia rating scale ICARS) Neuropsychological deficits (full scale IQ, verbal IQ or performance IQ, or both verbal and visual-spatial working memory functions below 1 SD for age) with suggestive radiological findings [17]	
Isolated tumorous CNS-LCH [18] Space-occupying lesions involving hypothalamic-pituitary region/pineal gland/meninges/choroid plexus	

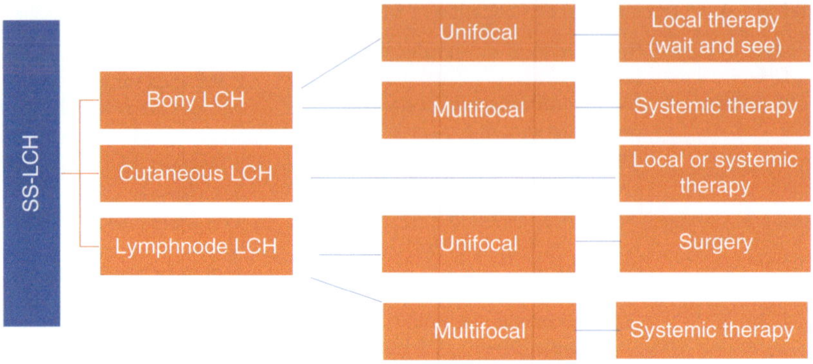

Fig. 1.2 Treatment approach to SS-LCH

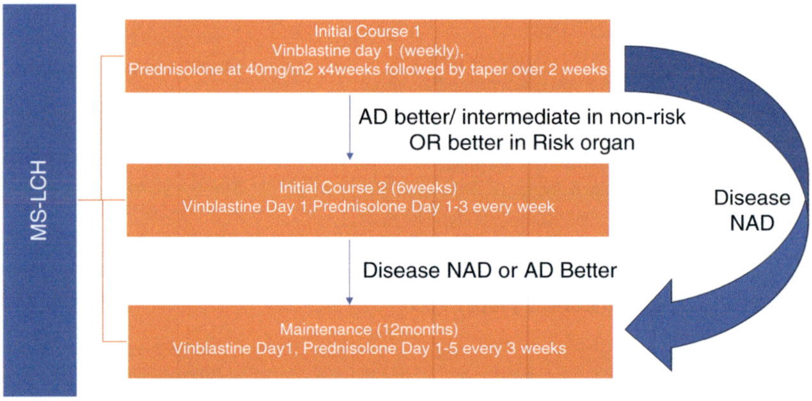

Fig. 1.3 Treatment approach to MS-LCH

1.4 Retinoblastoma

Retinoblastoma (RB) is the most common primary intraocular malignancy in children, accounting for 4% of all pediatric cancers [26]. It shows no geographic or racial predisposition [27]. Diagnosis and management can be challenging in developing countries due to late presentations and reluctance to perform enucleation, which may lead to extraocular metastasis. Children in these regions often present with invasion of critical eye structures, necessitating adjuvant therapy after enucleation to prevent relapse. Most retinoblastomas arise from complementary biallelic mutations of the RB1 gene, in line with Knudson's "2-hit" hypothesis, with mutations being sporadic or germline [28].

Radiology plays an important role not only in making diagnosis but also assessment of extent of disease along with response to treatment. Magnetic resonance imaging (MRI) is preferred over CT scan, if available, as it provides a more accurate imaging of the optic nerve extension [29]. A detailed ophthalmological examination under anesthesia including tonometry, slit lamp examination by an experienced ophthalmologist using indirect ophthalmoscopy should be done. Children with extraocular disease should also undergo CSF as well as bone marrow examination to differentiate stage iii (locoregional spread) from stage iv (metastatic) RB.

Treatment (Tables 1.6 and 1.7): For unilateral RB (intraocular group D/E or overt extraocular), enucleation of the affected eye is curative. In bilateral RB, the most affected eye is enucleated, while eye-conserving therapies are used for the other. Surgery is not recommended for children with stage III disease. Orbital exenteration is typically avoided unless there is a poor response to neoadjuvant chemotherapy; these patients should be treated aggressively with carboplatin-based regimens and orbital radiotherapy. For stage IV extraocular RB, neoadjuvant chemotherapy fol-

Table 1.6 Treatment of intraocular retinoblastoma [35]

Group	Definition	Treatment
A	Small tumors (≤3 mm) located away from the optic disc or fovea, confined to the retina.	Focal treatment
B	Tumors larger than 3 mm or those close to the optic disc or fovea, still confined to the retina.	Focal treatment ± Systemic chemotherapy up to 6 cycles
C	Well-defined tumors with minimal subretinal or vitreous seeding.	Unilateral: Enucleate Bilateral: Attempt 'second eye' salvage: Systemic chemotherapy 6 cycles ± focal treatment
D	Large or poorly defined tumors with extensive vitreous or subretinal seeding, with retinal detachment (>25%).	Unilateral: Enucleate Bilateral: Attempt 'second eye' salvage: Systemic chemotherapy ± focal treatment. If eye salvage fails: Enucleation. Post enucleation: If histopathological features are low risk, no further treatment is needed. If high risk, administer 6 cycles of chemotherapy.
E	Very large tumors that extend near the front of the eye, causing bleeding or glaucoma.	Enucleation. If low risk—No further treatment. If high-risk histopathological features—6 cycles of chemotherapy

Table 1.7 Treatment of extraocular retinoblastoma [35]

Stage	Definition	Treatment
0	Eye can be salvaged with focal treatment or systemic chemotherapy	Intraocular protocol
I	Enucleation with no tumor residue (low risk features on pathology)	
II	Enucleation is carried out, but there is tumor residue with high-risk pathology features, including: – Tumor at the cut end of the optic nerve – Extension into the sclera – Extra-scleral extension	Enucleation upfront. Histopathology-guided treatment. If no brain/ bone marrow metastases Chemotherapy: 12 cycles for tumor at optic nerve cut end or extraocular extension 6–12 cycles for scleral involvement. (clinical review & CSF analysis following every 3 cycles). External beam radiation therapy (EBRT) if available.
III	Regional extension	If the child presents with ophthalmitis, administer steroids for 3 days. If the child shows improvement and the globe appears normal, consider an examination under anesthesia (EUA) to evaluate for downstaging. 6 cycles of chemotherapy ↓ Enucleation (or exenteration) ↓ EBRT (45 Gy) ↓ 6 more cycles of chemotherapy (Total of 12 cycles). Clinical review & CSF analysis following every 3 cycles
IIIA	Overt orbital disease with optic nerve or extraocular extension	
IIIB	Regional lymph node extension	
IV	Metastatic disease	Consider palliation. Or, High-dose neoadjuvant chemotherapy ↓ ↓ Enucleation EBRT (45 Gy) ↓ Chemotherapy followed by ASCT
IVA	Hematogenous metastases	
IVB	CNS extension	

lowed by local control and high-dose chemotherapy with autologous stem cell rescue is the most effective approach. The cure rate can be as high as 70% without CNS involvement but drops to below 30% with CNS involvement [30–34].

1.5 Germ Cell Tumor

Germ cell tumors (GCTs) arise from primordial germ cells in the developing embryo, which are typically intended to form sperm or ova. These tumors represent approximately 3.5% of all pediatric cancers and exhibit a bimodal age distribution, with peaks occurring before age 4 and between 15 and 19 years [3]. Pediatric GCTs can be classified histologically into two main types: germinomas and non-germinomatous GCTs. The staging of malignant GCTs in children follows the system established by the Children's Oncology Group (COG). This staging system relies on imaging results, postoperative pathological findings, lymph node involvement, and the presence of metastasis (see Table 1.8) [36].

Table 1.8 The Children's Oncology Group (COG) staging of malignant germ cell tumors in children

Stage	Definition
I	Completely resected tumors
II	Microscopic residual disease or a persistently raised tumor marker after resection
III	Gross residual disease OR nodal involvement
IV	Distant metastasis

Certain tumor markers like alpha fetoprotein and beta HCG are used for diagnostic evaluation as well as to assess disease activity. Below 1 year, it becomes difficult to evaluate raised alpha fetoprotein levels as indicator of residual disease or its recurrence.

LDH can also be used to assess disease activity. It correlates with tumor bulk, response to chemotherapy/radiotherapy, and residual/recurrent disease.

Treatment (Fig. 1.4) The Malignant Germ Cell Tumors International Collaboration (MaGIC) risk group categorizes treatment based on factors such as age at diagnosis, tumor location, and

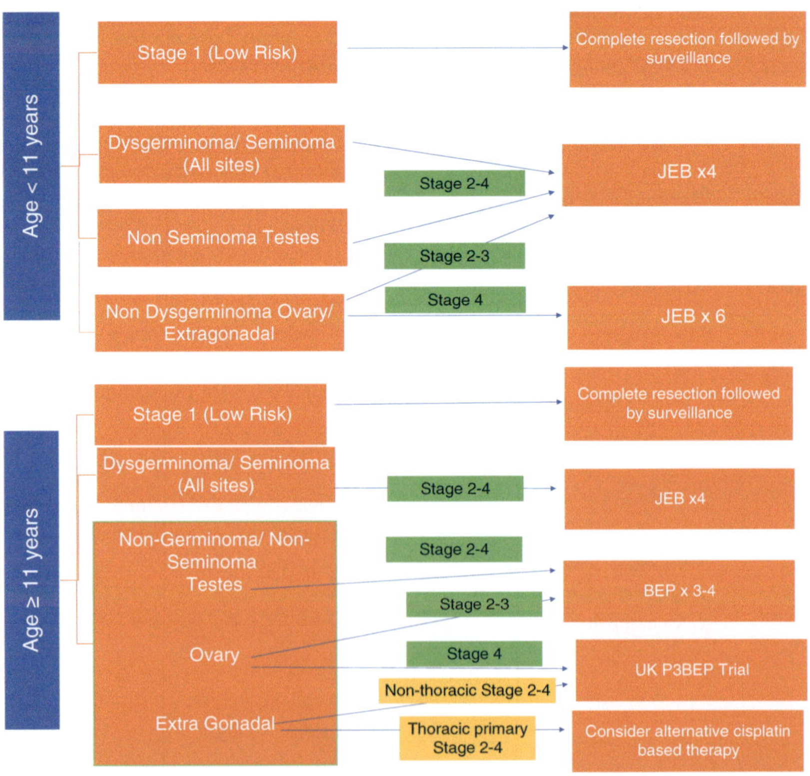

Fig. 1.4 Treatment schema as per CCLG, A. For children <11 yrs., B. For children ≥11 yrs.

COG staging [36, 37]. The primary treatment approach for pediatric germ cell tumors (GCTs) involves complete surgical resection, followed by adjuvant chemotherapy. If complete resection is not feasible at diagnosis, a biopsy is performed, and neoadjuvant chemotherapy is administered to facilitate the subsequent removal of any remaining tumor. However, certain subtypes of extracranial GCTs have shown resistance to platinum-based chemotherapy, which can adversely affect outcomes [37]. In adults with high-risk GCTs, high-dose chemotherapy (HDCT) combined with autologous stem cell transplantation (ASCT) has been employed, but there is currently no consensus on the use of this strategy in the pediatric population [38].

- JEB: Carboplatin, Etoposide, Bleomycin.
- UK P3BEP: accelerated BEP (bleomycin, etoposide, and cisplatin).

1.6 Wilms Tumor

Wilms tumor is the second most common intra-abdominal malignancy and ranks fifth among all pediatric cancers, comprising about 6% of pediatric malignancies. It is the predominant type of renal tumor in children, accounting for over 95% of such cases [39, 40]. The typical age of presentation is between 2 and 5 years, with approximately 95% of cases diagnosed before age 10 [41]. The most common initial symptom is the incidental discovery of an abdominal mass, followed by hematuria. In some instances, children may experience hypertension due to renal ischemia from the tumor's pressure on the renal artery. Systemic symptoms like fatigue, loss of appetite, weight loss, and fever may also occur. Dissemination is seen in 10–25% of cases, primarily affecting the lungs [42]. Recurrences most frequently happen in the lungs, abdomen, and liver.

1.6.1 Staging

Table 1.9 shows the staging system for renal tumors given by Children's Oncology Group Renal Tumors Committee.

Table 1.9 Staging system for renal tumors (Children's Oncology Group Renal Tumors Committee)

STAGE	
I	Completely resected tumor limited to kidney with intact capsule
II	Completely resected tumor without tumor at margins, regional lymph nodes negative, but with renal capsule penetration or vascular invasion.
III	Residual tumor present after surgery, confined to abdomen.
IV	Presence of metastasis or extra-abdominal lymph node
V	Bilateral Wilms tumor

Treatment Management of Wilms tumor is guided by two major collaborative groups: the National Wilms Tumor Study Group (NWTSG) (USA) and the International Society for Paediatric Oncology (SIOP) (Europe). The SIOP approach does not recommend confirmatory biopsy if clinical and radiological features suggest Wilms tumor, given that preoperative needle biopsies align with postoperative findings in 95% of cases [43, 44].

1.6.2 Prognostic Factors

Poor prognostic indicators include [45–53]:

- More than two-thirds of blastemal cells in the tumor post-induction chemotherapy.
- Anaplastic histology.
- Loss of heterozygosity (LOH) at chromosomes 1p and 16q.
- Persistent metastasis.
- Bilateral/recurrent Wilms tumor.

1.6.3 Risk Stratification

Treatment is based on risk categorization—low risk, intermediate risk, and high risk—according to histological features as per the SIOP approach (Table 1.10).

- Regimen EE-4A: vincristine, dactinomycin for 18 weeks.

Table 1.10 Summary of treatment approach SIOP and COG [54]

	NWTSG/COG	SIOP
Timing of surgery	Upfront nephrectomy for the purpose of histological diagnosis and accurate staging [5]	Preoperative chemotherapy, i.e., AV(stage I-III)/ AVD (stage IV) to shrink the tumor before surgery (within week 12 of therapy) and prevention of tumor rupture [1, 2, 5].
Postoperative chemotherapy		
Stage I	Tumors with favorable histology (FH) (age < 2 years) and tumor kidney weight < 550 g: Radical nephrectomy (RN) without further treatment. *For age > 2 years: Treatment same as stage 2*	Low-risk histology—No further treatment, Intermediate-risk tumors, tumor volume (TV) <500 ml—AV for 4 weeks High-risk tumors, TV >500 ml - AVD for 27 weeks
Stage II	Tumors with FH: *RN + adjuvant chemotherapy (EE-4A) FH and LOH 1p/16q: *RN + adjuvant chemotherapy (DD-4A)	Low and intermediate-risk tumors, TV <500 ml-AV for 27 weeks High-risk tumors with TV >500 ml—HR-1 for 34 weeks + flank RT
Stage III	Tumors with FH: RN + adjuvant chemotherapy with regimen (DD-4A) + flank RT; Tumors with FH and LOH 1p/16q: RN + adjuvant chemotherapy with regimen M for 31 weeks + flank RT	Low and intermediate-risk tumors, TV <500 ml—AV for 27 weeks High-risk tumors with TV >500 ml—HR-1@ for 34 weeks + flank RT
Stage IV	FH: RN + adjuvant chemotherapy DD-4A for 24 weeks + flank RT FH and LOH 1p/16q: RN + regimen M for 31 weeks + flank RT	Complete remission of metastasis: AVD for 27 weeks Incomplete response of metastasis: HR-1 for 34 weeks + RT of metastatic organ, surgical resection of metastatic lesions can be attempted when feasible without risk of organ morbidity High-risk histology of the primary tumor: HR-1 for 34 weeks + RT of metastatic organ
Stage V	Neoadjuvant chemotherapy with DD-4A for 6–12 weeks, partial nephrectomy, adjuvant chemotherapy depending on histologic response.	Neoadjuvant chemotherapy: AV for 4–6 weeks followed by surgery Aim of nephron-sparing surgery, adjuvant chemotherapy according to the histopathological subtype + abdominal/flank RT in appropriate cases.

- Regimen DD-4A: vincristine, dactinomycin, doxorubicin for 24 weeks.
- Regimen M: vincristine, dactinomycin, doxorubicin, cyclophosphamide, etoposide.
- Neoadjuvant chemotherapy.
  - Actinomycin D and Vincristine(AV) for 4 weeks (Stage I-III).
  - Actinomycin D, Vincristine, and Doxorubicin (AVD) for 6 weeks, for Stage IV.
- HR-1—etoposide, carboplatin, cyclophosphamide, doxorubicin.

Postoperative Radiotherapy: Those with stage III intermediate risk, and stage II-III high risk, i.e., those with diffuse anaplasia, clear cell sarcoma, and rhabdoid tumors require flank irradiation. Furthermore, blastemal histology in the high-risk group does not require radiotherapy if stage II. Current COG guidelines advocate omission of whole-lung irradiation if favorable histology (FH) without loss of heterozygosity at 1p and 16q, and complete response at 6 weeks after neoadjuvant chemotherapy [57].

The survival of patients with Wilms tumor is generally excellent, exceeding 90% [3]. The rate is 95% for patients with stages I and II Wilms tumor, 75–80% for patients with stage III, and 65–75% for patients with stage IV. Children with favorable histology experience recurrences in only 15% when compared to 50% in those with anaplastic histology. The prognosis is also poorer with liver metastases as compared to lung metastases. Most recurrences of Wilms tumor occur within 2 years of diagnosis [55]. Late recurrences (>5 years after diagnosis) are rare, i.e., 0.5% with prognosis similar to early recurrences [56].

1.7 Neuroblastoma

Neuroblastoma (NBL) is the most common extracranial solid tumor in children, accounting for 7% of all childhood malignancies and 15% of childhood cancer mortality worldwide. It is the most common malignancy in infants with an annual incidence of 10 per million live births. The peak age of incidence is 2 years [3]. It is the pediatric malignancy with the least favorable outcome and a cure rate that does not exceed 40% among the high-risk group in developing countries [58, 59].

It has been classified as per International Neuroblastoma Staging System traditionally. But with advances in neuroblastoma management currently, it is being classified based on International Neuroblastoma Risk Group staging system (INRGSS) as L1 (no imaging-defined risk factors (IDRFs), L2 (with IDRFs) and M (metastatic disease with exception of children <18 months with metastasis limited to skin, liver and bone marrow (stage MS) [60]. In addition to age at presentation, histology, and cytogenetic abnormalities, Children Oncology Group (COG) has also incorporated segmental chromosomal aberrations (SCA) like deletion of 1p and 11q, gain in chromosome 1q, 2p, and 17q as additional biomarker affecting risk group. Presence of SCA, MYCN, ALK, age at diagnosis >18 months, and advanced-stage disease are associated with poor prognosis [61–64]. As per COG, children with low and intermediate risk neuroblastoma have been reported to have 5-year overall survival >95%. However, the 5-year overall survival remains about 60%. Thus, appropriate risk stratification is important to identify those that require intensive multimodal treatment [64].

Treatment As per CCLG guidelines, risk stratification is used to guide treatment. The overview for treatment of low/intermediate risk neuroblastoma (Figs. 1.5 and 1.6) is as follows.

For numerical chromosomal aberration (NCA) or life-threatening symptoms (LTS): 2–4 courses of chemotherapy whereas for those with segmental chromosomal aberrations (SCA), 4 courses of chemotherapy are given.

1.7.1 High-Risk Neuroblastoma

Induction: The treatment approach varies among the COG and SIOPEN. COG advocates use of five cycles with topotecan, vincristine, doxorubicin, cyclophosphamide, cisplatin, and etoposide (NCT03126916). However,

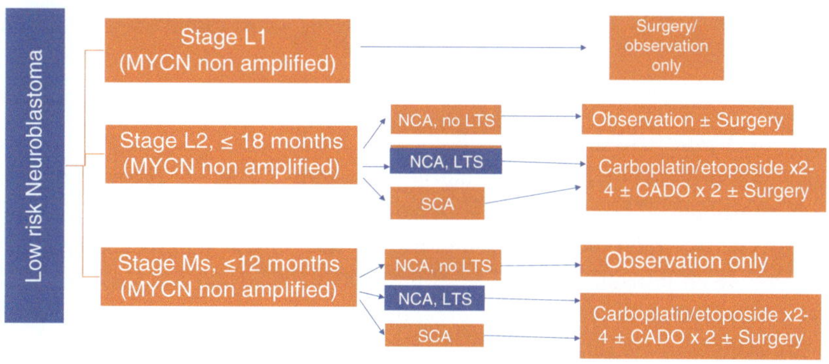

Fig. 1.5 Overview of treatment for low-risk neuroblastoma. *NCA* Numerical chromosomal aberration, life-threatening symptoms (LTS), segmental chromosomal aberrations (SCA)

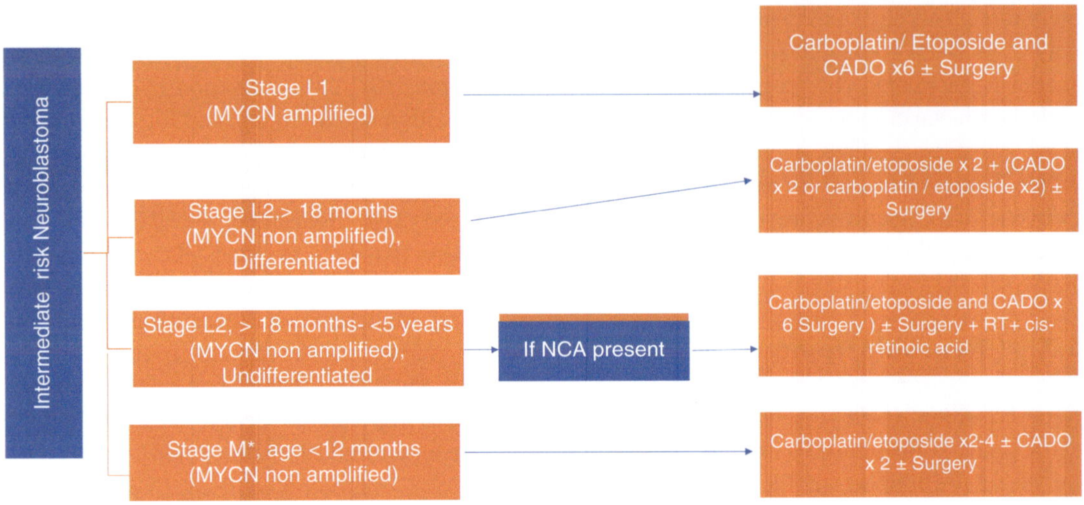

Fig. 1.6 Overview of treatment for intermediate-risk neuroblastoma. (*Stage M with age 12–18 months and NCA present, may be treated as high risk with rapid COJEC and surgery)

SIOPEN uses rapid COJEC that includes eight cycles of combination of vincristine, carboplatin, etoposide, cyclophosphamide, and cisplatin. Followed by appropriate chemotherapy, surgical excision of primary tumor (complete or gross total resection) is done [65]. Response to induction treatment, i.e., intensive chemotherapy followed by surgery should be done as per the updated 2017 International Neuroblastoma Response Criteria (INRC) (Table 1.11) [66].

It has been demonstrated that event-free survival (EFS) in those with PR or PD after induction treatment is better if bridging treatment, i.e., anti GD2 antibody (Dinutuximab) with temozolomide and irinotecan and/or ^{131}I-MIBG is given [67, 68].

Consolidation Children with high-risk NBL may then be taken up for ASCT (autologous stem cell transplant), if bone marrow is free of disease, followed by radiotherapy (preferably within 60 days from transplant) [69]. After the consolidation treatment, 6 cycles of 13-cis retinoic acid with/without anti-GD2 antibody (dinutuximab/naxitamab) have been observed to improve overall survival.

Table 1.11 2017 International Neuroblastoma Response Criteria (INRC)

Overall response	Response of components including primary tumor, metastatic disease, and bone marrow
Complete response (CR)	All disease indicators (primary tumor, metastases, and bone marrow) have fully resolved.
Partial response (PR)	At least one area shows improvement, while all other areas are better than stable disease.
Minor response (MR)	Improvement in one area, with at least one other area stable and no progression observed.
Stable disease (SD)	No areas show improvement or worsening, with all components remaining stable.
Progressive disease (PD)	At least one area demonstrates worsening or progression of the disease.

1.8 Rhabdomyosarcoma (RMS)

RMS comprises a heterogenous family of soft tissue cancers that arise from the mesenchymal cells that would give rise to striated muscle lineage cells. It is the most common pediatric soft tissue sarcoma with an incidence of 4.5 per million children per year [70, 71]. It is the third most common extracranial tumor following neuroblastoma and Wilms tumor. (3) There is a bimodal age distribution peaking at age 2–6 years and then at age 10–18 years. Tables 1.12 and 1.13 show staging and risk groups of RMS.

Treatment Protocol The COG protocol utilizes VAC (Vincristine, Actinomycin D, and Cyclophosphamide) for chemotherapy, followed by radiation therapy (RT) after 9–12 weeks, with additional chemotherapy based on risk group (Table 1.14) [72]. Exceptions to RT include:

- Low-risk localized fusion-negative RMS with initial R0 resection (IRS Group I).
- Localized fusion-negative RMS (vagina) achieving complete remission with induction chemotherapy.
- Standard-risk RMS at favorable sites with R0 resection after secondary surgery.

Both COG and EpSSG recommend delayed surgical excision post-induction chemotherapy to minimize organ impairment, though initial surgery may be considered for operable tumors in select cases [72, 73].

- Favorable sites — orbit, non-parameningeal head & neck, non-bladder/non prostate Genitourinary sites.
- Unfavorable sites—extremities, parameningeal, prostate, and bladder.
- Favorable pathology—embryonal, spindle, and botryoid RMS. Unfavorable pathology—alveolar RMS (including solid-alveolar variant).
- Favorable age & size —<10 years, and ≤ 5 cm.
- Unfavorable age & size—≥ 10 years, or > 5 cm.

Table 1.12 Staging and Clinical Grouping (COG)

Clinical group	Initial surgical findings
Group I	Localized disease with R0 resection (complete removal with clear margins)
A	Confined to the original site
B	Extends beyond the original site
Group II	Gross Total resection
A	R1 resection (microscopically positive margin)
B	R0 resection with lymph node involvement or invasion into adjacent organs
C	R1 resection with lymph node involvement
Group III	Gross residual disease
	R2 resection (remaining gross tumor) or biopsy only
Group IV	Metastasis at diagnosis

Table 1.13 Risk groups and treatment approach by COG

Risk group	Stage	Clinical group	Fusion status	Treatment (COG)
Low subset 1	1–2	I-II*	Fusion negative	0 Gy
	1	III (orbit only)		45 Gy (if CR to chemotherapy) or 50.4 Gy (if PR to chemotherapy)
Low subset 2	1	III(non-orbit)	Fusion negative	0 Gy
	3	I-II*		0 Gy
Intermediate	2–3	III	Fusion negative	50.4 Gy (if tumor ≤5 cm) or 59.4 Gy (if tumor >5 cm)
	4	IV < 10 years		
	1–3	I-III	Fusion positive	36 Gy
High	4	IV	Any	RT to metastatic sites should be done as consolidation at the end of planned chemotherapy Whole lung RT (15Gy) for patients with lung metastasis

*Clinical Group II receives 36–41.4Gy irrespective of fusion status

Table 1.14 Risk groups and treatment approach by EpSSG RMS 2005

Risk group	Site	IRS stage	Nodal stage	Pathology	Age and size	Treatment (EpSSG) (Chemotherapy)
Low	A	I	N0	F	F	8 cycles of low-dose VCR and Actinomycin D (VA)
Standard	A	I	N0	F	U	4 cycles of Ifosfamide, vincristine, and Actinomycin D (IVA)/5 cycles of VA
	F	II, III	N0	F	A	
	U	II, III	N0	F	F	
High	U	II, III	N0	F	U	9 cycles of IVA
	A	II, III	N1	F	A	
	A	I, II, III	N0	U	A	
Very high	A	I, II, III	N1	U	A	Ifosfamide vincristine, Actinomycin D, doxorubicin (IVADo)/IVA

A Any, *F* Favorable, *U* Unfavorable

1.9 Ewing's Sarcoma

Ewing's sarcoma (ES) is the second most prevalent primary malignant bone tumor in children and young adults, following osteosarcoma. It is part of a family of tumors that includes osseous Ewing's sarcoma, extraosseous ES, atypical ES, primitive neuroectodermal tumors (PNET), peripheral neuroepithelioma, and Askin tumors. Classified as one of the small round blue cell tumors of childhood, ES has an annual incidence of 2.9 per million in individuals under 20 years of age [74]. The most frequent primary sites for ES are the pelvic bones, followed by the long bones of the lower limbs and the chest wall. Lung metastasis is the most common, with bone and bone marrow also frequently involved; however, metastasis to the liver, lymph nodes, and central nervous system is uncommon.

Magnetic resonance imaging (MRI) is the preferred imaging technique for assessing the local extent of the tumor [75–78]. It is crucial for determining resection margins (T1 sequence), evaluating extraosseous tumor infiltration (T1/T2/post-contrast sequences), and identifying skip metastases (see Fig. 1.7).

Treatment (Fig. 1.8) The outcome of patients with localized extraosseous tumors is better as compared to osseous tumors. Interval compression, i.e., interval in between two cycles of chemotherapy, from initial 3 weeks to 2 weeks has been associated with better outcomes [76].

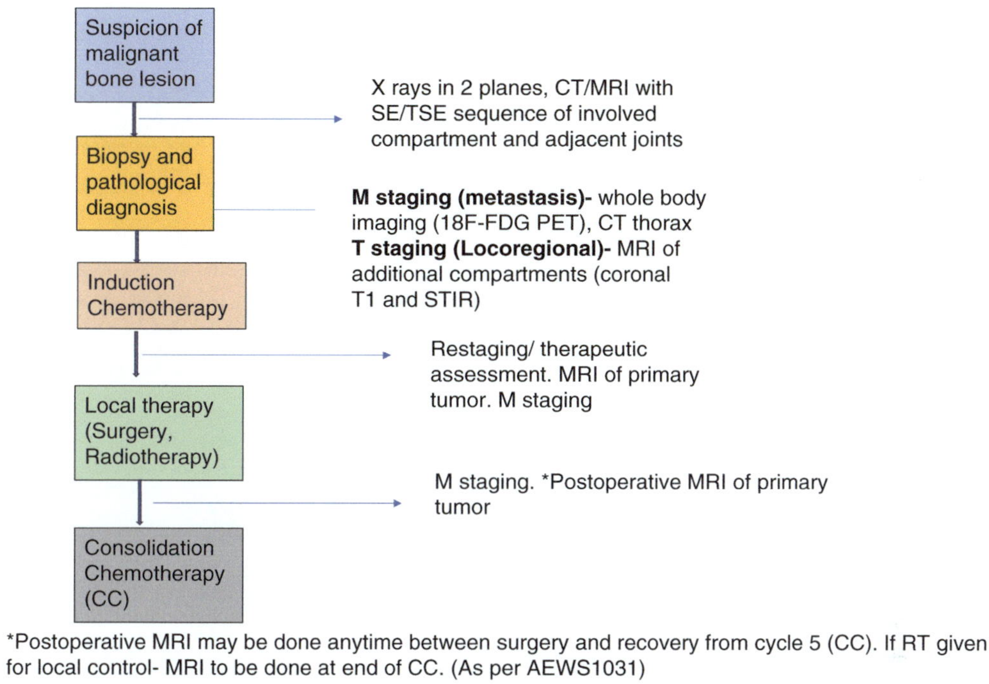

Fig. 1.7 Approach to diagnostic evaluation of child with Ewing's sarcoma. *SE* spin echo, *TSE* turbo spin echo, *STIR* short tau inversion recovery sequence

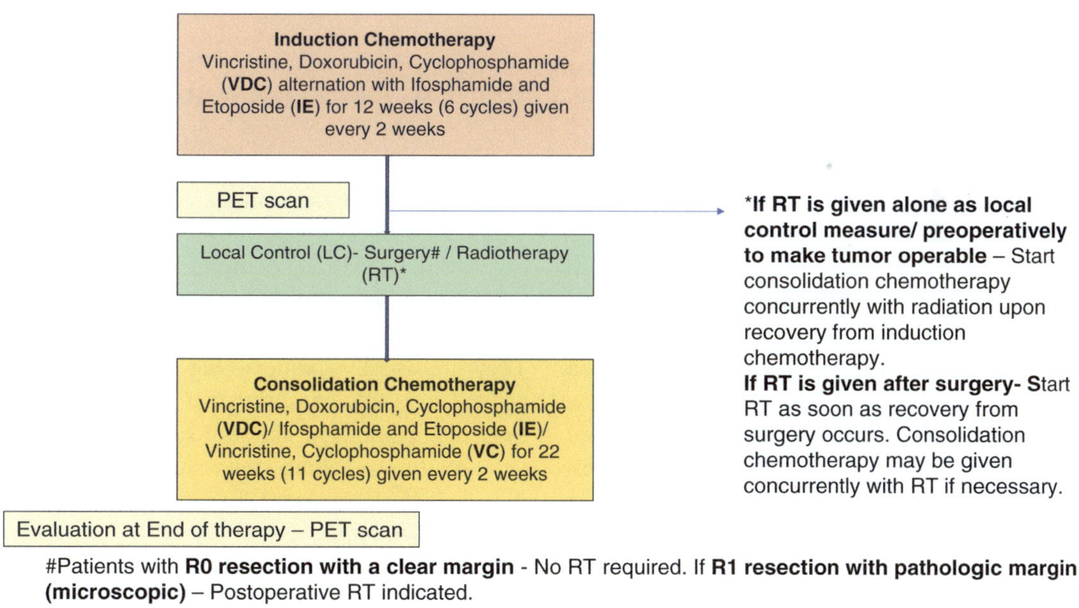

Fig. 1.8 Treatment of Ewing's sarcoma (as per COG AEWS1031 protocol)

1.10 Pediatric Brain Tumors

Pediatric brain tumors represent a diverse group with distinct developmental origins, genomic characteristics, treatment options, and outcomes. These tumors are the most common solid tumors in children, constituting approximately 20% of all childhood cancers [79]. In younger children (under 3 years), many brain tumors originate from embryonal cells, whereas tumors in older children are more likely to arise from glial cells [80, 81].

Average Risk MBL	High Risk MBL (≥1 of the following)
• Non metastatic MBL • With gross total resection • Without MYCN amplification • Without large cell/ anaplastic histology	• Metastatic MBL (chang stage M1-4, M+) • Significant residual disease after surgery (>1.5 cm^2, R+) • With MYCN amplification • With large cell/ anaplastic histology
Treatment • Craniospinal Irradiation to 23.4Gy with posterior fossa or involved field boost to 54 Gy followed by chemotherapy (Cyclophosphamide, cisplatin and vincristine)	**Treatment** • Craniospinal irradiation to 36- 39.6 Gy and a boost of upto 54 Gy to primary site. • Concurrent carboplatin is recommended in Group 3 HR MBL. • High dose chemotherapy followed by autologous stem cell transplant have also been used.

Fig. 1.9 Risk stratification and treatment approach in medulloblastoma

1.10.1 Medulloblastoma

Medulloblastoma (MBL) is the most prevalent malignant brain tumor in pediatric patients, accounting for 15% of all central nervous system tumors, 40% of tumors in the posterior fossa, and 90% of embryonal tumors [82]. The peak incidence occurs between ages 5 and 7, with a male-to-female ratio of 1.7:1 [83]. MBL is classified into four subtypes: wingless (WNT), sonic hedgehog (SHH), group 3, and group 4. Its risk stratification depends on factors such as age at diagnosis, metastatic status, extent of tumor resection, and the presence of large cell or anaplastic histology [84].

Current treatment for MBL focuses on achieving maximum safe resection, followed by chemotherapy and craniospinal irradiation. In older children, MBL is categorized into average-risk and high-risk groups to guide treatment decisions (see Fig. 1.9). In infants, due to the heightened sensitivity of the developing brain to radiation and the high rate of dissemination at diagnosis, alternative strategies are employed. These may include intraventricular or high-dose methotrexate (HDMTX), high-dose chemotherapy (carboplatin, thiotepa) followed by autologous stem cell transplantation (ASCT), or primary focal site radiation therapy. However, outcomes for infants remain poor, with low survival rates. A recent Children's Oncology Group (COG) trial indicated that after surgery, three cycles of induction chemotherapy (cyclophosphamide, cisplatin, vincristine, etoposide, plus HDMTX), followed by three cycles of consolidation chemotherapy (carboplatin, thiotepa) and ASCT, yielded a five-year overall survival rate of 80% in the HDMTX arm, compared to 40% in the non-HDMTX arm [85].

1.10.2 Pediatric Low-grade Glioma

Pediatric low-grade glioma (LGG) is the most frequent brain tumor encountered in children and young adults accounting for 40% of all reported cases [86]. This group comprises of spectrum of tumor subtypes with differing histopathological, demographic, and radiological features [87]. They are usually indolent (Fig. 1.10), however, prognosis is affected by extent of tumor resection, histopathology, and molecular characteristics of tumor along with dissemination at diagnosis (5–10% cases [88]) or concurrent diencephalic syndrome.

Neurofibromatosis Type I and tuberous sclerosis complex predispose for this entity [89].

Tumor resection is the treatment of choice for pediatric LGGs (Fig. 1.11). Following surgery, follow-up and observation are indicated in most cases.

Non-surgical treatment (Fig. 1.12): At diagnosis, all children with severe progressive neuro-

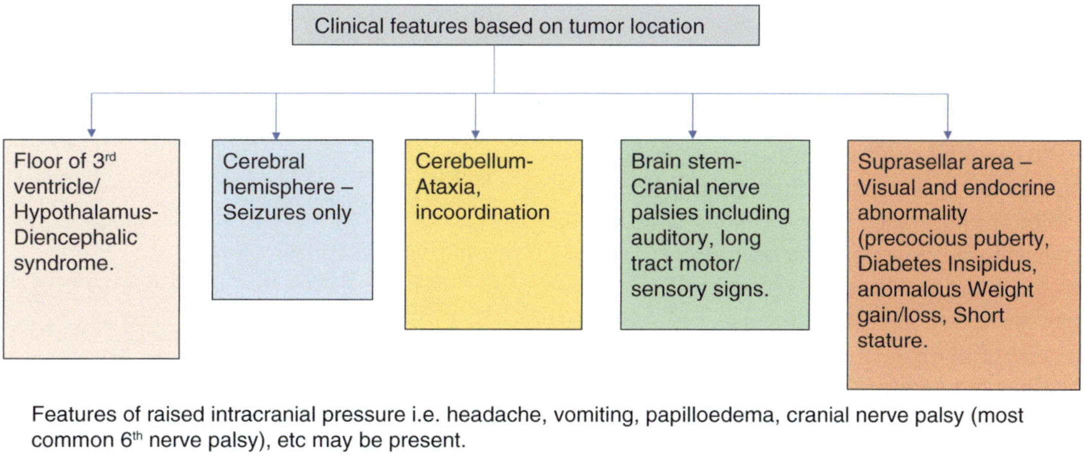

Fig. 1.10 Clinical features based on location of tumor

Fig. 1.11 Primary treatment strategy for pediatric low-grade gliomas (as adapted from Gnekow AK, Kandels D, van Tilburg C, et al. SIOP-E-BTG and GPOH Guidelines [90])

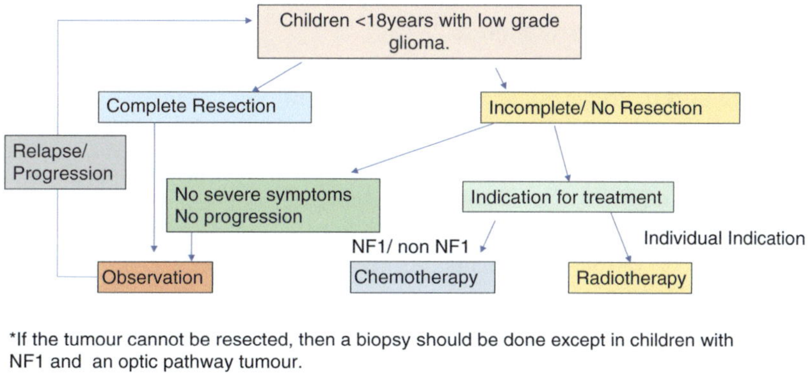

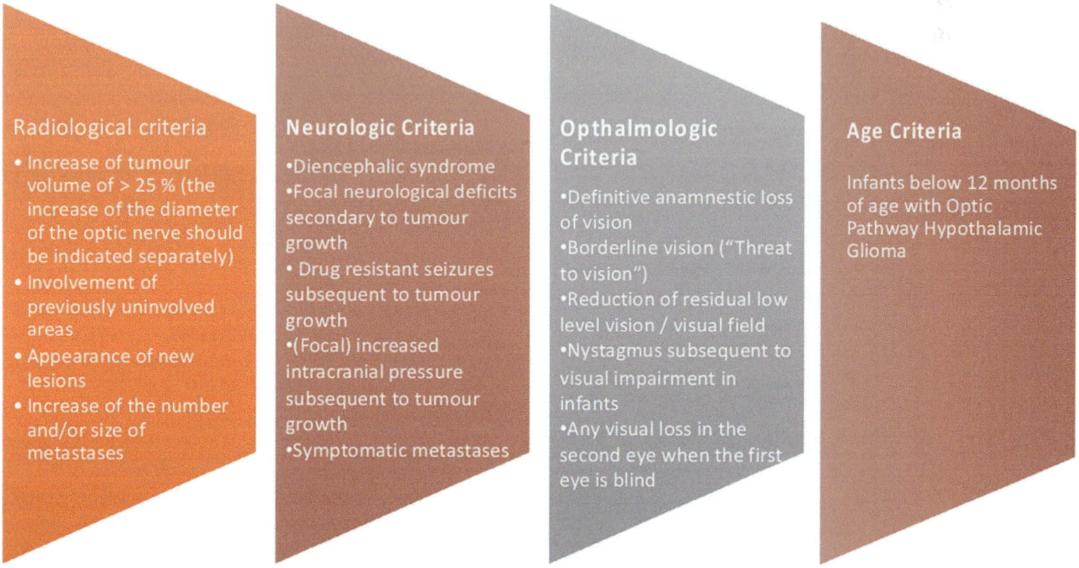

Fig. 1.12 Indications for non-surgical treatment of LGG according to SIOP-E-BTG guidelines [90]

logical/visual symptoms as well as infants with chiasmatic/hypothalamic glioma with or without diencephalic syndrome with metastasis or residual tumor should undergo treatment without period of observation. Furthermore, those with significant radiological progression of residual tumor or appearance of new lesions on MRI not amenable to surgery or those with severe progressive neurological/visual symptoms following initial observation, should also be offered non-surgical treatment.

Chemotherapy in pediatric LGG as per current UK CCLG guidelines includes vincristine and carboplatin. Children hypersensitive to carboplatin may be given vincristine and cisplatin alternating with vincristine and cyclophosphamide. Radiotherapy remains an alternative adjunct at any time point for these children.

In conclusion, having a comprehensive understanding of pediatric medical oncology treatment protocols is essential for radiologists involved in the care of young patients with cancer. This knowledge improves the accuracy of imaging interpretations and helps radiologists anticipate the effects of various treatments. As treatment approaches continue to change, incorporating radiological insights into clinical decision-making will be crucial for achieving better patient outcomes. Therefore, understanding these protocols allows radiologists to play an important role in the diagnosis and treatment of pediatric oncology.

References

1. Steliarova-Foucher E, Colombet M, Ries LAG, et al. International incidence of childhood cancer, 2001-10: a population-based registry study. Lancet Oncol. 2017;18(6):719–31.
2. World Health Organization. CureAll framework: WHO global initiative for childhood cancer: increasing access, advancing quality, saving lives. World Health Organization; 2021.
3. Lanzkowsky P, Lipton J, Fish JD. Lanzkowsky's manual of pediatric hematology and oncology. 6th ed; 2016.
4. Cheson BD, Fisher RI, Barrington SF, Cavalli F, Schwartz LH, Lister TA. Recommendations for initial evaluation, staging, and response assessment of Hodgkin and non-Hodgkin lymphoma: the Lugano classification. J Clin Oncol. 2014;32(27):3059–68.
5. Appel BE, Chen L, Buxton A, Wolden SL, Hodgson DC, Nachman JB. Impact of low-dose involved-field radiation therapy on pediatric patients with lymphocyte-predominant Hodgkin lymphoma treated with chemotherapy: a report from the children's oncology group. Pediatr Blood Cancer. 2012;59(7):1284!1289.
6. Kliegman R, Stanton B, et al. Nelson textbook of pediatrics. 21st ed; 2019.
7. Abdel Rahman H, Sedky M, Hamoda A, Raafat T, Youssef A, Omar W, et al. Role of FDG-PET scan in the management of pediatric mature B cell non-Hodgkin's lymphoma. CCHE experience. J Egypt Natl Canc Inst. 2016;28:95–9.
8. Bakhshi S, Radhakrishnan V, Sharma P, Kumar R, Thulkar S, Vishnubhatla S, et al. Pediatric nonlymphoblastic non-Hodgkin lymphoma: baseline, interim, and posttreatment PET/CT versus contrast-enhanced CT for evaluation—a prospective study. Radiology. 2012;262:956–68.
9. Sandlund JT, Pui CH, Zhou Y, et al. Effective treatment of advanced-stage childhood lymphoblastic lymphoma without prophylactic cranial irradiation: results of St Jude NHL13 study. Leukemia. 2009;23(6):1127–30.
10. Termuhlen AM, Smith LM, Perkins SL, et al. Disseminated lymphoblastic lymphoma in children and adolescents: results of the COG A5971 trial: a report from the children's oncology group. Br J Haematol. 2013;162(6):792–801.
11. Younes A, Bartlett NL, Leonard JP, et al. Brentuximab vedotin (SGN-35) for relapsed CD30-positive lymphomas. N Engl J Med. 2010;363(19):1812–21.
12. Mossé YP, Lim MS, Voss SD, et al. Safety and activity of crizotinib for paediatric patients with refractory solid tumours or anaplastic large-cell lymphoma: a children's oncology group phase 1 consortium study. Lancet Oncol. 2013;14(6):472–80.
13. Haupt R, Minkov M, Astigarraga I, Schafer E, Nanduri V, Jubran R, et al. Langerhans cell histiocytosis (LCH): guidelines for diagnosis, clinical work-up, and treatment for patients till the age of 18 years. Pediatr Blood Cancer. 2013;60(2):175–84.
14. Ronceray L, Potschger U, Janka G, Gadner H, Minkov M. Pulmonary involvement in pediatric-onset multisystem langerhans cell histiocytosis: effect on course and outcome. J Pediatr. 2012;161(1):129–33 e3.
15. Lahey ME. Prognostic factors in histiocytosis X. Am J Pediatr Hematol Oncol. 1981;3(1):57–60.
16. Minkov M, Grois N, Heitger A, Potschger U, Westermeier T, Gadner H. Response to initial treatment of multisystem Langerhans cell histiocytosis: an important prognostic indicator. Med Pediatr Oncol. 2002;39(6):581–5.
17. Prayer D, Grois N, Prosch H, Gadner H, Barkovich AJ. MR imaging presentation of intracranial disease

associated with Langerhans cell histiocytosis. AJNR Am J Neuroradiol. 2004;25(5):880–91.
18. Grois N, Fahrner B, Arceci RJ, Henter JI, McClain K, Lassmann H, et al. Central nervous system disease in Langerhans cell histiocytosis. J Pediatr. 2010;156(6):873–81, 81 e1.
19. Lau LM, Stuurman K, Weitzman S. Skeletal Langerhans cell histiocytosis in children: permanent consequences and health-related quality of life in long-term survivors. Pediatr Blood Cancer. 2008;50(3):607–12.
20. Womer RB, Raney RB Jr, D'Angio GJ. Healing rates of treated and untreated bone lesions in histiocytosis X. Pediatrics. 1985;76(2):286–8.
21. Cohen M, Zornoza J, Cangir A, Murray JA, Wallace S. Direct injection of methylprednisolone sodium succinate in the treatment of solitary eosinophilic granuloma of bone: a report of 9 cases. Radiology. 1980;136(2):289–93.
22. Egeler RM, Thompson RC Jr, Voute PA, Nesbit ME Jr. Intralesional infiltration of corticosteroids in localized Langerhans' cell histiocytosis. J Pediatr Orthop. 1992;12(6):811–4.
23. Gadner H, Grois N, Potschger U, Minkov M, Arico M, Braier J, et al. Improved outcome in multisystem Langerhans cell histiocytosis is associated with therapy intensification. Blood. 2008;111(5):2556–62.
24. Gadner H, Minkov M, Grois N, Potschger U, Thiem E, Arico M, et al. Therapy prolongation improves outcome in multisystem Langerhans cell histiocytosis. Blood. 2013;121(25):5006–14.
25. Morimoto A, Ikushima S, Kinugawa N, Ishii E, Kohdera U, Sako M, et al. Improved outcome in the treatment of pediatric multifocal Langerhans cell histiocytosis: results from the Japan Langerhans cell Histiocytosis study Group-96 protocol study. Cancer. 2006;107(3):613–9.
26. Moeez Uddin M, Farooque U, Aziz MZ, et al. Different types of clinical presentations and stages of retinoblastoma among children. Cureus. 2020;12(9):e10672.
27. Dimaras H, Corson TW, Cobrinik D, et al. Retinoblastoma Nat Rev Dis Primers. 2015;1(1):15021.
28. Mallipatna A, Marino M, Singh AD. Genetics of retinoblastoma. Asia Pac J Ophthalmol (Phila). 2016;5(4):260–4.
29. De Graaf P, GoÃàricke S, Rodjan F, et al. Guidelines for imaging retino- blastoma: imaging principles and MRI standardization. Pediatr Radiol. 2012;42(1):2–14.
30. Radhakrishnan V, Kashyap S, Pushker N, et al. Outcome, pathologic findings, and compliance in orbital retinoblastoma (international retinoblastoma staging system stage III) treated with neoadjuvant chemotherapy: a prospective study. Ophthalmology. 2012;119:1470–7.
31. Namouni F, Doz F, Tanguy ML, et al. High-dose chemotherapy with carboplatin, etoposide and cyclophosphamide followed by a haematopoietic stem cell rescue in patients with high-risk retinoblastoma: a SFOP and SFGM study. Eur J Cancer. 1997;33:2368–75.
32. Dunkel IJ, Aledo A, Kernan NA, et al. Successful treatment of metastatic retinoblastoma. Cancer. 2000;89:2117–21.
33. Cozza R, De Ioris MA, Ilari I, et al. Metastatic retinoblastoma: single institution experience over two decades. Br J Ophthalmol. 2009;93:1163–6.
34. Dunkel IJ, Chan HS, Jubran R, et al. High-dose chemotherapy with autologous hematopoietic stem cell rescue for stage 4B retinoblastoma. Pediatr Blood Cancer. 2010;55:149–52.
35. A resource material for the management of retinoblastoma in low & middle recource settings. September 2017.
36. Shaikh F, Murray MJ, Amatruda JF, Coleman N, Nicholson JC, Hale JP, Pashankar F, Stoneham SJ, Poynter JN, Olson TA, et al. Paediatric extracranial germ-cell tumours. Lancet Oncol. 2016;17:e149–62.
37. Frazier AL, Hale JP, Rodriguez-Galindo C, Dang H, Olson T, Murray MJ, Amatruda JF, Thornton C, Arul GS, Billmire D, et al. Revised risk classification for pediatric extracranial germ cell tumors based on 25 years of clinical trial data from the United Kingdom and United States. J Clin Oncol. 2015;33:195–201.
38. Lew C-Z, Liu H-C, Hou J-Y, Huang T-H, Yeh T-C. Pediatric Extracranial germ cell tumors: review of clinics and perspectives in application of autologous stem cell transplantation. Cancers. 1998;2023:15.
39. Dome JS, Fernandez CV, Mullen EA, Kalapurakal JA, Geller JI, Huff V, et al. Children's oncology group's 2013 blueprint for research: renal tumors. Pediatr Blood Cancer. 2013;60:994–1000.
40. Varan A. Wilms' tumor in children: an overview. Nephron-Clin Pract. 2008;108:83–90.
41. Davidoff AM. Wilms tumor. Adv Pediatr Infect Dis. 2012;59:247–67.
42. Kaste SC, Dome JS, Babyn PS, Graf NM, Grundy P, Godzinski J, et al. Wilms tumour: prognostic factors, staging, therapy and late effects. Pediatr Radiol. 2008;38:2–17.
43. Dome JS, Graf N, Geller JI, Fernandez CV, Mullen EA, Spreafico F, et al. Advances in wilms tumor treatment and biology: progress through international collaboration. J Clin Oncol. 2015;33:2999–3007.
44. Acha T, Calvo C, Alfaro J, Galarón P. Wilms tumor: what's new? Clin Transl Oncol. 2005;7:81–94.
45. Grundy PE, Breslow NE, Li S, Perlman E, Beckwith JB, Ritchey ML, et al. Loss of heterozygosity for chromosomes 1p and 16q is an adverse prognostic factor in favorable-histology Wilms tumor: a report from the national Wilms tumor study group. J Clin Oncol. 2005;23:7312–21.
46. Grundy PE, Telzerow PE, Breslow N, Moksness J, Huff V, Paterson MC. Loss of heterozygosity for chromosomes 16q and 1p in Wilms' tumors predicts an adverse outcome. Cancer Res. 1994;54:2331–3.

47. Brok J, Lopez-Yurda M, Tinteren HV, Treger TD, Furtwängler R, Graf N, et al. Relapse of Wilms' tumor and detection methods: a retrospective analysis of the 2001 renal tumor study group-international society of pediatric oncology Wilms' tumor protocol database. Lancet Oncol. 2018;19:1072–81.
48. Daw NC, Chi YY, Kalapurakal JA, Kim Y, Hoffer FA, Geller JI, et al. Activity of vincristine and irinotecan in diffuse anaplastic Wilms tumor and therapy outcomes of stage II to IV disease: results of the children's oncology group AREN0321 study. J Clin Oncol. 2020;38:1558–68.
49. Charlton J, Irtan S, Bergeron C, Pritchard-Jones K. Bilateral Wilms tumor: a review of clinical and molecular features. Expert Rev Mol Med. 2017;19:e8.
50. Ehrlich P, Chi YY, Chintagumpala MM, Hoffer FA, Perlman EJ, Kalapurakal JA, et al. Results of the first prospective multi-institutional treatment study in children with bilateral Wilms tumor (AREN0534): a report from the children's oncology group. Ann Surg. 2017;266:470–8.
51. Verschuur A, Van Tinteren H, Graf N, Bergeron C, Sandstedt B, de Kraker J. Treatment of pulmonary metastases in children with stage IV nephroblastoma with risk-based use of pulmonary radiotherapy. J Clin Oncol. 2012;30:3533–9.
52. Grundy PE, Green DM, Dirks AC, Berendt A, Breslow NE, Anderson JR, et al. Clinical significance of pulmonary nodules detected by CT and not CXR in patients treated for favorable histology Wilms tumor on national Wilms tumor studies-4 and–5: a report from the children's oncology group. Pediatr Blood Cancer. 2012;59:631–5.
53. Warmann SW, Furtwangler R, Blumenstock G, Armeanu S, Nourkami N, Leuschner I, et al. Tumor biology influences the prognosis of nephroblastoma patients with primary pulmonary metastases: results from SIOP 93-01/GPOH and SIOP 2001/GPOH. Ann Surg. 2011;254:155–62.
54. Theilen TM, Braun Y, Bochennek K, Rolle U, Fiegel HC, Friedmacher F. Multidisciplinary treatment strategies for Wilms tumor: recent advances, technical innovations and future directions. Front Pediatr. 2022 Jul;14(10):852185.
55. Furtwängler R, Nourkami N, Alkassar M, von Schweinitz D, Schenk JP, Rübe C, et al. Update on relapses in unilateral nephroblastoma registered in 3 consecutive SIOP/GPOH studies-a report from the GPOH-nephroblastoma study group. Klin Padiatr. 2011;223:113–9.
56. Malogolowkin M, Spreafico F, Dome JS, van Tinteren H, Pritchard-Jones K, van den Heuvel-Eibrink MM, et al. Incidence and outcomes of patients with late recurrence of Wilms' tumor. Pediatr Blood Cancer. 2013;60:1612–5.
57. Fernandez CV, Perlman EJ, Mullen EA, et al. Clinical outcome and biological predictors of relapse after nephrectomy only for very low-risk Wilms tumor: a report from children's oncology group AREN0532. Ann Surg. 2017;265(4):835–40.
58. Bansal D, Totadri S, Chinnaswamy G, Agarwala S, Vora T, Arora B, Prasad M, Kapoor G, Radhakrishnan V, Laskar S, Kaur T, Rath GK, Bakhshi S. Management of Neuroblastoma: ICMR consensus document. Indian J Pediatr. 2017 Jun;84(6):446–55.
59. Nelson WE. In: Kliegman R, Stanton B, St Geme JW, Schor NF, Behrman RE, editors. Nelson textbook of pediatrics. 21st ed. Elsevier Inc; 2020.
60. Monclair T, Brodeur GM, Ambros PF, et al. The international Neuroblastoma risk group (INRG) staging system: an INRG task force report. J Clin Oncol. 2009;27:298–303.
61. Schleiermacher G, Mosseri V, London WB, et al. Segmental chromosomal alterations have prognostic impact in neuroblastoma: a report from the INRG project. Br J Cancer. 2012;107:1418–22.
62. Ambros PF, Ambros IM, Brodeur GM, et al. International consensus for neuroblastoma molecular diagnostics: report from the international neuroblastoma risk group (INRG) biology committee. Br J Cancer. 2009;100:1471–82.
63. Liang WH, Federico SA, London WB, et al. Tailoring therapy for children with neuroblastoma based on risk group classification: past, present, and future. JCO Clin Cancer Inform. 2020;4:895–905.
64. Irwin MS, Naranjo A, Zhang FF, Cohn SL, London WB, Gastier-Foster JM, Ramirez NC, Pfau R, Reshmi S, Wagner E, Nuchtern J, Asgharzadeh S, Shimada H, Maris JM, Bagatell R, Park JR, Hogarty MD. Revised Neuroblastoma risk classification system: a report from the children's oncology group. J Clin Oncol. 2021;39(29):3229–41.
65. Peinemann F, van Dalen EC, Berthold F. Rapid COJEC induction therapy for high-risk Neuroblastoma patients—Cochrane review. Klin Padiatr. 2016;228:130–4. https://doi.org/10.1055/s-0042-103158.
66. Barr EK, Laurie K, Wroblewski K, Applebaum MA, Cohn SL. Association between end-induction response according to the revised international Neuroblastoma response criteria (INRC) and outcome in high-risk neuroblastoma patients. Pediatr Blood Cancer. 2020;67:e28390.
67. Desai AV, Applebaum MA, Karrison TG, Oppong A, Yuan C, Berg KR, MacQuarrie K, Sokol E, Hall AG, Pinto N, et al. Efficacy of post-induction therapy for high-risk neuroblastoma patients with end-induction residual disease. Cancer. 2022;128:2967–77.
68. Federico SM, Naranjo A, Zhang F, Marachelian A, Desai AV, Shimada H, Braunstein SE, Tinkle CL, Yanik GA, Asgharzadeh S, et al. A pilot induction regimen incorporating dinutuximab and sargramostim for the treatment of newly diagnosed high-risk neuroblastoma: a report from the children's oncology group. J Clin Oncol. 2022;40:10003.

69. Mazloom A, Louis CU, Nuchtern J, Kim E, Russell H, Allen-Rhoades W, Krance R, Paulino AC. Radiation therapy to the primary and Postinduction chemotherapy MIBG-avid sites in high-risk Neuroblastoma. Int J Radiat Oncol Boil Phys. 2014;90:858–62.
70. Yu AL, Gilman AL, Ozkaynak MF, London WB, Kreissman SG, Chen HX, Smith M, Anderson B, Villablanca JG, Matthay KK, et al. Anti-GD2 antibody with GM-CSF, interleukin-2, and isotretinoin for neuroblastoma. N Engl J Med. 2010;363:1324–34.
71. Rajagopalan A, Christenberry SC. Venkataraman Ramachandran. Rhabdomyosarcoma Pediatr Rev October. 2022;43(10):599–600.
72. Yechieli RL, Mandeville HC, Hiniker SM, et al. Rhabdomyosarcoma. Pediatr Blood Cancer. 2021;68(Suppl. 2):e28254.
73. Malempati S, Hawkins DS. Rhabdomyosarcoma: review of the children's oncology group (COG) soft-tissue sarcoma committee experience and rationale for current COG studies. Pediatr Blood Cancer. 2012;59(1):5–10.
74. PizzoPA PDG. Principles and practice of pediatric oncology. 5thed ed. Philadelphia: Lippincott Williams & Wilkins; 2006.
75. Thompson MJ, Shapton JC, Punt SE, Johnson CN, Conrad EU 3rd. MRI identification of the osseous extent of pediatric bone sarcomas. Clin Orthop Relat Res. 2018;476:559–64.
76. Shahid M, Albergo N, Purvis T, Heron K, Gaston L, Carter S, Grimer R, Jeys L. Management of sarcomas possibly involving the knee joint when to perform extra-articular resection of the knee joint and is it safe? Eur J Surg Oncol. 2017;43:175–80.
77. Enneking WF, Kagan A. "Skip" metastases in osteosarcoma. Cancer. 1975;36:2192–205.
78. Harrison DJ, Parisi MT, Shulkin BL. The role of (18) F-FDG-PET/CT in pediatric sarcoma. Semin Nucl Med. 2017;47:229–41.
79. Hwang EI, Sayour EJ, Flores CT, Grant G, Wechsler-Reya R, Hoang-Minh LB, Kieran MW, Salcido J, Prins RM, Figg JW, et al. The current landscape of immunotherapy for pediatric brain tumors. Nat Cancer. 2022;3:11–24. https://doi.org/10.1038/s43018-021-00319-0.
80. Udaka YT, Packer RJ. Pediatric brain tumors. Neurol Clin. 2018;36:533–56.
81. MacDonald TJ. Aggressive infantile embryonal tumors. J Child Neurol. 2008;23:1195–204.
82. Ostrom QT, Cioffi G, Waite K, Kruchko C, Barnholtz-Sloan JS. CBTRUS statistical report: primary brain and other central nervous system tumors diagnosed in the United States in 2014-2018. Neuro-Oncology. 2021;23(12 Suppl 2):iii1–105.
83. Sun T, Plutynski A, Ward S, Rubin JB. An integrative view on sex differences in brain tumors. Cell Mol Life Sci. 2015;72:3323–42.
84. Choi JY. Medulloblastoma: current perspectives and recent advances. Brain Tumor Res Treat. 2023;11(1):28–38.
85. Lafay-Cousin L, Dufour C. High-dose chemotherapy in children with newly diagnosed medulloblastoma. Cancers (Basel). 2022;14:837.
86. Kleihues P, Louis DN, Scheithauer BW, et al. The WHO classification of tumors of the nervous system. J Neuropathol Exp Neurol. 2002;61(3):215–225; discussion 226–219.
87. Gnekow AK, Falkenstein F, von Hornstein S, et al. Long-term follow-up of the multicenter, multidisciplinary treatment study HIT-LGG-1996 for low-grade glioma in children and adolescents of the German speaking Society of Pediatric Oncology and Hematology. Neuro-Oncology. 2012;14(10):1265–84.
88. von Hornstein S, Kortmann RD, Pietsch T, et al. Impact of chemotherapy on disseminated low-grade glioma in children and adolescents: report from the HIT-LGG 1996 trial. Pediatr Blood Cancer. 2011;56(7):1046–54.
89. Hernaiz Driever P, von Hornstein S, Pietsch T, et al. Natural history and management of low-grade glioma in NF-1 children. J Neuro-Oncol. 2010;100(2):199–207.
90. Gnekow AK, Kandels D, van Tilburg C, et al. SIOP-E-BTG and GPOH guidelines for diagnosis and treatment of children and adolescents with low grade glioma. Klin Padiatr. 2019;231(3):107–35.

Basic Principles of Pediatric Surgical Oncology: What Radiologist Should Know

2

Kanika Sharma, Sarita Chowdhary, Shiv Prasad Sharma, and Ishan Kumar

2.1 Introduction

Tumors are staged according to their extents, capsular invasion, vascularity, and various other parameters. However, most of these factors are decided based on the available imaging. The role of initial imaging cannot be undermined since these guides for planning the upfront surgeries in selected cases or initiation of radiotherapy/chemotherapy [1]. Radiologists are prime members of tumor boards across the globe, where they actively participate in diagnosis and management of pediatric surgical malignancies.Within the context of pediatric surgical oncology, the role of a radiologist is crucial in both diagnosis and treatment planning [2]. Radiologists utilize advanced imaging techniques such as MRI, CT scans, and ultrasound to accurately identify and characterize tumors in children. Their expertise in interpreting these images plays a significant role in guiding surgical interventions and determining the best course of treatment for the young patients.

Moreover, radiologists collaborate closely with pediatric oncologists and surgeons to ensure that the imaging findings are integrated into the overall management of the patient's condition. This collaboration enhances the precision of surgical procedures and aids in monitoring the effectiveness of treatment over time.

2.2 General Consideration for Imaging

Age It is of paramount importance for radiologists to be well-versed with the age-wise distribution of pediatric tumors and their specific characteristics.

Image-Guided Biopsy Integration of tumor biology with radiological findings is collaborative for high diagnostic accuracy of tumors [3]. Often, needle biopsy can miss anaplasia, therefore it is mandatory to take 8–10 cores of tumor needle biopsy from different quadrants of tumor.

Invasion It is important to differentiate whether a tumor is invading the surrounding structures or just pushing the structures. The compressive mass effect on the surrounding structures can be responsible for clinical and radiological interpretation of involvement of peri-tumor structure. A close examination and definition of tumor wall/capsule with surrounding structures and vessels

K. Sharma · S. Chowdhary · S. P. Sharma
Department of Pediatric Surgery, Institute of Medical Sciences, Banaras Hindu University, Varanasi, India
e-mail: Kanikasharma@bhu.ac.in

I. Kumar (✉)
Department of Radiodiagnosis and Imaging, Institute of Medical Sciences, Banaras Hindu University, Varanasi, Uttar Pradesh, India

I. Kumar et al. (eds.), *Practical Approach to Imaging in Pediatric Oncology*,
https://doi.org/10.1007/978-981-96-8158-7_2

can guide this decision. A well-defined tumor capsule and preserved wall of surrounding structure with a defined plane in-between rules out tumor invasion. Similarly, a collapsed lumen of vessels of surrounding structure rules out invasion.

Encasement This term is used to describe the alignment of tumors along the major vessels. The term "Encasement" is commonly used for neuroblastoma in describing vascular involvement according to Image-defined risk factors (IDRF). If a tumor encases a vital structure, it implies that structure maybe transversing through the content of tumor, while structure may still not be infiltrated by the tumor. However, this poses a serious risk of damage to the vital structure during the surgery.

Resectability A well-delineated lesion is a blessing for surgeons. Tumors which are localized and encapsulated with no involvement or extension to vessels have a tendency to get resected without any tumor spill or rupture. All surgeons prefer to do a gross total resection of tumor (GTR). On the other hand, when there is infiltration into surrounding structures or vascular extension, then complete resection becomes difficult and surgeons may have to resort to other maneuvers to ensure complete tumor resection. For most of the unresectable tumor at presentation, the neoadjuvant chemotherapy can be advised as per the type and staging of tumor. Post-neoadjuvant chemotherapy, depending upon the response of tumor, resectability has to be assessed and surgical plan has to be devised. In cases where a tumor is extending into a large vessel, the surgical team plans for advanced vascular control.

Tumor Response In solid tumors, the tumor response following neoadjuvant chemotherapy or radiotherapy is evaluated commonly with the help of RECIST criteria [4]. RECIST criteria utilize one-dimensional criteria or parameters, acquired from the cross-sectional serial images. Also, other criteria like 3-D volumetric assessment of tumor response have also been used. Radiologist should be aware of post-chemotherapy changes such as fibrosis and calcification. These changes can alter signals in MRI which can cause low signals in T1 and T2 images leading to underestimation of extent of disease. Though MRI is preferred cross-sectional imaging for response assessment, CT is preferred over MRI in immediate preoperative phase.

Surveillance Surveillance imaging focus on detection of recurrences. Surveillance protocols of pediatric tumors are formulated to assess the locoregional as well as common metastatic sites for recurrences [1, 2]. These protocols are proposed based on the stage at presentation, response to treatment, residual disease, and grade of tumor. Often depending upon the risk-stratification of tumor type, intensity and frequency of follow-up visits and investigations are decided. USG and MRI have gained popularity in surveillance protocols. While high-definition USG can detect small recurrences in expert hands, MRI has been implemented in various protocols for its advantage of being radiation-free and excellent delineation of organs. A retrospective study conducted by the NWTS-5 group suggested comparable overall survival after recurrence in Wilms tumor, when compared with chest x-ray and abdominal ultrasound as surveillance modality [5]. The study also highlighted that surveillance imaging was superior to clinical presentation for diagnosing the recurrences, and recurrences diagnosed by CT had the shortest time from diagnosis to recurrence. The tumor biology is proposed to be the main determinant of outcome rather than the frequency and modality of surveillance imaging.

2.3 Renal Masses

Most common pediatric renal malignancy is Wilms tumor. Non-Wilms renal tumors include CCSK, RTK, renal cell carcinoma (RCC), and other rare tumors (lymphoma, germ cell tumor, neuroblastoma, rhabdomyosarcoma, or sarcoma). The two important international groups, i.e., The North American—Children's Oncology Group (COG) and the European group—International Society of Pediatric Oncology-Renal Tumor Study Group (SIOP-RTSG) have their imaging protocols defined for diagnosis, staging, and surveillance [6]. Beek et al. have highlighted the similarities and differences of imaging (USG, CT, and MRI) protocol of the two groups under the global initiative of HARMONICA along with their technical requirements [6–9]. The outcomes of treatment of these groups are comparable [6, 7]. COG prefers upfront nephrectomy while SIOP favors preoperative chemotherapy. The risk group in WT is done based on the histology. COG considers presence or absence of anaplasia (very low, low, intermediate, and high risk group); while SIOP assesses based on the percentage of preoperative chemotherapy-induced changes and viable tumor components (low, intermediate, and high-risk group). An overview to approach to renal masses is given in Fig. 2.1.

It is important to differentiate nephrogenic rest from small WT, especially in cases of predisposing syndromes like WAGR, Beckwith-Wiedemann syndrome. While imaging and needle biopsy are not very effective in identifying the pseudocapsule, thereby less sensitive in differentiating nephrogenic rest with WT [10]. MRI has higher sensitivity to detect nephrogenic rest. COG proposed a cut-off of 1.75 cm for differentiating the two entities. Nephrogenic rests can have varied biological nature according to which management is planned. These may remain dormant, involute spontaneously, proliferate to hyperplastic nephrogenic rest forming a thick rind of nephroblastic cells, and only a small number of nephrogenic rest undergo clonal transformation to WT. Thus, for tumor specimens with presence of nephrogenic rests, it is advisable to monitor contralateral kidney for malignant transformation. As such for isolated lesion, no therapy is given, however for diffuse and multifocal lesions (nephroblastomatosis), chemotherapy is administered (Fig. 2.2).

COG defines pulmonary metastasis, CT thorax with or without contrast, as round, sharply marginated with lack of calcification and located outside a fissure. SIOP-RTSG defines pulmonary nodules ≥3 mm as lung metastases on plain CT thorax [6]. Presence of intra-cranial involvement or early pulmonary metastasis is suggestive of rhabdoid tumor of kidney (RTK). Presence of bony metastasis with renal masses is characteristic of clear-cell sarcoma of kidney (CCSK).

SIOP advocates percutaneous core-needle biopsy for patients aged 7 or above presenting with renal masses or for those with unusual imaging findings (such as calcification, lymphadenopathy, vessel encasement, psoas muscle infiltration, or near complete extrarenal tumor) [11].

For upfront tumor resection, cross-sectional imaging (CT/MRI) details the extent of tumor and resectability; while patients receiving neoadjuvant chemotherapy, the post-chemotherapy response is evaluated with cross-sectional imaging where size, necrosis, vascular extension, and invasion of tumor are assessed. Surgical resection includes nephrouretectomy with lymphnode sampling (from hilar, suprahilar, infrahilar, paracaval (for right masses), para-aortic (for left masses), aorto-caval, iliac, and mesenteric lymphnodes). While standard nephrouretectomy is the treatment of choice, in some cases (such as solitary kidney, bilateral renal tumor), nephron-sparing surgery or partial nephrectomy with lym-

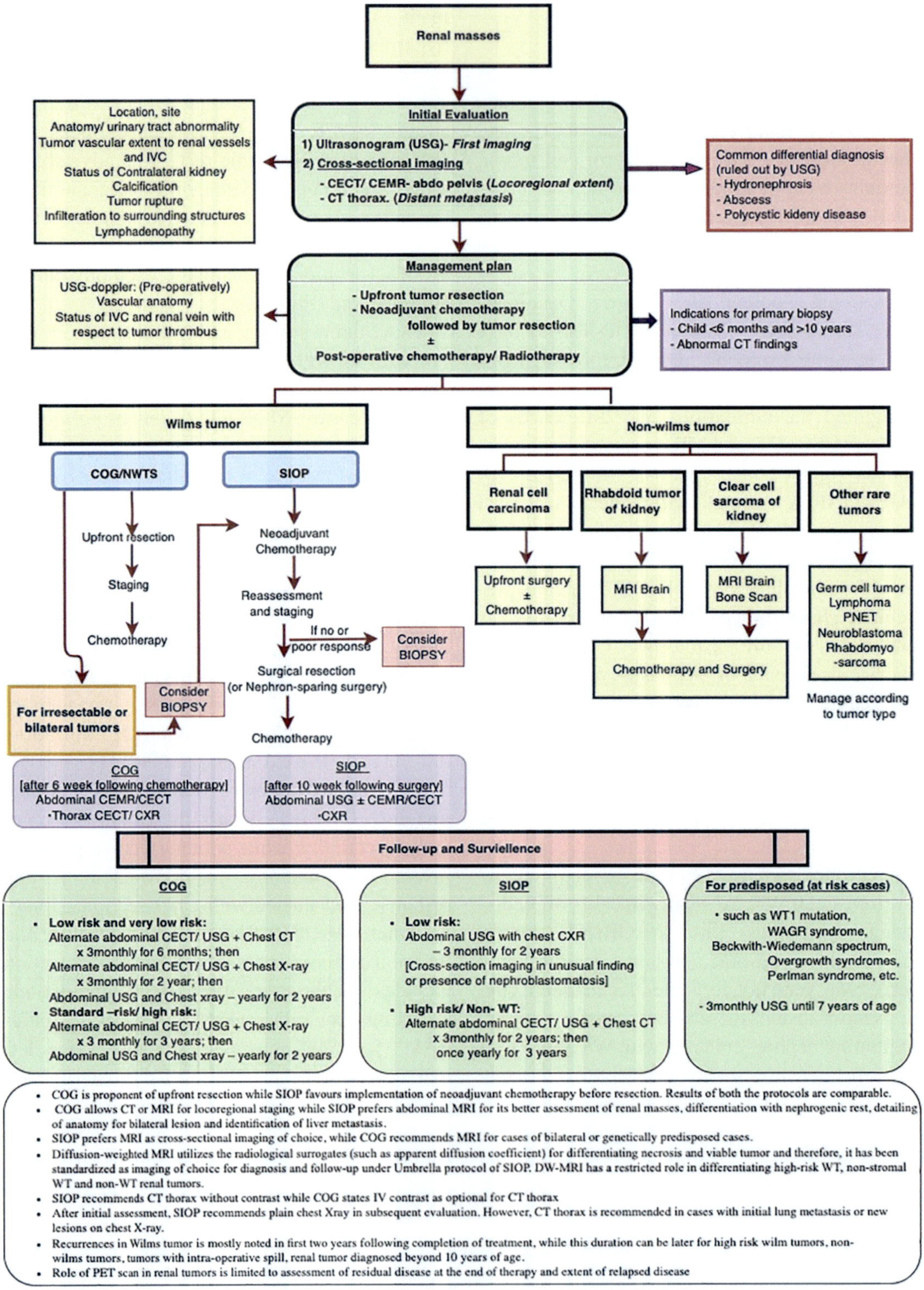

Fig. 2.1 Management outline of renal masses

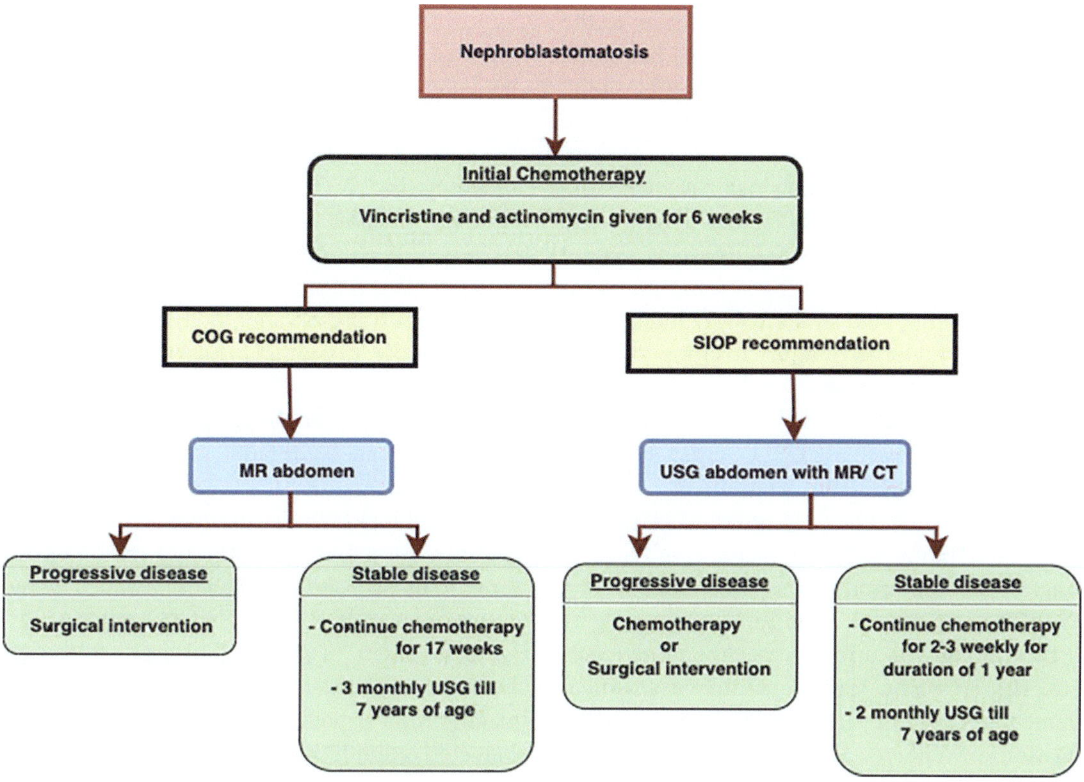

Fig. 2.2 Management outline of nephroblastomatosis

phnode sampling can also be planned. For masses which shrink sparing pelvis and majority of renal parenchyma, nephron-sparing surgery can be planned.

During surveillance, for locoregional assessment, abdominal USG is the standard of investigation for both COG and SIOP [6]. Cross-sectional imaging (CECT or CE MRI) is advised for all follow-up if renal mass is in COG, while SIOP reserves cross-sectional imaging (CEMRI preferred over CECT) for cases suggestive of recurrence on abnormal abdominal USG. Since pulmonary metastasis is the most common site of recurrence, radiological surveillance of the thoracic cavity is of paramount importance after complete remission of tumor. COG protocols have both CXR and CT thorax after completion of treatment while SIOP uses CXR only. Since most of the recurrence in renal tumors is evident within 2 years of treatment completion, both the protocols implement 3–6 monthly review for the first 2 years followed by yearly visit till a minimum of 5 years of treatment completion. A surveillance 3-monthly ultrasound is suggested for patients with predisposition syndrome (WAGR, Denys-Drash, hemihypertrophy, or Beckwith-Wiedemann syndrome) [12].

2.4 Neuroblastoma

Neuroblastoma (NB) is the most common extracranial tumor of childhood. Commonly, neurogenic tumors are described under three histological types, i.e., ganglioneuroblastoma, neuroblastoma, and ganglioneuroma [13]. These tumors can arise from the cervical region to the pelvis with suprarenal location (50%) being the most common site. International Neuroblastoma Risk Group (INRG) Task Force and International Neuroblastoma Risk Group Staging System (INRGSS) are two common risk grouping systems. Image-defined risk factors (IDRF) are important for the INRGSS risk grouping system [14]. IDRFs describe the relationship of tumor with surrounding vital structures, such that these highlight the high risk of injury to or involvement of vital structures during surgery.

For diagnosis and staging, important imaging modality involves USG, cross-sectional imaging (CT/MRI for anatomical details), nuclear medicine imaging (meta-[123I] iodobenzylguanidine (MIBG) scintigraphy, 3-D single-photon emission computed tomography (SPECT), positron emission tomography (PET)) along with urinary catecholamine levels [15, 16]. However, for preoperative assessment immediately before surgery, CECT is the investigation of choice as vascular relations are appreciated better on CECT while MRI may underestimate the exact disease extent [17]. Radiologists should clearly define adhesion, invasion, encasement, and infiltration for vascular or organ involvement [13].

Tumor biology plays a very important role in disease prognosis. Of this, N-MYC and segmental chromosomal aberrations are indicative of poor prognosis. Image-guided core needle biopsy is commonly used for tissue diagnosis of NB [18]. Surgical Complexity Index (SCI) has recently been proposed to define weightage to IDRF items which can be predictive or indicative of surgical complexity during NB resection [19].

Current treatment protocols for NB consist of a combination of intensive multi-agent induction chemotherapy, surgery, radiation, myeloablative consolidation therapy with stem cell rescue and transplantation, 13-cis retinoic acid, and immunotherapy (Fig. 2.3). Complete surgical resection improves outcome in low-risk as well as high-risk NB [20]. Surgical resection of >90% of all macroscopic disease is recommended for neuroblastoma with preservation and management of encased major vessel [21]. En-bloc resection of surrounding structures and organs is not indicated. In cases of very large tumor mass, debulking surgery can be offered to relieve pressure from vital organs.

International neuroblastoma response criteria have been proposed for assessing the treatment response in NB, which also takes into account the reassessment of IDRFs and RECIST criteria [22]. For assessment of residual disease, following chemotherapy and surgery, among cross-sectional imaging MRI is preferred due to its better tissue characterization [23]. MIBG has proven to be of superior diagnostic value in the identification of early metastasis and recurrence of bony metastasis.

The important differential diagnosis is Wilms tumor, which is also a retroperitoneal tumor found in the same age group as NB [24]. Table 2.1 provides the clues to differentiate between neuroblastoma and Wilms tumor.

The timing of surveillance in neuroblastoma is intensive for N-MYC amplification and high-risk cases [16]. While there is no consensus or guideline available among the societies, a comprehensive layout of surveillance can be seen summarized in Fig. 2.2.

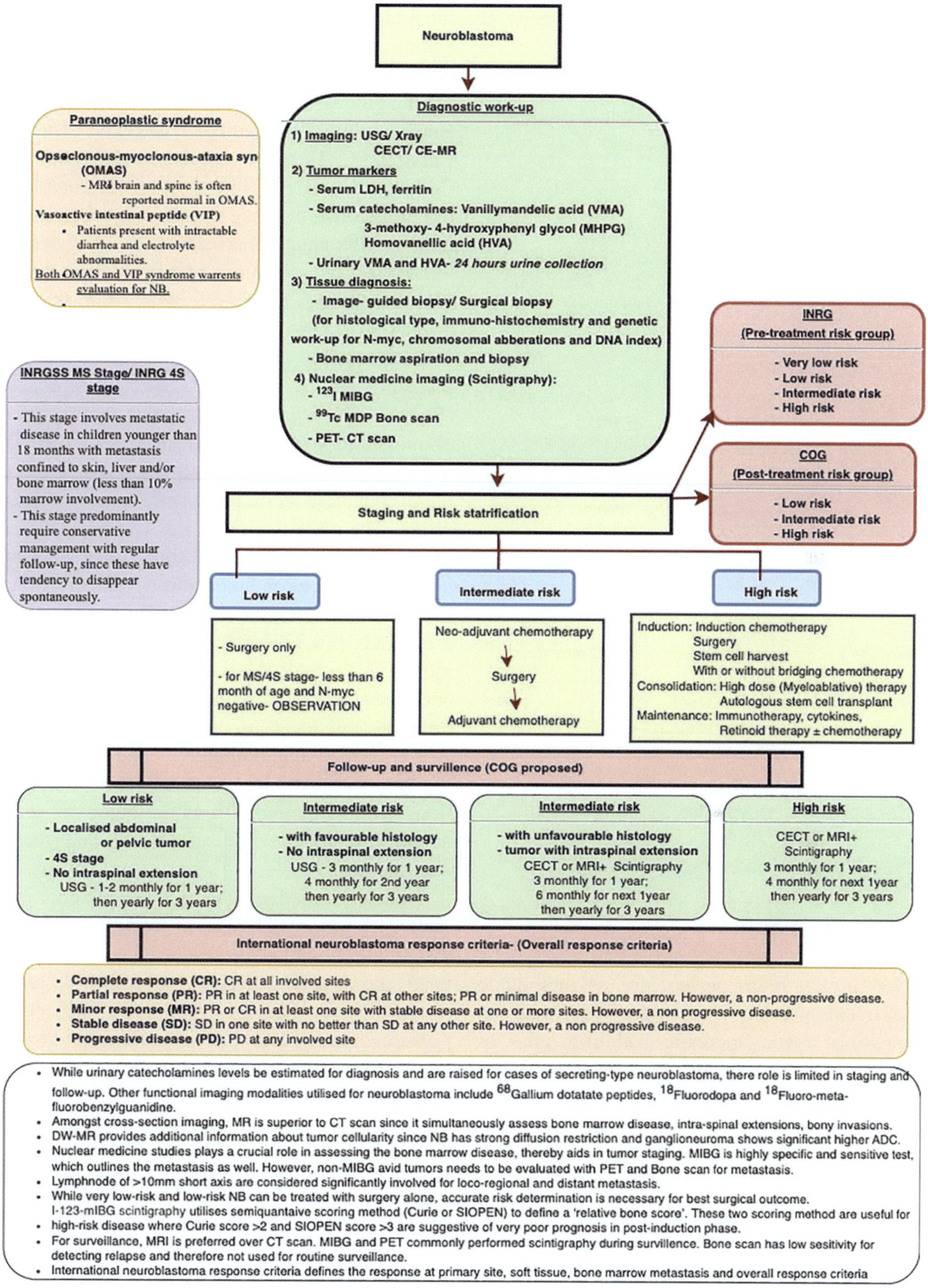

Fig. 2.3 A brief outline of management plan of neuroblastoma

Table 2.1 Difference between neuroblastoma and Wilms tumor

	Neuroblastoma	Wilms tumor
General condition	Emaciated child Poor growth and development	Healthy child Well-nourished child
Presenting complains	Abdominal mass Opsoclonus-myoclonus <5% Diarrhea, VIP syndrome <1%	Abdominal mass 25–30% – abdominal pain, fever, hematuria, anemia, or hypertension
Imaging- site °°capsule °°vascular involvement °°calcification	Suprarenal No capsule Encasement of major vessels Calcification ++ (90%)	Renal cortex and / or pelvis Pseudocapsule ++ Invasion++ Calcification ± (< 10%) Claw sign +
Common metastasis sites	Bone/ bone marrow> lung> liver	Lung > Liver
Commonly associated genetic aberrations	N-MYC amplification ALK amplification DNA ploidy Gain of chromosome 17 q Deletion of 11q, 1p	Wt-1 mutation IGF-2 mutation 11p loss

2.5 Liver Tumors

Liver tumors can present as asymptomatic abdominal masses with other constitutional symptoms (fever, anorexia, vomiting, etc.) or respiratory distress in cases of abdominal distension [25]. The important marker for liver malignancy in the pediatric age group is serum alpha-fetoprotein. For hepatoblastoma and HCC, PRETEXT (pre-treatment extent of tumor) for primary assessment of disease and POSTTEXT (post-treatment extent of tumor) for response following neoadjuvant chemotherapy are assessed on cross-sectional imaging (CT or MRI) for defining the resectability of tumor [26]. Pediatric Hepatic International Tumor Trial (PHITT) under Children's Hepatic tumors International Collaboration (CHIC) is a recent international trial which will evaluate the role of pretreatment radio-pathological characteristics of hepatic tumors and revise the treatment guidelines [27]. Fig. 2.4 outlines the working algorithm for the evaluation of hepatic masses.

Surgical resection and chemotherapy are the mainstay of treatment of liver malignancy (Fig. 2.5) [28]. Upfront resection is only recommended for very-low risk PRETEXT I and II under COG guidelines; and for PRETEXT I under Japanese Pediatric Liver Tumor (JPLT) group. The prerequisite for upfront resection is to attain at least 1 cm margin from middle hepatic vein and/or main portal vein division. International Childhood Liver Tumor strategy group (SIOPEL) recommends neoadjuvant chemotherapy for all. Reassessment for response and resectability is done with cross-sectional imaging and levels of alpha-fetoprotein after 2–8 cycles of chemotherapy depending upon the protocol. Atypical, non-anatomical resections are associated with worse outcome, thus to be reserved for multifocal or metastatic disease.

RELIVE initiative (international collaboration under PHITT), which aims to study the relapses and progression of pediatric hepatic tumor, facilitated the protocol design for follow-up and response assessment of liver tumor [29]. The post-treatment surveillance of hepatoblastoma is guided by the level of alpha-fetoproteins, while for cases of hepatocellular carcinoma surveillance imaging is required irrespective of alpha-fetoprotein levels [30]. The relapsed or progressive disease requires advanced treatment regimen.

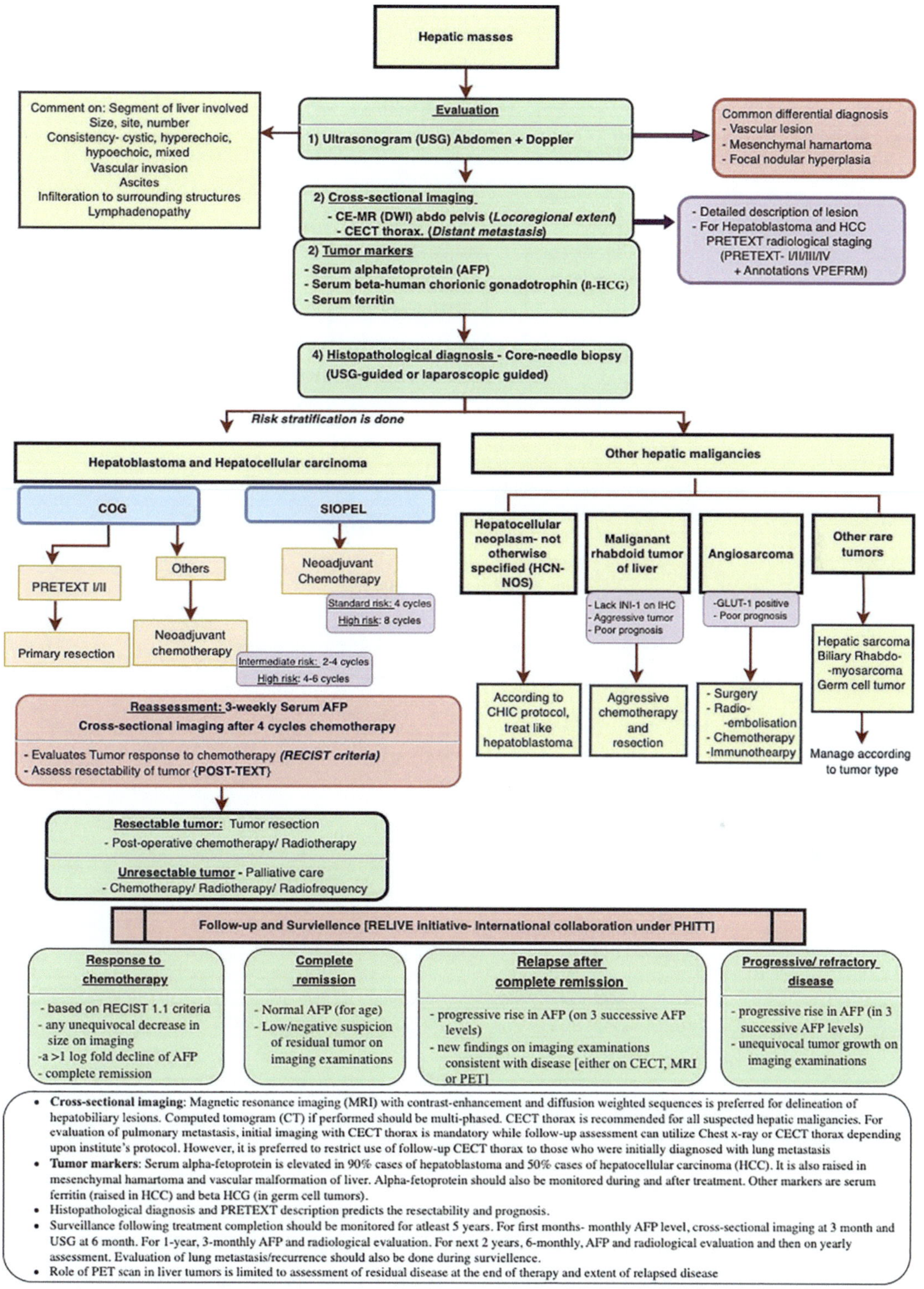

Fig. 2.4 Outlines the management of liver masses

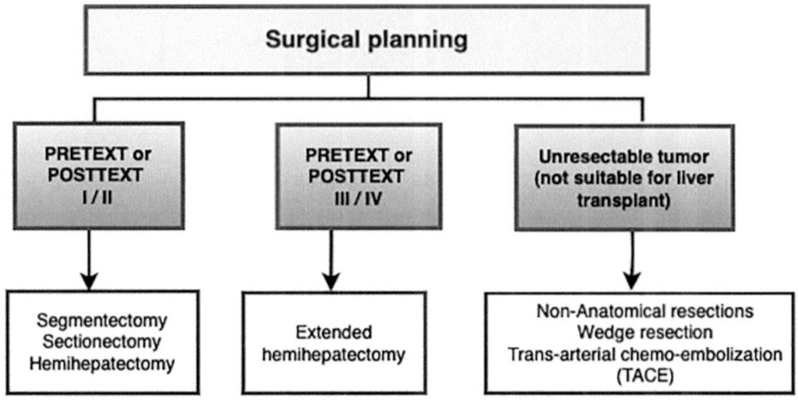

Indication for liver transplantation

- Multifocal PRETEXT IV
- Solitary PRETEXT IV
- PRETEXT III with vascular involvement (V+, P+)
- Tumor adjoining major vessels or invading major vessels
- Central tumor [Segment Iv, V VIII] involvement in close proximity to major vessels

Indication of upfront resection in CHIC

- PRETEXT I and II with M-, VPEFR-
- PRETEXT II with age <8 years; AFP >100ng/dL

Nomenclature of anatomical resection

Segmentectomy	Any 1 segment 1-8
Bisegmentectomy	Any 2 segment 1-8
Right hepatectomy or hemihepatectomy	Segments 5-8 ± Segment 1
Left hepatectomy or hemihepatectomy	Segments 2-4 ± Segment 1
Right anterior sectionectomy	Segments 5,8
Right posterior sectionectomy	Segments 6,7
Left medial sectionectomy	Segment 4
Left lateral sectionectomy	Segments 2,3
Extended Right hepatectomy or hemihepatectomy (Right trisectionectomy)	Segments 5-8+ Segment 4 ± Segment 1
Extended Left hepatectomy or hemihepatectomy (Left trisectionectomy)	Segments 2-5+ Segment 8 ± Segment 1

Fig. 2.5 Surgical plan for liver masses

2.6 Germ Cell Tumors

Germ cell tumors (GCT) arise from primordial germ cells [31]. They usually present at various locations and behave differently clinically. Pediatric GCTs will develop in the gonads or along the midline structures of the body. Any alteration in molecular signaling causes the development of GCT in extragonadal location (cervical, mediastinal, retroperitoneal, and sacrococcygeal region). Alpha-fetoprotein, beta-HCG, and LDH are common tumor markers used to differentiate types of GCT. Benign tumors are more common in prepubertal children with teratoma being the most common histological type.

Ovarian GCT: Ovarian GCT are usually benign in adults; however, in children and adolescents one-third cases of GCT are malignant [32].

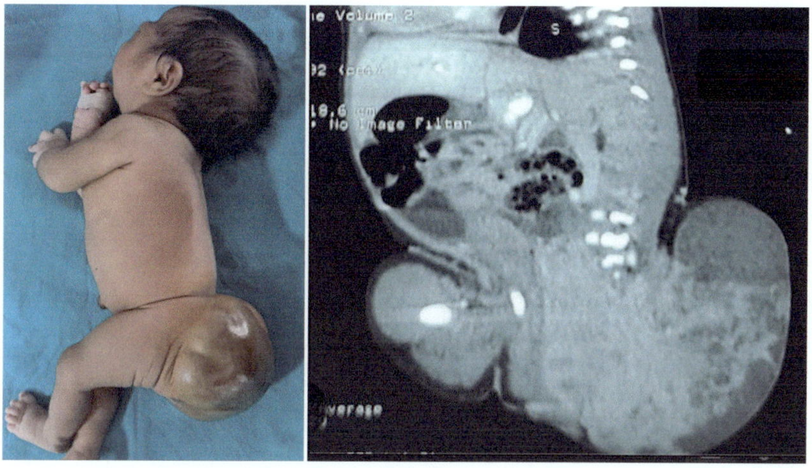

Fig. 2.6 Altman type 1 sacrococcygeal teratoma in 10-day-old with a large exophytic mass at lower back with multilobulated irregular surface extending gluteal region (outside the body) and displacing the anus anteriorly. Imaging shows a heterogenous multicystic exophytic growth arising from sacrococcygeal region. No intraperitoneal extension is noted

Clinical features, tumor markers, and imaging of GCT help in diagnosis and further planning of types of GCT. Mature teratoma with negative tumor marker is treated with ovarian sparing surgery while oophorectomy is done in immature teratoma with suspicion of malignancy. Complete tumor resection with ipsilateral oophorectomy with or without salpingectomy is performed for suspected malignancies. Complete intraperitoneal staging at the time of initial tumor resection is essential [33].

Testicular GCT: Testicular germ cell tumors (TGCTs), which are the most common testicular neoplasms, commonly occur in young and middle-aged men [34]. Evolving knowledge of genetics, pathogenesis, and immunohistochemical markers of TGCTs led to the updated 2016 World Health Organization (WHO) classification system, which has substantial diagnostic and treatment implications. Rarely, teratomas and choriocarcinomas commonly regress and form a fibrotic scar-like area with calcifications which is termed as Burned-out TGCT. Testicular sparing surgery (tumorectomy or tumor enucleation) can be done in a patient where USG shows salvageable testicular tissue and tumor markers are normal [35]. The tumors with raised tumor markers or post-pubertal masses require high inguinal orchidectomy. For malignant histology, chemotherapy is required.

Sacrococcygeal tumors (SCT) can be diagnosed antenatally and may warrant ex-utero intrapartum treatment (EXIT) procedure for massive tumors causing vascular steal phenomenon [36]. Altman classification is described to define the extent of intracorporeal and extracorporeal involvement of tumor (Fig. 2.6). This helps to plan the approach of surgery and counsel the guardians of child accordingly. Most of these tumors are benign. However, with the advancing age, the unresected tumors can undergo malignant transformation, so early resection is preferred.

Imaging defines the resectability of tumor, especially in cases of non-testicular GCT. For testicular tumor, scrotal USG, clinical examination, and tumor markers guide the decision for testis-sparing surgery or orchidectomy [34, 35]. MR provides better assessment of tumor response and is utilized as support tool for discriminating benign from malignant GCT [37]. If imaging shows a resectable well well-encapsulated tumor, upfront surgery should be done with complete tumor resection. If gross total resection is not feasible or imaging suggests infiltrative tumor, then one has to resort to biopsy with neoadjuvant chemotherapy. Unlike adults, there is no role of retroperitoneal lymphnode dissection in pediatric GCT. For follow-up and surveillance, tumor markers are monitored predominantly (Fig. 2.7).

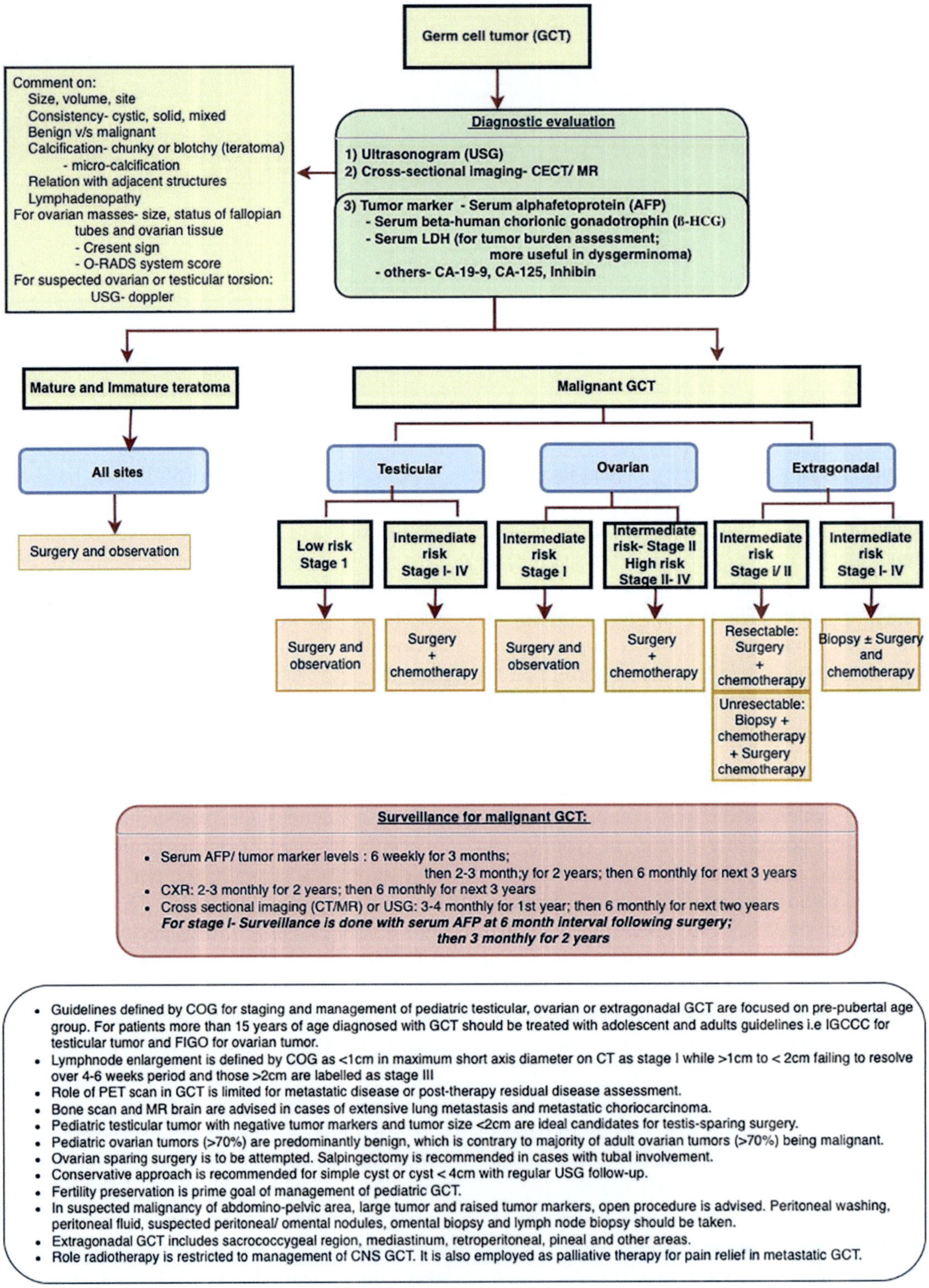

Fig. 2.7 Concise management plan of germ cell tumor

2.7 Soft-Tissue Sarcoma

Soft-tissue sarcomas are rare tumors accounting for less than 10% of all pediatric tumors [38]. Of these, 50% constitute rhabdomyosarcomas (RMS) (third most common extracranial solid-tumor of pediatric age), while rest are non-rhabdomyosarcoma soft tissue sarcoma (NRSTS) (Table 2.2).

RMS is a malignant lesion with tendency to differentiate to skeletal muscle from pluripotent mesenchymal cells [38]. Tumor spreads via lymphnodes, and thus, sentinel lymphnodes sampling is important in RMS. The two major histological types of RMS include alveolar and embryonal, where PAX-FOX fusion-positive alveolar RMS has poorer prognosis than embryonal RMS and fusion-negative alveolar RMS. Local recurrences are attributed to pathological sentinel lymphnodes or microscopic residual disease [39]. The risk stratification of RMS is done utilizing pre-treatment TNM staging, group of the site, age of presentation, identification of PAX-FOX fusion for COG; while EpSSG (European Pediatric Soft tissue sarcoma group) incorporates age, tumor size, histological subtype, and nodal involvement in risk stratification.

The management plan for soft tissue sarcoma is outlined in Fig. 2.8. The prime objective of the treatment is to achieve R0 resection margins and maintain the local control without relapse.

MRI is the imaging of choice for head and neck, parameningeal, paraspinal, genitourinary, and extremities masses; while CECT is preferred for thoracic and abdominal masses [40]. However, EpSSG/ESPR oncology taskforce emphasized on acquiring MRI (T1, T2, and post contrast with DWI) for all suspected RMS, with exception of those where bone erosion or involvement is suspected such as RMS near skull base [41]. Tumor volume and size should be well documented for response assessment following therapy. The biopsy of lesion assesses histopathology and chromosomal aberrations [38]. If there are no neurovascular bundle involved or surrounding infiltration, and R0 resection is possible without debilitating surgery, then upfront surgery is planned, else neoadjuvant chemotherapy with locoregional radiation is given. Tumor involving vital structures (such as head and neck RMS) often chemotherapy and local irradiation is

Table 2.2 Basic differences between rhabdomyosarcoma and non-rhabdomyosarcoma soft-tissue sarcoma

	Rhabdomyosarcoma (RMS)	Non-RMS Soft-tissue sarcoma
Age of presentation	Bimodal [2–6 years; adolescent]	Bimodal [infant; 15–19 years]
Common sites	Head and neck; genitourinary	Extremities; trunk
Histological types	– Embryonal – Alveolar – Botryoidal spindle cell	Many variants: Infantile fibrosarcoma; Neurofibrosarcoma; synovial sarcoma; Hemangiopericytoma; Leiomyosarcoma; solitary fibrous tumor; Malignant fibrous histiocytoma; etc.
Treatment	Chemotherapy+ radiotherapy + surgery	Surgical excision
Response to chemotherapy	Chemo-sensitive	Chemoresistance
Sites of metastasis	Lung, lymphnode, bone marrow, liver	Lung
Common genetic aberrations	PAX/FOX fusion Loss of heterozygosity 11p 15	Translocations, deletions EWS-WT1 fusion

Sarcoma commonly presents as painless enlarging masses, which may become symptomatic due to compression of neurovascular bundle or invasion of surrounding structures

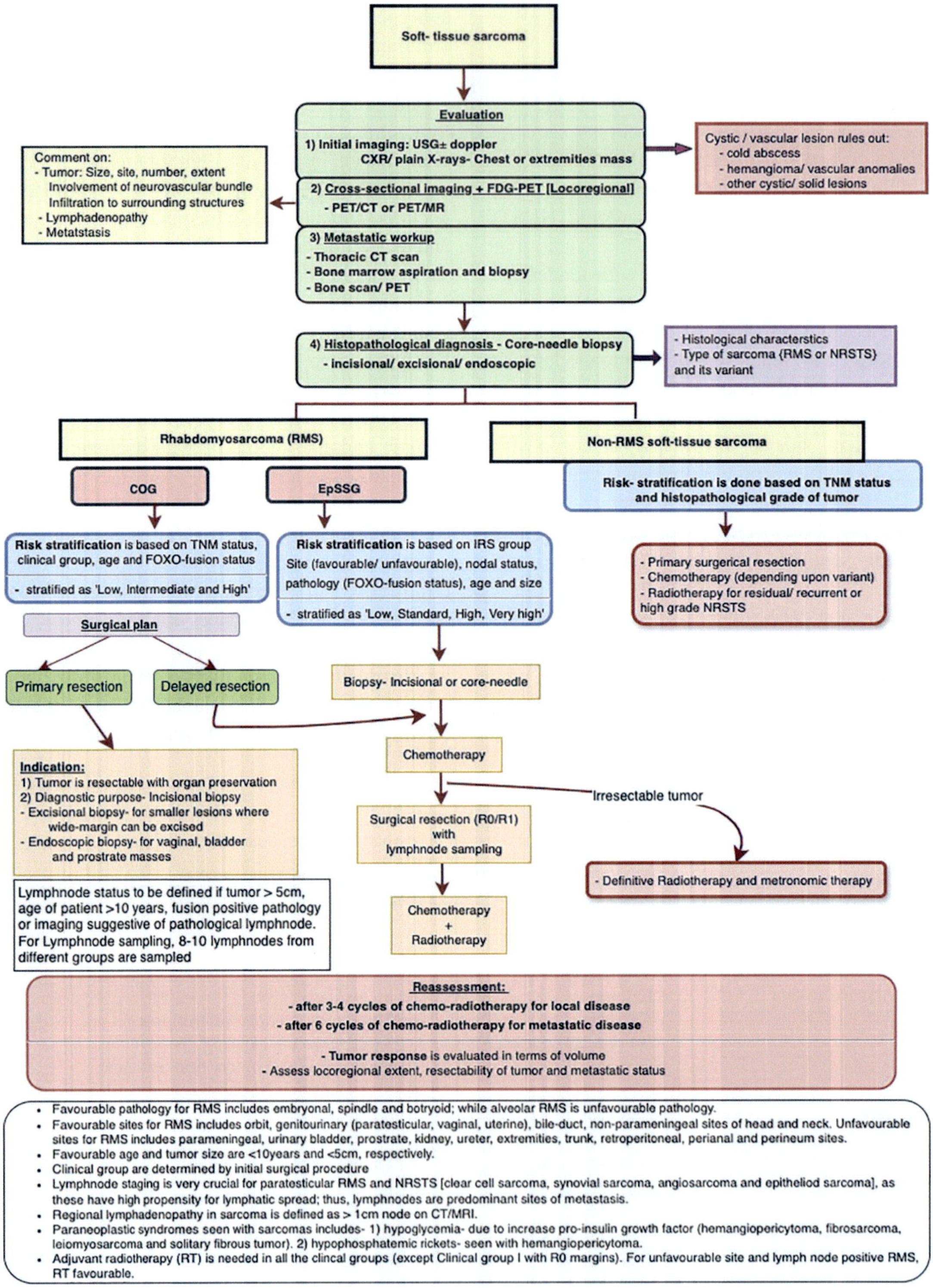

Fig. 2.8 Management of soft-tissue sarcoma in pediatric patients

offered as primary treatment. Reassessment with cross-sectional imaging (MRI preferred) is done after 3–4 cycles of chemotherapy. In cases of only biopsy, imaging of biopsy tract should also be taken into account while reporting; similarly, during surgery, the biopsy tract should be excised to avoid recurrences. If no excision is possible, then definitive radiotherapy is to be offered. There is no role of debulking surgery or residual excision at the end of therapy. For metastatic disease, high-risk and very-high-risk groups are usually managed with definitive radiotherapy and may require metronomic therapy. Tumor response is assessed with cross-sectional imaging and PET [41]. Definition of primary response is given as per RECIST 1.1 or 3-D volumetric assessment. SUV_{max} of more than 4.35 correlates with distant metastasis and poorer outcomes.

For NRSTS, standard staging workup includes TNM with histological grading. CECT thorax is done in addition to locoregional imaging. Enlarged lymphnode requires FNAC or excisional biopsy. Surgery is the mainstay of treatment for NRSTS, since these tumors are chemoresistant and radiotherapy is reserved for residual, relapse, and high-grade cases. Sentinel lymphnode biopsy is advised for NRSTS due to high risk for lymphnode metastasis (synovial sarcoma, epithelioid sarcoma, clear cell sarcoma, and angiosarcoma).

The surveillance should continue for 5 years post-treatment completion to look for any relapse. Apart from relapses, surveillance predominantly takes into account the toxicity of radiotherapy to the concerned area [42]. Imaging of primary site and chest radiograph is commonly done during the surveillance period. However, recent studies don't state any benefit of surveillance imaging on survival of relapsed cases [43]. Currently, an undergoing multinational FaR-RMS trial by EpSSG/CWG will further provide insight into relapsing RMS.

2.8 Bone Tumors

Among pediatric bone tumors, skeletal metastasis involving bone marrow and bone is frequently seen with neuroblastoma, clear-cell sarcoma of kidney, rhabdomyosarcoma, and other pediatric malignancies, an indicator of poorer prognosis [44]. Primary bone tumors are rare in the pediatric age group (3–5% of all pediatric tumors), and among them osteosarcoma and Ewing's sarcoma/primary neuroectodermal tumor (EW/PNET) are common [45]. Since osteosarcoma is radiotherapy-resistant, multimodal chemotherapy and wide resection are the treatment of choice for osteosarcoma. Ewing sarcoma requires chemo-radiation therapy with wide surgical resection. Radiotherapy in EW/PNET alone is reserved for patients with unresectable disease following neoadjuvant chemotherapy or those refusing surgery. Biopsy is recommended for histopathological diagnosis and staging. Musculoskeletal Tumor Society (MSTS) and The American Joint Committee on Cancer (AJCC) are two staging systems. Since surgical resection may involve the growing areas of long bones, there is a high risk of limb length discrepancy in growing children. Surgeons need to plan alternative resection methods, such as to prepare for limb salvage surgery, joint-sparing surgery, use of intercalary allografts, various osseointegration methods, rotationplasty, etc. Amputation is reserved for selected cases, to avoid simultaneous psychosocial impairments in child.

Recurrence occurs in more than one-third cases of high-grade OS and EWS within the first 2 years after therapy. Therefore, for these, the recommended surveillance intervals are every 3 months for the first 2 years, every 6 months for the next 3 years, and every year for the next 5 years [45]. For low-risk tumor, annual ressessment for two years is recommended. MRI is the investigation of choice for local surveillance. For limb salvage surgery, MARS technique is utilized. CT chest is required in high-risk cases, while plain chest radiograph is used for monitoring in low-risk cases. PET CT/MRI is recommended for whole-body evaluation of extrapulmonary metastases for new clinical symptoms or imaging findings.

2.9 Thoracic Masses

Pediatric thoracic neoplasms are very rare, yet these are difficult to diagnose owing to non-specific presentation (Fig. 2.9) [46]. Pulmonary secondaries (metastatic from other primary tumors) are more common than primary lung malignancy [47]. Minimally invasive surgery has revolutionized the surgical approach for thoracic masses, where thoracoscopically guided needle biopsies, excisional/incisional biopsies, tumor resection in selected cases, and resection of nodules can be done [48]. Lung secondaries, indicative of poorer prognosis, are managed with the advanced chemo-radiotherapy for the specific primary malignancy, yet resection of these secondary malignancies is rarely required for tumors [49]. Increased survival with metastatectomy is observed in osteosarcoma, hepatoblastoma, synovial sarcoma (NRSTS), and adrenocortical tumors [50]. Further, the size and number of nodules help in deciding the certainty for pulmonary metastasis and guide the planning for resection of secondaries. While plain CXR maybe needed in follow-up and surveillance of non-metastatic disease, CT scan becomes mandatory in case of documented malignancy at initiation or suspicion during follow-up.

Pleuropulmonary blastoma (PPB), inflammatory myofibroblastic tumor, and carcinoid tumor are common primary pediatric malignancy [47]. CXR is done for initial evaluation followed by CT or MRI for diagnosis, staging, response evaluation, and surveillance, and PET/CT is reserved predominantly for assessment of treatment response in advanced cases. Surgical resection is the treatment of choice followed by chemo-radiotherapy for PPB.

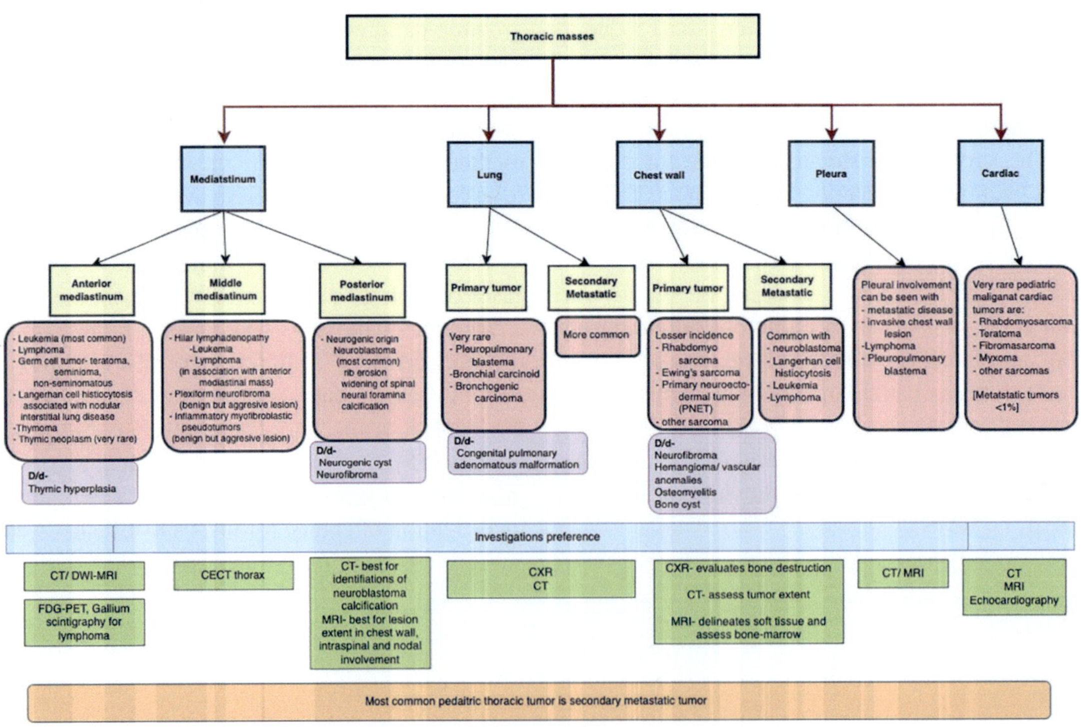

Fig. 2.9 Overview of pediatric thoracic malignancies

Special caution should be exercised while reporting an anterior mediastinal mass since these tumors may compress the tracheobronchial tree or interrupt venous return, and this compression becomes apparent during sedation or general anesthesia leading to catastrophic consequences [51]. Therefore, it is imperative to document the anteroposterior diameter of trachea [percentage of tracheal cross-sectional area; %TCA] along with the extent of anterior mediastinal masses [mediastinal mass ratio; MMR] and tracheal shift [52]. More than 50% reduction of tracheal anteroposterior diameter is associated with more intraoperative complication and risk during anesthesia. It is important to counsel and discuss this high-risk situation with the patient's family, surgeon, and anesthesiologists to plan for biopsy with safe alternatives (i.e., local anesthesia; upright positioning; utilizing newer safer anesthetic drugs such as ketamine, dexmedetomodine).

- The smallest anteroposterior tracheal diameter is measured at the level of the thoracic inlet at a segment of trachea with no evidence of extrinsic compression by the tumor.
- %TCA is calculated by the cross-sectional area (CSA) of a dimension of the trachea at its smallest and largest lumina using the following formula of an ellipse -axial image. CSA = (widest diameter/2 × narrowest diameter/2) × π.%TCA = (the smallest CSA)/(the largest CSA).
- MMR is defined as the maximum width of the mediastinal mass divided by the maximum intrathoracic width (at the level of diaphragm) on the CT image.

Table 2.3 Ultrasonographic characteristics of cervical lymphadenopathy

Oval shaped Minimal hilar vascularity Echogenic fatty hilum	Reactive lymphnode
Increased hilar vascularity Central necrosis Inflammation of surrounding tissues Edema Abscess—'Swirling debris pattern'	Infective or inflamed lymphnode
Absent/eccentric hilum Displacement of hilar vasculature Central necrosis Matted/aggregation of nodes into mass Irregular borders Irregular capsular blood flow patterns	Malignant lymphnode
Presence of hilum Matted nodes Sharp margins Strong internal echoes/hyperechogenic	Tubercular lymphnode

Table 2.4 Reporting protocol for cervical lymphadenopathy. (Adapted from Fraser et al. [55])

S.no	Lymphnode characteristics	Marking
1.	Involved nodes	Right: I II III IV V VI VII left: I II III IV V VI VII
2.	Echogenicity of nodes	Hypoechoic hyperechoic
3.	Largest size of nodes	
4.	Shape of nodes	Oval Round
5.	Intranodal necrosis	Yes No
6.	Calcification	Present Absent
7.	Edema	Yes No
8.	Vascularity	Normal Irregular Avascular
9.	Hilar echogenicity	Normal linear diffuse
Conclusion		

2.10 Cervical Lymphadenopathy

Palpable cervical lymphadenopathy is a very common presentation to the pediatric outpatient department. While most of them are reactive or infective, the other may be malignant (Tables 2.3, and 2.4). Lymphoma is the common malignancy in the pediatric age group presenting with generalized or cervical lymphadenopathy [53]. Children with infective pathology may have a preceding history of head and neck infection with fever, sore throat, cough, or cold. However, prolonged history of fever, associated with weight loss, anorexia, presence of persistent or unexplained palpable nodes, is suggestive of a serious underlying pathology such as tuberculosis, Langerhans cell histiocytosis, or lymphoma (Hodgkin lymphoma or non-Hodgkin lymphoma). The required laboratory workup includes basic blood test (CBC, ESR, LDH) with serology testing of suspected organisms. High-resolution USG with B-mode and Doppler helps in differentiating benign and malignant neck pathology [54]. A standardized protocol had been proposed for USG reporting of cervical lymphadenopathy (Fig. 2.5) [55]. The virtual touch imaging quantification shear wave elastography (VTIQ SWE) provides a quantitative assessment of tissue stiffness [56]. CXR is commonly advised for the evaluation of infection, tuberculosis, and to rule out mediastinal involvement [57]. Mediastinal widening is suggestive of mediastinal mass or hilar lymphadenopathy; further, cross-sectional imaging (CT or MRI) has to be considered for anatomical delineation and further planning for anesthesia and surgery. MRI is preferred for the evaluation of neck masses with intracranial and intraspinal extensions.

Since the sensitivity of FNAC is variable (67% to 100%), a negative FNAC report is not reliable for ruling out malignancy [58]. Thus, an excisional biopsy, which is the gold standard for tissue diagnosis, is helpful for precise histopathological diagnosis with details of exact type and subset of pathology. Biopsy is done under local anesthesia or sedation, where 2 or more lymphnodes are excised with their capsules intact and sent for histopathology with immunohistochemistry and GeneXpert (for tuberculosis). Depending upon the tissue diagnosis, definitive treatment can be planned.

2.11 Recent Advances and Updates

Artificial Intelligence (AI)

AI assists radiologists in interpreting complex imaging studies by providing automated analysis of lesions, tumor characteristics, and treatment response.

- **Radiomics** utilizes radiological imaging to pathologically classify tumor type as well as predict the anaplasia, thereby allowing the risk-stratification of tumor [59]. It can serve as 'virtual biopsy' where entire tumor can be assessed. An important example is utilization of CT-based radiomics signals and markers to predict the N-myc amplification in tumor burden [60].
- **Augmented reality (AR)** helps in planning the surgical excision with simultaneous early differentiation of healthy and malignant tissues [61]. There have been AR navigation system based on preoperative CT and MRI imaging for use in endoscopic surgery for pediatric tumors.
- **3D models** have been utilized for preparation of surgery, deciding the course of action by simulating and practicing the intra-operative scenario in a laboratory set-up [62]. 3-D visualization and simulation of tumor resection help to plan a successful total tumor resection, especially for complex masses.

Advances in Functional Imaging

The continued development of advanced functional imaging modalities such as diffusion-weighted imaging (DWI), dynamic contrast-enhanced imaging (DCE), and positron emission tomography (PET) provides detailed insights into tumor microenvironments, metabolic activity, and treatment response, enabling more personalized and targeted therapeutic strategies [63]. Some other advancements in cross-sectional images are dual-energy CT, blood oxygenation level-dependent (BOLD) MRI, and arterial spin labelling (ASL) which help in further characterization of tumor.

Enhanced Imaging for Minimal Residual Disease Detection

Further advancements in imaging technology aim to improve the detection of minimal residual disease (MRD) in pediatric oncology patients [64]. High-resolution imaging methods, including advanced molecular imaging and next-generation radiotracers, are being developed to detect and monitor residual cancer cells at subsistent levels, contributing to more accurate assessment and management of treatment response and relapse risk.

Interventional Radiology
This newer and rapidly advancing field in radiology provides an important extension to the armamentarium of pediatric onco-surgery [65]. Especially for highly vascular and poorly chemo-responsive tumors, preoperative tumor embolization can be used to curtail the blood supply to large tumor, thereby shrinking it for safer tumor resection with controlled blood loss. For inoperable cases, this has been used as palliative care. Another method, tumor angio-chemo-embolization (TACE), which is extensively used for adult hepatocellular carcinoma (HCC), has shown promising results in pediatric hepatic malignancy.

Others MRI machines are now available with higher tesla programs and set-ups with the availability of more sequences. This provides quicker and higher spatial resolution images, which is very useful in pediatric cases. Child needs shorter or no sedation for the acquisition of images under these processors.

Further, with the advent of newer anesthesia workstation, monitors that are compatible with MRI suite as well as safer anesthesia options, MRI can be done in pediatric patients with ease in a well-monitored manner.

References

1. Weiser DA, Kaste SC, Siegel MJ, et al. Imaging in childhood cancer: a Society for Pediatric Radiology and Children's oncology group joint task force report. Pediatr Blood Cancer. 2013;60:1253–60.
2. Frush DP, Callahan MJ, Coley BD, et al. Comparison of the different imaging modalities used to image pediatric oncology patients: A COG diagnostic imaging committee/SPR oncology committee white paper. Pediatr Blood Cancer. 2023;70(Suppl 4):e30298.
3. Jackson TJ, Williams RD, Brok J, et al. Children's cancer and Leukaemia group (CCLG) renal Tumours group. The diagnostic accuracy and clinical utility of pediatric renal tumor biopsy: report of the UK experience in the SIOP UK WT 2001 trial. Pediatr Blood Cancer. 2019;66:e27627.
4. Schwartz LH, Litière S, de Vries E, et al. RECIST 1.1-update and clarification: from the RECIST committee. Eur J Cancer. 2016;62:132–7.
5. Mullen EA, Chi YY, Hibbitts E, et al. Impact of surveillance imaging modality on survival after recurrence in patients with favorable-histology Wilms tumor: A report from the children's oncology group. J Clin Oncol. 2018;18(36):JCO1800076.
6. van der Beek JN, Artunduaga M, Schenk JP, et al. Similarities and controversies in imaging of pediatric renal tumors: A SIOP-RTSG and COG collaboration. Pediatr Blood Cancer. 2023;70(Suppl 2):e30080.
7. Spreafico F, Fernandez CV, Brok J, et al. Wilms tumour. Nat Rev Dis Primers. 2021;7:75.
8. Watson T, Oostveen M, Rogers H, et al. The role of imaging in the initial investigation of paediatric renal tumours. Lancet Child Adolesc Health. 2020;4:232–41.
9. Hötker AM, Lollert A, Mazaheri Y, et al. Diffusion-weighted MRI in the assessment of nephroblastoma: results of a multi-center trial. Abdom Radiol (NY). 2020;45:320212.
10. Fialkowski E, Sudour-Bonnange H, Vujanic GM, et al. The varied spectrum of nephroblastomatosis, nephrogenic rests, and Wilms tumors: review of current definitions and challenges of the field. Pediatr Blood Cancer. 2023;70(Suppl 2):e30162.
11. Brisse HJ, de la Monneraye Y, Cardoen L, et al. From Wilms to kidney tumors: which ones require a biopsy? Pediatr Radiol. 2020;50:1049–51.
12. Artunduaga M, Eklund M, van der Beek JN, et al. Imaging of pediatric renal tumors: A COG diagnostic imaging committee/SPR oncology committee white paper focused on Wilms tumor and nephrogenic rests. Pediatr Blood Cancer. 2023;70(Suppl 4):e30004.
13. Lanza C, Galeazzi V, Carboni N, et al. Neuroblastoma image-defined risk factors in adrenal neuroblastoma: role of radiologist. Gland Surg. 2019;8:S168–77.
14. Brisse HJ, McCarville MB, Granata C, et al. International Neuroblastoma risk group project. Guidelines for imaging and staging of neuroblastic tumors: consensus report from the international Neuroblastoma risk group project. Radiology. 2011;261:243–57.
15. Littooij AS, de Keizer B. Imaging in neuroblastoma. Pediatr Radiol. 2023;53:783–7.
16. Lai HA, Sharp SE, Bhatia A, et al. Imaging of pediatric neuroblastoma: A COG diagnostic imaging committee/SPR oncology committee white paper. Pediatr Blood Cancer. 2023;70(Suppl 4):e29974.
17. Burnand K, Barone G, McHugh K, et al. Preoperative computed tomography scanning for abdominal neuroblastomas is superior to magnetic resonance imaging for safe surgical planning. Pediatr Blood Cancer. 2019;66:e27955.
18. Pio L, Brisse HJ, Alaggio R, et al. Image-guided core-needle or surgical biopsy for neuroblastoma

diagnosis in children: A systematic review and meta-analysis from the International Society of Pediatric Surgical Oncology (IPSO). Pediatr Blood Cancer. 2024;71:e30789.
19. Avanzini S, Dall'Igna P, Bjornland K, et al. Beyond image defined risk factors (IDRFs): a delphi survey highlighting definition of the surgical complexity index (SCI) in neuroblastoma. Pediatr Surg Int. 2023;39:191.
20. Seemann NM, Erker C, Irwin MS, et al. Survival effect of complete surgical resection of the primary tumor in patients with metastatic, high-risk neuroblastoma in a large Canadian cohort. Pediatr Blood Cancer. 2023;70:e30286.
21. Shaffiey SA, Le HD, Christison-Lagay E, et al. Critical elements of pediatric neuroblastoma surgery. Semin Pediatr Surg. 2023;32:151338.
22. Orr KE, McHugh K. The new international neuroblastoma response criteria. Pediatr Radiol. 2019;49:1433–40.
23. Chung C, Boterberg T, Lucas J, et al. Neuroblastoma. Pediatr Blood Cancer. 2021;68(Suppl 2):e28473.
24. Dumba M, Jawad N, McHugh K. Neuroblastoma and nephroblastoma: a radiological review. Cancer Imaging. 2015;15:5.
25. Dong Y, Cekuolis A, Schreiber-Dietrich D, et al. Review on pediatric malignant focal liver lesions with imaging evaluation: part I. Diagnostics (Basel). 2023;13:3568.
26. Towbin AJ, Meyers RL, Woodley H, et al. 2017 PRETEXT: radiologic staging system for primary hepatic malignancies of childhood revised for the Paediatric hepatic international tumour trial (PHITT). Pediatr Radiol. 2018;48:536–54.
27. Meyers RL, Maibach R, Hiyama E, et al. Risk-stratified staging in paediatric hepatoblastoma: a unified analysis from the children's hepatic tumors international collaboration. Lancet Oncol. 2017;18:122–31.
28. Murawski M, Weeda VB, Czauderna P. Surgical management in hepatoblastoma: points to take. Pediatr Surg Int. 2023;39:81.
29. O'Neill AF, Trobaugh-Lotrario A, Geller JI, et al. The RELIVE consortium for relapsed or refractory pediatric hepatoblastoma and hepatocellular carcinoma: a scoping review of the problem and a proposed solution. EClinicalMedicine. 2024;69:102446.
30. Schooler GR, Infante JC, Acord M, et al. Imaging of pediatric liver tumors: A COG diagnostic imaging committee/SPR oncology committee white paper. Pediatr Blood Cancer. 2023;70(Suppl 4):e29965.
31. Jezierska M, Gawrychowska A, Stefanowicz J. Diagnostic, prognostic and predictive markers in pediatric germ cell tumors-past, present and future. Diagnostics (Basel). 2022;12:278.
32. Behr GG, Morani AC, Artunduaga M, et al. Imaging of pediatric ovarian tumors: A COG diagnostic imaging committee/SPR oncology committee white paper. Pediatr Blood Cancer. 2023;70(Suppl 4):e29995.
33. Weil BR, Rich BS, Madenci AL, et al. Critical elements in the operative management of pediatric malignant ovarian germ cell tumors. Semin Pediatr Surg. 2023;32:151342.
34. Sangüesa C, Veiga D, Llavador M, Serrano A. Testicular tumours in children: an approach to diagnosis and management with pathologic correlation. Insights Imaging. 2020;11:74.
35. Aldrink JH, Glick RD, Baertschiger RM, et al. Update on pediatric testicular germ cell tumors. J Pediatr Surg. 2021;57:690–9.
36. Phi JH. Sacrococcygeal Teratoma: a tumor at the center of embryogenesis. J Korean Neurosurg Soc. 2021;64:406–13.
37. Cavalcante CEB, Magalhães Pereira Souza F, Eiras Martins G, et al. Diffusion-weighted imaging in pediatric extracranial germ cell tumors. PLoS One. 2023;18:e0294976.
38. Yechieli RL, Mandeville HC, Hiniker SM, et al. Rhabdomyosarcoma. Pediatr Blood Cancer. 2021;68(Suppl 2):e28254.
39. Terwisscha van Scheltinga S, Rogers T, Smeulders N, et al. Developments in the surgical approach to staging and resection of rhabdomyosarcoma. Cancers (Basel). 2023;15:449.
40. Acord MR, Pace E, El-Ali A, Chaturvedi A, Iyer RS, Navarro OM, Pandit-Taskar N, Parikh K, A, Schechter A, Shaikh R, McCarville MB. Imaging of pediatric extremity soft tissue tumors: a COG diagnostic imaging committee/SPR oncology committee white paper. Pediatr Blood Cancer. 2023;70(Suppl 4):e29944.
41. de Vries ISA, van Ewijk R, Adriaansen LME, et al. Imaging in rhabdomyosarcoma: a patient journey. Pediatr Radiol. 2023;53:788–812.
42. Panda SP, Chinnaswamy G, Vora T, et al. Diagnosis and Management of Rhabdomyosarcoma in children and adolescents: ICMR consensus document. Indian J Pediatr. 2017;84:393–402.
43. Fetzko S, Fonseca A, Frances Wedekind M, et al. Is detection of relapse by surveillance imaging associated with longer survival in patients with rhabdomyosarcoma? J Pediatr Hematol Oncol. 2022;44:305–12.
44. Salom M, Chiari C, Alessandri JMG, et al. Diagnosis and staging of malignant bone tumours in children: what is due and what is new? J Child Orthop. 2021;15:312–21.
45. Cederberg KB, Iyer RS, Chaturvedi A, et al. Imaging of pediatric bone tumors: a COG diagnostic imaging committee/SPR oncology committee white paper. Pediatr Blood Cancer. 2022;70(Suppl 4):e30000.
46. Biko DM, Lichtenberger JP 3rd, Rapp JB, et al. Mediastinal masses in children: radiologic-pathologic correlation. Radiographics. 2021;41:1186–207.
47. Thacker PG, Iyer RS, Pace E, et al. Imaging of pediatric pulmonary tumors: A COG diagnostic imaging committee/SPR oncology committee white paper. Pediatr Blood Cancer. 2023;70(Suppl 4):e29964.

48. Meazza C, Gattuso G. Multidisciplinary team approach for pediatric thoracic tumors: new horizons and oldies but goldies. Pediatr Med. 2019;2:14.
49. Cruz-Conde MC, Gallego Herrero C, Rasero Ponferrada M, et al. Practical management of pulmonary nodules in the most common pediatric tumors. Radiologia (Engl Ed). 2021;63:245–51.
50. Heaton TE, Davidoff AM. Surgical treatment of pulmonary metastases in pediatric solid tumors. Semin Pediatr Surg. 2016;25:311–7.
51. Halepota HF, Tan JSK, Reddy SK, et al. Association of anesthetic and surgical risk factors with outcomes of initial diagnostic biopsies in a current cohort of children with anterior mediastinal masses. World J Pediatr Surg. 2021;4:e000303.
52. Honda M, Yuki A, Takahiro H, et al. Predictive risk score of respiratory complications in children with mediastinal tumors: A case-control study. Cancer Med. 2023;12:1167–76.
53. Weinstock MS, Patel NA, Smith LP. Pediatric cervical lymphadenopathy. Pediatr Rev. 2018;39:433–43.
54. Papakonstantinou O, Bakantaki A, Paspalaki P, et al. High-resolution and color Doppler ultrasonography of cervical lymphadenopathy in children. Acta Radiol. 2001;42:470–6.
55. Fraser L, O'Neill K, Locke R, Attaie M, Irwin G, Kubba H, MacGregor FB. Standardising reporting of cervical lymphadenopathy in paediatric neck ultrasound: a pilot study using an evidence-based reporting protocol. Int J Pediatr Otorhinolaryngol. 2013;77:1248–51.
56. Kılıç A, Çolakoğlu EH. Virtual touch tissue imaging quantification shear wave elastography for determining benign versus malignant cervical lymph nodes: a comparison with conventional ultrasound. Diagn Interv Radiol. 2019;25:114–21.
57. Chong V. Cervical lymphadenopathy: what radiologists need to know. Cancer Imaging. 2004;4:116–20.
58. Locke R, Comfort R, Kubba H. When does an enlarged cervical lymph node in a child need excision? A systematic review. Int J Pediatr Otorhinolaryngol. 2014;78:393–401.
59. Shur JD, Doran SJ, Kumar S, et al. Radiomics in oncology: a prac-tical guide. Radiographics. 2021;41:1717–32.
60. Qian LD, Zhang SX, Li SQ, et al. Predicting MYCN amplification in paediatric neuroblastoma: development and validation of a 18F-FDG PET/CT-based radiomics signature. Insights Imaging. 2023;14:205.
61. Privitera L, Paraboschi I, Cross K, et al. Above and beyond robotic surgery and 3D modelling in paediatric cancer surgery. Front Pediatr. 2021, 9:777840.
62. Shah NR, Weadock WJ, Williams KM, et al. Use of modern three-dimensional imaging models to guide surgical planning for local control of pediatric extracranial solid tumors. Pediatr Blood Cancer. 2024;71:e30933.
63. Kurz FT, Schlemmer HP. Imaging in translational cancer research. Cancer Biol Med. 2022;19:1565–85.
64. Fonseca R, Arribas M, Wiedmeier-Nutor JE, et al. Integrated analysis of next generation sequencing minimal residual disease (MRD) and PET scan in transplant eligible myeloma patients. Blood Cancer J. 2023;13:32.
65. Zambaiti E, Siles Hinojosa A, Montano V, Mutanen A, Glenisson M, Sarnacki S, Franchi Abella S, Pariente D, Pio L. Interventional radiology-guided procedures in the treatment of pediatric solid tumors: A systematic review and meta-analysis. Eur J Pediatr Surg. 2020;30:317–25.

Complications and Imaging Considerations with Cancer Treatment

3

Shivi Jain, Kajal Kumari, and Ashish Verma

3.1 Introduction

Advancements in cancer treatment have improved survival rates for children, but all therapies carry the risk of toxic effects, impacting various organ systems. Radiologists play a key role in identifying these complications, which can arise during diagnosis, initial treatment, or after therapy completion. Early complications include oncologic emergencies like superior vena cava syndrome, metabolic disturbances, and infections. Later effects include leukoencephalopathy, cataracts, cardiomyopathy, hepatic fibrosis, renal dysfunction, scoliosis, hypothyroidism, and secondary malignancies. Awareness of these issues enhances patient surveillance and timely intervention, improving long-term outcomes and quality of life.

3.1.1 Thoracic and Pulmonary Complications

Pulmonary complications frequently arise early in cancer treatment, often as a result of chemotherapy, radiation, or hematopoietic cell transplants. However, identifying these issues can be difficult for radiologists, as pre-existing conditions and the simultaneous presence of infectious and non-infectious causes can produce similar imaging findings. Early recognition of pulmonary abnormalities, particularly those with distinct radiologic appearances, is crucial for accurate diagnosis and timely intervention, which can improve patient outcomes.

Pulmonary complications can be divided into infectious and non-infectious causes which further can be divided into early and late complications.

In the early phase post-hematopoietic cell transplant (HCT), both infectious and non-infectious complications are equally prevalent [1]. Common early infections include bacterial pneumonia, respiratory viruses, and invasive fungal pneumonia [2]. Bacterial pneumonia typically manifests as lobar opacities [2], while respiratory viruses like rhinovirus and parainfluenza exhibit a variety of imaging findings, ranging from normal CT scans to ground-glass opacities. Aspergillosis (Figs. 3.1, 3.2, and 3.3) is distinguished by CT findings such as a halo or air crescent sign.

S. Jain (✉) · K. Kumari · A. Verma
Department of Radiodiagnosis and Imaging, Institute of Medical Sciences, Banaras Hindu University, Varanasi, Uttar Pradesh, India
e-mail: averma@bhu.ac.in

I. Kumar et al. (eds.), *Practical Approach to Imaging in Pediatric Oncology*,
https://doi.org/10.1007/978-981-96-8158-7_3

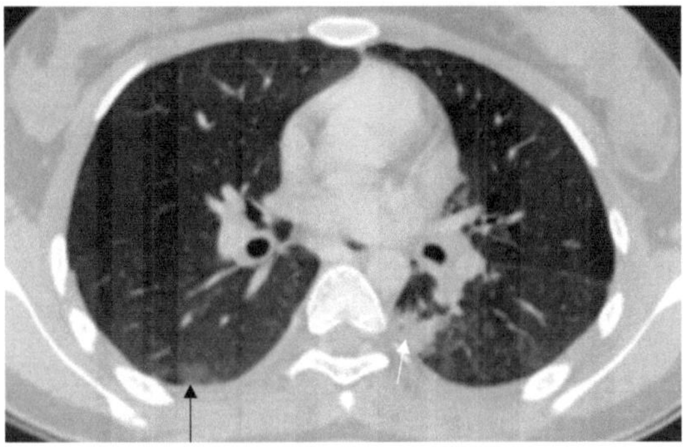

Fig. 3.1 Axial CT chest of 10-year-old boy showing an area of consolidation (white arrow) with surrounding patchy areas of ground glass opacities (black arrow) in left lower lobe of lung 2 months after radiotherapy suggestive of acute radiation

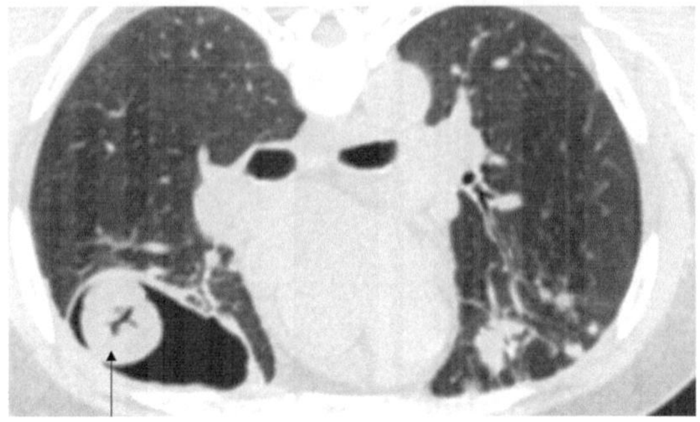

Fig. 3.3 Aspergilloma in a 14-year-old boy, 1 year after bone marrow transplantation for acute lymphoblastic leukemia. The CT scan reveals a large cavity in the right upper lobe containing a fungus ball (arrow). Aspergillus species were identified in the laboratory culture of a lobectomy specimen

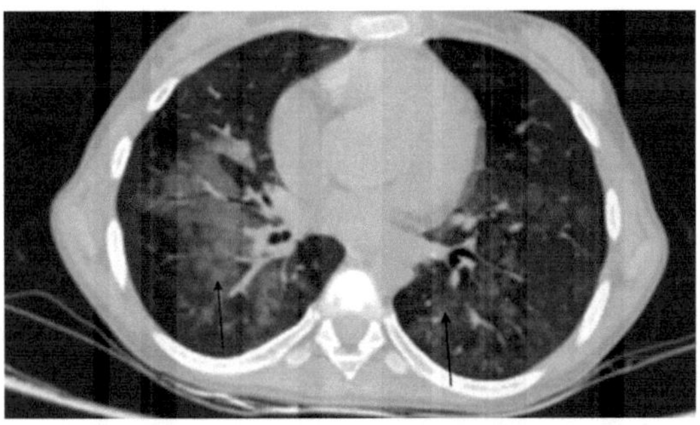

Fig. 3.2 Pulmonary hemorrhage in a 10-year-old girl occurs 3 weeks after bone marrow transplantation for acute lymphoblastic leukemia. The CT scan reveals ground-glass opacities and patchy consolidations (black arrows) in both lung fields

In the late phase, infections like herpes viruses and Pneumocystis jiroveci pneumonia (PJP) become more frequent [2]. These late infections may present as diffuse ground-glass opacities [4]. Despite prophylaxis, breakthrough PJP cases continue to occur, and invasive fungal infections are common in severe GVHD (graft-versus-host disease) patients [3, 4] According to time of onset, microbial agents, imaging characteristics, clinical signs, and symptoms associated with infectious complications are summarized in Table 3.1 [5].

Non-infectious pulmonary complications following hematopoietic cell transplant are common and carry poor prognoses [6, 7]. These complications occur in 12–30% of pediatric patients, contributing to 16% of transplant-related deaths [8, 9]. Non-infectious pulmonary complications that arise early include conditions like pulmonary edema, idiopathic pneumonia syndrome, diffuse alveolar hemorrhage (Fig. 3.2), peri-engraftment respiratory distress syndrome (PERDS), pulmonary veno-occlusive disease (PVOD), and acute radiation pneumonitis (Fig. 3.1).

Late non-infectious complications include fibrosis and progressive pulmonary disease, BOOP (bronchiolitis obliterans organizing

Table 3.1 Onset of infection with its common etiologic agent, clinical signs, and symptoms with radiological findings [5]

Onset	Entity	Clinical signs/symptoms	Radiological findings
Early	Bacterial pneumonia	Fever, hypoxia, cough	Focal segmental or lobar pulmonary opacities
	Respiratory viruses	Fever, cough, increased work of breathing, hypoxia	Normal to a range of findings such as nodules, ground-glass attenuation, or consolidation
	Invasive fungal pneumonia	Fever, chest pain, hemoptysis, hypoxia	Pulmonary aspergillosis: dense, well-circumscribed lesion(s), halo sign, air crescent sign, or wedge-shaped segmental/lobar consolidation
Late	Herpes virus (HSV, VZV, CMV, HHV6)	Fever, tachypnea	Pulmonary hyperinflation, along with bilateral perihilar opacities, may progress into diffuse airspace disease or present as patchy areas of ground-glass opacity
	Pneumocystis jiroveci pneumonia	Tachypnea, hypoxemia	Bilateral, diffuse ground-glass opacities with interstitial opacities, miliary pattern
	Respiratory viruses	Fever, cough, increased work of breathing, hypoxia	Combination of nodules, ground-glass attenuation, or consolidation

pneumonia), and radiation recall pneumonitis (Fig. 3.1). According to time of onset, imaging characteristics and agents associated with non-infectious complications are summarized in Table 3.2 [5].

Lung fibrosis is a significant late effect in children treated for cancer, particularly with radiotherapy, busulfan, bleomycin, and lomustine/carmustine, which can damage lung tissue. High-resolution CT (HRCT) is the gold standard for detecting fibrosis, showing reticular opacities and honeycombing, while pulmonary function tests (PFTs) reveal reduced FVC and DLCO. These findings correlate with symptoms like dyspnoa and restrictive lung disease. The risk is dose-dependent, with higher radiation doses increasing fibrosis severity. Long-term follow-up with HRCT and PFTs, as recommended by groups like SKION LATER, is essential. Survivors should avoid smoking and get annual flu vaccinations [10].

Late pulmonary complications after hematopoietic stem cell transplantation (HSCT) include chronic GVHD, infections, BOOP, fibrosis, and lymphoid interstitial pneumonitis. Chronic GVHD, common in long-term survivors, raises the risk of bacterial, fungal, and viral pneumonias, as well as obstructive lung diseases like bronchiolitis obliterans (BO), seen as mosaic attenuation and air trapping on high-resolution CT.

BOOP (Fig. 3.4) is a rare post-engraftment complication, often linked to chronic GVHD, while obliterative bronchiolitis is a leading cause of obstructive lung disease in HSCT survivors, typically showing hyperinflation on chest X-rays. Thin-section CT scans improve diagnostic accuracy, revealing air trapping, decreased vessel size (mosaic perfusion), bronchial dilation, and wall thickening. Cryptogenic organizing pneumonia (COP) is another HSCT complication, manifesting as patchy peripheral infiltrates on imaging, particularly in children.

Table 3.2 Non-infectious pulmonary complications, their radiological findings with description and associated chemotherapeutic agents [5]

Pulmonary complication	Radiological findings	Chemotherapeutic agents	Description
Early-onset			
Inflammatory interstitial pneumonitis	Ground-glass opacities and patchy consolidation indicative of interstitial edema and/or alveolar consolidation [13]	Methotrexate, bleomycin, procarbazine, carmustine, mitoxantrone, paclitaxel (due to Cremophor EL vehicle)	Nonproductive cough, dyspnea, low-grade fever, and fine crackles.
Pulmonary edema	Cardiomegaly, pleural effusion, pulmonary vessel prominence, diffuse ground-glass opacities, and septal thickening	Cytosine arabinoside (Ara-C), interleukin-2 (IL-2), all-trans-retinoic acid (ATRA)	Noncardiogenic pulmonary edema due to endothelial inflammation and vascular leak.
Capillary leak syndrome	Pleural effusions in 52% of IL-2 cases, interlobular septal thickening, ground glass opacities	Interleukin-2, all-trans-retinoic acid	Vascular leak syndrome, especially in the lungs, associated with IL-2 and ATRA..
Pulmonary veno-occlusive disease	Diffuse ground-glass opacities, septal and peribronchial thickening, soft-tissue edema around the hila and mediastinum, small pleural effusions, and dilatation of the central pulmonary arteries [14].	Bleomycin	Gradual occlusion of postcapillary pulmonary venules, resulting in increased resistance and eventual right ventricular failure [14].
Diffuse alveolar hemorrhage (DAH)	Diffuse ground-glass opacities, crazy-paving pattern (related to intra- and interlobular septal thickening). No cardiomegaly or effusions, differentiating it from pulmonary edema	Conditioning regimen, thrombotic microangiopathy, occult infection	Occurs in 2% of pediatric HCT recipients, characterized by fever, dyspnea, hypoxia, and hemoptysis. Blood and inflammatory cells in alveoli lead to impaired gas exchange
Peri-engraftment respiratory distress syndrome (PERDS)	Diffuse ground-glass opacification, interlobular septal thickening, perihilar or peribronchial consolidation, pleural effusions. No cardiomegaly or signs of pulmonary edema.	Post HSCT	Occurs during neutrophil engraftment (days 5–21 post-transplant). Involves cytokine release causing pulmonary edema, rash, fever, and acute respiratory failure.
Late-onset			
Fibrosis and progressive pulmonary disease	Reticular opacities (interlobular and intralobular septal thickening) honeycombing and volume loss	Bleomycin, methotrexate, carmustine	Chronic, progressive dyspnea and restrictive lung disease.
Bronchiolitis obliterans	Air trapping, decreased vessel size (mosaic perfusion), bronchial dilation, and wall thickening	Carmustine, busulfan	Progressive airway obstruction, cough, dyspnea, and wheezing due to fibrotic scarring of small airways.
Radiation recall pneumonitis	Well-defined alveolar consolidation, ground-glass opacity, or infiltrates aligned with radiation portals [11, 12].	Dactinomycin, doxorubicin, paclitaxel	Inflammatory reaction within a previously irradiated area, triggered by chemotherapy, typically manifests with cough and dyspnea about 3–4 months post-radiotherapy..

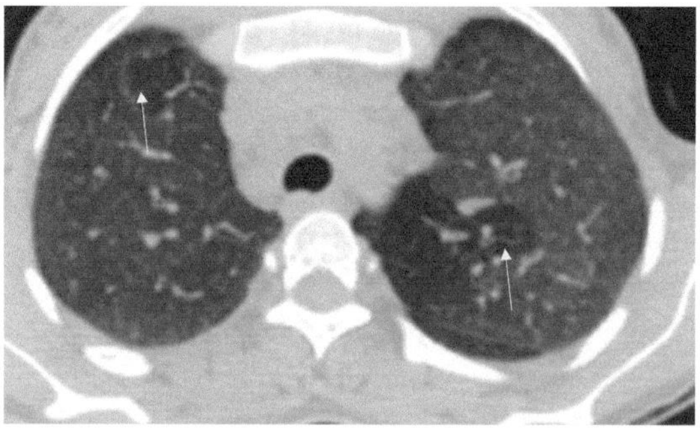

Fig. 3.4 Bronchiolitis obliterans in a 13-year-old boy with acute myeloid leukemia, following hematopoietic stem cell transplantation and graft-versus-host disease. The CT scan in the expiratory phase shows patchy areas of air trapping in both lungs (arrows)

3.2 Cardiovascular Complications

Cardiovascular complications, particularly heart failure, are major concerns in pediatric cancer patients treated with anthracyclines or radiation. Cardiotoxicity prevalence varies, with systolic dysfunction reported from 0.0% to 56.4% and diastolic dysfunction from 30.0% to 100%, reflecting study differences. Screening typically uses echocardiography, measuring systolic function through fractional shortening (FS) and ejection fraction (EF), though these can be inconsistent. Global longitudinal strain (GLS), an echocardiographic measure of the heart muscle's deformation during contraction, assesses longitudinal shortening of the left ventricle and may provide more sensitive detection of cardiac injury. The cumulative dose of anthracyclines is a key risk factor, correlating with declines in FS, EF, and GLS, suggesting GLS inclusion in screening protocols. Uniform guidelines based on treatment doses would improve identification of at-risk patients and preventive care [11].

3.2.1 Gastrointestinal Complications

Gastrointestinal complications of cancer therapy in children include radiation enteropathy, neutropenic colitis, and GVHD. Other therapy-related issues affecting the abdomen include gastrointestinal perforations, fistulas, small bowel intussusceptions, and capillary-leak related effusions and ascites.

3.2.1.1 Radiation Enteropathy

Radiation enteropathy affects the small bowel mucosa, which is highly sensitive to radiation due to its rapid cell turnover [12]. Radiation exposure accelerates apoptosis and impairs mitosis, resulting in denudation of intestinal crypts and truncation of villi. Acute radiation enteropathy typically manifests as self-limiting diarrhea due to malabsorption a few days to weeks after exposure [13].

Imaging findings include mucosal hyperenhancement and thickening of the bowel wall [12]. Life-threatening radiation-related enteropathies, such as radiation proctitis previously seen in children with abdominopelvic tumors, are now rare due to advancements in radiation therapy and the use of tissue expanders and mesh for bowel protection during pelvic radiation [14].

3.2.1.2 Neutropenic Colitis

Neutropenic colitis, or typhlitis, is a severe inflammation of the cecum and colon walls in children with profound neutropenia, posing a life-threatening condition. It primarily affects the cecum but can extend into the distal colon. In contrast, Clostridium difficile infection typically involves the entire colon, while graft-versus-host disease (GVHD) affects both the large and small bowel, characterized by mucosal enhancement in fluid-filled, distended bowel loops. Pseudomembranous colitis due to C. difficile may show marked nodularity of the thickened colon with an "accordion sign" [15].

Imaging plays a critical role in diagnosing neutropenic colitis, revealing thickening of the cecal wall that may extend into the terminal ileum and ascending colon, potentially involving the entire colon. In cases where neutropenic colitis is suspected, abdominal ultrasound serves as the primary imaging modality and is often adequate for both diagnosis and follow-up. Common symptoms include abdominal pain, tenderness, fever, and diarrhea, with an incidence of approximately 2.6% among children treated for cancer, notably more prevalent in those over 16 years of age [16].

Additional signs may include pneumatosis, peri-cecal inflammatory changes, and varying degrees of ascites. Imaging reveals bowel wall thickening ≥3 mm in size, measured by ultrasound or CT scan, which is crucial for diagnosis and follow-up. Ultrasound and CT scans are useful for excluding other conditions that mimic typhlitis, such as appendicitis and bowel perforation.

3.2.1.3 Benign Pneumatosis Intestinalis

Pneumatosis intestinalis, which can occur alongside complications such as neutropenic colitis in children who have undergone cancer therapy or HSCT, is frequently observed as an isolated condition without additional issues like free air or portal venous gas. Unlike cases requiring surgical intervention, benign pneumatosis does not necessitate surgical treatment.

Benign pneumatosis is typically identified through abdominal radiographs, with the theory proposing that loss of bowel wall integrity and mucosal disruption contribute to its development.

3.2.1.4 Fungal Esophagitis

Esophageal candidiasis, commonly seen in children undergoing cancer treatment, is predominantly caused by *Candida albicans*, although non-albicans strains are becoming increasingly important. Fungal infections, including esophagitis, frequently occur in patients with severe neutropenia receiving chemotherapy, with most drugs being implicated, and additional risk factors such as prolonged hospital stays, radiation therapy, and broad-spectrum antibiotic use [16]. The fungi most commonly responsible for esophagitis are *Candida* and *Aspergillus* [16]. Symptoms include dysphagia, odynophagia, nausea, vomiting, and fever. Imaging, particularly CT scans, often shows diffuse, nonspecific esophageal wall thickening, with diagnosis confirmed via endoscopy and biopsy.

3.2.1.5 Graft Versus Host Disease (GVHD)

Gastrointestinal complications following HSCT often present as GVHD, with CT findings showing abnormal enhancement of the bowel wall, affecting both the small bowel and colon, with or without thickening [17]. MRI studies have confirmed this, correlating with mucosal destruction and replacement by granulation tissue. Similar enhancement may be seen in the gallbladder and urinary bladder walls reflecting a comparable histopathological process [18].

3.3 Hepatobiliary and Pancreatic Complications

Therapy-induced effects on the hepatobiliary system include hepatic fungal disease/microabscesses, chemotherapy-related hepatic steatosis, hepatic veno-occlusive disease, focal nodular hyperplasia (FNH), hemochromatosis from multiple transfusions, and hepatic fibrosis. Chronic effects comprise FNH, hemochromatosis, and hepatic fibrosis.

3.3.1 Hepatotoxicity and Liver Parenchymal Disease

Chemotherapy-induced liver injury in adults can cause conditions such as steatosis, steatohepatitis, sinusoidal obstructive syndrome, nodular regenerative hyperplasia, hepatic veno-occlusive disease, and peliosis [19]. Hepatic veno-occlusive disease is a notable complication of HSCT, chemotherapy, and radiation, with an incidence of 5–60%, and can be fatal in up to 40% of affected children, depending on severity [20].

Some authors view sinusoidal obstructive syndrome, nodular regenerative hyperplasia, hepatic veno-occlusive disease, and peliosis as a continuum resulting from chemotherapy-induced microvascular injury, leading to obstruction of sinusoids and small venules, along with vascular congestion [21].

Parenchymal disease, comprising steatosis (fatty infiltration), fibrosis, and siderosis (iron

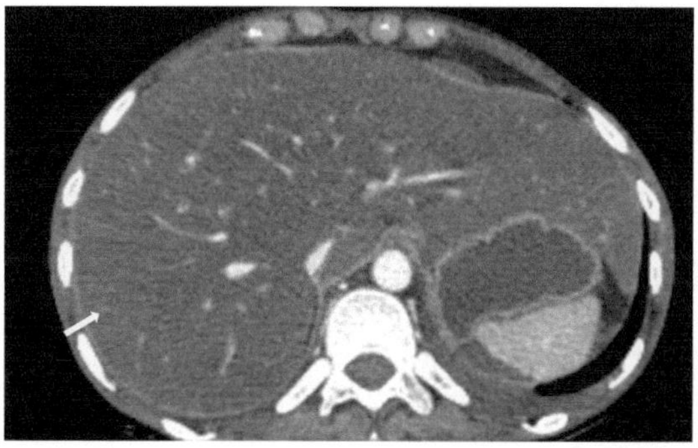

Fig. 3.5 Hepatomegaly with steatosis on a CT scan of a 16-year-old boy with ALL, 2 weeks after the start of therapy. The liver is significantly hypodense (arrow)

accumulation), can be attributed to the hepatotoxic effects of numerous medications.

Steatosis (Fig. 3.5) results from hepatocyte triglyceride accumulation, often occurring in acute lymphocytic leukemia (ALL) patients treated with L-asparaginase [22]. Although a few pediatric cancer patients develop fibrosis or cirrhosis, the overall incidence of acute and chronic liver injury in this group is unknown [23].

Ultrasound typically depicts increased liver echotexture relative to kidneys in both steatosis and fibrosis cases [24]. Nonenhanced CT scans reveal distinct liver parenchyma and hepatic vessels contrast [24]. Intravenous-enhanced CT scans show hypodense liver compared to spleen [24]. Hepatic fibrosis lacks correlation with CT changes. MR imaging diagnoses steatosis effectively through proton chemical shift imaging, with signal subtraction on opposed-phase images.

3.3.2 Siderosis

Siderosis, also known as secondary hemochromatosis, results from iron accumulation in reticuloendothelial cells and sometimes hepatocytes [25].

Pathological evidence shows siderosis in 14–70% of patients treated for ALL [22, 25]. Frequent blood transfusions can also lead to siderosis. On imaging, the liver appears enlarged with diffuse increased density on nonenhanced CT scans, exceeding 75 Hounsfield units [26]. MRI reveals diffuse low signal intensity due to the paramagnetic effect of ferritin and ferric ions, resulting in shortened T1 and T2 relaxation times [26].

3.3.3 Hepatic Veno-Occlusive Disease

Hepatic veno-occlusive disease (VOD) affects hepatic sinusoids, causing endothelial inflammation and obstruction of terminal hepatic and sublobular venules [27]. Local hypercoagulable state leads to fibrin and debris aggregates, occluding endothelium pores and resulting in postsinusoidal portal hypertension [27].

VOD can complicate various chemotherapy regimens, primarily caused by dactinomycin, vincristine, and cyclophosphamide combination [27]. Portal vein thrombosis may rarely follow or associate with VOD [27].

Clinically, VOD presents with painful hepatomegaly, jaundice, and ascites [27].

Diagnosis is confirmed by biopsy [28]. Imaging reveals hepatomegaly, periportal edema, and ascites on both sonography and CT scans [27]. Ultrasound is the preferred imaging modality, demonstrating an increased intrahepatic resistive index (>0.8), reduced or reversed portal venous flow, patent but attenuated hepatic veins, gallbladder wall edema, ascites, and hepatomegaly (Fig. 3.6) [27].

3.3.4 Chemotherapy-Related Pancreatitis

Pancreatitis induced by chemotherapy is observed particularly with l-asparaginase administration in the treatment of acute lymphoblastic leukemia in children. The incidence of asparaginase-associated

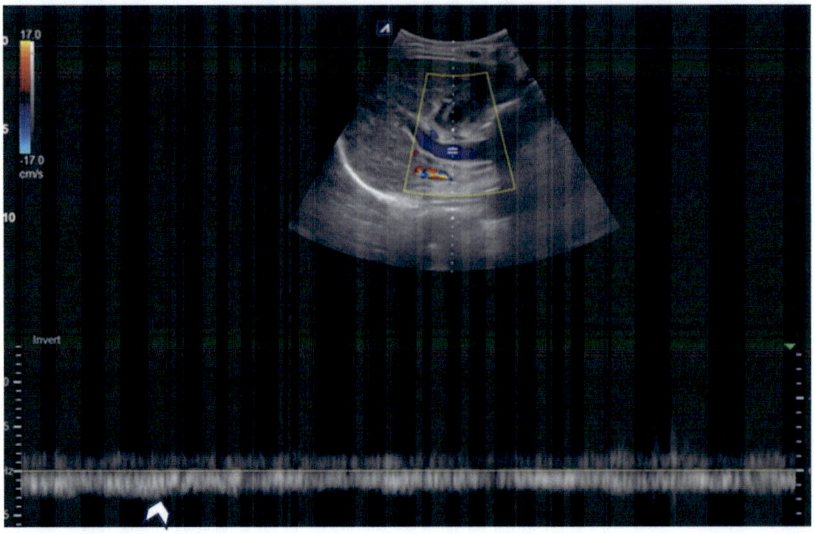

Fig. 3.6 Hepatic veno-occlusive disease in a 12-year-old girl who received hematopoietic stem cell transplantation for myelodysplasia. The color and spectral waveforms indicate a reversal of portal venous flow (arrowhead)

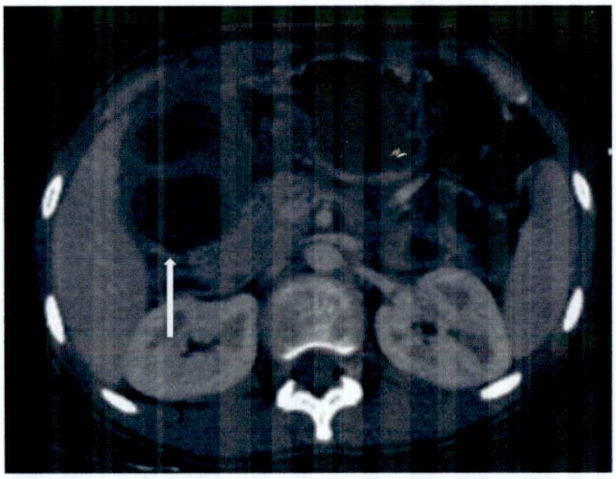

Fig. 3.7 Asparaginase-associated pancreatitis in a 15-year-old girl with acute lymphoblastic leukemia who has a history of receiving l-asparaginase. The CECT of the abdomen shows the presence of a multiloculated pseudocyst (arrow) in the right upper quadrant, located anterior to the head of the pancreas

pancreatitis ranges from 7% to 18% [46]. This condition can result in acute pancreatitis, serving as a reason for discontinuing the treatment.

Imaging reveals diffuse pancreatic enlargement, peripancreatic fat streaking, and fluid on ultrasound and CT scans [27]. Diagnosis is confirmed by elevated blood levels of amylase and lipase. Asparaginase-related pancreatitis may present complications such as pseudocyst formation (Fig. 3.7) and necrosis.

3.3.5 Gallstones, Pseudolithiasis, Crystals, and Sludge

Gallstones, pseudolithiasis, crystals, and sludge are uncommon in pediatric patients, with chemotherapeutic agents accounting for around 7.4% of cases [29].

Gallstones are primarily associated with high doses of cytarabine and asparaginase, and they may resolve spontaneously. Other factors in cancer patients that increase the risk of gallstones include systemic infection, prolonged fasting, total parenteral nutrition, bone marrow transplantation, and radiotherapy [30]. Although the exact mechanisms are not always clear, various molecular targeted therapies have been linked to biliary complications, ranging from mild cholestasis, cholelithiasis, and gallbladder edema to cholangitis and severe cholecystitis [30].

Imaging modalities reveal gallbladder crystals and sludge as echogenic foci without posterior shadowing on sonography and as mildly dense material on CT scans.

Acalculous cholecystitis, which can occur due to chemotherapeutic agents like vincristine, cyclophosphamide, and cytosine-arabinoside, is characterized by painful gallbladder showing wall edema with or without overdistention, and it lacks stones [31].

3.3.6 Neurological Complications

Neurological complications from chemotherapy and radiation therapy can lead to leukoencephalopathy and neurocognitive issues. These complications are especially severe in patients receiving high doses or those under 5 years old, making it essential for radiologists to recognize these potential effects.

Neurological complications due to cancer treatment can be divided into acute and delayed. Acute neurological complications are broadly divided into infectious or non-infectious causes.

Infections from viruses, bacteria, fungi, and parasites account for 35% of acute neurotoxicity in pediatric ALL patients post-HSCT. Infections, the most common complication, vary based on post-transplantation stages. Pre-engraftment sees heightened risk of sepsis from Gram-negative bacteria, fungi, and viruses. Early post-engraftment is marked by depressed cellular immunity, leading to cytomegalovirus (CMV), fungal, and Gram-positive bacterial infections. Late post-engraftment sees infections from encapsulated bacteria and herpes zoster virus [32, 33]. Aspergillus commonly causes focal infective cerebral lesions post-HSCT, visible as low-attenuation foci on CT and hyperintensity on T2-weighted MR images. Herpes encephalitis and Epstein-Barr virus infections exhibit specific MR imaging changes [32, 34]. Due to immunosuppression, symptoms may be absent, necessitating vigilance for new neurological signs [35]. Emerging techniques like next-generation sequencing can be used to identify the pathogens.

Non-infectious etiology of acute neurotoxicity largely relates to drug toxicities, vascular events, and metabolic and immune-mediated (CNS GvHD) [36]. Acute drug toxicity commonly presents as aseptic meningitis (chemical meningitis or arachnoiditis) and leukoencephalopathy (LE), and common cerebrovascular complications can be sinus thrombosis and posterior reversible encephalopathy syndrome (PRES).

Posterior Reversible Encephalopathy Syndrome (PRES) (Fig. 3.10) is a complication of pediatric cancer treatment, especially leukemia, linked to loss of cerebral autoregulation, hypertension, and drugs like steroids, L-asparaginase, and immunosuppressants [37]. Mean arterial blood pressure at onset of PRES was noticed to be 140/85 mmHg by Siebert et al. Imaging shows symmetric edema in parietal, occipital, and frontal lobes, with FLAIR and T2W highlighting vasogenic edema. ADC values can help distinguish infarcts [38]. Three primary variations of the traditional PRES imaging pattern [38] are:

1. **Holohemispheric watershed pattern—** Vasogenic edema in a linear pattern spanning the frontal, parietal, and occipital lobes, with lesser involvement of the temporal lobes.
2. **Dominant parietal/occipital—**Typical "posterior" pattern involving parietal and occipital cortex and white matter with variable involvement of the temporal lobes.
3. **Superior frontal sulcus—**Frontal abnormality located along the mid to posterior aspect of the superior frontal sulcus.

Although PRES is generally known to be fully reversible, persistent lesions such as infarction or hemorrhage are well recognized. Contrast enhancement is seen in about 20% of patients with PRES. Intraparenchymal or subarachnoid hemorrhage around cortical or subcortical lesions is seen in 10–25% of cases [39]. Additionally, temporal lobe involvement, restricted diffusion on MRI, and associated multi-organ failure are more frequent in pediatric PRES compared with adults (Fig. 3.8) [40].

Cerebral Venous Thrombosis (CVT) presents with symptoms such as headaches, seizures, loss of consciousness, and visual abnormalities. Imaging findings for CVT include non-visualization of occluded veins or sinuses due to absent signals and flow defects on MRI. Gadolinium-enhanced T1-weighted imaging (T1WI) is sensitive for diagnosing CVST, with a sensitivity of 82%. Among the non-enhanced sequences, gradient-recalled echo (GRE) is sensitive at 77.4% during the acute stage. T1WI (69.6%), FLAIR (34.4%), and diffusion-weighted imaging (DWI) (18.8%)

demonstrate lower sensitivity. Overall, nonenhanced MRI sequences have a relatively lower diagnostic performance compared to gadolinium-enhanced T1WI. The crucial role of chemotherapy in the development of CVST associated with ALL is underscored by the observation that more than 90% of these cases happen during induction therapy. As a result, studies have focused on the chemotherapeutic drugs administered, particularly asparaginase, and their impact on hemostasis [41].

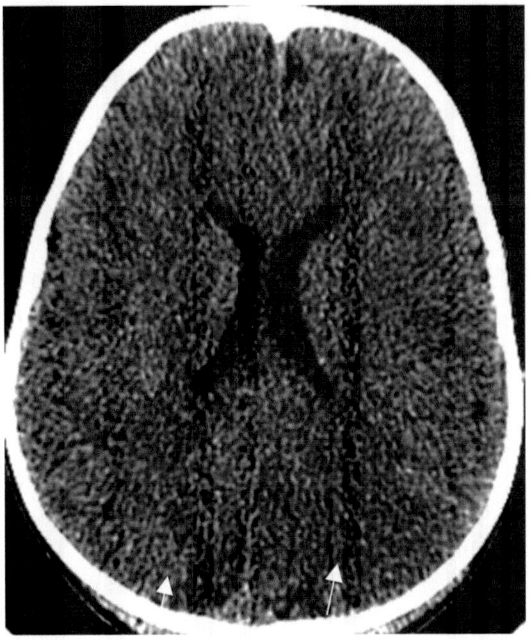

Fig. 3.8 Axial nonenhanced CT scan of the brain in a 5-year-old girl after HSCT who developed hypertension and headache reveals decreased attenuation of the posterior parietal regions consistent with posterior reversible encephalopathy syndrome (arrows). These regions did not enhance after contrast material administration

Trousseau's syndrome refers to a hypercoagulable state associated with malignancy, and it shares similarities with cancer-associated thrombosis. In pediatric patients, particularly those with leukemia, it can manifest in various ways, including deep vein thrombosis (DVT), pulmonary embolism (PE), chronic disseminated intravascular coagulation (DIC) related to nonbacterial thrombotic endocarditis (NBTE), and arterial thrombosis. Trousseau's syndrome should be considered, particularly in cases where cerebral infarctions occur in three or more vascular territories. Microemboli are often dispersed across multiple vascular regions [42]. Additionally, MRI combined with MR venography can be effective in diagnosing dural sinus thrombosis, as MR venography may reveal a loss of the flow void in the affected dural sinus [43]. Since there are no definitive diagnostic criteria for Trousseau's syndrome, it is crucial to investigate for malignant tumors when unexplained cerebral infarctions or sinus thrombosis are detected.

Hippocampal sclerosis is a neuropathological condition marked by significant neuronal loss and gliosis, primarily in the cornu ammonis area 1 and subiculum of the hippocampus. While often linked to infantile seizures, cerebritis, or trauma, it has also been reported in hematological malignancies due to factors like methotrexate neurotoxicity, radiation, or bone marrow transplantation [44]. It is a major cause of refractory temporal lobe epilepsy in children but the exact relationship between hippocampal sclerosis and epilepsy remains unclear. MRI, especially coronal FLAIR and STIR images, can reveal hippocampal atrophy and high signal intensity, aiding early diagnosis [45]. Rare neurological complications like radiation necrosis, cerebrovascular accident, and mineralizing angiopathy are usually linked to high-dose radiation.

Radiation-induced focal hemosiderin deposition (RIFHD) is a late complication of radiation therapy, characterized by hemorrhagic microangiopathies like capillary telangiectasias and cavernous malformations. These two malformations differ by the presence of brain parenchyma between the dilated vessels, though they likely share a common pathway [46]. RIFHD involves vascular injury, endothelial proliferation, and vessel wall necrosis, leading to ischemia and infarction [47]. The minimum radiation dose threshold is 6–12 Gy, with higher doses increasing RIFHD frequency [48]. While often asymptomatic, symptomatic bleeding is more common in infratentorial RIFHD [49]. MRI reveals mixed intensity lesions, best seen on iron-sensitive sequences [47].

Radiation-induced white matter injury, an another late complication of radiotherapy which may appear months to years post-therapy, resulting from vascular damage. MRI reveals T1 hypointensity and T2 hyperintensity in affected areas, particularly in the periventricular region [50]. White matter volume loss may occur, though central necrosis is rare in children [50].

Cataracts may develop following orbital or cranial irradiation for conditions like rhabdomyosarcoma and leukemia. Formation is common, affecting up to 90% of patients receiving doses over 750 rad (7.5 Gy) to the lens, typically occurring within 12–18 months post-treatment. Radiation therapy-related changes in the pediatric brain mirror those in adults, with acute effects appearing within 6 weeks, characterized by T1 and T2 prolongation with edema but no enhancement.

In pediatric cancer patients, various neurological complications occur due to chemotherapy, radiotherapy, and immunotherapy which present with distinct clinical pictures and imaging findings. Therefore, common complications are discussed with each in detail.

3.4 Chemotherapy-Induced Complications

Neurotoxicity poses a significant challenge in the treatment of pediatric cancers with conventional chemotherapy. Numerous chemotherapeutic agents can lead to central nervous system (CNS) side effects, especially when given intrathecally or in high doses. Common adverse effects include encephalopathy, cerebellar degeneration, myelopathy, as well as impacts on vision, hearing, and taste [51]. Chemotherapy-induced brain infections are rare but serious complications resulting from the immunosuppressive effects of chemotherapy, which can make the brain more vulnerable to infections by pathogens (Fig. 3.9). Additionally, the risk of CNS neurotoxicity increases when these drugs are used alongside other medications or in combination with radiotherapy. Common complications of some drugs are illustrated in Table 3.3.

3.4.1 Methotrexate Neurotoxicity

Methotrexate-induced central neurotoxicity affects 3–7% of children undergoing treatment for ALL [52]. Methotrexate-induced neurotoxic-

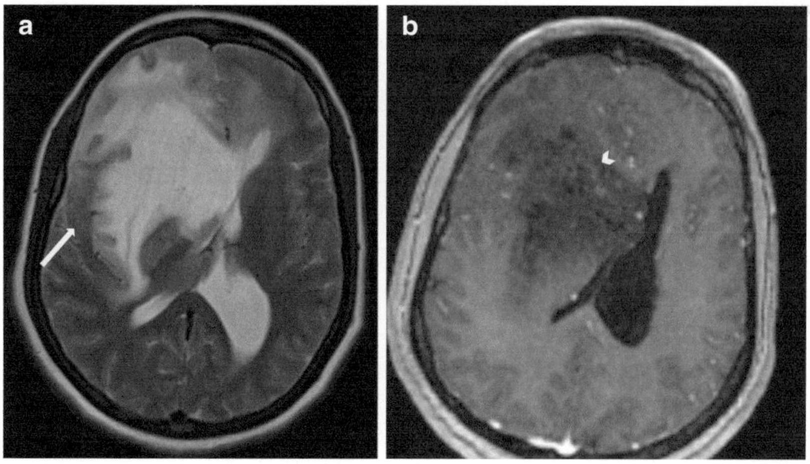

Fig. 3.9 Radiation-induced cerebral malignancy in an 18-year-old boy, 10 years after bone marrow transplantation for acute lymphoblastic leukemia. (**a**) The T2-weighted MR image reveals a lesion exhibiting significant mass effect, loss of gray matter–white matter differentiation, and edema (arrow). (**b**) The contrast-enhanced T1-weighted MR image displays a lesion with minimal heterogeneous enhancement in the right frontal lobe (arrowhead). A biopsy confirmed the diagnosis of high-grade glioma

Table 3.3 Drugs, its class, and its associated neurological complications

Drug class	Drug	Neurologic symptoms
Alkylating agents	Cyclophosphamide	Reversible encephalopathy: dizziness, blurred vision
	Ifosfamide	Encephalopathy: confusion, hallucinations, psychosis, disorientation, memory loss, seizure, delirium (10–30% of pediatric patients) Myoclonus, focal deficits
	Busulfan	Headaches Dizziness
Platinum compounds	Cisplatin	SIADH Cranial neuropathies: ototoxicity, ageusia
Antimetabolites	Cytarabine	Pancerebellar syndrome: dysarthria, dysmetria, ataxia, nystagmus Seizures and confusional syndromes
	Methotrexate	Chemical meningitis Leukoencephalopathy: stroke-like episodes
Natural products	Asparaginase	Cerebral sinovenous thrombosis Encephalopathy, seizures, coma (rare)
Immunosuppressants	Cyclosporine A	Metabolic encephalopathies: paresthesia, headache, seizures, confusion PRES
	Tacrolimus	Vascular endothelial damage: seizures, headache, confusion Encephalopathy (uncommon)

ity can manifest with acute, subacute, and chronic symptoms, such as alterations in mental status, neurological deficits, seizures, and cognitive impairments. The clinical feature may develop at 2 days to 2 weeks after administration, may develop over minutes to hours and eventually the clinical features fluctuate over the course of the disease. One of the frequent findings associated with this neurotoxicity is leukoencephalopathy, which is identified by white matter hyperintensity on T2/FLAIR (Fig. 3.10). The characteristic imaging finding is restriction in diffusion-weighted images which is reversible after symptom resolution [53]. The changes may be unilateral or bilateral or may be alternating between the two sides. Post contrast enhancement may be present.

Mateos et al. studied the largest cohort of children treated for acute lymphoblastic leukemia (ALL) and lymphoblastic lymphoma (LBL) to assess methotrexate (MTX) neurotoxicity. They identified key risk factors, including age $\geq$ 10 at diagnosis and grade 3+ elevation of AST. Discontinuing intrathecal (IT) MTX after neurotoxicity increased CNS relapse rates, while continuing IT MTX led to a low recurrence risk (<13%). Their findings highlight the need for further research into clinical and genetic risk factors to mitigate neurotoxicity while supporting ongoing IT MTX use.

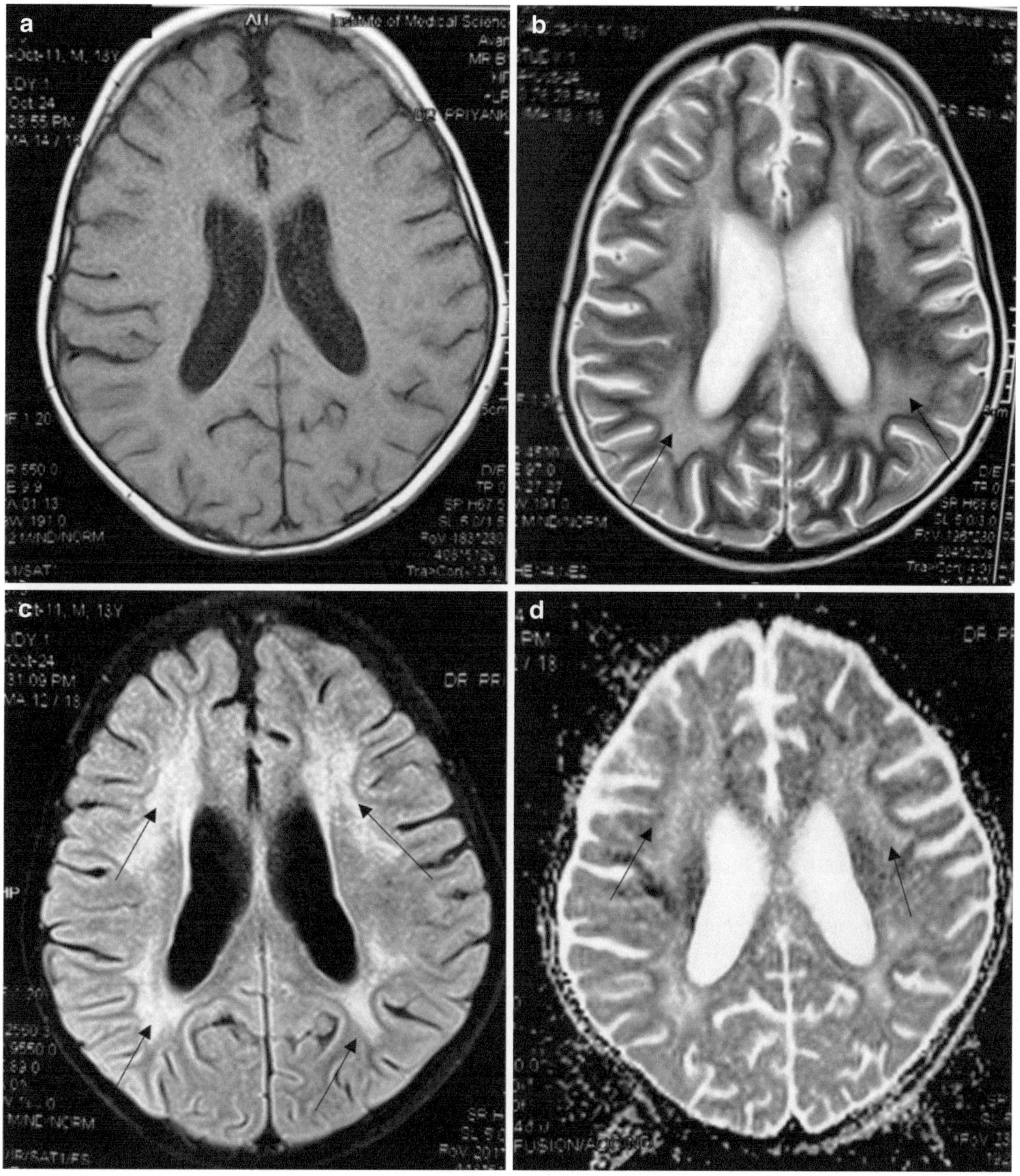

Fig. 3.10 (**a**–**d**) Leukoencephalopathy in a 13-year-old child 2 weeks after intrathecal methotrexate. (**a**) T1W image shows no significant changes. (**b**) T2W image shows symmetrical hyperintensity in bilateral centrum semiovale with relative sparing of subcortical U fibers. (**c**, **d**) Corresponding areas show hyperintensity in FlAIR image with T2 shine through on ADC image

3.5 Radiation Therapy-Induced Complications

Radiation therapy can lead to various neurotoxic effects. Pediatric patients are particularly vulnerable to neurocognitive impairment due to brain radiotherapy, with cognitive dysfunction emerging years post-treatment. The proton beam therapy may reduce late effects, especially in pediatric brain tumors [54].

Stroke-like migraine attacks after radiation therapy (SMART syndrome) present with headaches and other neurological symptoms, often years after treatment [55]. A radiation dose of >50 Gy has been suggested as a threshold, but lower doses have also been reported. Imaging is essential in diagnosing SMART syndrome, with brain MR imaging as the preferred method [56]. In the acute phase, it typically shows unilateral gyriform enhancement and T2/FLAIR hyperintense cortical swelling, unrelated to vascular territories [56]. This usually reflects the high-dose radiation field but can occasionally be bilateral. The temporal and parietal lobes are most commonly affected, followed by the occipital and frontal lobes [57].

Secondary brain tumors can arise from radiation, particularly in children receiving high doses. Additionally, radiation-induced cerebrovascular disease may develop years later, leading to complications like moyamoya syndrome [58]. Factors influencing these conditions include age, radiation dose, and concurrent chemotherapy [59].

3.5.1 Immunotherapy-Induced Complications

Immunotherapy, particularly in pediatric oncology, presents a promising alternative to traditional chemotherapy, targeting resistant cancers with potentially reduced toxicity. However, data on CNS toxicity remain sparse. Notably, therapies like Blinatumomab and CAR T cells are associated with significant neurotoxic effects, while agents such as Rituximab show less impact [60]. Severe neurotoxicity is a negative prognostic factor for survival. CAR T cell therapy has demonstrated effectiveness in refractory ALL but can lead to complications like cytokine release syndrome (CRS) and immune effector cell-associated neurotoxicity syndrome (ICANS), with symptoms often emerging 4–5 days post-infusion [61].

3.6 Genitourinary Complications

Genitourinary complications from cancer therapy include kidney involvement due to infections (especially fungal), tumor lysis syndrome, and prolonged renal dysfunction. Radiation exposure can cause focal or diffuse kidney damage, leading to functional decline.

3.6.1 Tumor Lysis Syndrome

Tumor lysis syndrome (TLS) is a metabolic disruption occurring shortly after the start of cancer treatment.

Tumor lysis syndrome (TLS) results from the release of ions and metabolic byproducts into the blood after rapid cancer cell death, causing hyperuricemia, hyperkalemia, hyperphosphatemia, hypocalcemia, and acute renal failure. Diagnosis is based on clinical and lab assessments, with imaging used to detect obstructive causes like nephrolithiasis from uric acid crystals. Nephromegaly and striated nephrogram may also appear in TLS.

3.6.2 Hemorrhagic Cystitis

Hemorrhagic cystitis may arise from both infectious and non-infectious causes, with its incidence reported to reach up to 25% in children following hematopoietic stem cell transplantation (HSCT) [62].

Cyclophosphamide and total-body irradiation, commonly used in HSCT preparation, are often associated with hemorrhagic cystitis in children [63].

Severe hemorrhagic cystitis, associated with being over 5 years old, HSCT, and the presence of BK virus in the urine, heightens the risk of complications like bladder perforation, hydronephrosis, and renal impairment [64].

Ultrasound is the preferred method for diagnosing hemorrhagic cystitis, revealing bladder wall thickening, hyperemia, and intraluminal clots [65]. BK virus-associated hemorrhagic cystitis in HSCT recipients may show vascular mural nodules amidst diffuse bladder wall thickening on imaging [66]. Other causes of non-hemorrhagic cystitis include GVH and radiation cystitis.

3.7 Musculoskeletal Complications

Musculoskeletal complications resulting from cancer treatment can impact bones, bone marrow, muscles, and soft tissues. Many bone-related complications, such as bone atrophy, scoliosis, metaphyseal alterations, and osteochondroma development, tend to develop gradually over time.

3.7.1 Bone Changes

Osteonecrosis is a common complication following hematopoietic stem cell transplantation (HSCT), often resulting from cancer treatments such as steroid use, bone marrow transplantation, and radiation therapy. It occurs in approximately 6% of children with acute lymphocytic leukemia and up to 13.8% of pediatric HSCT survivors, regardless of symptoms [67].

Within 2–5 years post-HSCT, patients frequently experience a significant decline in bone mineral density, leading to osteoporosis, osteopenia, and avascular necrosis, especially in weight-bearing joints like the hip and knee, affecting around 20% of patients [68].

Conventional radiographs are less sensitive for early osteonecrosis detection, while MRI can identify it sooner. Whole-body MRI is useful in children with leukemia, showing affected areas as geographic regions with serpiginous borders—dark on T1-weighted and bright on T2-weighted or STIR images. Central regions may lose signal on fat-saturated images, with border enhancement indicating inflammation and hyperemia [69] (Fig. 3.11).

Skeletal abnormalities linked to total body irradiation post-HSCT include enchondromas, metaphyseal abnormalities, and osteochondromas, with younger children being particularly susceptible to these anomalies [70]. Rarely, cases of radiation-induced malignant exostoses and simultaneous occurrences of osteochondroma and osteosarcoma have been reported after HSCT.

3.7.2 Marrow Changes

Radiation therapy induces fatty marrow replacement, observable on MRI as hyperintensity of the marrow on T1-weighted images, appearing as early as 1–2 weeks post-radiation and more noticeably at 6–8 weeks [71]. Recovery back to red marrow depends on radiation dose, noted by reduced signal intensity on T1-weighted images. Hematopoietic growth factors like G-CSF stimu-

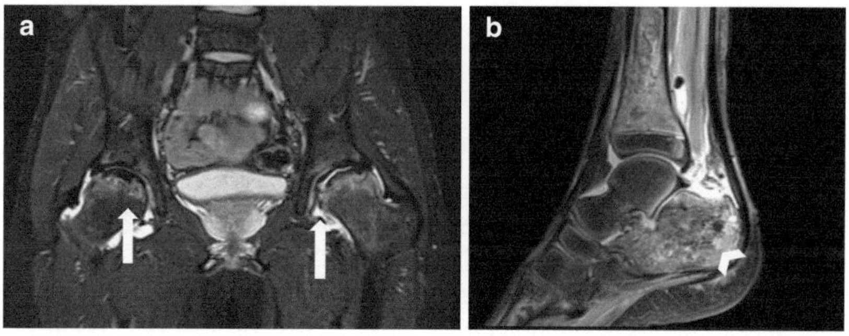

Fig. 3.11 (**a, b**) Avascular necrosis. (**a**) Avascular necrosis of the bilateral hip (arrow) is observed in a 17-year-old boy 4 months after bone marrow transplantation for acute myeloid leukemia. Geographic areas of avascular necrosis in both femoral heads are shown on the T2-weighted MR image. (**b**) Calcaneal avascular necrosis (arrowhead) is noted in a 10-year-old boy 10 months post-HSCT for leukemia

late marrow recovery, leading to the reconversion of yellow to red marrow, which appears as low signal on T1-weighted images and mildly hyperintense signal on T2-weighted images [72]. On PET-CT scans, GCSF administration may cause transiently increased FDG uptake in bone marrow and spleen, which can mimic bone metastases [73].

3.7.3 Soft Tissue Changes

Soft tissue changes such as myositis are a result of chemotherapy and radiation therapy, showing as abnormal increased T2 signal in irradiated muscles. This condition, called radiation recall myositis, is triggered by chemotherapeutic agents like vincristine, cyclophosphamide, doxorubicin, and etoposide, resembling radiation recall pneumonitis [74]. Radiation recall myositis often occurs alongside recall dermatitis and typically manifests within days to weeks after the triggering agent is administered, with a shorter interval between radiotherapy and chemotherapy increasing the likelihood of its occurrence.

3.8 Endocrine Complications

Thyroid nodules, multinodular goiter, and thyroid carcinoma are common complications observed in children post-HSCT [75]. Diagnostic imaging plays a limited role in evaluating endocrine abnormalities following HSCT, with ultrasound (US) being primarily used to assess the thyroid and hand radiographs employed to gauge the extent of delayed skeletal maturation.

3.9 Paranasal Sinus

Paranasal sinusitis is a common complication following bone marrow transplantation, occurring in more than one-third of patients within 2 years post-transplantation. It is often an underrecognized cause of fever in this population [76].

CT screening of the sinuses in children before bone marrow transplantation is recommended due to the risk of sinus abnormalities leading to sinusitis [76]. Key radiographic and CT findings of paranasal sinusitis include air-fluid levels and soft-tissue thickening, with direct coronal CT preferred for its higher sensitivity.

Invasive sinusitis, often caused by Aspergillus species, can affect the mucosa, submucosa, bone, or vascular structures. Common CT findings for both invasive and bacterial sinusitis include mucosal thickening, sinus opacification, and facial soft-tissue swelling. Classic signs of invasive sinusitis—like periantral soft-tissue invasion and bone erosion—are not always observed. Recent evidence suggests that significant unilateral thickening of the paranasal sinus mucosa is the most common early CT sign of invasive sinusitis [77].

3.10 Secondary Malignancies

The reported incidence of secondary malignancies after allogeneic HSCT varies widely, potentially due to differences in underlying disease, initial treatment, and immunosuppression. Thus, determining the exclusive role of HSCT in secondary malignancy development is challenging.

Secondary malignancies after HSCT fall into three categories: (1) Myelodysplasia and acute myeloid leukemia, which occur after autologous HSCT. (2) Lymphoma and post-transplantation lymphoproliferative disorder (PTLD), occurring after allogeneic HSCT. (3) Solid tumors with longer latency, which can occur in any post-HSCT patients (Fig. 3.11) [78].

Children under 10 years old have the highest overall risk of developing post-transplantation malignancies, with up to a 60-fold increased risk.

3.11 Post-transplant Lymphoproliferative Disorder (PTLD)

Imaging findings of post-transplantation lymphoproliferative disorder (PTLD) include lymphadenopathy, focal parenchymal masses, and nodules. Focal masses and nodules can develop within

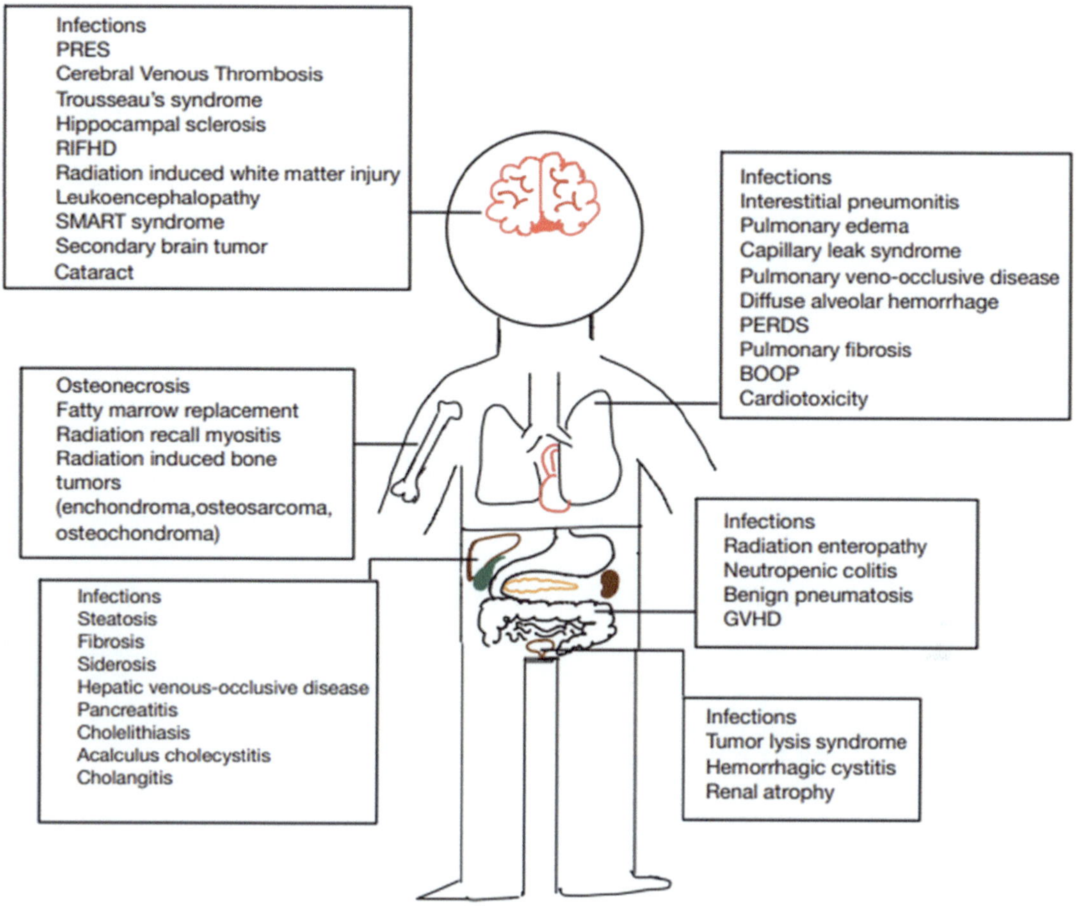

Fig. 3.12 Summary of complications in post chemoradiotherapy and post HSCT

various organs. PTLD can also manifest as diffuse infiltration of organs without distinct focal masses (Fig. 3.12).

References

1. Peña E, Souza CA, Escuissato DL, Gomes MM, Allan D, Tay J, Dennie CJ. Noninfectious pulmonary complications after hematopoietic stem cell transplantation: practical approach to imaging diagnosis. Radiographics. 2014;34(3):663–83. https://doi.org/10.1148/rg.343135080. PMID: 24819788.
2. Gertz SJ, McArthur J, Hsing DD, Nitu ME, Smith LS, Loomis A, Fitzgerald JC, Duncan CN, Mahadeo KM, Moffet J, Hall MW, Pinos EL, Cheifetz IM, Rowan CM; Pediatric acute lung injury, sepsis investigators (PALISI) network. Respiratory pathogens associated with intubated pediatric patients following hematopoietic cell transplant. Transpl Infect Dis. 2020;22(4):e13297. https://doi.org/10.1111/tid.13297. Epub 2020 Apr 28. PMID: 32306533.
3. Alexander BD, Lamoth F, Heussel CP, Prokop CS, Desai SR, Morrissey CO, Baddley JW. Guidance on imaging for invasive pulmonary Aspergillosis and Mucormycosis: from the imaging working group for the revision and update of the consensus definitions of fungal disease from the EORTC/MSGERC. Clin Infect Dis. 2021;72(Suppl 2):S79–S88. https://doi.org/10.1093/cid/ciaa1855. PMID: 33709131.
4. Escuissato DL, Gasparetto EL, Marchiori E, Rocha Gde M, Inoue C, Pasquini R, Müller NL. Pulmonary infections after bone marrow transplantation: high-resolution CT findings in 111 patients. AJR Am J Roentgenol. 2005;185(3):608–15. https://doi.org/10.2214/ajr.185.3.01850608. PMID: 16120907.
5. Morin CE, McBee MP, Elbahlawan L, Griffin LM, Maron GM, Nguyen HN, Sharma A, Snyder EJ, Jeudy J. Early pulmonary complications related to cancer treatment in children. Pediatr Radiol.

2022;52(10):2017–28. https://doi.org/10.1007/s00247-022-05403-w. Epub 2022 Jul 2. PMID: 35778572.
6. Kaya Z, Weiner DJ, Yilmaz D, Rowan J, Goyal RK. Lung function, pulmonary complications, and mortality after allogeneic blood and marrow transplantation in children. Biol Blood Marrow Transplant. 2009;15(7):817–26. https://doi.org/10.1016/j.bbmt.2009.03.019. Erratum in: Biol Blood Marrow Transplant. 2009;15(9):1141. PMID: 19539213
7. Rowan CM, Gertz SJ, McArthur J, Fitzgerald JC, Nitu ME, Loomis A, Hsing DD, Duncan CN, Mahadeo KM, Smith LS, Moffet J, Hall MW, Pinos EL, Cheifetz IM, Tamburro RF, Investigators of the Pediatric Acute Lung Injury and Sepsis Network. Invasive mechanical ventilation and mortality in pediatric hematopoietic stem cell transplantation: a multicenter study. Pediatr Crit Care Med. 2016;17(4):294–302. https://doi.org/10.1097/PCC.0000000000000673. PMID: 26910477
8. Broglie L, Fretham C, Al-Seraihy A, George B, Kurtzberg J, Loren A, MacMillan M, Martinez C, Davies SM, Pasquini MC. Pulmonary complications in pediatric and adolescent patients following allogeneic hematopoietic cell transplantation. Biol Blood Marrow Transplant. 2019;25(10):2024–30. https://doi.org/10.1016/j.bbmt.2019.06.004. Epub 2019 Jun 12. PMID: 31201861; PMCID: PMC7262781
9. Elbahlawan L, Galdo AM, Ribeiro RC. Pulmonary manifestations of hematologic and oncologic diseases in children. Pediatr Clin N Am. 2021;68(1):61–80. https://doi.org/10.1016/j.pcl.2020.09.003. PMID: 33228943
10. Versluys AB, Bresters D. Pulmonary complications of childhood cancer treatment. Paediatr Respir Rev. 2016;17:63–70. https://doi.org/10.1016/j.prrv.2015.09.004. Epub 2015 Sep 26. PMID: 26531217
11. Kouwenberg TW, van Dalen EC, Feijen EAM, Netea SA, Bolier M, Slieker MG, Hoesein FAAM, Kremer LCM, Grotenhuis HB, Mavinkurve-Groothuis AMC. BMC Cancer. 2023;23:866. Published online 2023 Sep 14. https://doi.org/10.1186/s12885-023-11353-9. PMCID: PMC10500898.
12. Maturen KE, Feng MU, Wasnik AP, Azar SF, Appelman HD, Francis IR, Platt JF. Imaging effects of radiation therapy in the abdomen and pelvis: evaluating "innocent bystander" tissues. Radiographics. 2013;33(2):599–619. https://doi.org/10.1148/rg.332125119. PMID: 23479716
13. MacNaughton WK. Review article: new insights into the pathogenesis of radiation-induced intestinal dysfunction. Aliment Pharmacol Ther. 2000;14(5):523–8. https://doi.org/10.1046/j.1365-2036.2000.00745.x. PMID: 10792113
14. Ransom JL, Novak RW, Kumar AP, Hustu HO, Pratt CB. Delayed gastrointestinal complications after combined modality therapy of childhood rhabdomyosarcoma. Int J Radiat Oncol Biol Phys. 1979;5(8):1275–9. https://doi.org/10.1016/0360-3016(79)90653-9. PMID: 528277
15. Kirkpatrick ID, Greenberg HM. Gastrointestinal complications in the neutropenic patient: characterization and differentiation with abdominal CT. Radiology. 2003;226(3):668–74. https://doi.org/10.1148/radiol.2263011932. Epub 2003 Jan 24. PMID: 12601214
16. McCarville MB, Adelman CS, Li C, Xiong X, Furman WL, Razzouk BI, Pui CH, Sandlund JT. Typhlitis in childhood cancer. Cancer. 2005;104(2):380–7. https://doi.org/10.1002/cncr.21134. PMID: 15952190
17. Worawattanakul S, Semelka RC, Kelekis NL, Sallah AS. MR findings of intestinal graft-versus-host disease. Magn Reson Imaging. 1996;14(10):1221–3. https://doi.org/10.1016/s0730-725x(96)00245-7. PMID: 9065914
18. Donnelly LF, Morris CL. Acute graft-versus-host disease in children: abdominal CT findings. Radiology. 1996;199(1):265–8. https://doi.org/10.1148/radiology.199.1.8633157. PMID: 8633157
19. Khoury NJ, Kanj V, Abboud M, Muwakkit S, Birjawi GA, Haddad MC. Abdominal complications of chemotherapy in pediatric malignancies: imaging findings. Clin Imaging. 2009;33(4):253–60. https://doi.org/10.1016/j.clinimag.2008.10.029. PMID: 19559346
20. Robinson PJ. The effects of cancer chemotherapy on liver imaging. Eur Radiol. 2009;19(7):1752–62. https://doi.org/10.1007/s00330-009-1333-6. PMID: 19238392
21. Czauderna P, Katski K, Kowalczyk J, Kurylak A, Lopatka B, Skotnicka-Klonowicz G, Sawicz-Birkowska K, Godziński J. Venoocclusive liver disease (VOD) as a complication of Wilms' tumour management in the series of consecutive 206 patients. Eur J Pediatr Surg. 2000;10(5):300–3. https://doi.org/10.1055/s-2008-1072380. PMID: 11194540
22. DeLeve LD, Shulman HM, McDonald GB. Toxic injury to hepatic sinusoids: sinusoidal obstruction syndrome (veno-occlusive disease). Semin Liver Dis. 2002;22(1):27–42. https://doi.org/10.1055/s--2002-23204. PMID: 11928077
23. Castellino S, Muir A, Shah A, Shope S, McMullen K, Ruble K, Barber A, Davidoff A, Hudson MM. Hepatobiliary late effects in survivors of childhood and adolescent cancer: a report from the children's oncology group. Pediatr Blood Cancer. 2010;54(5):663–9. https://doi.org/10.1002/pbc.22265. PMID: 19890896; PMCID: PMC2838980
24. Bardi E, Mulder RL, van Dalen EC, Bhatt NS, Ruble KA, Burgis J, Castellino SM, Constine LS, den Hoed CM, Green DM, Koot BGP, Levitt G, Szonyi L, Wallace WH, Skinner R, Hudson MM, Kremer LCM, Effinger KE, Bresters D. Late hepatic toxicity surveillance for survivors of childhood, adolescent and young adult cancer: recommendations from the international late effects of childhood cancer guideline harmonization group. Cancer Treat Rev. 2021;100:102296.

https://doi.org/10.1016/j.ctrv.2021.102296. PMID: 34571378
25. MacKenzie JR. Complications of treatment of paediatric malignancies. Eur J Radiol. 2001;37(2):109–19. https://doi.org/10.1016/s0720-048x(00)00292-8. PMID: 11223477
26. Joy D, Thava VR, Scott BB. Diagnosis of fatty liver disease: is biopsy necessary? Eur J Gastroenterol Hepatol. 2003;15(5):539–43. https://doi.org/10.1097/01.meg.0000059112.41030.2e. PMID: 12702913
27. Kawamoto S, Soyer PA, Fishman EK, Bluemke DA. Nonneoplastic liver disease: evaluation with CT and MR imaging. Radiographics. 1998;18(4):827–48. https://doi.org/10.1148/radiographics.18.4.9672968. PMID: 9672968
28. Day DL, Carpenter BL. Abdominal complications in pediatric bone marrow transplant recipients. Radiographics. 1993;13(5):1101–12. https://doi.org/10.1148/radiographics.13.5.8210593. PMID: 8210593
29. Raja RA, Schmiegelow K, Frandsen TL. Asparaginase-associated pancreatitis in children. Br J Haematol. 2012;159(1):18–27. https://doi.org/10.1111/bjh.12016. PMID: 22909259
30. Sandoval C, Katz B, Stringel G, Jayabose S, Lebovics E. Cholelithiasis and choledocholithiasis after sequential cytarabine and asparaginase. J Pediatr Hematol Oncol. 2003;25(8):637–9. https://doi.org/10.1097/00043426-200308000-00010. PMID: 12902918
31. Büyükaşik Y, Koşar A, Demiroğlu H, Altinok G, Ozcebe OI, Dündar S. Acalculous acute cholecystitis in leukemia. J Clin Gastroenterol. 1998;27(2):146–8. https://doi.org/10.1097/00004836-199809000-00009. PMID: 9754777
32. Coley SC, Jäger HR, Szydlo RM, Goldman JM. CT and MRI manifestations of central nervous system infection following allogeneic bone marrow transplantation. Clin Radiol. 1999;54(6):390–7. https://doi.org/10.1053/crad.1999.0200. PMID: 10406341
33. Wiznitzer M, Packer RJ, August CS, Burkey ED. Neurological complications of bone marrow transplantation in childhood. Ann Neurol. 1984;16(5):569–76. https://doi.org/10.1002/ana.410160507. PMID: 6391364
34. Miaux Y, Ribaud P, Williams M, Guermazi A, Gluckman E, Brocheriou C, Laval-Jeantet M. MR of cerebral aspergillosis in patients who have had bone marrow transplantation. AJNR Am J Neuroradiol. 1995;16(3):555–62. PMID: 7793381; PMCID: PMC8337670
35. Dulamea AO, Lupescu IG. Neurological complications of hematopoietic cell transplantation in children and adults. Neural Regen Res. 2018;13(6):945–54. https://doi.org/10.4103/1673-5374.233431. PMID: 29926815; PMCID: PMC6022482
36. Gabriel M, Hoeben BAW, Uhlving HH, Zajac-Spychala O, Lawitschka A, Bresters D, Ifversen M. A review of acute and long-term neurological complications following haematopoietic stem cell transplant for paediatric acute lymphoblastic leukaemia. Front Pediatr. 2021;9:774853. https://doi.org/10.3389/fped.2021.774853. PMID: 35004543; PMCID: PMC8734594
37. Morris EB, Laningham FH, Sandlund JT, Khan RB. Posterior reversible encephalopathy syndrome in children with cancer. Pediatr Blood Cancer. 2007;48(2):152–9. https://doi.org/10.1002/pbc.20703. PMID: 16317748
38. Bartynski WS, Boardman JF. Distinct imaging patterns and lesion distribution in posterior reversible encephalopathy syndrome. AJNR Am J Neuroradiol. 2007;28(7):1320–7. https://doi.org/10.3174/ajnr.A0549. PMID: 17698535; PMCID: PMC7977645
39. Okabe T, Nozaki T, Aida N, Starkey J, Enokizono M, Niwa T, Handa A, Numaguchi Y, Kurihara Y. MR imaging findings in some rare neurological complications of paediatric cancer. Insights Imaging. 2018;9(3):313–24. https://doi.org/10.1007/s13244-018-0628-z. Epub 2018 May 15. PMID: 29766473; PMCID: PMC5991004
40. Habetz K, Ramakrishnaiah R, Raina SK, Fitzgerald RT, Hinduja A. Posterior reversible encephalopathy syndrome: a comparative study of pediatric versus adult patients. Pediatr Neurol. 2016;65:45–51. https://doi.org/10.1016/j.pediatrneurol.2016.09.001. Epub 2016 Sep 13. PMID: 27720711
41. Wani NA, Kosar T, Pala NA, Qureshi UA. Sagittal sinus thrombosis due to L-asparaginase. J Pediatr Neurosci. 2010;5(1):32–5. https://doi.org/10.4103/1817-1745.66683. PMID: 21042505; PMCID: PMC2964787
42. Finelli PF, Nouh A. Three-territory DWI acute infarcts: diagnostic value in cancer-associated hypercoagulation stroke (trousseau syndrome). AJNR Am J Neuroradiol. 2016;37(11):2033–6. https://doi.org/10.3174/ajnr.A4846. Epub 2016 Jun 30. PMID: 27365322; PMCID: PMC7963789
43. Vázquez E, Delgado I, Sánchez-Montañez A, Barber I, Sánchez-Toledo J, Enríquez G. Side effects of oncologic therapies in the pediatric central nervous system: update on neuroimaging findings. Radiographics. 2011;31:1123–39.
44. Kasai-Yoshida E, Ogihara M, Ozawa M, Nozaki T, Morino M, Manabe A, Hosoya R. Temporal lobe epilepsy with hippocampal sclerosis in acute lymphoblastic leukemia. Pediatrics. 2013;132(1):e252–6. https://doi.org/10.1542/peds.2012-1420. Epub 2013 Jun 17. PMID: 23776122
45. Adachi Y, Yagishita A, Arai N. White matter abnormalities in the anterior temporal lobe suggest the side of the seizure foci in temporal lobe epilepsy. Neuroradiology. 2006;48(7):460–4. https://doi.org/10.1007/s00234-006-0092-1. Epub 2006 Apr 28. PMID: 16645843
46. Rigamonti D, Johnson PC, Spetzler RF, Hadley MN, Drayer BP. Cavernous malformations and capillary telangiectasia: a spectrum within a single pathologi-

cal entity. Neurosurgery. 1991;28(1):60–4. PMID: 1994283
47. Jain R, Robertson PL, Gandhi D, Gujar SK, Muraszko KM, Gebarski S. Radiation-induced cavernomas of the brain. AJNR Am J Neuroradiol. 2005;26(5):1158–62. PMID: 15891176; PMCID: PMC8158583
48. Koike T, Yanagimachi N, Ishiguro H, Yabe H, Yabe M, Morimoto T, Shimizu T, Takakura H, Kato S. High incidence of radiation-induced cavernous hemangioma in long-term survivors who underwent hematopoietic stem cell transplantation with radiation therapy during childhood or adolescence. Biol Blood Marrow Transplant. 2012;18(7):1090–8. https://doi.org/10.1016/j.bbmt.2011.12.582. Epub 2011 Dec 23. PMID: 22198541
49. Abla AA, Turner JD, Mitha AP, Lekovic G, Spetzler RF. Surgical approaches to brainstem cavernous malformations. Neurosurg Focus. 2010;29(3):E8. https://doi.org/10.3171/2010.6.FOCUS10128. PMID: 20809766
50. Ball WS Jr, Prenger EC, Ballard ET. Neurotoxicity of radio/chemotherapy in children: pathologic and MR correlation. AJNR Am J Neuroradiol. 1992;13(2):761–76. PMID: 1566726; PMCID: PMC8333213
51. Weaver L, Samkari A. Neurological complications of childhood cancer. Semin Pediatr Neurol. 2017;24(1):60–9. https://doi.org/10.1016/j.spen.2016.12.005. Epub 2016 Dec 23. PMID: 28779867
52. Badke C, Fleming A, Iqbal A, Khilji O, Parhas S, Weinstein J, Morgan E, Hijiya N. Rechallenging with intrathecal methotrexate after developing subacute neurotoxicity in children with hematologic malignancies. Pediatr Blood Cancer. 2016;63(4):723–6. https://doi.org/10.1002/pbc.25850. Epub 2015 Dec 18. PMID: 26681571
53. Abdou MAA, El Kiki HA, Madney Y, et al. Chemotherapy-related neurotoxicity in pediatric cancer patients: magnetic resonance imaging and clinical correlation. Egypt J Radiol Nucl Med. 2021;52:230. https://doi.org/10.1186/s43055-021-00606-x.
54. Mabbott DJ, Spiegler BJ, Greenberg ML, Rutka JT, Hyder DJ, Bouffet E. Serial evaluation of academic and behavioral outcome after treatment with cranial radiation in childhood. J Clin Oncol. 2005;23(10):2256–63. https://doi.org/10.1200/JCO.2005.01.158. PMID: 15800316
55. Brown WR, Thore CR, Moody DM, Robbins ME, Wheeler KT. Vascular damage after fractionated whole-brain irradiation in rats. Radiat Res. 2005;164(5):662–8. https://doi.org/10.1667/rr3453.1. PMID: 16238444
56. Dominguez M, Malani R. Stroke-like migraine attacks after radiation therapy (SMART) syndrome: a comprehensive review. Curr Pain Headache Rep. 2021;25(5):33. https://doi.org/10.1007/s11916-021-00946-3. PMID: 33761013
57. Singh TD, Hajeb M, Rabinstein AA, et al. SMART syndrome: retrospective review of a rare delayed complication of radiation. Eur J Neurol. 2021;28:1316–23.
58. Remes TM, Suo-Palosaari MH, Heikkilä VP, Sutela AK, Koskenkorva PKT, Toiviainen-Salo SM, Porra L, Arikoski PM, Lähteenmäki PM, Pokka TM, Arola MO, Riikonen VP, Sirkiä KH, Lönnqvist TRI, Rantala HMJ, Ojaniemi MK, Harila-Saari AH. Radiation-induced meningiomas after childhood brain tumor: a magnetic resonance imaging screening study. J Adolesc Young Adult Oncol. 2019;8(5):593–601. https://doi.org/10.1089/jayao.2019.0010. Epub 2019 May 7. PMID: 31063432
59. Peiffer AM, Leyrer CM, Greene-Schloesser DM, Shing E, Kearns WT, Hinson WH, Tatter SB, Ip EH, Rapp SR, Robbins ME, Shaw EG, Chan MD. Neuroanatomical target theory as a predictive model for radiation-induced cognitive decline. Neurology. 2013;80(8):747–53. https://doi.org/10.1212/WNL.0b013e318283bb0a. Epub 2013 Feb 6. PMID: 23390169; PMCID: PMC3589296
60. von Stackelberg A, Locatelli F, Zugmaier G, Handgretinger R, Trippett TM, Rizzari C, Bader P, O'Brien MM, Brethon B, Bhojwani D, Schlegel PG, Borkhardt A, Rheingold SR, Cooper TM, Zwaan CM, Barnette P, Messina C, Michel G, DuBois SG, Hu K, Zhu M, Whitlock JA, Gore L. Phase I/phase II study of Blinatumomab in pediatric patients with relapsed/refractory acute lymphoblastic leukemia. J Clin Oncol. 2016;34(36):4381–9. https://doi.org/10.1200/JCO.2016.67.3301. Epub 2016 Oct 31. PMID: 27998223
61. Grupp SA, Kalos M, Barrett D, Aplenc R, Porter DL, Rheingold SR, Teachey DT, Chew A, Hauck B, Wright JF, et al. Chimeric antigen receptor–modified T cells for acute lymphoid leukemia. N Engl J Med. 2013;368:1509–18. https://doi.org/10.1056/NEJMoa1215134.
62. Miano M, Faraci M, Dini G, Bordigoni P, Paediatric Working EBMT, Party. Early complications following haematopoietic SCT in children. Bone Marrow Transplant. 2008;41(Suppl 2):S39–42. https://doi.org/10.1038/bmt.2008.53. PMID: 18545243
63. McCarville MB, Hoffer FA, Gingrich JR, Jenkins JJ 3rd. Imaging findings of hemorrhagic cystitis in pediatric oncology patients. Pediatr Radiol. 2000;30(3):131–8. https://doi.org/10.1007/s002470050031. PMID: 10755748
64. Riachy E, Krauel L, Rich BS, McEvoy MP, Honeyman JN, Boulad F, Wolden SL, Herr HW, La Quaglia MP. Risk factors and predictors of severity score and complications of pediatric hemorrhagic cystitis. J Urol. 2014;191(1):186–92. https://doi.org/10.1016/j.juro.2013.08.007. Epub 2013 Aug 13. PMID: 23954584
65. Cartoni C, Arcese W, Avvisati G, Corinto L, Capua A, Meloni G. Role of ultrasonography in the diagnosis and follow-up of hemorrhagic cystitis after bone

marrow transplantation. Bone Marrow Transplant. 1993;12(5):463–7. PMID: 8298557
66. Schechter T, Liebman M, Gassas A, Ngan BY, Navarro OM. BK virus-associated hemorrhagic cystitis presenting as mural nodules in the urinary bladder after hematopoietic stem cell transplantation. Pediatr Radiol. 2010;40(8):1430–3. https://doi.org/10.1007/s00247-010-1556-3. Epub 2010 Mar 11. PMID: 20221593
67. te Winkel ML, Pieters R, Hop WC, de Groot-Kruseman HA, Lequin MH, van der Sluis IM, Bökkerink JP, Leeuw JA, Bruin MC, Egeler RM, Veerman AJ, van den Heuvel-Eibrink MM. Prospective study on incidence, risk factors, and long-term outcome of osteonecrosis in pediatric acute lymphoblastic leukemia. J Clin Oncol. 2011;29(31):4143–50. https://doi.org/10.1200/JCO.2011.37.3217. Epub 2011 Sep 26. PMID: 21947829
68. Kaste SC, Shidler TJ, Tong X, Srivastava DK, Rochester R, Hudson MM, Shearer PD, Hale GA. Bone mineral density and osteonecrosis in survivors of childhood allogeneic bone marrow transplantation. Bone Marrow Transplant. 2004;33(4):435–41. https://doi.org/10.1038/sj.bmt.1704360. PMID: 14716354
69. Sharma S, Leung WH, Deqing P, Yang J, Rochester R, Britton L, Neel MD, Ness KK, Kaste SC. Osteonecrosis in children after allogeneic hematopoietic cell transplantation: study of prevalence, risk factors and longitudinal changes using MR imaging. Bone Marrow Transplant. 2012;47(8):1067–74. https://doi.org/10.1038/bmt.2011.234. Epub 2011 Dec 12. PMID: 22158389; PMCID: PMC3310343
70. Taitz J, Cohn RJ, White L, Russell SJ, Vowels MR. Osteochondroma after total body irradiation: an age-related complication. Pediatr Blood Cancer. 2004;42(3):225–9. https://doi.org/10.1002/pbc.10426. PMID: 14752859
71. Fletcher BD. Effects of pediatric cancer therapy on the musculoskeletal system. Pediatr Radiol. 1997;27(8):623–36. https://doi.org/10.1007/s002470050201. PMID: 9252425
72. Fletcher BD, Wall JE, Hanna SL. Effect of hematopoietic growth factors on MR images of bone marrow in children undergoing chemotherapy. Radiology. 1993;189(3):745–51. https://doi.org/10.1148/radiology.189.3.7694312. PMID: 7694312
73. Ulaner GA, Lyall A. Identifying and distinguishing treatment effects and complications from malignancy at FDG PET/CT. Radiographics. 2013;33(6):1817–34. https://doi.org/10.1148/rg.336125105. PMID: 24108564
74. Hattangadi J, Esty B, Winey B, Duigenan S, Huang M, Yock T. Radiation recall myositis in pediatric Ewing sarcoma. Pediatr Blood Cancer. 2012;59(3):570–2. https://doi.org/10.1002/pbc.23374. Epub 2011 Oct 20. PMID: 22021129
75. Gallardo D, Ferrà C, Berlanga JJ, Banda ED, Ponce C, Salar A, Alonso E, Español I, Riu C, Grañena A. Neurologic complications after allogeneic bone marrow transplantation. Bone Marrow Transplant. 1996;18(6):1135–9. PMID: 8971384
76. Billings KR, Lowe LH, Aquino VM, Biavati MJ. Screening sinus CT scans in pediatric bone marrow transplant patients. Int J Pediatr Otorhinolaryngol. 2000;52(3):253–60. https://doi.org/10.1016/s0165-5876(00)00296-2. PMID: 10841955
77. DelGaudio JM, Swain RE Jr, Kingdom TT, Muller S, Hudgins PA. Computed tomographic findings in patients with invasive fungal sinusitis. Arch Otolaryngol Head Neck Surg. 2003;129(2):236–40. https://doi.org/10.1001/archotol.129.2.236. PMID: 12578456
78. Baker KS, DeFor TE, Burns LJ, Ramsay NK, Neglia JP, Robison LL. New malignancies after blood or marrow stem-cell transplantation in children and adults: incidence and risk factors. J Clin Oncol. 2003;21(7):1352–8. https://doi.org/10.1200/JCO.2003.05.108. Erratum in: J Clin Oncol. 2003 Aug 15;21(16):3181. PMID: 12663726

Oncological Emergencies

4

Gaurav Raj and Kaustubh Gupta

4.1 Introduction

Primary tumour and its metastasis with associated secondary paraneoplastic syndromes along with treatment complications of reactions to chemo-radiotherapy constitute common causative factors for various oncological emergencies with imaging playing an important role for early detection as well as for guiding therapy. This chapter will focus on paediatric oncological emergencies which are mostly encountered in the emergency department (ED). While major portion of oncological emergencies are due to long-standing primary cancers with only a few patients presenting with such emergencies having a previously unknown primary tumour. Every radiologist must be having a thorough knowledge of such acute emergencies in the paediatric population in which early diagnosis and management is lifesaving as due to the different biological nature of paediatric malignancies vs adult malignancies.

Metabolic oncological emergencies are mostly diagnosed initially based on the clinical symptoms and laboratory parameters with no initial role of imaging. Structural oncological emergencies due to anatomical distortion by the tumour require emergent imaging for diagnosis and treatment planning. Oncological emergencies presenting in the central nervous, cardio-thoracic, and abdomino-pelvic systems can be diagnosed easily when there is a combination of characteristic patho-physiological findings and imaging findings are seen which helps in patient care. Oncological emergencies secondary to complications of radiotherapy and chemotherapy also show characteristic imaging finding which aid in early diagnosis.

Knowledge of complications such as raised intracranial pressure, malignant spinal cord compression, acute airway compromise, SVC syndrome, abdominal compartment syndrome, bowel obstruction and bowel perforation should be immediately communicated to the clinician as per ACR guidelines of non-routine and emergent communication.

G. Raj (✉) · K. Gupta
Department of Radiology, Dr. Ram Manohar Lohia Institute of Medical Sciences (Dr. RMLIMS), Lucknow, Uttar Pradesh, India

I. Kumar et al. (eds.), *Practical Approach to Imaging in Pediatric Oncology*,
https://doi.org/10.1007/978-981-96-8158-7_4

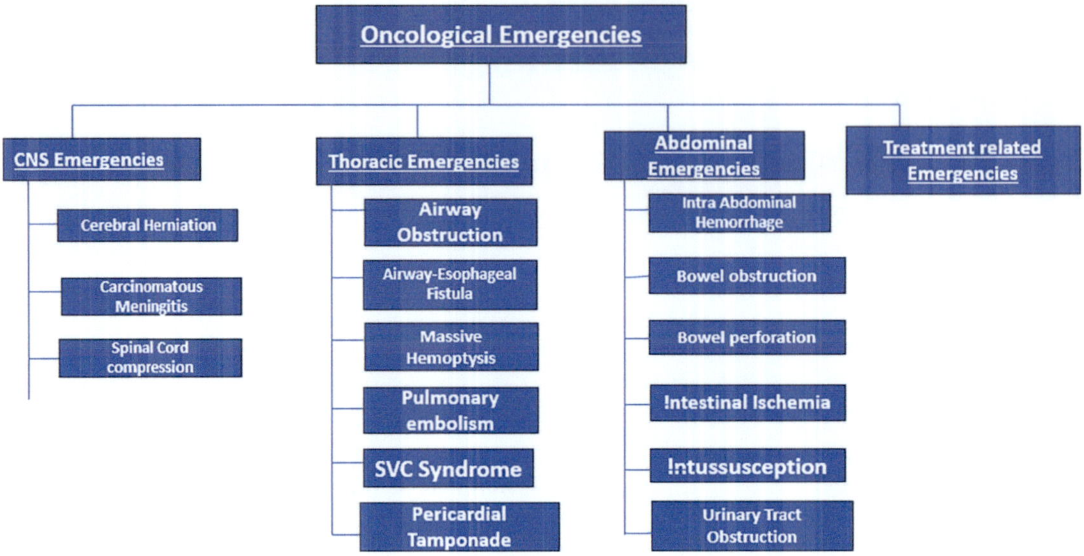

Overview of oncological emergencies

4.2 Central Nervous System

Clinical symptoms are highly variable with differing presentation depending on the age and the characteristics of lesion making a clinical diagnosis difficult due to non-specific nature of the symptoms with sub-acute onset being the most common. Headache and intermittent seizures are the most common presenting symptoms[1]with neurological symptoms mimicking strokes being associated with tumoral haemorrhage or with lesions causing intracranial venous sinus thrombus.

Imaging protocols are the same as used for paediatric cases without oncological emergencies [1] and consist of trans-fontanelle ultrasound which is quick and easily accessible screening modality for cases with a patent fontanel. It is sensitive in demonstrating ventricular dilatation, mass, focal parenchymal abnormality with the Doppler tool easily assessing for any venous thrombosis [2]. CT is the first-line modality in oncology patients with clinical suspicion of emergencies with CEMRI being reserved as the imaging test of choice in difficult cases. Both cross-sectional modalities easily demonstrate displacement of intracranial structures, midline shift and any ventricular compression and assessing the severity of compression. Both imaging modalities help in evaluating the type of brain herniation.

NCCT allows prompt identification of intracranial shift, oedema, haemorrhage, hydrocephalus which helps the neurosurgeon in deciding the type of treatment required and to rule out any need for emergent surgery. NCCT can also be used for demonstrating cerebral venous sinus thrombosis and any haemorrhage. MR imaging is mainly used for meningeal carcinomatosis and spinal cord compression and for the evaluation of posterior fossa lesions which are better characterized on MR with the modality also being used for further lesion characterization when neurosurgical opinion is required.

Posterior fossa intracranial masses are the most common intracranial neoplasm causing deaths in children with the most common oncological emergency being acute hydrocephalus which is irrespective of tumour grade and is seen due to extrinsic compression and obstruction to CSF flow and due to intraventricular infiltration of tumour in late cases. Obstruction of foramen of Monro, cerebral aqueduct, fourth ventricle and the outlet foramen are also seen [2, 3].

Most common posterior fossa low-grade tumour is the pilocytic astrocytoma with ependymoma and tumours of embryonal origin (medulloblastomas, atypical teratoid rhabdoid tumour, embryonal tumours with multilayered rosettes) being relatively less common. During an emergency presentation, the role of radiologist however is limited to tumour localization and detecting any local complications such as haemorrhage and hydrocephalous which are vital for the neurosurgeon in surgical planning and is lifesaving.

Specific complications include Cushing's triad due to raised intracranial pressure, stroke due to vascular occlusion and various complications presenting as emergencies which have been discussed in detail in this chapter.

4.2.1 Cerebral Herniation

Cerebral herniation is frequently seen as a complication of brain tumours and presents with a wide spectrum of clinical presentations depending upon the type of herniation [4]. Primary mass or metastasis causing direct mass effect on the brain parenchyma is the most common causative factor with associated effects also acting as an important cause for herniation. Peritumoral oedema also causes significant mass effect on the parenchyma and causes significant herniation syndromes and can be easily differentiated from primary tumour on post contrast images. Intratumoral changes such as haemorrhage and abscess formation can cause mass effect which causes cerebral herniation and can be differentiated based on a combination of characteristic clinical and imaging features [5, 6].

Radiological approach to cerebral herniation should include details such as anatomical landmarks, direction of mass effect and should include details about displaced structures, any indirect sign and the subsequent complications secondary to compromise of vital structures which presents as an emergency.

Types of herniation include subfalcine herniation, ascending and descending trans tentorial herniation which are further subdivided into anterior, posterior, central and lateral hernias, tonsillar and transalar hernias [4].

Mandatory reporting checklist in such cases must include the type of herniation, the degree of displacement of displaced structures with respect to the bony landmark should be mentioned as its quantification helps in determining the prognosis and for assessing the patient as a candidate for decompressive craniotomy and craniectomy. Decompressive craniectomy being the most common emergent surgical procedure done in such patients, common complications include haemorrhage, external cerebral herniation, wound complications and CSF leak/fistulae, knowledge of which is important as such patients frequently require serial imaging to monitor for progression and course of these complications.

External cerebral herniation is also a type of herniation frequently encountered in such patients [4]. Craniectomy defect allows for expansion of the underlying brain parenchyma and in cases where the craniectomy defect is small, the externally herniated parenchyma may cause pressure on the cortical veins which causes focal parenchymal ischemia along the craniectomy sites. Paradoxical hernia is seen in rare cases of craniectomy in which there is inward depression of brain parenchyma due to negative air pressure when the atmospheric pressure exceeds the intracranial pressure [4] (Table 4.1).

Large, iso to hyperdense mass located within the posterior fossa in a central location causing mass effect on the fourth ventricle with secondary obstructive hydrocephalus with trans ependymal periventricular ooze seen along the fronto-occipital horns of bilateral lateral ventricles (Fig. 4.1a).

Large mass (medulloblastoma) situated in the middle of the posterior fossa showing high intensity on T2 imaging and low intensity on T1 imaging, with only subtle and patchy post-contrast enhancement (Fig. 4.1b.). Vermis cannot be seen separately and mass is likely originating from it and fully obliterating the fourth ventricle with secondary obstructive hydrocephalus (Fig. 4.1c.) and is in close proximity to the dorsal brainstem, without clear signs of extension into pons.

Table 4.1 Overview of cerebral herniation [4]

Type	Landmark	Prognosis	Displaced structures	Complications
Subfalcine	Septum Pellucidum	Shift<5 mm: Good Shift>15 mm: Poor	Cingulate gyrus and corpus callosum	Cingulate gyrus necrosis-hypobulia, apathy, indifference Pericallosal artery compression and infarct
Descending transtentorial	Tentorial notch	Poor prognosis especially in late stages secondary to brainstem haemorrhage	Uncus, parahippocampal gyrus, isthmus of fornical gyrus, diencephalon, midbrain and pons	3rd cranial nerve compression, posterior cerebral artery, and midbrain compression
Ascending transtentorial	Tentorial incisura, Quadrigeminal plate cistern	Poor prognosis due to compression of cerebellar hemispheres and vermis	Superior cerebellar hemispheres and vermis	Brainstem compression and compromise of respiratory Centre
Tonsillar	Foramen of Monroe, mc Rae's line	Good prognosis with timely intervention	Cerebellar tonsils, pons, medulla	Cerebellar infarcts, obstructive supratentorial hydrocephalus
Transalar	Sphenoid ridge	Poor prognosis	Frontal lobe, temporal lobe	MCA territory infarction due to compression of ICA and MCA

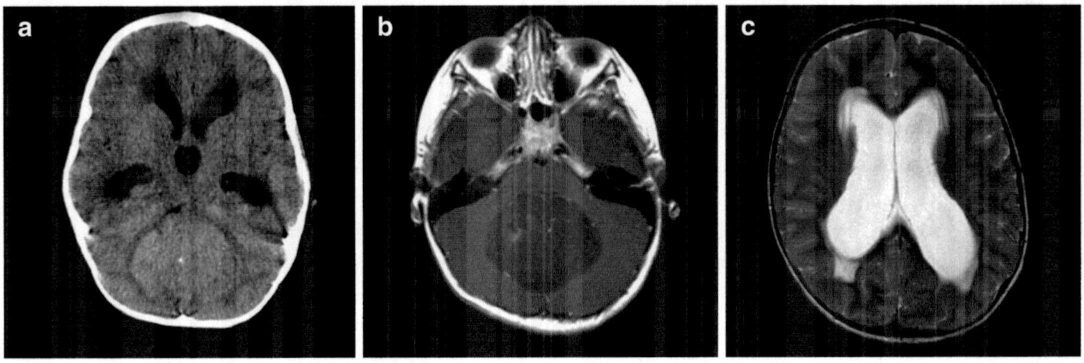

Fig. 4.1 Medulloblastoma

Choroid plexus papilloma presenting as a heterogeneous (partly cystic with areas of calcification) lesion located in the atrium, occipital horn, and posterior aspect of body of the right lateral ventricle (Fig. 4.2a, b, c). The satellite lesions in the right lateral ventricle and temporal and frontal horns suggest CSF dissemination with obstruction of the temporal horn of the right lateral ventricle. Additional secondary changes of vasogenic oedema in the surrounding brain parenchyma are seen with mass effect seen in the form of medial deviation of the right uncus, effacement of the basilar cisterns, midline shift of 12 mm towards the left side and deformity of the midbrain (Fig. 4.2d, e, f).

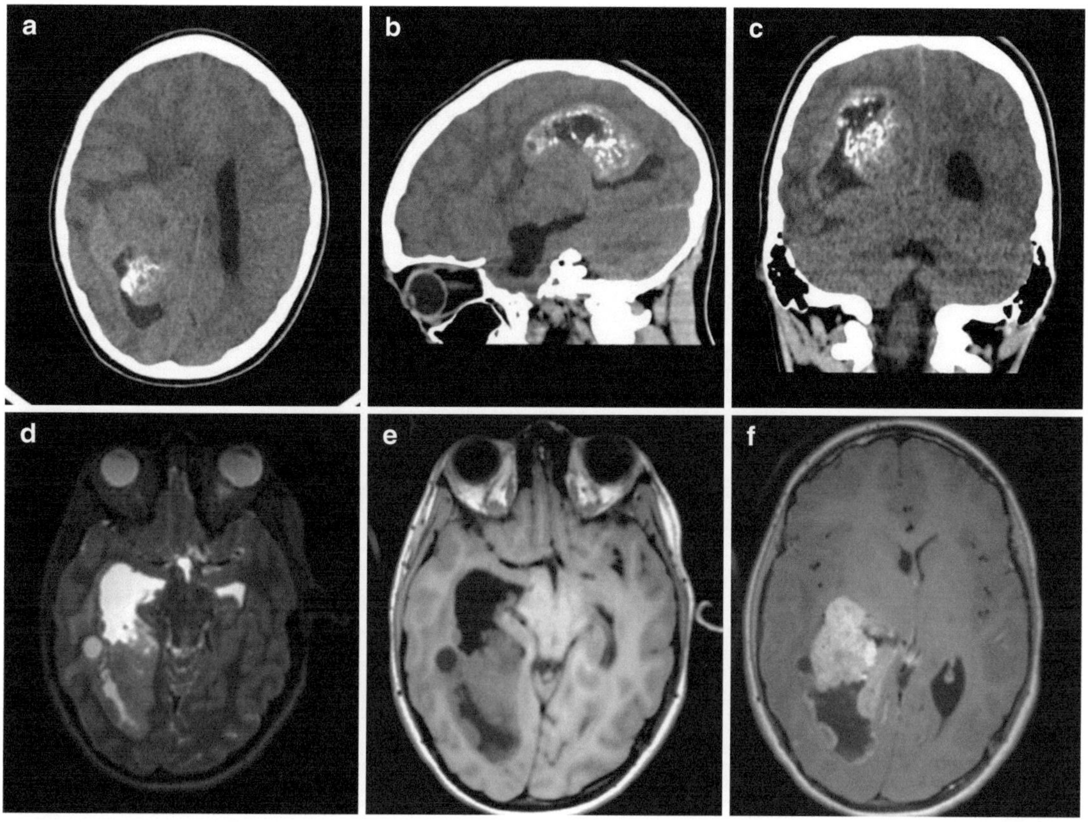

Fig. 4.2 Choroid Plexus papilloma

4.3 Carcinomatous Meningitis

Mostly seen due to hematogenous dissemination with direct spread from contiguous effected parenchyma, choroid plexus metastasis, epidural and subdural spread from vertebral metastasis and iatrogenic secondary to neurosurgical intervention being causative factors in carcinomatous meningitis [7, 8].

Carcinomatous meningitis presents clinically as an emergency depending upon the site of involvement with most common general clinical symptoms requiring prompt ER referral being severe headache, raised ICP and subsequent confusion and altered mentation. Involvement of posterior fossa structures, as seen in pediatric subgroup, presents as cerebellar symptoms such as ataxia and nystagmus while distant involvement of the neuraxis and the spinal cord in particular presents as hemi or quadriparesis with bladder bowel dysfunction. Such patients are candidates for imaging of the entire neuraxis to localize the site of involvement to guide focal radiotherapy as it is required for reducing the bulk of plaque-like deposits in the spinal cord [8].

Tumour deposits at the brainstem and the spinal cord require urgent clinical referral for imaging and subsequent chemotherapy and focal radiotherapy to reduce bulk as these deposits can compromise the respiratory centre and limb/ extremity weakness respectively. Imaging follow-up of all these patients is recommended to monitor the treatment response.

MRI imaging is the gold standard with contrast imaging of the entire neuraxis with or without analgesia for optimal patient positioning [7]. MR imaging helps in clinical decision making in suspected cases of meningeal carcinomatosis with CSF negative of malignant cells but presenting with most common imaging presentations—

Fig. 4.3 Carcinomatous meningitis

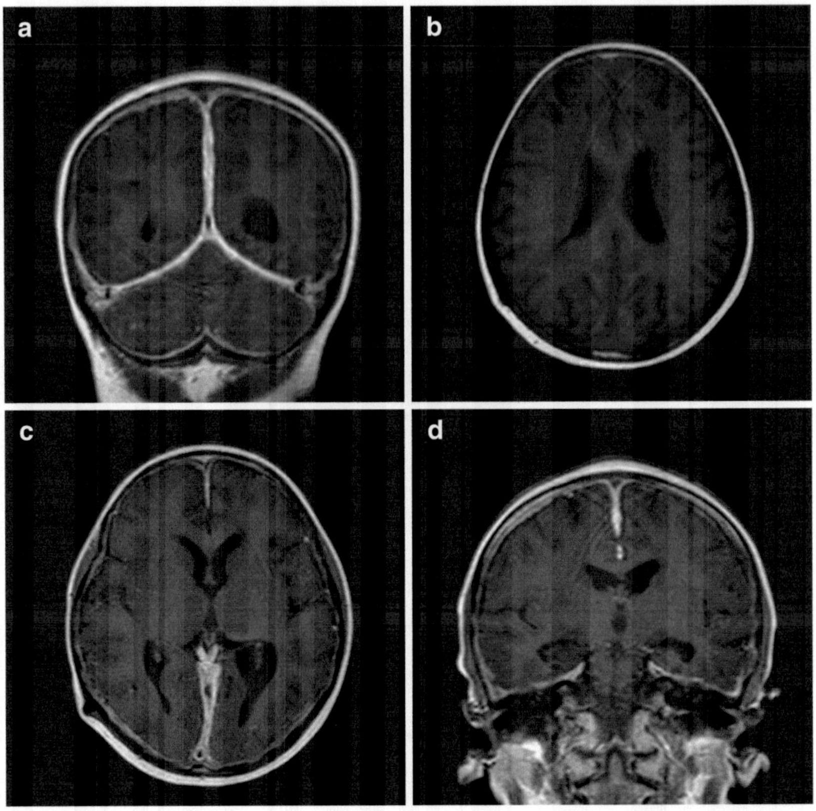

linear or nodular meningeal enhancement with ventricular effacement. Diffuse or asymmetrical nodular enhancement can be appreciated [8].

Seizures in patient treated for acute lymphoblastic leukaemia (ALL). Leukemic meningitis with Fig. 4.3a–d showing nodular meningeal enhancement.

4.4 Compression of Spinal Cord and Cauda Equina

4.4.1 Spinal Cord Compression

External compression of the cord with secondary compressive myelopathy is the most frequent causative factor for neurological emergency in paediatric oncology patients, most commonly via paravertebral mass with imaging playing a vital role in early detection as prolonged compression progresses to irreversible neurological damage within a short time. Imaging of the entire spine is recommended to detect multifocal spread [9, 10].

Neuroblastoma is most important causative lesion with other causes being sarcomas and Hodgkin's lymphoma.

Leptomeningeal metastatic spread is rare and carries a better prognosis in the paediatric population as compared to the adults with imaging helping in early identification and thus allowing for curated chemotherapy and radiotherapy regime [9].

CECT images demonstrate a heterogeneously enhancing mass in the mediastinum at a paraspinal location (Fig. 4.4a Axial and Fig. 4.4b. Coronal reformat).

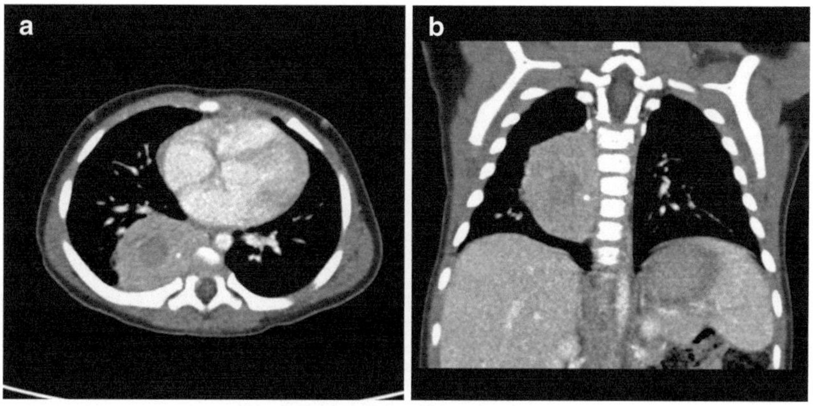

Fig. 4.4 Thoracic neuroblastoma

4.5 Orbit

Proptosis is the most prevalent clinical manifestation of orbital pathology which can be benign or malignant. Cross-sectional imaging plays an important role as it helps in differentiation between the benign and malignant causes and evaluates the extension. MRI is helpful as MR appearances of common benign pathologies—orbital haemangioma and orbital pseudo tumour have characteristic imaging features and help in differentiation of these common benign pathologies from malignant causes of proptosis.

Rhabdomyosarcoma (RMS) is the most common primary malignancy [11] of the orbit presenting as an emergency due to its high incidence (4%) in pediatric population with an associated risk of blindness on delay in diagnosis. 10% cases of RMS are seen within the orbit in the first decade of life [12] and MRI is very accurate for local staging of lesions less than 5 cm which have been proven to be embryonal type on histology. Lesions larger than 5 cm or showing alveolar type histopathology are locally staged by PET-CT. Malignant rhabdoid tumour is one of the most common causes of orbital metastasis in infants presenting as rapidly progressive proptosis and imaging should include not only the orbits but the entire neuraxis to rule out an associated primary or secondary lesion.

An exophytic soft tissue signal intensity mass appearing isointense to muscle on T1 (Fig. 4.5b), hyperintense on T2 (Fig. 4.5a, d) with diffusion restriction and post contrast enhancement is seen centred in the extraconal compartment of left orbit (Fig. 4.5c) seen arising from the superior part of the orbital cavity. The superior oblique muscle is not visualized separately (Fig. 4.5b, c) and the lesion is causing mass effect in the form of anteroinferior displacement of the ocular muscles causing proptosis of the globe with associated deformity of the superior part of orbital cavity with extension into the preseptal compartment. No obvious bony involvement or extension to posterior orbit is seen. There is associated stretching of the optic nerve which is also seen due to mass effect. Final diagnosis of anaplastic rhabdomyosarcoma (Fig. 4.5e).

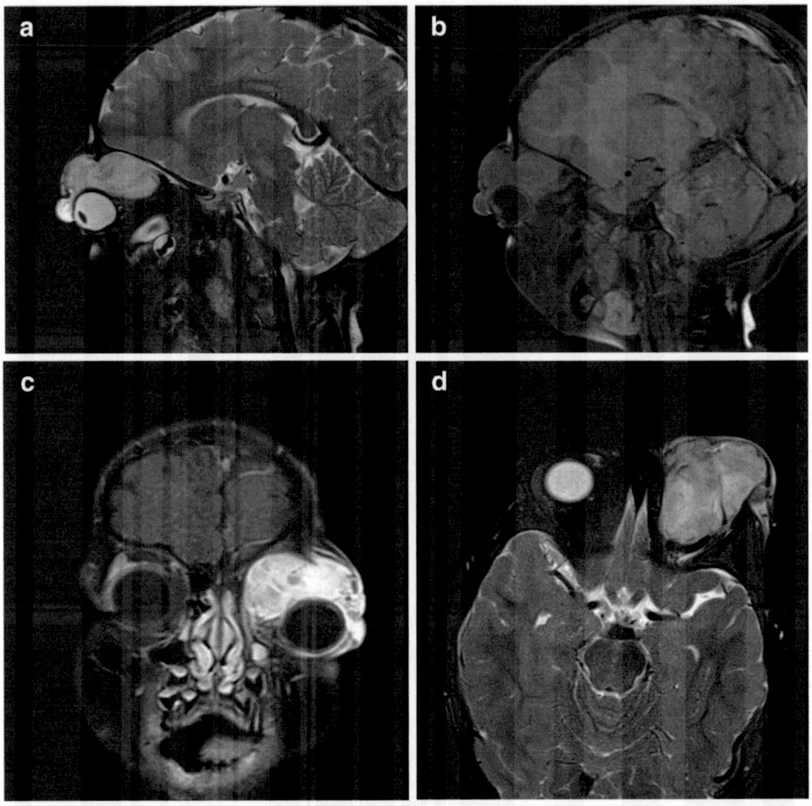

e

PATHOLOGY REPORT

CLINICAL INFORMATION	Upper eyelid mass, Excision, UNDIFFERENTIATED SPINDLE AND ROUND CELL TUMOR.
NATURE OF SPECIMEN	Immunohistochemistry.

GROSS

Sections are prepared from the paraffin block of the lesion no. S10883-22 for immunohistochemistry.

MICROSCOPIC

Section examined from specimen received reveals portion of tumor tissue formed of cellular proliferation of spindle and round cells showing moderate nuclear anaplasia. There are scattered atypical multipolar mitosis are seen. Tumor is involving surgical margins.

Examination of the immunostained sections shows:

- Desmin = STRONG POSITIVE.
- Myogenin = PATCHY POSITIVE.
- CD99 = WEAK POSITIVE.
- TLE1, SMA, CD34, S100 = NEGATIVE.
- Ki67 = HIGH PROLIFERATION INDEX (MORE THAN 80%).

FINAL DIAGNOSIS

Upper eyelid mass, Immunohistochemistry, **ANAPLASTIC RHABDOMYOSARCOMA**.

Fig. 4.5 Orbital rhabdomyosarcoma

4.6 Emergencies of the Thorax

4.6.1 Compression of the Airway and SVC Syndrome

Common malignancies of childhood which involve the mediastinum—Lymphoma, Leukaemia, Germ cell tumours and anterior mediastinal masses [13, 14] predispose to compression syndromes of the superior vena cava (SVC) and the trachea secondary to increased pliability of the structures to compression in the paediatric population resulting in SVC syndrome and airway compromise respectively. Imaging helps in identifying the cause, site and the severity of the compression as majority presents with respiratory distress in the emergency setting where swift diagnosis is required which can be easily done via plain radiograph and Multidetector CT with sagittal and coronal reformations which are easily available with an added benefit of evaluation of the lung parenchyma. Upper airway obstruction presents as acute respiratory failure whereas lower respiratory compromise causes subacute symptoms like dyspnoea, cough and in a few cases, as fever secondary to obstructive pneumonia. Multi-detector CT evaluation has an added benefit of intra-luminal evaluation of the trachea-bronchial tree via CT virtual bronchoscopy and helps in planning for conventional fibreoptic bronchoscopy which is an invasive procedure and is comparatively difficult in children [15].

Large mediastinal mass (Fig. 4.6a, b) with significant external compression of the SVC (Fig. 4.6b). A case of mediastinal lymphoma—large B-cell.

4.6.2 Superior Vena Cava Syndrome

Carcinoma lung and lymphoma are the most common cancers causing SVC syndrome [13, 14, 16] with other common causes being metastasis, mediastinal germ cell tumour and thymomas. The reduced and obstructed blood supply from the upper extremities is secondary to direct invasion of the SVC by the tumour or secondary tumour thrombus which causes intra-luminal narrowing with progressive complete luminal obstruction. Clinical symptoms depend upon the nature of malignancies, the rapidity of involvement of SVC as well as presence of thrombus with the patency and status of the collaterals.

Multi-detector chest CT with iodinated contrast media and option of multiplanar reconstruction is preferred modality for evaluation which helps in identification of the exact point and severity of flow compromise, evaluation of the thrombus for its extent and status of collateral vessels with associated evaluation of the underlying tumour.

Role of interventional radiology in management of such cases in adults has proven to be effective, especially with percutaneous stenting having the advantages of shorter recovery period of surgical thrombectomy [16, 17], however in the paediatric age group, current body of evidence states that SVC stenting has proven to be highly efficacious in relieving SVC obstruction in non-malignant causes [17] despite the more difficult procedure vs adults due to a smaller luminal calibre, role in treating malignant SVC obstruction in this age group is under evaluation.

4.6.3 Pleural Effusion

Rare complication in the paediatric population heralding poor prognosis and is a sign of suboptimal treatment response (15%) [18] with non-Hodgkin's lymphoma being one of the frequent causes with underlying pathophysiology being obstruction to or reduced venous return to the

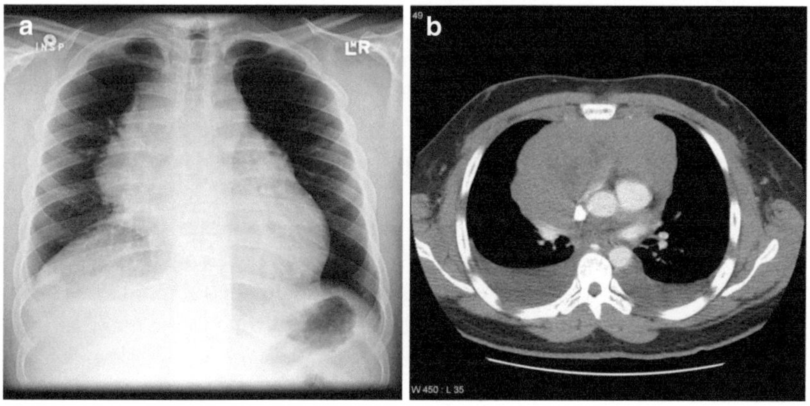

Fig. 4.6 Mediastinal lymphoma

heart with or without associated lymphatic obstruction secondary to bulky disease. Effusions are easily detected on X-ray and ultrasound of the chest with ultrasound having the added advantage of demonstrating the nature and complexity of the fluid and with advantage of image-guided drainage catheter placement for relieving large effusion which may be causing respiratory compromise.

4.6.4 Esophago-Respiratory Fistula

An extremely rare complication secondary to radiotherapy of thoracic paediatric malignancies. Mostly seen in adults secondary to radiotherapy of advanced oesophageal carcinomas, as the complication is almost insidious and fatal, a level of suspicion should be kept by the clinician as well as the radiologist whenever a child undergoing radiotherapy presents with symptoms of respiratory tract infection which are refractory to antimicrobial therapy. MDCT is the modality of choice for evaluation as the modality along with the option of minimum intensity projection gives highly detailed evaluation of the bronchial tree and allows for the evaluation of small defects [19].

4.6.5 Haemoptysis

As compared to adults haemoptysis is rare in the paediatric age group, especially in small children who tend to swallow blood and not clinically apparent. The most common cause of haemoptysis is non-malignant cystic fibrosis. In children the cut off for massive life-threatening haemoptysis in a 24-h window has been kept as >8 ml/kg body weight [20]. Additional clinical symptoms include chest pain and refractory cough with air trapping on auscultation.

Tumours in paediatric population can cause haemoptysis via compression of the bronchial vessels or directly when presenting as an endobronchial mass [21]. Atypical chest carcinoid has been reported to cause massive haemoptysis in a 6-year-old child. Bronchial artery embolization is effective with a cure rate of 85% [20] but is limited to cases where endobronchial treatment options like octreotide and vasopressors administered via the endobronchial route have failed [22].

4.6.6 Pericardial Effusion and Tamponade

A variety of factors are responsible for pericardial effusion seen in the paediatric oncology patients and mostly include medical causes like cardiac failure and secondary to side effects of chemo and radiotherapy. A rare cause includes hematopoietic stem cell transplant with associated secondary pericardial infiltration from leukemic cells [23]. Imaging plays a role as large pericardial effusion causing tamponade can be assessed by ultrasound which also evaluates the extent of narrowing of cardiac chambers. CT can also be used for evaluation of cardiac chambers and for assessment of the degree of tamponade not only secondary to pericardial effusion but also via a cardiac mass which may be causing compression of the chambers. However, despite the advantages offered by cross-sectional imaging, 2D Echo remains the first modality used in this age group.

4.7 Abdominal Emergencies

4.7.1 Uncontrolled Intra-Abdominal Haemorrhage

Rare and fatal complication [24, 25] seen in paediatric cancer patients with hypervascular malignancies being the most common cause with patient presenting in the emergency setting with a large spontaneous hemoperitoneum. Lymphoma and leukaemia which also present as visceral masses most commonly involving the liver and spleen can also cause fatal haemorrhage secondary to spontaneous rupture [24] of these organs due to the mass with risk factors being bulk of the mass, a subcapsular location and excessive vascularity.

Ultrasound can be used for evaluation as the first-line modality and demonstrates echogenic complex fluid.

NCCT shows high attenuation ascites with clotted blood showing HU values ranging between 45 and 70 HU with the added advantage of visualizing a high attenuation hematoma which may be the sentinel clot and indicates the source of bleed. On CECT active bleed can be seen as an area of contrast blush and indicates a need for vascular embolization or an emergent exploratory laparotomy.

Pelvic soft tissue opacity displaces bowel superiorly indicative of a lesion. Calcification was not apparent (Fig. 4.7a).

MR images of abdominal MRI show a large heterogenous signal intensity mass within the pelvis showing high signal on T2 (Fig. 4.7b, d). On T1 the lesion is predominantly isointense with some areas of high signal which could be indicative of intralesional fat (Fig. 4.7c). Postoperative diagnosis of a teratoma was confirmed.

4.7.2 Abdominal Compartment Syndrome

Primarily a clinical diagnosis however imaging and the radiologist plays a key role by helping raise awareness in a clinically suspected case as diagnosis is made by assessing venous compression. Imaging evaluation of the IVC plays a key role as abdominal ultrasound helps in assessing the caval index and post post-contrast CT study in the venous phase shows the extent of compression. As the underlying mechanism is secondary to rapid elevation in intra-abdominal compartment volume beyond the capacity of expansion of anterior abdominal wall, there is a decrease in blood flow to the organs, resulting in impaired organ function and eventual organ failure [26], hence the condition is potentially fatal with a high mortality (~60%) and a swift diagnosis is of the essence as an emergent decompressive laparotomy is required in most cases. Aetiology includes large (bilateral) Wilm's tumour, proliferating lymphoblastic and leukemic infiltrates and giant ovarian masses.

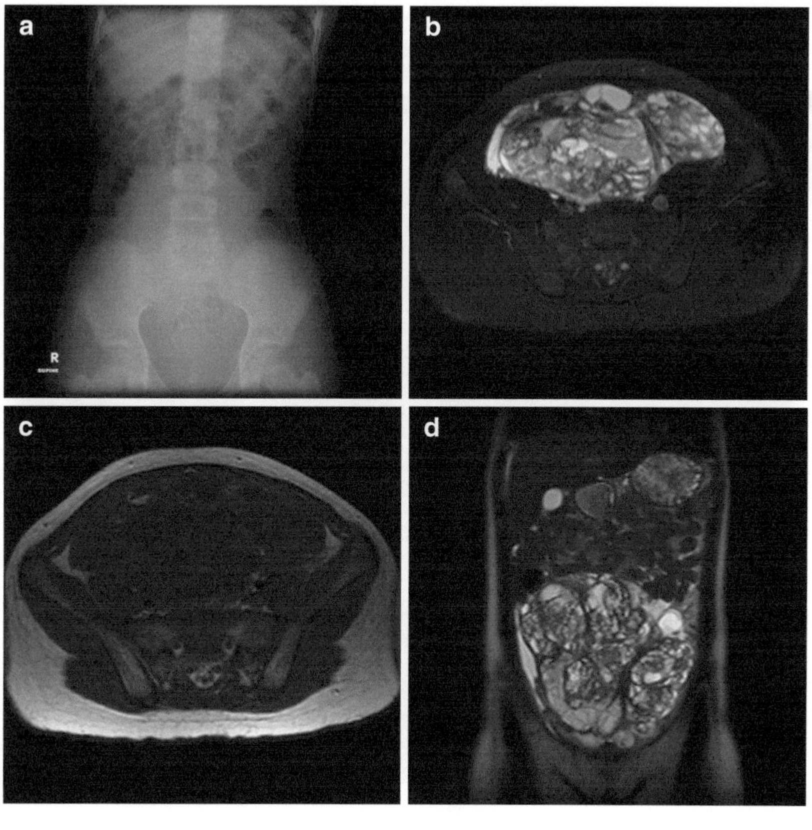

Fig. 4.7 Large abdominal teratoma

As the entity is predominantly a clinical diagnosis knowledge of radiological features is imperative and a few have been documented based on study by Pickhardt et al. who described radiological features of abdominal compartment syndrome on CT, namely a round abdominal contour with loss of ovoid shape with AP to transverse abdominal ratio > 0.8, frank compression of kidneys and retroperitoneal structures and diffuse generalized bowel wall thickening due to reperfusion oedema secondary to hypovolemia due to vascular compression [27].

4.8 Intestinal Emergencies

Acute bowel perforation, ischemia, intussusception and bowel obstruction are frequent causes of emergency in paediatric oncology.

4.8.1 Bowel Obstruction

In paediatric population intussusception is frequent reason of bowel obstruction and is also reported in healthy children with mean age of presentation being 1 year however it's incidence in children more 2 years should warrant suspicion of an underlying malignant causative lead point (Burkitt's lymphoma is most common cause with incidence of 18%) [20, 21]. Ultrasound is the first line modality which is also helpful in identifying and in localizing the lead point which may be asymmetrical bowel wall thickening, tumour or neoplastic lymph node [28].

History of abdominal distension with blood PR.

Small bowel loops are abnormal on imaging which show significant wall thickening with inter bowel fluid (Fig. 4.8a, b) with differentials being infective, inflammatory, and neoplastic aetiologies after MRI Abdomen (Fig. 4.8c, d) which was confirmed at colonoscopic biopsy as Burkitt lymphoma with chemotherapy done following diagnosis. There was adequate treatment response with remission and no incidence of recurrence.

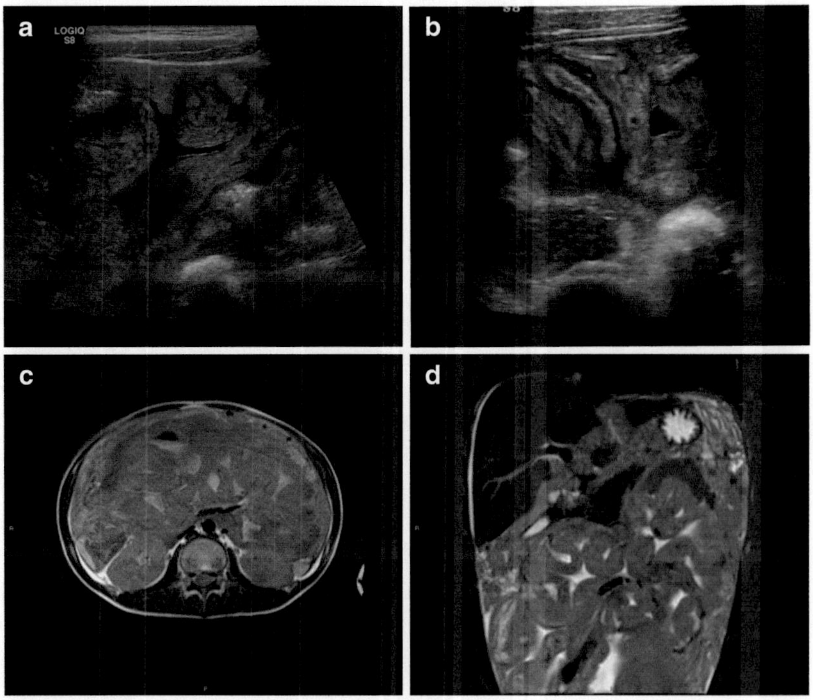

Fig. 4.8 Burkitt Lymphoma

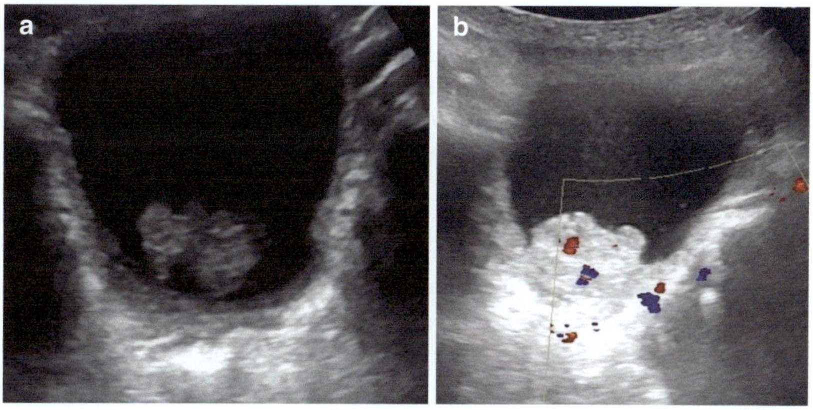

Fig. 4.9 Embryonal Botryoid Rhabdomyosarcoma

4.8.2 Bowel Perforation

Obstruction of bowel by malignant lesion most commonly results in perforation in long-standing cases with some cases seen secondary to post radio-chemotherapy for a bowel malignancy [29]. Demonstration of free air under diaphragm and the peritoneal cavity is pathognomic and can be easily done by erect abdominal radiographs with multi-detector CT being very sensitive for pneumoperitoneum with added advantage of identifying the site of perforation.

4.8.3 Urinary Tract Obstruction

Most commonly occurs due to large pelvic masses which cause extrinsic compression of the distal ureter with subsequent upstream urinary tract dilatation and hydronephrosis most commonly by large mass forming, neuroblastoma, teratoma of the sacrococcygeal region and germ cell tumours of the ovary in females. Lymphomas can also present with urinary tract obstruction due to mass effect from enlarged lymph nodes which is seen in 20% of the cases [26]. Direct invasion of the urinary tract by an enlarged intrarenal mass is also seen.

Obstruction usually resolves itself after treatment of primary lesion with a minority of cases (13%) requiring an intervention [26] in which ureteric stenting is the intervention of choice over nephrostomy via percutaneous route due to significant reduction in risk of urinary tract infections. Ultrasound is the primary and first-line imaging modality of choice with MRI being reserved for difficult cases and in cases requiring further lesion characterization.

A 3-year-old boy presenting with acute pain with episodic macroscopic haematuria with history of passage of clots and maintained renal function tests.

Lobulated well-defined echogenic mass measuring is seen at the bladder base (Fig. 4.9a) showing mild vascularity (Fig. 4.9b) was seen attached to the bladder wall. The mass was non-mobile on dynamic and decubitus scanning with no definite extravesical extension and diagnosis was confirmed on tissue biopsy as that of a rare Embryonal Botryoid Rhabdomyosarcoma.

4.9 Treatment-Related Emergencies—Haematological and Vascular

4.9.1 Venous Thromboembolism

A rarer complication in comparison to adults with incidence higher in comparison to healthy subjects [29–31].

Most common cause is complication of therapy which includes chronic indwelling catheters and treatment with steroids, L-asparaginase specially in cases of ALL. Primary malignancy causing venous thromboembolism includes ALL which causes hyperleukocytosis, soft tissue and bone sarcomas causing reduced mobility and blood stasis and tumour thrombosis as in 4–8% cases of Wilm's tumour. Imaging assessment includes duplex ultrasound assessment of the limbs with probe compression in all cases where deep vein thrombosis of the extremities is clinically suspected, pulmonary CT angiography (CTPA) dislodged thrombus which may cause embolism of the pulmonary circulation and multiphase CT evaluation with dedicated venous phase for assessing for venous thrombus of large systemic veins. Venous thromboembolism as a complication of an oncologic process is more frequently seen in the pediatric population in comparison to the adult group.

4.9.2 Haemorrhage and Disseminated Intravascular Coagulopathy

Excessive activation of blood coagulation factors and their consumption is seen secondary to diffusely disseminated metastasis or advanced AML in the paediatric population with high mortality. Other causes include cases of Kasabach-Merritt syndrome (KMS) and excessive vascular tumours such as Kaposiform haemangioendothelioma (KHE) [32]. CECT with arterial, venous with or without delayed phases in the acute setting confirms the site of the acute haemorrhage for guiding intervention with tailored protocol for paediatric population by removing the NCCT and acquiring only arterial and portal phases to reduce the radiation exposure.

4.9.3 Hypertension

Haemorrhagic stroke with irreversible end organ damage may be the only presenting symptom of some paediatric malignancies which cause hypertension [33, 34] and are seen largely in cases of tumours producing excessive catecholamine as in neuroblastoma and phaeochromocytomas or secondary to mass effect on the aorta and renal arteries.

While biochemical evaluation is the mainstay for the evaluation of tumours producing excessive catecholamine, imaging ultimately plays a role as these lesions are visualized on cross-sectional imaging. Definitive diagnosis on imaging is seen in cases of vascular compressive tumours initially by ultrasound and then followed by cross-sectional imaging which is imperative for preoperative evaluation and image-guided endovascular therapeutic intervention.

4.10 Conclusion

Through this chapter, an attempt has been made to provide an overview of the oncological complications, their manifestations, and their imaging considerations. Such children are ultimately managed by a multidisciplinary team and require prompt action and informative diagnostic imaging which helps in formulating treatment strategies. A good communication becomes mandatory between the team of treating physicians and imaging and diagnostics play a pivotal role in this.

Because such children with acute complications will not present to a tertiary care centre with access to a multidisciplinary team, all radiologists must have knowledge of such complications as it is imperative in contributing to the low rates of morbidity and mortality in all such cases.

4.11 Summary

- *Primary tumour and its metastasis with associated secondary paraneoplastic syndromes and treatment complications constitute common causative factors.*
- *Headache and intermittent seizures are the most common presenting symptoms in CNS Oncological emergencies.*
- *Emergencies of the spinal cord and orbits are extremely debilitating and warrant imaging and diagnosis on an emergent basis because of sudden unsettling symptoms.*
- *Compression of the airway and SVC syndrome, pleural effusion, pericardial effusion with cardiac tamponade, massive haemoptysis and esophago-respiratory fistulas are the thoracic oncological emergencies.*

- *Abdominal emergencies include abdominal compartment syndrome, uncontrolled abdominal haemorrhage, gastrointestinal include bowel obstruction and perforation and obstruction of the urinary tract.*
- *Haematological emergencies are mostly secondary to treatment-related complications and include venous thromboembolism, haemorrhage and disseminated intravascular coagulation and hypertension.*

References

1. Siegel R, Naishadham D, Jemal A. Cancer statistics, 2012. CA Cancer J Clin. 2012;62(1):10–29.
2. Jaff MR, McMurtry MS, Archer SL, et al. Management of massive and submassive pulmonary embolism, iliofemoral deep vein thrombosis, and chronic thromboembolic pulmonary hypertension: a scientific statement from the American Heart Association. Circulation. 2011;123(16):1788–830.
3. Shepard JA, Moore EH, Templeton PA, McLoud TC. Pulmonary intravascular tumor emboli: dilated and beaded peripheral pulmonary arteries at CT. Radiology. 1993;187(3):797–801.
4. Riveros Gilardi B, Muñoz López JI, Hernández Villegas AC, Garay Mora JA, Rico Rodríguez OC, Chávez Appendini R, et al. Types of cerebral herniation and their imaging features. Radiographics. 2019;39(6):1598–610.
5. McCurdy MT, Shanholtz CB. Oncologic emergen cies. Crit Care Med. 2012;40(7):2212–22.
6. Fagedet D, Thony F, Timsit JF, et al. Endovascular treatment of malignant superior vena cava syndrome: results and predictive factors of clinical efficacy. Cardiovasc Intervent Radiol. 2013;36(1):140–9.
7. Refaat MM, Katz WE. Neoplastic pericardial effusion. Clin Cardiol. 2011;34(10):593–8.
8. Anwar A, Gudlavalleti A, Ramadas P. Carcinomatous Meningitis [Internet]. PubMed. Treasure Island (FL): StatPearls Publishing; 2020. Available from: https://www.ncbi.nlm.nih.gov/books/NBK560816/
9. Ahn S, Lee YS, Lim KS, Lee JL. Emergency department cancer unit and management of oncologic emergencies: experience in Asan medical center. Support Care Cancer. 2012;20(9):2205–10.
10. Cook AM, Lau TN, Tomlinson MJ, Vaidya M, Wakeley CJ, Goddard P. Magnetic resonance imaging of the whole spine in suspected malignant spinal cord compression: impact on management. Clin Oncol (R Coll Radiol). 1998;10(1):39–43.
11. Higdon ML, Higdon JA. Treatment of oncologic emergencies. Am Fam Physician. 2006;74(11):1873–80.
12. Morcos SK. Review article: effects of radiographic contrast media on the lung. Br J Radiol. 2003;76(905):290–5.
13. Wang GR, Ensor JE, Gupta S, Hicks ME, Tam AL. 25 bronchial artery embolization for the management of hemoptysis in oncology patients: utility and prognostic factors. J Vasc Interv Radiol. 2009;20(6):722–9.
14. Kwek JW, Iyer RB, Dunnington J, Faria S, Silverman PM. Spectrum of imaging findings in the abdomen after radiotherapy. AJR Am J Roentgenol. 2006;187(5):1204–11.
15. Chen K, Varon J, Wenker OC. Malignant airway obstruction: recognition and management. J Emerg Med. 1998;16(1):83–92.
16. Nossair F, Schoettler P, Starr J, Chan AKC, Kirov I, Paes B, et al. Pediatric superior vena cava syndrome: an evidence-based systematic review of the literature. Pediatr Blood Cancer. 2018;65(9):e27225.
17. Laha S, Gangopadhyay D, Roy M, Mazumdar J, Das M, Das P. Transcatheter stenting of superior vena cava to treat postoperative SVC syndrome in a child: a case report. The Egyptian Heart Journal [Internet] 2024 [cited 2024 Oct 7];76(1).
18. Eastridge BJ, Lefor AT. Complications of indwelling venous access devices in cancer patients. J Clin On- col. 1995;13(1):233–8.
19. Balazs A, Galambos Z, Kupcsulik PK. Characteristics of esophagorespiratory fistulas resulting from esophageal cancers: a single-center study on 243 cases in a 20-year period. World J Surg. 2009;33(5):994–1001.
20. Roebuck DJ, Barnacle AM. Haemoptysis and bronchial artery embolization in children. Paediatr Respir Rev. 2008;9(2):95–104.
21. Bennett J. ClinicalKey [Internet]. Clinicalkey.com. Elsevier; 2020. Available from: https://www.clinicalkey.com/#
22. Zhao QM, Zhao L, He L, Wu L, Lu Y, Chu C, et al. Bronchial artery embolization in pediatric pulmonary hemorrhage: a single-center experience. J Vasc Interv Radiol. 2020;31(7):1103–9.
23. Katabathina VS, Restrepo CS, Martinez-Jimenez S, Riascos RF. Nonvascular, nontraumatic mediastinal emergencies in adults: a comprehensive review of imaging findings. Radiographics. 2011;31(4):1141–60.
24. Cascino TL. Neurologic complications of systemic cancer. Med Clin North Am. 1993;77(1):265–78.
25. Coburn MW, Rodriguez FJ. Cerebral herniations. Appl Radiol. 1998;27(5):10–6.
26. Giglio P, Gilbert MR. Neurologic complications of cancer and its treatment. Curr Oncol Rep. 2010;12(1):50–9.
27. Pickhardt PJ, Shimony JS, Heiken JP, Buchman TG, Fisher AJ. The abdominal compartment syndrome: CT findings. Am J Roentgenol. 1999;173(3):575–9.
28. Sze G, Soletsky S, Bronen R, Krol G. MR imaging of the cranial meninges with emphasis on contrast

enhancement and meningeal carcinomatosis. AJR Am J Roentgenol. 1989;153(5):1039–49.
29. Ara C, Coban S, Kayaalp C, Yilmaz S, Kirimlioglu V. Spontaneous intestinal perforation due to non-Hodgkin's lymphoma: evaluation of eight cases. Dig Dis Sci. 2007;52(8):1752–6.
30. Bassiri AG, Haghighi B, Doyle RL, Berry GJ, Rizk NW. Pulmonary tumor embolism. Am J Respir Crit Care Med. 1997;155(6):2089–95.
31. Roberts KE, Hamele-Bena D, Saqi A, Stein CA, Cole RP. Pulmonary tumor embolism: a review of the literature. Am J Med. 2003;115(3):228–32.
32. Shin JH, Kim JH, Song HY. Interventional management of esophagorespiratory fistula. Korean J Radiol. 2010;11(2):133–40.
33. Zhao W, Yang Z, Chen LA. Etiological diagnosis and treatment of central airway obstruction: report of 40 cases and review of the literature [in Chinese]. Zhonghua Jie He He Hu Xi Za Zhi. 2011;34(8):590–4.
34. Crocker M, Anthantharanjit R, Jones TL, et al. An extended role for CT in the emergency diagnosis of malignant spinal cord compression. ClinRadiol. 2011;66(10):922–7.

Artificial Intelligence: Applications in Pediatric Oncology Imaging

5

Harsimran Bhatia, Anmol Bhatia, Anirudh Gupta, and Kushaljit Singh Sodhi

5.1 Introduction

Artificial intelligence (AI) is a rapidly emerging field of computer science that simulates human brain function and can design algorithms to perform human-like cognitive functions [1–3].

Majority of the applications of AI in the real world, including the medical field, are based on the concept of machine learning (ML). ML is a subset of AI that enables the learning or training of computers. In other words, the machine can train itself to make decisions based on the input data and make predictions, based on the basis of input or training data provided. Deep learning (DL) is further a sub-domain of ML, where the algorithms are structured like neural networks [1–5]. Convolutional neural networks (CNNs) are multi-layered algorithms that process complex large amounts of data, to generate appropriate desired outputs.

H. Bhatia · A. Bhatia · K. S. Sodhi (✉)
Department of Radiodiagnosis & Imaging, Post Graduate Institute of Medical Education & Research (PGIMER), Chandigarh, India

A. Gupta
All India Institute of Medical Sciences, Kalyani, India
e-mail: anirudh.mbbs-2020@aiimskalyani.edu.in

Use of AI in Healthcare and Oncology The immense utility of AI-based applications in medicine, nursing, and other healthcare-related sciences stems from the ability of these methods to efficiently generate electronic medical records instead of paper-based data. Advanced computer informatics and software analysis contributed to the processing of a large amount of patient data and integration of all records [6, 7]. Of particular interest in the field of imaging and healthcare has been the use of ML-based methods in oncology. Cancer contributes to a major burden of mortality and morbidity in the present times. The presence of various cancer-related genes and their potential to serve as targets of specific therapeutic drugs has paved a path for extensive research and applications of AI in this field. ML has immense application in the field of oncology, beginning from cancer detection and diagnosis to analyzing results of treatment and predicting prognosis [8–10]. Thus, with the advancements in imaging technologies and the field of radiology and pathology, AI can contribute a lot in pediatric cancer staging and management.

5.2 AI in Pediatric Oncology: Need and Utility

Pediatric oncology represents a dynamic research domain, with giant progress being made in the field of molecular genetics and subtyping as well

I. Kumar et al. (eds.), *Practical Approach to Imaging in Pediatric Oncology*,
https://doi.org/10.1007/978-981-96-8158-7_5

as development of anti-cancer drugs. When compared to the adults, cancer therapeutics carry more importance in children due to different immune levels in the pediatric population, and children are also more susceptible to the adverse effects of cytotoxic drugs [11].

Machine learning-based models help in establishing algorithms for appropriate diagnosis by feeding large data sets as inputs that help in pattern recognition and training [12].

With integrated clinical data, these softwares can serve as comprehensive analytical tools that aid in the detection and characterization of tumors. By feeding features specific to each tumor and its various subtypes, better characterization and early diagnosis can be made [13–15]. After an accurate diagnosis is made, these algorithms contribute to plan personalized treatment regimens for children by analyzing their clinical and genetic data and comparing it with the large input data fed previously. On the same lines, drug sensitivities and toxicities to various chemo and radiotherapeutic regimes can be predicted accurately beforehand. In healthy children, these analytical tools offer appropriate screening tools and imaging tests to detect early-stage tumors in susceptible populations [10].

Most of the computational strategies to diagnose and predict tumors have been based and applied on adult populations. Since the genetic basis, molecular mechanisms, presentations, and treatment regimens differ considerably between adult and pediatric cancers, such AI-based models with respect to pediatric cancers are still in research or in the early phases of development. A relatively lesser number of cases or input data also contributes to slow progress and understanding of these computer-based models [10].

The most important practical aim of AI in pediatric oncology is to ensure early diagnosis, offer better treatment plans to allow reduced mortality, and ensure a longer cancer-free survival [10]. Also, machine learning tools may help in identifying high-risk patient groups and thus suggesting appropriate screening tests for these patients.

5.3 AI in Pediatric Oncology: General Applications

The various applications of AI in pediatric oncology are summarized below:

1. ***Selection of Appropriate Test***

One of the essential components in this is to identify blood biomarkers for specific cancers. Extensive research on the same has already been accomplished in the adult population with respect to colon, lung, hepatocellular, and breast cancers [16–20]. Patients with positive blood biomarkers can then be assigned proper screening and imaging tests to narrow down a differential diagnosis of the possible cancers. For example, increased urinary Vanillylmandelic acid (VMA) levels have been linked to neural crest tumors and thus patients with elevated levels of the same should be referred for an abdominal sonography. Similarly, a child with a mediastinal mass should undergo serum lactate dehydrogenase (LDH) level testing for prognostication in lymphoma cases and this must be incorporated into the imaging report.

In addition, ML-based algorithms can help in establishing imaging protocols that are best suited for screening patients with familial cancer syndromes to detect early-stage tumors [21, 22]. This is because there is still no universal consensus amongst radiologists concerning the best suited imaging techniques and protocols to be used as surveillance screening tools [21, 22].

2. ***Acquisition and Reconstruction of Image***

Radiation exposure remains a persistent concern in pediatric imaging. Deep CNN-based models can be exquisitely used to differentiate high-dose and low-dose images. The second step involves creation of standard dose images from low dose images. Researchers have used CNN-based models to denoise low-dose CT scans for appropriate image equality. Also, multiple successful studies have generated standard dose PET images from low dose scans [10]. Newer ML-based algorithms are being increasingly used to accelerate acquisition times of MRI scans and also reduce dose of gadolinium-based contrast agents [23, 24].

3. ***Detection and Characterization of Malignancy***

A number of CN-based models to detect various non-malignant pathologies are now in use. This includes the role of AI in detecting pneumonia in children and using hand radiographs to detect bone age of children [10]. Once these algorithms differentiate abnormal from normal scans, tumor lesions need to be identified. After identification, ML-based algorithms help in segmentation and quantification of these tumors (Fig. 5.1). Various studies have shown the utility of AI in the detection of liver tumors, breast tumors, and malignant pulmonary nodules on chest CT [25–27].

Radiomics refers to this specific application of AI in extracting quantitative features exclusive to each tumor thus aiding in early and accurate diagnosis.

In addition, tumor characterization has been done with much accuracy by using these ML-based algorithms. Examples include classification of glioblastoma multiforme (GBM) and rhabdomyosarcoma into various subtypes [10].

ML-based techniques have also been used to attribute or link various genetic mutations to various tumor subtypes. Radiomics analysis has been used to classify various pediatric brain tumors as discussed ahead [28–30].

4. ***Selection of Therapy and Its Monitoring***

Deep CNN-based models can help the clinicians in predicting the impact of genomic variations in determining the sensitivity of tumor cells to chemotherapy [31]. 18-Fluorodeoxyglucose Positron Emission Tomography (18-FDG-PET) is one of the most commonly used studies to assess the tumor response to chemo or radiotherapy. Since the tumor cells show a significant decrease in the metabolism prior to a visible

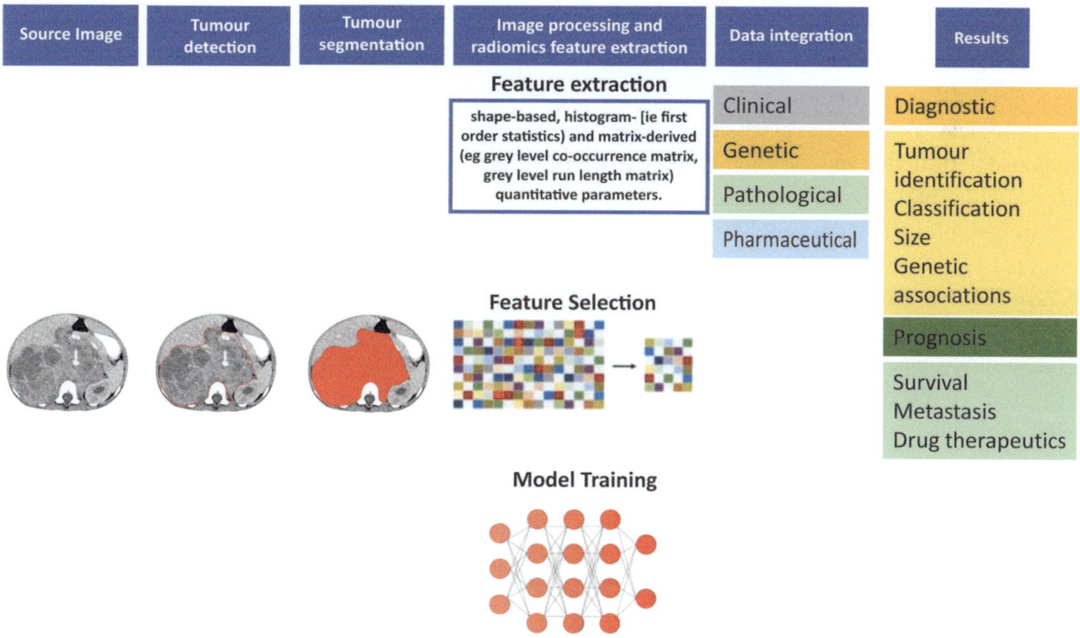

Fig. 5.1 A schematic diagram denoting the basic steps/components and the workflow involved in generating results from patient's data using an AI-based algorithm. (For reference, contrast-enhanced CT image of a 2-year-old child with neuroblastoma is used)

Table 5.1 Important applications of AI in pediatric oncology

1.	Selection of appropriate test	Use of blood biomarkers to help assign imaging tests
		Assess and score the genetic predisposition and clinical symptoms
2.	Image reconstruction and quality control	Reduction in scan times
		Reduction in radiation dose
		Reduction in contrast dosage
		Reduction in image noise and artifacts
3.	Tumour detection	Differentiate normal and abnormal scans
		Differentiate benign from malignant lesions
		Provide tumor measurements and staging
4.	Tumour classification and characterization	Use of radiogenomics
		Classify various tumors based on blood biomarkers
		Predict survival and tumor prognosis
5.	Selection of treatment	Select appropriate treatment regimen
		Predict tumor drug sensitivities and drug toxicities
6.	Assessment of response to therapy	Provide automated tumor measurements
		Assess response based on tumor regression
		Provide tumor therapy response scores
7.	Communication of test results	Provide standardized results and reports
		Inform patient and clinicians about test results

decrease in size, 18-FDG PET is often used as a marker to assess tumor response. CNN-based models can easily identify responders from non-responders [32, 33]. ML-based algorithms can also help in determining the response of tumors to various drugs [34]. In future, these shall potentially contribute toward expanding our understanding of various molecular, genetic, and physiological factors in assessing the tumor response to drug therapy. Further, these may help in predicting the survival in children with cancer and thus improve outcomes.

5. ***Facilitation and Communication of Results***

Radiology workflow can be better organized by collaborating clinical as well as radiological data (including abnormal case detection, quantitative tumor analysis, and prioritizing cases with exceptional findings) finally providing appropriate staging of the tumor [10]. AI algorithms, in addition, can help in better communicating the test results to the patients and healthcare providers with appropriate reminders and subsequent follow-up visits and tests.

These general applications are summarized in Table 5.1.

5.4 AI in Pediatric Oncology: Specific Applications

The specific tumor-wise applications of AI are discussed below.

1. ***General Role in Neuro-oncology***

Initial radiomics-related research was carried out extensively in lung cancer. Similar radiomics-based models have been used features extracted from MRI to create specific signature models, especially for various subtypes of GBM [29, 35].

Multiple studies have used radiomics-based features in pre-operatively diagnosing the genotype of tumor, which has immense therapeutic and prognostic implications [29, 35]. Not only diagnosis, radiomics models have also been able to accurately differentiate primary GBM from other metastatic brain tumors [36]. In addition, features extracted from ML algorithms have also proven to be helpful in predicting tumor response to therapy, determining molecular profiles of tumors, and differentiating pseudo-progression from true tumor progression [37]. Similar research is being carried out in the field of pediatric brain tumors as discussed below.

2. ***Posterior Fossa Tumors***

A qualitative review of MRI images is routinely done by radiologists in order to classify various pediatric posterior fossa tumors in children. Although many advanced techniques like spectroscopy and MR perfusion (in addition to routine sequences) help in better characterization of these tumors, accurate classification is not possible due to considerable overlap of features. Recently, radiomics-based analysis using T2WI, post-contrast T1W1, and Apparent Diffusion Coefficient (ADC) values incorporating various clinical variables has been used to detect medulloblastoma, ependymoma, and pilocytic astrocytoma with high accuracy [38–40]. Recent studies have further attempted to classify medulloblastoma into various molecular subtypes, based on various ML-based models [41].

3. ***Osteosarcoma***

Pediatric osteosarcoma (OS) contributes to a large burden of cancer disease in children. Early and prompt diagnosis can reduce mortality and morbidity associated with the disease [42]. As previously discussed, machine learning and CNN-based models aid in every step of diagnosis and treatment. The primary task in osteosarcoma imaging is twofold. The first being detection of the lesion, on various modalities including MRI, PET-CT, and PET-MRI. In addition, quantification of the tumor by delineating its borders has important diagnostic and therapeutic implications [43]. This quantitative information can be provided by the use of automated segmentation models today, the most popular being U-Net, which is an efficient CNN-based model that uses steps of encoding and subsequent decoding to reconstruct images that correspond with the input [43–49].

4. **Neuroblastoma**

Neuroblastoma is the most common extracranial solid tumor in the pediatric population and accounts for about 15% of cancer-related mortality in this population [50, 51]. The tumor is known to have extensive clinical heterogeneity with diverse clinical manifestations. Given the complexity of oncogenesis of the tumor and specific genotypes associated with adverse disease (MYCN, ALK), a large amount of data is being acquired from animal-based models as well as machine learning to further explore the genetic etiology of this tumor in order to create newer targets for drug therapy [52–54].

5.5 Future Perspectives

Radiomics As the term states, radiomics refers to the use of AI in extracting quantitative features from radiology data and scans as has been discussed previously. Specifically, this refers to the development of specific imaging biomarkers that can be considered global signature models of various tumors so that ML-based models can easily detect, classify, and characterize various tumors with the help of available imaging data. This is done by complex mathematical and computational analysis of hundreds of parameters derived from imaging data including shape and voxel intensity [14, 15, 55].

Flowchart 5.1 *denotes the various steps involved in a typical radiomics-based model.*

Radio Genomics This broad term in addition to radiomics also incorporates various genetic and molecular features. It explores the relationships between the quantitative features derived from radiological data at the tissue level and other biological characteristics at genomic or proteomic level. These features in turn help in correlating a relationship between the clinical diagnosis, therapeutic options, and patient prognosis [56].

Texture Analysis This refers to the analysis of the tumor at tissue level with the help of available features that can be analyzed extensively by ML-based methods. By extrapolating information from hundreds of quantitative features, tumoral behaviors can be accurately predicted [57–60].

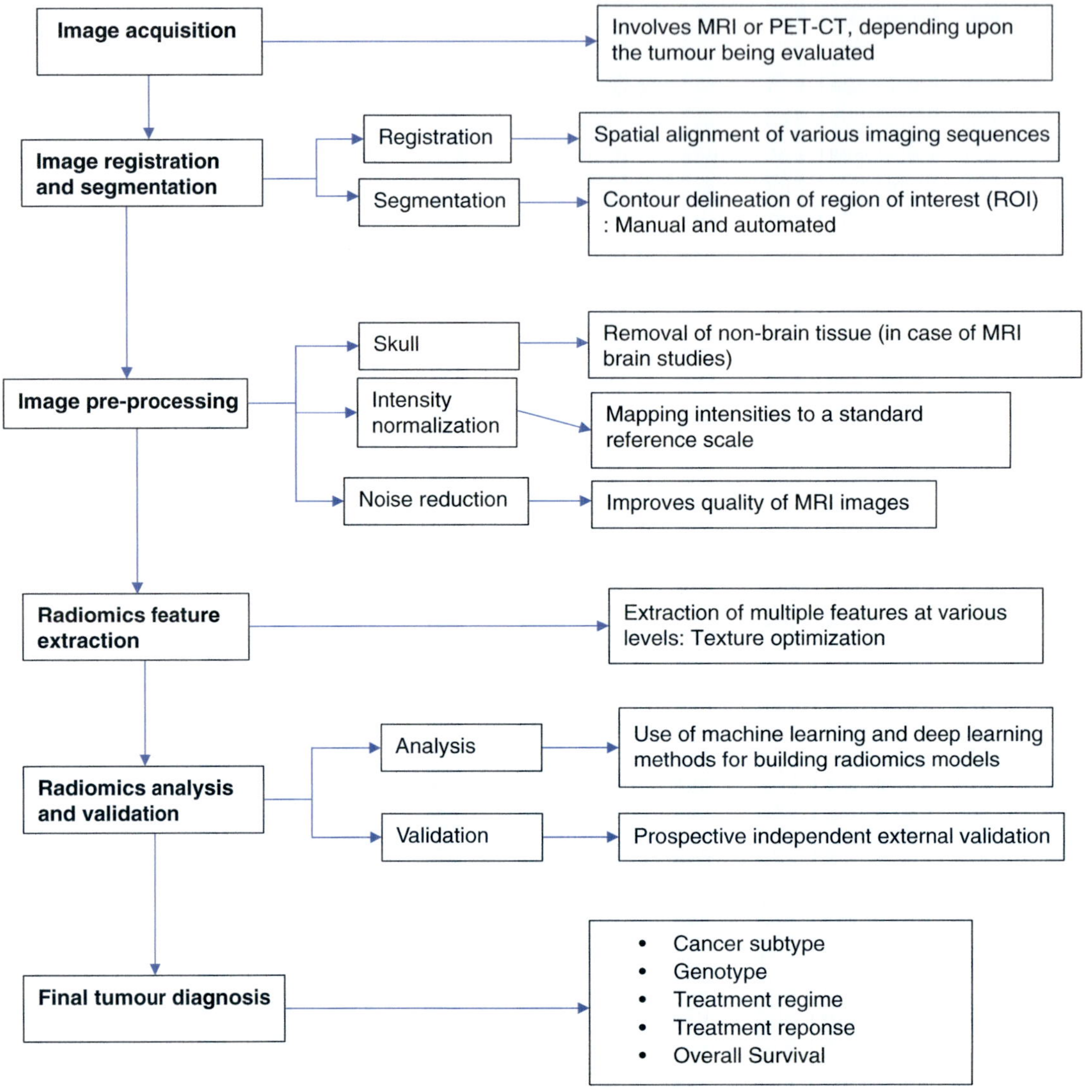

Flowchart 5.1 Flowchart denoting the basic steps in the use of radiomics

Currently, a lot of work is in progress in the field of pediatric oncology with the latest research model being the PRIMAGE project which is a European multi-center research initiative that utilizes AI in medical imaging to facilitate the management of two specific pediatric cancers; namely neuroblastoma and diffuse intrinsic pontine glioma [58]. Comprehensive analysis of imaging features is done with clinical and molecular data on an open-cloud platform, to ensure reliable predictions and thus enhance the decision-making power and support system of the involved clinicians [58].

5.6 Limitations of AI

Although ML-based algorithms have revolutionized the field of adult oncology, applications in pediatric oncology imaging are still limited. This is attributed to limited data sets due to the lesser availability of cases of pediatric cancers. Though adult data has been often extrapolated to train ML-based softwares by the transfer learning approach, most CNNs are not generalizable from adults to children. Therefore, further research and insight into AI algorithms for pediatric oncology are required to develop better computational analysis.

The second major drawback is a roadblock for radiomics in general. The reproducibility and repeatability of radiomics is still questionable because these factors depend upon technical factors like size and quality of image, imaging sequence used, image artifacts as well as software used for image reconstruction. One of the major issues in this aspect can be image segmentation, which when using the manual technique leads to many interobserver variations. This can still be overcome by using DL-based technique of automated segmentation. Thus, large data sets are required to validate the reliability of radiomics-based models. Another potential challenge is the difficulty in interpreting the results of radiomics [55].

The applications and utility of AI in pediatric oncology are ever growing. However, compared to adults, the data on pediatric cancers to generate data sets as input models for computational analysis and ML models is scarce in comparison to adults. This is because the number of patients with pediatric cancers is proportionately less and has different spectrum [54]. To ensure better training of CNN-based computational analysis, data from multiple institutions can be pooled together and these deep CNNs can be cross-linked to help in better analysis and to ensure accurate diagnosis [10].

5.7 Conclusion

A lot of progress has been made in the field of AI, related to pediatric oncology, with many applications available today, in clinical workflow and management protocols. Radiomics-based models can help in detecting the tumor early, and also help to monitor the entire treatment period and prognosis with a customized case-based approach. Although AI has been widely used in diagnosing many pediatric tumors like medulloblastoma and neuroblastoma, further research and data in this field are essential for advanced accuracy, predictability, and extrapolation to other pediatric tumors while keeping in mind the limitations.

References

1. Ardahan Sevgili S, Şenol S. Prediction of chemotherapy-related complications in pediatric oncology patients: artificial intelligence and machine learning implementations. Pediatr Res. 2023;93(2):390–5. https://doi.org/10.1038/s41390-022-02356-6.
2. Jordan MI, Mitchell TM. Machine learning: trends, perspectives, and prospects. Science. 2015;349:255–60. https://doi.org/10.1126/SCIENCE.AAA8415.
3. Ghahramani Z. Probabilistic machine learning and artificial intelligence. Nature. 2015;521:452–9. https://doi.org/10.1038/nature14541.
4. Deo RC. Machine learning in medicine. Circulation. 2015;132:1920–30. https://doi.org/10.1161/CIRCULATIONAHA.115.001593.
5. Bhatia H, Bhatia A, Ahuja C, Singh A, Sodhi KS. Artificial intelligence: a primer for the radiologists. Indographics. 2022;1:215–21.
6. Bertsimas D, Wiberg H. Machine learning in oncology: methods, applications, and challenges. JCO Clin Cancer Inform. 2020;4:885–94. https://doi.org/10.1200/CCI.20.00072.
7. D'Amore B, Smolinski-Zhao S, Daye D, Uppot RN. Role of machine learning and artificial intelligence in interventional oncology. Curr Oncol Rep. 2021;23(6):70. Published 2021 Apr 20. https://doi.org/10.1007/s11912-021-01054-6.
8. Elemento O, Leslie C, Lundin J, Tourassi G. Artificial intelligence in cancer research, diagnosis and therapy. Nat Rev Cancer. 2021;21(12):747–52. https://doi.org/10.1038/s41568-021-00399-1.
9. Huynh E, Hosny A, Guthier C, et al. Artificial intelligence in radiation oncology. Nat Rev Clin Oncol. 2020;17(12):771–81. https://doi.org/10.1038/s41571-020-0417-8.
10. Daldrup-Link H. Artificial intelligence applications for pediatric oncology imaging. Pediatr Radiol. 2019;49(11):1384–90. https://doi.org/10.1007/s00247-019-04360-1.
11. Marshall GM, Carter DR, Cheung BB, et al. The prenatal origins of cancer. Nat Rev Cancer. 2014;14(4):277–89. https://doi.org/10.1038/nrc3679.
12. Chartrand G, Cheng PM, Vorontsov E, et al. Deep learning: a primer for radiologists. Radiographics. 2017;37(7):2113–31. https://doi.org/10.1148/rg.2017170077.

13. Martí Bonmatí L, Alberich-Bayarri A, García-Martí G, et al. Biomarcadores de imagen, imagen cuantitativa y bioingeniería [Imaging biomarkers, quantitative imaging, and bioengineering]. Radiologia. 2012;54(3):269–78. https://doi.org/10.1016/j.rx.2010.12.013.
14. European Society of Radiology (ESR). White paper on imaging biomarkers. Insights. Imaging. 2010;1(2):42–5. https://doi.org/10.1007/s13244-010-0025-8.
15. European Society of Radiology (ESR). What the radiologist should know about artificial intelligence – an ESR white paper. Insights. Imaging. 2019;10(1):44.
16. Fortunato O, Boeri M, Verri C, et al. Assessment of circulating microRNAs in plasma of lung cancer patients. Molecules. 2014;19(3):3038–54. Published 2014 Mar 10. https://doi.org/10.3390/molecules19033038.
17. Zhang B, Liang XL, Gao HY, Ye LS, Wang YG. Models of logistic regression analysis, support vector machine, and back-propagation neural network based on serum tumor markers in colorectal cancer diagnosis. Genet Mol Res. 2016;15(2) https://doi.org/10.4238/gmr.15028643.
18. Hornbrook MC, Goshen R, Choman E, et al. Early colorectal cancer detected by machine learning model using gender, age, and complete blood count data [published correction appears in Dig Dis Sci. 2017 Nov 27;]. Dig Dis Sci 2017;62(10):2719–27. https://doi.org/10.1007/s10620-017-4722-8.
19. Lü L, Sun J, Shi P, et al. Identification of circular RNAs as a promising new class of diagnostic biomarkers for human breast cancer. Oncotarget. 2017;8(27):44096–107. https://doi.org/10.18632/oncotarget.17307.
20. Patterson AD, Maurhofer O, Beyoglu D, et al. Aberrant lipid metabolism in hepatocellular carcinoma revealed by plasma metabolomics and lipid profiling. Cancer Res. 2011;71(21):6590–600. https://doi.org/10.1158/0008-5472.CAN-11-0885.
21. Kumar P, Gill RM, Phelps A, Tulpule A, Matthay K, Nicolaides T. Surveillance screening in li-fraumeni syndrome: raising awareness of false positives. Cureus. 2018;10(4):e2527. Published 2018 Apr 24. https://doi.org/10.7759/cureus.2527.
22. Schooler GR, Davis JT, Daldrup-Link HE, Frush DP. Current utilization and procedural practices in pediatric whole-body MRI. Pediatr Radiol. 2018;48(8):1101–7. https://doi.org/10.1007/s00247-018-4145-5.
23. Zhu B, Liu JZ, Cauley SF, Rosen BR, Rosen MS. Image reconstruction by domain-transform manifold learning. Nature. 2018;555(7697):487–92. https://doi.org/10.1038/nature25988.
24. Gong E, Pauly JM, Wintermark M, Zaharchuk G. Deep learning enables reduced gadolinium dose for contrast-enhanced brain MRI. J Magn Reson Imaging. 2018;48(2):330–40. https://doi.org/10.1002/jmri.25970.
25. Bi L, Kim J, Kumar A, Wen L, Feng D, Fulham M. Automatic detection and classification of regions of FDG uptake in whole-body PET-CT lymphoma studies. Comput Med Imaging Graph. 2017;60:3–10. https://doi.org/10.1016/j.compmedimag.2016.11.008.
26. Helm EJ, Silva CT, Roberts HC, et al. Computer-aided detection for the identification of pulmonary nodules in pediatric oncology patients: initial experience. Pediatr Radiol. 2009;39(7):685–93. https://doi.org/10.1007/s00247-009-1259-9.
27. Linguraru MG, Richbourg WJ, Liu J, et al. Tumor burden analysis on computed tomography by automated liver and tumor segmentation. IEEE Trans Med Imaging. 2012;31(10):1965–76. https://doi.org/10.1109/TMI.2012.2211887.
28. Fetit AE, Novak J, Rodriguez D, et al. Radiomics in paediatric neuro-oncology: a multicentre study on MRI texture analysis. NMR Biomed. 2018;31(1) https://doi.org/10.1002/nbm.3781.
29. Kickingereder P, Bonekamp D, Nowosielski M, et al. Radiogenomics of glioblastoma: machine learning-based classification of molecular characteristics by using multiparametric and multiregional MR imaging features. Radiology. 2016;281(3):907–18. https://doi.org/10.1148/radiol.2016161382.
30. Zarinabad N, Wilson M, Gill SK, Manias KA, Davies NP, Peet AC. Multiclass imbalance learning: improving classification of pediatric brain tumors from magnetic resonance spectroscopy. Magn Reson Med. 2017;77(6):2114–24. https://doi.org/10.1002/mrm.26318.
31. Kang J, Rancati T, Lee S, et al. Machine learning and radiogenomics: lessons learned and future directions. Front Oncol. 2018;8:228. Published 2018 Jun 21. https://doi.org/10.3389/fonc.2018.00228.
32. Kleis M, Daldrup-Link H, Matthay K, et al. Diagnostic value of PET/CT for the staging and restaging of pediatric tumors. Eur J Nucl Med Mol Imaging. 2009;36(1):23–36. https://doi.org/10.1007/s00259-008-0911-1.
33. McCarville MB. New frontiers in pediatric oncologic imaging. Cancer Imaging. 2008;8(1):87–92. Published 2008 Mar 25. https://doi.org/10.1102/1470-7330.2008.0012.
34. Cairns J, Ung CY, da Rocha EL, et al. A network-based phenotype mapping approach to identify genes that modulate drug response phenotypes. Sci Rep. 2016;6:37003. Published 2016 Nov 14. https://doi.org/10.1038/srep37003.
35. Li J, Liu S, Qin Y, et al. High-order radiomics features based on T2 FLAIR MRI predict multiple glioma immunohistochemical eatures: a more precise and personalized gliomas management. PLoS One. 2020;15:e0227703.
36. Chen C, Ou X, Wang J, et al. Radiomics-based machine learning in differentiation between glioblastoma and metastatic brain tumors. Front Oncol. 2019;9:806.

37. Ak M, Toll SA, Hein KZ, Colen RR, Khatua S. Evolving role and translation of radiomics and radiogenomics in adult and pediatric neuro-oncology. AJNR Am J Neuroradiol. 2022;43(6):792–801. https://doi.org/10.3174/ajnr.A7297.
38. Zwanenburg A, Vallieres M, Abdalah MA, et al. The image bio- marker standardization initiative: standardized quantitative radiomics for high-throughput image-based phenotyping. Radiology. 2020;295:328–38.
39. Vallieres M, Kay-Rivest E, Perrin LJ, et al. Radiomics strategies for risk assessment of tumour failure in head-and-neck cancer. Sci Rep. 2017;7:10117.
40. Zhou H, Hu R, Tang O, et al. Automatic machine learning to differentiate pediatric posterior fossa tumors on routine MR imaging. AJNR Am J Neuroradiol. 2020;41(7):1279–85. https://doi.org/10.3174/ajnr.A6621.
41. Iv M, Zhou M, Shpanskaya K, et al. MR imaging-based radiomic signatures of distinct molecular subgroups of medulloblastoma. AJNR Am J Neuroradiol. 2019;40:154–61.
42. Silva RS, Guilhem DB, Batista KT, Tabet LP. Quality of life of patients with sarcoma after conservative surgery or amputation of limbs. Acta Ortopedica Brasileira. 2019;27(5):276–80.
43. Rich JM, Bhardwaj LN, Shah A, et al. Deep learning image segmentation approaches for malignant bone lesions: a systematic review and meta-analysis. Front Radiol. 2023;3:1241651. https://doi.org/10.3389/fradi.2023.1241651.
44. Minaee S, Boykov Y, Porikli F, Plaza A, Kehtarnavaz N, Terzopoulos D. Image segmentation using deep learning: a survey. IEEE Trans Pattern Anal Mach Intell. 2022;44(7):3523–42. https://doi.org/10.1109/TPAMI.2021.3059968.
45. Luo D, Zeng W, Chen J, Tang W. Deep learning for automatic image segmentation in stomatology and its clinical application. Front Med Technol. 2021;3:767836. Published 2021 Dec 13. https://doi.org/10.3389/fmedt.2021.767836.
46. Keiron O, Nash R. An introduction to convolutional neural networks. ArXiv 2015; abs/1511.08458. https://doi.org/10.48550/arXiv.1511.08458
47. Isensee F, Jaeger PF, Kohl SAA, Petersen J, Maier-Hein KH. nnU-Net: a self-configuring method for deep learning-based biomedical image segmentation. Nat Methods. 2021;18(2):203–11. https://doi.org/10.1038/s41592-020-01008-z.
48. Kirillov A, Mintun E, Ravi N, et al. Segment anything. arXiv. 2023. arXiv:2304.02643. https://doi.org/10.48550/arXiv.2304.02643.
49. Wu J, Zhou L, Gou F, Tan Y. A residual fusion network for osteosarcoma MRI image segmentation in developing countries. Comput Intell Neurosci. 2022;2022:7285600. Published 2022 Aug 3. https://doi.org/10.1155/2022/7285600.
50. Salazar BM, Balczewski EA, Ung CY, Zhu S. Neuroblastoma, a paradigm for big data science in pediatric oncology. Int J Mol Sci. 2016;18(1):37. Published 2016 Dec 27. https://doi.org/10.3390/ijms18010037.
51. Maris JM, Hogarty MD, Bagatell R, Cohn SL. Neuroblastoma. Lancet. 2007;369:2106–210.
52. Cheung NK, Dyer MA. Neuroblastoma: developmental biology, cancer genomics and immunotherapy. Nat Rev Cancer. 2013;13:397–411.
53. De Preter K, Vandesompele J, Heimann P, et al. Human fetal neuroblast and neuroblastoma transcriptome analysis confirms neuroblast origin and highlights neuroblastoma candidate genes. Genome Biol. 2006;7:R84.
54. Adamson PC, Houghton PJ, Perilongo G, Pritchard-Jones K. Drug discovery in paediatric oncology: roadblocks to progress. Nat Rev Clin Oncol. 2014;11:732–9.
55. Barredo Arrieta A, Díaz-Rodríguez N, Del Ser J, et al. Explainable Artificial Intelligence (XAI): concepts, taxonomies, opportunities and challenges toward responsible AI. Inf Fusion. 2020;58:82–115.
56. Li R. Radiomics and radiogenomics. In: El Naqa I, Murphy MJ, editors. Machine and deep learning in oncology, medical physics and radiology. Cham: Springer; 2022. https://doi.org/10.1007/978-3-030-83047-2_16.
57. Voss SD. Pediatric oncology and the future of oncological imaging. Pediatr Radiol. 2011;41(Suppl 1):S172–85. https://doi.org/10.1007/s00247-011-2008-4.
58. Martí-Bonmatí L, Alberich-Bayarri Á, Ladenstein R, et al. PRIMAGE project: predictive in silico multi-scale analytics to support childhood cancer personalised evaluation empowered by imaging biomarkers. Eur Radiol Exp. 2020;4(1):22. Published 2020 Apr 3. https://doi.org/10.1186/s41747-020-00150-9.
59. Peschmann AL, Beer M, Ammann B, et al. Quantitative DWI predicts event-free survival in children with neuroblastic tumours: preliminary findings from a retrospective cohort study. Eur Radiol Exp. 2019;3(1):6.
60. van Timmeren JE, Cester D, Tanadini-Lang S, Alkadhi H, Baessler B. Radiomics in medical imaging-"how-to" guide and critical reflection. Insights Imaging. 2020;11(1):91. https://doi.org/10.1186/s13244-020-00887-2.

6 Nuclear Medicine in Paediatric Oncology

Varun Shukla and Abhishek Uppal

6.1 Introduction

Nuclear medicine is a modality that utilizes radioisotopes for imaging. It extrapolates the principle that nuclei achieve stability through radioactive decay, emitting gamma rays, positrons, beta particles, and alpha particles.

In contrast to radiology, which predominantly delineates anatomical structures, nuclear medicine is oriented towards the exploration of physiological, pathophysiological, and functional dimensions.

Nuclear medicine imaging evolved from an analogue rectilinear whole-body scanner to a digital gamma camera, where gamma-emitting isotopes were used. An inherent limitation of this planar imaging was spatial resolution; however, with improvements in machines capable of obtaining tomography (known as SPECT or Single Photon Emission Computed Tomography), providing three-dimensional information with or without fusion X-ray-based conventional computed tomography (CT) the sensitivity of the modality increased by many folds.

V. Shukla (✉)
Department of Nuclear Medicine, Homi Bhabha Cancer Hospital and Research Centre, Tata Memorial Centre, New Chandigarh, India

A. Uppal
Department of Nuclear Medicine, Tata Memorial Hospital, Tata Memorial Centre, Mumbai, India

With the advent of hybrid PET/CT (Positron Emission Tomography/Computed Tomography) scanners, imaging provided higher sensitivity and resolution, and anatomical details were provided simultaneously. Studies identified the significant impact PET/CT made in the management of various malignancies and hence it has been incorporated into the workup of various malignancies.

Nuclear medicine diagnostic techniques involve the injection of a specific radiotracer, which is a compound made up of radioisotope conjugated with peptides, antibodies, or analogous entities. The movement of the radiotracer facilitates the visualization of biological processes through the detection of emitted gamma rays or positrons. A semi-quantitative data of standardized uptake value (SUV), a ratio of uptake in a lesion relative to the administered activity normalized for patient body weight, is a useful tool in oncology, especially for response assessment.

Therapeutic nuclear medicine utilizes radioisotopes that have the potential of cell kill utilizing particulate radiation, e.g. beta or alpha emissions, which are labelled to carriers like peptides, antibodies, or analogues specific for tumours.

Thus, radionuclide therapy is also a form of targeted therapy, the concept of a paired radioisotope, one diagnostic and other therapeutic using the same carrier targeting a specific region of the

I. Kumar et al. (eds.), *Practical Approach to Imaging in Pediatric Oncology*,
https://doi.org/10.1007/978-981-96-8158-7_6

tumour is termed as theranostics, e.g. Gallium 68 (Ga68) and Lutetium177 (Lu177) pair used in neuroendocrine tumours.

In this chapter, we shall discuss radionuclide procedures, both diagnostic and therapeutic available for the management of common paediatric malignancies.

Before we discuss the indications of NM studies in different common cancers, we shall look into the characteristics of the common radiotracers used in paediatric malignancies.

- Iodine labelled metaiodobenzylguanidine (MIBG): A norepinephrine (NE) analogue is used as a carrier to bind with the NE receptors which are expressed in abundance in neuroblastoma tumours. MIBG is commonly labelled with I 123, in the Western world. This, being cyclotron produced is an expensive radioisotope, and not easily available in most developing countries. The alternate isotope used is the 131 iodine a beta emitter, a therapeutic radiotracer but a small dose is used for diagnostic purposes. Physiological uptake of MIBG is seen in the salivary glands, heart, base of lungs, liver, kidneys, urinary bladder, and bowel (Fig. 6.1).
- Fluorodeoxyglucose (FDG): This tracer extrapolates the increased glucose utilization of cancer cells due to the Warburg effect, labelled glucose or its analogue would identify sites of increased glucose utilization, a surrogate marker for cell proliferation.
- Physiological FDG uptake is seen in areas of high glucose metabolism or areas where FDG is excreted in, such as the brain, salivary glands, Waldeyer's lymphatic ring, heart, bowel, kidneys, ureters, and urinary bladder (Fig. 6.2). FDG is also seen in infective tissue due to the high uptake by macrophage and hence can be a reason for false-positive findings.
- Methylene Di Phosphonate (MDP): Technetium 99 m labelled Methylene Di Phosphonate (Tc99m MDP) is a radiotracer

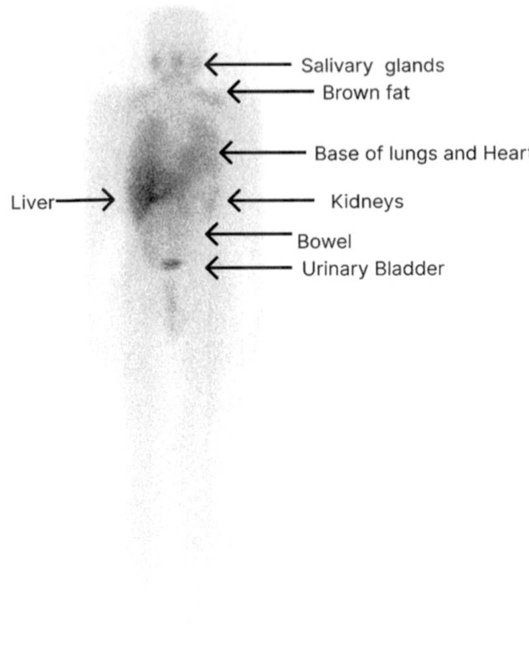

Fig. 6.1 Physiological radiotracer distribution of I-131 Metaiodobenzylguanidine

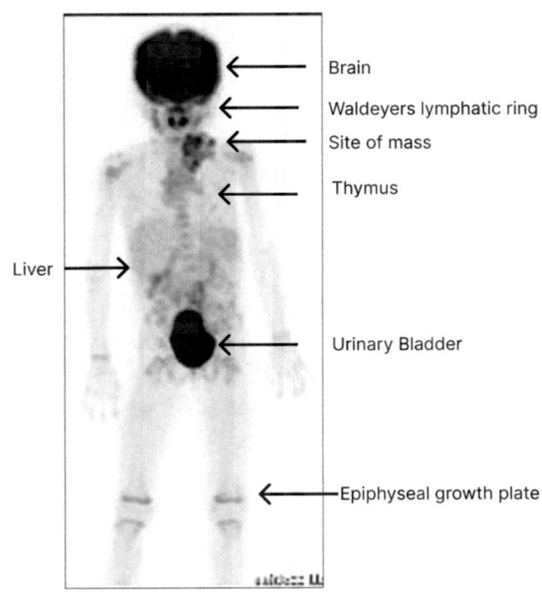

Fig. 6.2 Physiologic distribution of FDG, note the supraclavicular mass on the left side in this child with neuroblastoma

targeting increased osteoblastic activity. It is very sensitive in early detection of osteoblastic bone lesions such as metastases from osteogenic sarcomas.
- Fluro Ethyl L-Tyrosine (FET): This is a radiopharmaceutical targeting amino acid metabolism; glial tissue shows increased amino-acid utilization and hence FET is a good marker of glial tissue proliferation.

6.2 Lymphoma

Hodgkin's lymphomas are a common paediatric malignancy. The commonest type of non-Hodgkins's lymphoma in the paediatric population are Burkitt's lymphoma, lymphoblastic lymphoma, and anaplastic large cell lymphoma. Clusters of cells in different stages of maturation mean that the very high glucose metabolism in them can be targeted [1, 2].

6.2.1 Guidelines and Indications

The Lugano conference established the role of FDG PET/CT for lymphoma imaging. It recommends FDG PET/CT at baseline, interim, and end of treatment for Hodgkin's and certain FDG avid aggressive NHL. The NCCN guidelines too support these indications [3].

FDG PET/CT for staging is useful as it locates all the nodal stations. The highest impact of FDG is in identifying extra-nodal sites of involvement including liver, spleen, and marrow lesions with reasonable sensitivity and specificity. In Hodgkin's lymphomas, the absence of marrow disease on PET/CT obviates the need for a marrow biopsy. Disease involvement on CT images is based on the size criteria, often nodes may not be enlarged but may show FDG uptake suggestive of involvement, leading to altered staging [3, 4].

6.2.2 Response Assessment

FDG PET CT plays a crucial role in response assessment (Fig. 6.3). The Deauville scoring has been advocated for interim and end-of-treatment assessment. Deauville's score is a five-point visual score. The Deauville's score is given based on relative uptake in the lesion compared to the mediastinal blood pool and liver, a score of 1 is

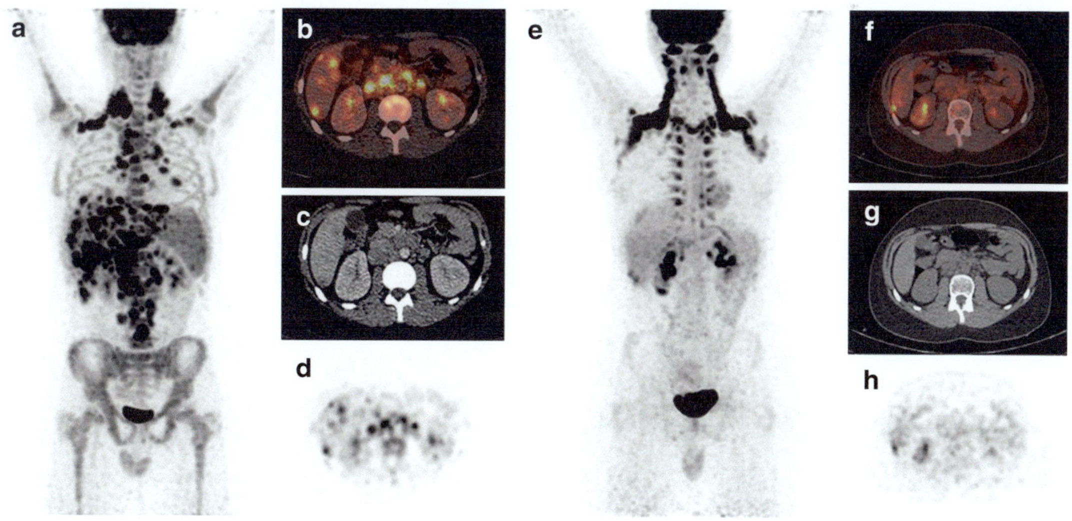

Fig. 6.3 Pre and post chemotherapy comparison 18F FDG PET/CT in a 12-year-old boy with non-Hodgkin's lymphoma, (**a**), (**e**) MIP, (**b**), (**f**) Fused PET/CT, (**c**), (**g**) CT and (**d**), (**h**) PET images; note the supra and infra-diaphragmatic adenopathy, liver and marrow involvement, post therapy images (**f**), (**g**) show morphologically visible nodes with complete metabolic response

uptake less than mediastinal blood pool, 2 is equal to the mediastinal blood pool, 3 is more than blood pool and equal to or less than liver, 4 and 5 are mildly and markedly more than the liver (Table 6.1) [3].

The scores have been incorporated into the Lugano classification of response assessment—a score of 1–3 is considered as a complete metabolic response while 4 & 5 suggest partial response (PR) if uptake is reduced from baseline, stable disease (SD) if tracer shows no change in intensity or progressive disease (PD) if uptake greater than baseline or one or more new FDG avid lesions (Table 6.2).

In this era of treatment of paediatric cancers where the emphasis is on reducing the late effects of treatment in children, studies have proved PET scans as a useful tool to limit the treatment, reduce the number of chemotherapy cycles, or avoid RT to tumour site if the interim scan shows complete metabolic response (CMR). Treatment de-escalation regimes are under trial to look at PET-adapted management protocols [5].

Since FDG targets metabolism, false-positive findings on PET/CT for lymphoma include foci of infection or inflammation or even post-chemotherapy marrow stimulation. False-negative findings may also be due to the low avidity of the disease in general. It may be helpful to look at the corresponding CT and be aware of patterns of FDG uptake to avoid these pitfalls. In diagnostic dilemmas where patient outcomes may be adversely affected, pathologic correlation is always helpful [5, 6].

Table 6.1 Deauville's five-point scale

Deauville's score	Assessment
1	No uptake on FDG PET/CT
2	Uptake ≤ mediastinum
3	Mediastinum uptake < tumour uptake < liver uptake
4	Uptake > liver (moderately high uptake)
5	New lesion and/or uptake ≫ liver (markedly high)

6.2.3 Recent Updates

PET/CT may be used for RT field planning and may yield better results as compared to CT-based planning. Targeted radiation therapy fields such as involved field radiation therapy or involved node radiation therapy use PET data for limiting radiation dose to non-target organs [7].

6.3 Langerhans Cell Histiocytosis

Langerhans cell histiocytosis (LCH) is a histiocytic disorder, in which Langerhans cells show clonal proliferation in various organ systems.

There are two types of LCH, first being single-system disease, one or multiple lesions of one system, or second being, multi-system disease. The treatment of each varies and it is crucial to differentiate the type. PET/CT is advantageous in evaluating newly diagnosed cases of LCH due to its ability to scan the entire body and detect disease involvement in non-skeletal regions, the risk organs namely neurological, endocrine, liver, spleen, or nodal involvement.

Table 6.2 Response assessment using Deauville's score after FDG PET/CT

Modality	Clinical application	Complete response	Partial response	Stable disease	Progressive disease
FDG PET/CT	FDG-avid lymphoma (including Hodgkin lymphoma and diffuse large B-cell lymphoma)	Score of 1, 2, 3 in nodal or extra nodal sites with or without a residual mass	Score of 4 or 5 with reduced uptake compared with baseline and residual mass of any size	Score of 4 or 5 with no obvious change in uptake in FDG PET/CT	Score of 4 or 5 in any lesion with increased intensity of uptake from baseline and/or new FDG avid lesion consistent with lymphoma

Often, FDG PET/CT helps identify the site of biopsy for histological confirmation of the disease.

Few studies have shown that FDG scans delineate more lesions than conventional imaging modalities. The reduction in FDG uptake due to treatment makes it a good method for assessing response. A study utilized FDG PET/CT as a tool for PET-adapted treatment alteration and has shown a good outcome in those receiving additional therapy due to positive PET/CT [8].

6.4 Neuroblastoma

Neuroblastoma is a common round blue cell tumour of the paediatric age group. It frequently arises from the autonomic ganglia. MIBG and FDG are used to image neuroblastomas. MIBG or meta-iodo benzyl Guanidine labelled with I 131 uses the active sodium transport mediated uptake-1 mechanism for localization onto tumour cells.

Certain precautions to be considered before the patient is injected with MIBG:

1. Ensure thyroid blockade before administering the radiopharmaceutical to the patient.
2. Many pharmaceuticals targeting the autonomic system might interfere with the uptake of MIBG and need to be stopped before administration of MIBG.

6.4.1 Guidelines and Indications

I 123 MIBG has a sensitivity and specificity of 85–96 and 95–99% respectively for the diagnosis of neuroblastoma. Both the SIOP and INRG recommend MIBG as a staging investigation [9–11]. At staging it helps not only in establishing the extent of disease but also in cases of diagnostic dilemmas to establish the nature of a mass. Physiological areas of uptake such as the liver, heart, bowel, bladder, etc. might lead to diagnostic pitfalls, SPECT/CT may be helpful in such cases.

In developing countries like India 123 I MIBG is not available and hence a small dose of 131 I MIBG is used for diagnostic purposes (Fig. 6.4). This could reduce the sensitivity and resolution of the images.

FDG PET/CT has the added advantage of improved spatial resolution (Fig. 6.5). Areas of metastatic involvement in the hepatic region and pericardiac region which can be missed on MIBG scans can be identified on these scans easily.

Both MIBG and FDG PET/CT complement each other, especially in MIBG-negative tumours. Studies have shown MIBG to be better in stage IV disease, whereas FDG may be better in stage I and II disease [12].

6.4.2 Post-treatment Imaging

Post-treatment response evaluation may be done with MIBG. Many prognostic scores based on MIBG scans are available. Curie's and SIOPEN scores are the commonly used scores [13, 14]. A reduction of the scores to 2 in post-therapy response assessment prognosticates a good outcome.

6.4.3 Therapeutic Role of Radioactive Iodine MIBG

Higher doses of MIBG have been used as therapy in refractory, metastatic, or recurrent neuroblastoma. This therapy provides adequate palliation.

Frontline use of MIBG in the conventional therapy regime has shown to be useful in high-risk neuroblastoma with better progression-free survival and overall survival. Some trials have shown no additional toxicity with the addition of higher doses of MIBG in conjunction with high-dose chemotherapy before stem cell harvest and transplant [16, 17].

6.4.4 Recent Updates

Few new tracers are available in the management of neuroblastoma. Somatostatin receptor imaging (SSTR) using Ga68 labelled DOTANOC is being frequently used for staging neuroblastoma, this targets somatostatin receptors on tumour cells. This

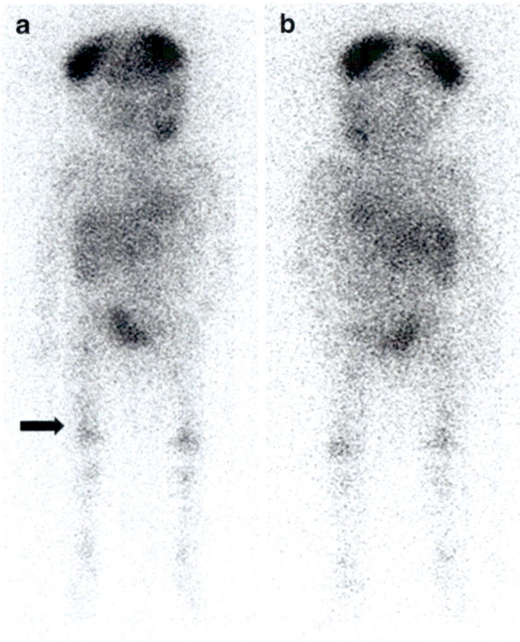

Fig. 6.4 (**a**) Anterior and (**b**) Posterior images of 131-I MIBG planar scan in a 2-year-old child with neuroblastoma, note the extensive marrow disease (black arrow)

has theranostic applications as there are encouraging reports on the use of beta emitter Lutetium177 labelled with TATE (somatostatin receptor analogue) to treat refractory neuroblastoma.

Another tracer with potential for use in neuroblastoma is a PET/CT scan done with labelled Dopa, which targets dopamine metabolism. The advantage of this tracer is its ability to accurately assess residual marrow disease in post-induction scans [18].

6.5 Bone and Soft Tissue Sarcomas

Primary bone tumours in the paediatric population commonly include osteogenic sarcoma, Ewing's sarcoma, chondrosarcomas, and soft tissue sarcomas of mesenchymal origin.

Osteogenic sarcoma (OGS) is a common malignancy afflicting children, especially young adults. It typically involves the distal femoral epiphysis with extension into meta and diaphysis,

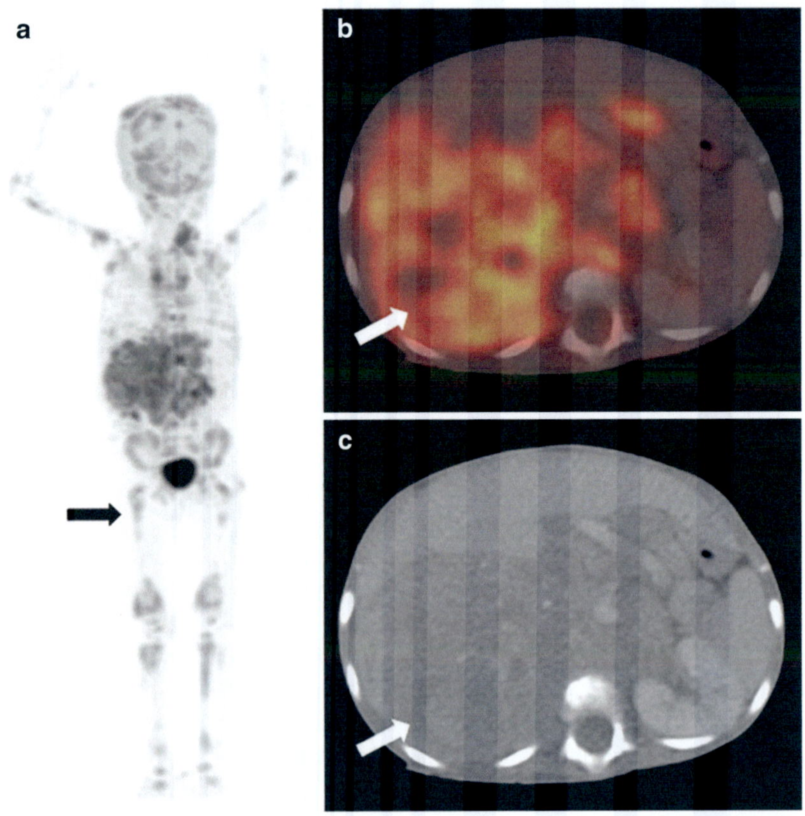

Fig. 6.5 (**a**) MIP, (**b**) PET/CT fusion, (**c**) CT of 3-year-old child with neuroblastoma, note the large hypermetabolic retroperitoneal soft tissue mass (white arrow) and extensive marrow lesions (black arrow)

it is an aggressive lesion with an osteoid matrix, typically its metastasis may also show an osteoid matrix. Therefore, targeting this process, i.e. the osteoid matrix may be a helpful strategy to visualize the disease and stage it.

Technetium 99 m labelled Methylene diphosphonate (Tc99m MDP) conventional bone scan locates areas of increased osteoblastic activity and osteoid matrix. The labelled phosphonate will show increased uptake at the primary site and will also show abnormal uptake in osteoblastic metastatic skeletal lesions (Fig. 6.6). Hence this modality was used to stage OGS.

Unfortunately, this tracer does not get adsorbed at non-skeletal sites and hence, may fail to detect malignant tissue in the marrow or regions of low to poor osteoblastic activity like in

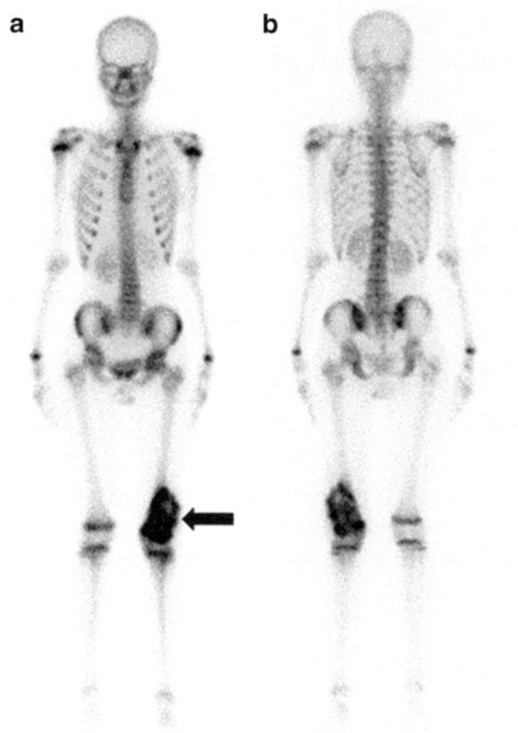

Fig. 6.6 (**a**) Anterior and (**b**) Posterior images of Technetium99m Methylene Di Phosphonate (Tc99m MDP) scan, note the left distal femoral primary mass (black arrow)

lytic lesions. This type of metastatic involvement, however, is not commonly encountered.

FDG PET/CT with its ability to detect metastases based on identifying sites of increased glucose turnover, delineates metastatic involvement in skeletal and non-skeletal areas.

6.5.1 Guidelines and Indications

NCCN recommends FDG PET/CT under three scenarios in sarcomas.

1. Malignancies with a potential of nodal metastases: such as clear cell sarcoma, epithelioid sarcoma, rhabdomyosarcoma, and angiosarcoma. In such cases, FDG PET/CT may help image the nodal basins.
2. At baseline in those cases where FDG PET/CT is intended to be used to assess response to neoadjuvant therapy.
3. In intra-abdominal/retroperitoneal sarcomas, where focal intense uptake within a large tumour helps in locating a site for biopsy (may help differentiate well-differentiated and undifferentiated sarcomas) [19].

6.5.2 Post-treatment Imaging

Various studies have used FDG PET/CT as a tool to assess response to neoadjuvant chemotherapy, as it acts as a prognosticator in OGS, and responders show good outcomes with prolonged overall survival [20].

6.5.3 Recent Advances

Recently, PETMRI utilizing integrated PET and MRI has been extremely useful in bone and soft tissue tumours as it integrates the fine resolution of the MRI in detecting adjacent neurovascular bundle involvement and infiltration into surrounding soft tissue with the metabolic information of FDG at locoregional and distant sites in one imaging modality. Emerging data reveals it to be useful not only in staging but also in prognostication of tumours [21].

6.6 Paediatric Thyroid Cancer

Paediatric thyroid cancer differs from adults in certain aspects. Although the management of paediatric cancer is a therapeutic domain and typically outside the scope of a diagnostic textbook, a brief mention of the same is made.

6.6.1 Guidelines and Indications

Radioactive Iodine ablation is indicated in high-risk thyroid cancers. RAI therapy is not used in low-risk patients and is decided on a case-to-case basis in intermediate and high-risk patients.

The American Thyroid Association recommends post-treatment radio-iodine scans only in intermediate and high-risk thyroid cancer patients. Often post-therapy scans unearth metastatic sites not detected on pre-treatment lower-dose iodine whole-body scans. The commonest site of metastatic involvement could be micro-pulmonary metastases not detected on conventional imaging [22].

6.7 Paediatric Brain Tumours

Although brain tumours are typically the domain of an MRI, nuclear medicine may play a complimentary role in certain indications, especially post-treatment response and recurrence.

6.7.1 Guidelines and Indications

The Response Assessment in Neuro-Oncology Group gives recommendations on the potential use of PET/CT in brain tumours. They suggest the use of amino acid tracers such as Fluoroethyl Tyrosine (FET) and F dopa and glucose metabolism tracers such as FDG.

The most important role of a PET/CT is in locating the site of biopsy where conventional imaging is equivocal at diagnosis.

Another emerging role of PET/CT at staging is its role in tumour volume and extent delineation helping in RT planning.

6.7.2 Post-treatment Imaging

The commonest dilemma in post-RT response assessment is in deciphering necrosis versus recurrence. FET or DOPA has better sensitivity in localizing regions of recurrence [23].

6.7.3 Recent Updates

SSTR imaging plays a complementary role in the diagnosis of atypical skull base and dural lesions on Conventional imaging. The presence of SSTR helps in confirming meningioma.

There is also a consensus guideline on the use of diagnostic and Lu177 labelled somatostatin (TATE) for therapy of refractory, recurrent, or inoperable meningiomas [24, 25].

6.8 Conclusion

Overall nuclear medicine primarily helps in the management of various paediatric malignancies predominantly using FDG PET/CT. The hybrid imaging modality provides both anatomical and functional information, reducing the radiation burden in children and also the time to initiate therapy. This can thus work as a one-stop-shop modality. With the advent of PET/MR machines, the radiation burden will be further reduced.

In neuroblastoma MIBG continues to play a crucial role however due to the lack of availability of 123 labelled MIBG, FDG can play an important role in overcoming the limitation of 131 MIBG currently used for diagnostic purposes.

Various malignancies can also be offered theranostic options using labelled beta or alpha emitters.

References

1. Benamor M, Ollivier L, Brisse H, Moulin-Romsee G, Servois V, Neuenschwander S. PET/CT imaging: what radiologists need to know. Cancer Imaging. 2007;7(Special issue A):S95–9.

2. Guja KE, Nadel H, Iagaru A. Overview and recent advances in 18F-FDG PET/CT for evaluation of pediatric lymphoma. Semin Nucl Med. 2023;53(3):400–12.
3. Cheson BD, Fisher RI, Barrington SF, Cavalli F, Schwartz LH, Zucca E, et al. Recommendations for initial evaluation, staging, and response assessment of Hodgkin and non-Hodgkin lymphoma: the Lugano classification. J Clin Oncol. 2014;32(27):3059–67.
4. Agrawal A, Rangarajan V, Puranik AD. PET/CT in non-Hodgkin lymphoma. Cham: Springer Nature; 2021. 115p.
5. Gallamini A, Zwarthoed C. Interim FDG-PET imaging in lymphoma. Semin Nucl Med. 2018;48(1):17–27.
6. Han S. 18F-FDG PET/CT: normal variants, artefacts and pitfalls in lymphoma. In: Kayani I, editor. PET/CT in Hodgkin's lymphoma [internet]. Cham: Springer; 2017 [cited 2024 Jan 26]. p. 41–53. (Clinicians' Guides to Radionuclide Hybrid Imaging). Available from: https://doi.org/10.1007/978-3-319-57225-3_6
7. Pepper NB, Oertel M, Rehn S, Kobe C, Eich HT. Modern PET-guided radiotherapy planning and treatment for malignant lymphoma. Semin Nucl Med. 2023;53(3):389–99.
8. Luo ZH, Lu PX, Qi WL, Liao FX, Jin AF, Zen QY. Role of 18F-FDG PET/CT in the diagnosis and management of patients with Langerhans cell histiocytosis. Quant Imaging Med Surg. 2022;12(6):3351–63.
9. Parikh NS, Howard SC, Chantada G, Israels T, Khattab M, Alcasabas P, et al. SIOP-PODC adapted risk stratification and treatment guidelines: recommendations for neuroblastoma in low- and middle-income settings. Pediatr Blood Cancer. 2015;62(8):1305–16.
10. Monclair T, Brodeur GM, Ambros PF, Brisse HJ, Cecchetto G, Holmes K, et al. The International Neuroblastoma Risk Group (INRG) staging system: an INRG task force report. J Clin Oncol. 2009;27(2):298–303.
11. Shapiro B. Summary, conclusions, and future directions of [131I]metaiodobenzylguanidine therapy in the treatment of neural crest tumors. J Nucl Biol Med Turin Italy 1991. 1991;35(4):357–63.
12. Sharp SE, Shulkin BL, Gelfand MJ, Salisbury S, Furman WL. 123I-MIBG scintigraphy and 18F-FDG PET in neuroblastoma. J Nucl Med. 2009;50(8):1237–43.
13. Suc A, Lumbroso J, Rubie H, Hattchouel JM, Boneu A, Rodary C, et al. Metastatic neuroblastoma in children older than one year: prognostic significance of the initial metaiodobenzylguanidine scan and proposal for a scoring system. Cancer. 1996;77(4):805–11.
14. Ady N, Zucker JM, Asselain B, Edeline V, Bonnin F, Michon J, et al. A new 123I-MIBG whole body scan scoring method—application to the prediction of the response of metastases to induction chemotherapy in stage IV neuroblastoma. Eur J Cancer Oxf Engl 1990. 1995;31A(2):256–61.
15. He H, Xu Q, Yu C. The efficacy and safety of Iodine-131-metaiodobenzylguanidine therapy in patients with neuroblastoma: a meta-analysis. BMC Cancer. 2022;22:216.
16. Hoefnagel CA, de Kraker J, Voûte PA, Valdés Olmos RA. Preoperative [131I]metaiodobenzylguanidine therapy of neuroblastoma at diagnosis ("MIBG de novo"). J Nucl Biol Med Turin Italy 1991. 1991;35(4):248–51.
17. Feng J, Cheng FW, Leung AW, Lee V, Yeung EW, Ching Lam H, et al. Upfront consolidation treatment with 131I-mIbG followed by myeloablative chemotherapy and hematopoietic stem cell transplantation in high-risk neuroblastoma. Pediatr Investig. 2020;4(3):168–77.
18. Feng L, Li S, Wang C, Yang J. Current status and future perspective on molecular imaging and treatment of neuroblastoma. Semin Nucl Med. 2023;53(4):517–29.
19. NCCN clinical practice guidelines in oncology (NCCN guidelines®) soft tissue sarcoma version 3.2023—December 12, 2023.
20. Hongtao L, Hui Z, Bingshun W, Xiaojin W, Zhiyu W, Shuier Z, et al. 18F-FDG positron emission tomography for the assessment of histological response to neoadjuvant chemotherapy in osteosarcomas: a meta-analysis. Surg Oncol. 2012;21(4):e165–70.
21. Buchbender C, Heusner TA, Lauenstein TC, Bockisch A, Antoch G. Oncologic PET/MRI, part 2: bone tumors, soft-tissue tumors, melanoma, and lymphoma. J Nucl Med. 2012;53(8):1244–52.
22. Francis GL, Waguespack SG, Bauer AJ, Angelos P, Benvenga S, Cerutti JM, et al. Management guidelines for children with thyroid nodules and differentiated thyroid cancer. Thyroid. 2015;25(7):716–59.
23. Law I, Albert NL, Arbizu J, Boellaard R, Drzezga A, Galldiks N, et al. Joint EANM/EANO/RANO practice guidelines/SNMMI procedure standards for imaging of gliomas using PET with radiolabelled amino acids and [18F]FDG: version 1.0. Eur J Nucl Med Mol Imaging. 2019;46(3):540–57.
24. Cornelius JF, Langen KJ, Stoffels G, Hänggi D, Sabel M, Jakob SH. Positron emission tomography imaging of meningioma in clinical practice: review of literature and future directions. Neurosurgery. 2012;70(4):1033–41. discussion 1042.
25. Filippi L, Palumbo I, Bagni O, Schillaci O, Aristei C, Palumbo B. Somatostatin receptor targeted PET-imaging for diagnosis, radiotherapy planning and Theranostics of Meningiomas: a systematic review of the literature. Diagnostics. 2022;12(7):1666.

7 Whole-Body MRI in Pediatric Oncology

Deeksha Bhalla and Manisha Jana

7.1 Introduction

Whole-body MRI (WB-MRI) has emerged as a valuable tool for comprehensive head-to-toe evaluation of various pediatric systemic disorders. The unique ability of whole-body imaging combined with lack of ionizing radiation make it an attractive option for staging and follow-up of malignancies as well. There is, however, the challenge of long acquisition time, which requires that protocols be tightly tailored as per patient age and the expectation from the examination. Due to large variability in institutional experience and preferences, currently high-quality evidence for standardization of both indications and protocols does not exist in literature. The Oncology task force of the European Society for Pediatric Radiology has recently released guidelines based on consensus opinion for common malignancies encountered in childhood [1]. In this chapter, we aim to summarize the available evidence on current practices in whole-body MRI in pediatric oncology.

D. Bhalla
Department of Radiodiagnosis, Postgraduate Institute of Child Health, Noida, India

M. Jana (✉)
Department of Radiodiagnosis and Interventional Radiology, All India Institute of Medical Sciences, New Delhi, India

7.2 Consensus Guidelines

The applications of whole-body MRI in pediatric oncology are twofold. It may be used in a diagnostic setting, for staging, post-therapy restaging, or follow-up of known malignancy patients, which is the most common application. Another important application has emerged in recent years, which is screening in patients with hereditary tumor predisposition syndromes.

7.2.1 Diagnostic Applications

1. **Pediatric Lymphoma**

Lymphoma in children can be of the Hodgkin (HL) or non-Hodgkin (NHL) variety. Hodgkin lymphoma is staged as per the Ann Arbor staging system with the Cotswald modification, while NHL is staged according to the revised International Pediatric Non-Hodgkin lymphoma staging system.

Staging

For diagnosis of lymphoma, only abdominal ultrasonography and/or chest radiography is recommended. However, for staging, the current recommendation differs among HL and NHL. For HL, since these are uniformly FDG-avid tumors, whole body PET-CT from skull base to mid-thigh remains the first-line imaging modality [1, 2]. For

I. Kumar et al. (eds.), *Practical Approach to Imaging in Pediatric Oncology*,
https://doi.org/10.1007/978-981-96-8158-7_7

NHL, the modalities are more varied. CT of the neck, chest, abdomen, and pelvis along with cranial/spinal MRI (if indicated) is performed. There is also a recommendation to perform additional PET-CT from vertex to toe in patients with B cell NHL, since NHL has a propensity for bony metastases [3].

In this setting, whole-body MRI is a useful alternative, and there has been increasing interest in using this modality for staging. A recent meta-analysis comparing WB MRI with PET-CT found that the pooled sensitivity of WB MRI was 95.8%, while for extra-nodal disease it was 88.9% [4]. As per the ESPR recommendations, WB MRI can be a useful alternative to contrast CT, however for FDG avid lymphomas, FDG-PET-CT is still to be preferred.

Post-treatment Imaging

FDG PET has been extensively studied for the assessment of interim as well as post-therapy response, in children with lymphoma. While some studies have attempted to compare ADC values on WB MRI with SUV [5, 6] values at FDG PET, no conclusive results have been found. The role of WB MRI in interim assessment therefore, is still under investigation.

2. **Neuroblastoma**

NB is the second most common extracranial solid tumor in children, with 70% children showing metastases at the time of presentation. The staging of neuroblastoma is based on the International Neuroblastoma Staging System (INSS), which is predominantly surgical staging and not routinely performed on imaging. The International Neuroblastoma Risk Group Staging System, which defines staging based on the presence of one or more image-defined risk factors (IDRFs), is relevant for radiologists to know and accurately define.

Staging

Due to its origin from neural crest-derived cells, NB displays avidity for meta-iodo-benzyl-guanidine (MIBG) and thus, radiolabeled I123 MIBG is the mainstay of imaging metastatic disease in children, with FDG-PET reserved for the 10% of these tumors that are non-MIBG avid [7].

In children with NB, the primary metastatic sites are liver, lymph nodes, bone marrow, and skin. Among these, WB MRI shows high sensitivity for detecting marrow metastases, which was established in the study by Kembhavi et al. [8]. Further, Ishiguchi et al. [9] also established similar sensitivity for whole-body MRI using diffusion-weighted imaging versus FDG-PET for detection of lymphadenopathy.

For local staging of tumor as well, CT or MRI are to be performed [10]. Therefore, the Oncology Working group recommends exploiting the combination of MRI for local staging with WB MRI for detection of skeletal metastases [1].

Post-treatment Imaging

I123 MIBG or PET-CT based on avidity is the current imaging recommendation for interim assessment, and MRI plus functional imaging is recommended at the end of therapy in patients who undergo surgery. The role of WB MRI in response assessment is unclear at present.

3. **Sarcomas**

Sarcomas account for ~10–15% of malignant solid tumors in children and adolescents. Head-to-toe imaging is essential for small primary in the extremities, skeletal, or other distant metastasis. The delineation of metastases is of utmost importance, since surgical resection of metastatic lesions is also recommended.

Staging

Soft Tissue Sarcoma

Rhabdomyosarcoma is the most common soft tissue sarcoma in children.

High-resolution MRI for local disease and loco-regional lymph nodes and CT for lung metastases are recommended. Bone scan, whole-body MRI, and PET scan are optional [11].

Bone Tumors

Osteogenic sarcoma is the most common malignant bone tumor in children, followed by Ewing's sarcoma. The local staging is based on radiographs as well as MRI of the involved bone, including the adjoining joints. Chest CT is performed for pulmonary and bone scintigraphy for bone metastases. PET-CT and WB-MRI are being increasingly used, but are optional in current guidelines [12]. Skeletal metastases have a worse prognosis than pulmonary metastases [13]. WB-MRI has shown higher accuracy than PET-CT for detection of skeletal metastases. In a study performed by Bosma et al., the sensitivity and specificity of PET-CT (62% and 100% respectively) were far exceeded by WB MRI (99% and 100% respectively). Thus, WB MRI may be used as a combined modality for local staging as well as detection of skeletal metastases (Figs. 7.1 and 7.2).

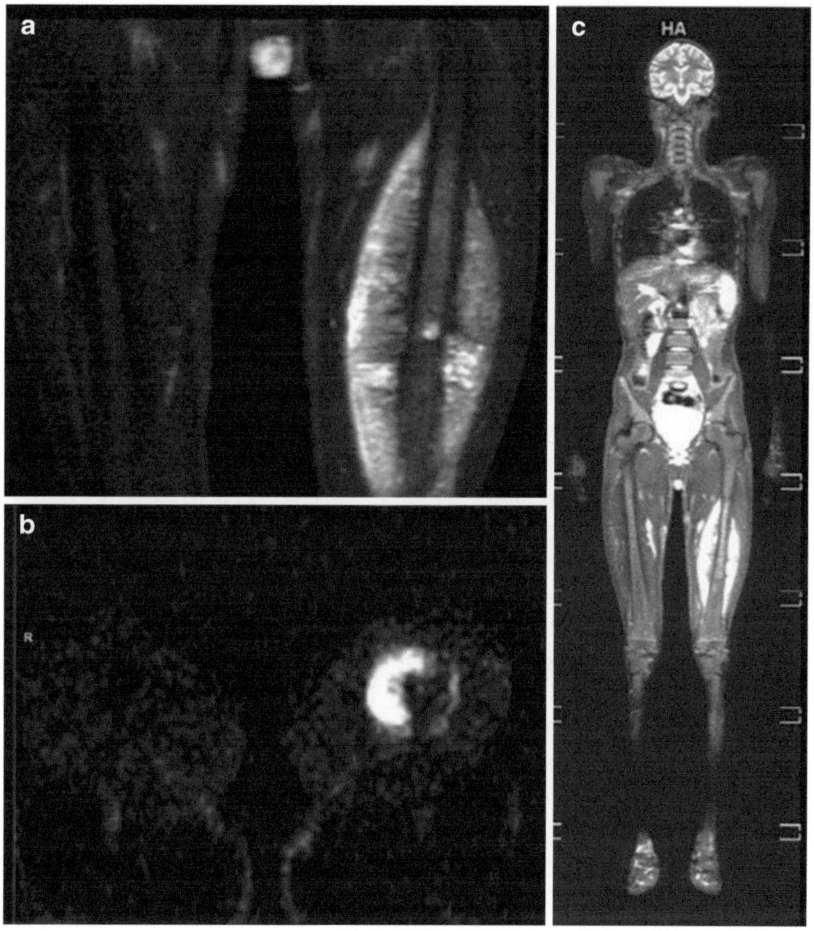

Fig. 7.1 Whole-body MRI in osteosarcoma. (**a**) STIR coronal of the thigh shows a hyperintense lesion with soft tissue component and spiculated periosteal reaction. (**b**) On the axial DWI images, intense diffusion restriction is seen. (**c**) WB MRI from vertex to toe shows the lesion in left thigh. No metastases are seen

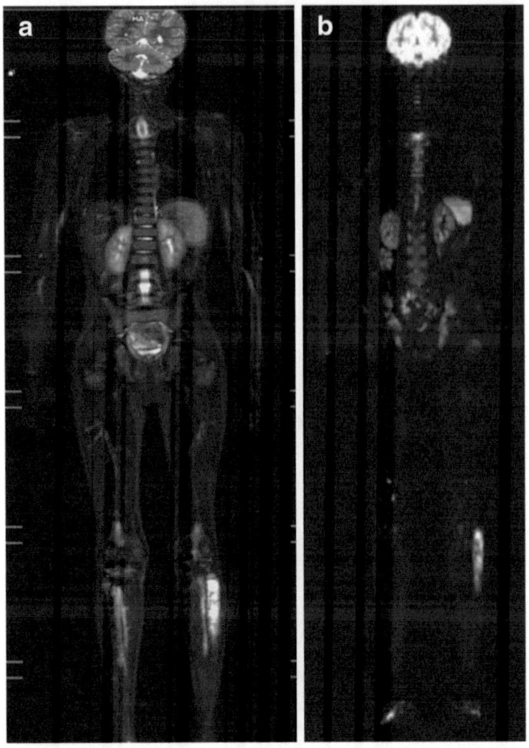

Fig. 7.2 WB MRI in Ewing's sarcoma. (**a**) STIR coronal image shows marrow hyperintensity along with soft tissue in the left fibula with no lesion elsewhere in the body. (**b**) On the coronal DWIBS image, diffusion restriction is seen within the lesion, as well as physiological sites such as the brain and spleen

Post-treatment Imaging

Clinical assessment and chest radiographs/CT are currently used. The role of WB MRI, though being used at multiple centers, has not been evaluated in sufficient studies.

4. Langerhans Cell Histiocytosis

The revised classification of Langerhans cell histiocytosis (LCH) is based on extent of disease involvement. It is classified into unifocal, single-system multifocal and multi-system (with or without risk organ involvement) forms. The prognosis of children with single-system disorders is uniformly better than those with multisystem involvement.

Staging

Current imaging guidelines are given in the LCH-IV International Collaborative Treatment Protocol for Children and Adolescents with Langerhans cell histiocytosis (EudraCT Nr.: 2011–001699-20).

The imaging protocol for staging includes a radiographic skeletal survey, abdominal US for liver and spleen involvement, and a chest radiograph. Additional imaging may be performed as indicated, chest CT for lung involvement, head CT for craniofacial lesions, brain MRI for neurological involvement, and spine MRI for suspicious vertebral lesions.

A study by Kim et al. showed that WB-MRI is an excellent imaging method to assess disease extent, with significantly higher sensitivity for detecting both skeletal and extra-skeletal lesions (99%), without an increase in false-positive results in this patient population [14]. Goo et al. also showed WB MRI identified additional skeletal lesions in three (38%) of eight patients, compared with plain radiography, and in two (25%) of eight, compared with bone scintigraphy highlighting the advantage of the lack of ionizing radiation [15].

The Oncology group advises that WB MRI *should* be performed in children at disease onset, particularly if sedation is not required.

Post-treatment Imaging

In assessing response to chemotherapy, Mueller et al. compared PET-CT and WB MRI. They found that persistent signal abnormality was seen on T2-weighted and contrast enhancement on ceT1, even in lesions that were not FDG avid. These findings may be present due to tissue reorganization post chemotherapy. No advantage was found in reducing the false negatives as well in this study [16]. Thus, the role of WB MRI in post-therapy evaluation remains controversial.

7.3 Diagnostic Imaging Protocols

A 'modular' approach to whole-body magnetic resonance imaging protocol has been proposed by Schafer et al. [17], consisting of basic sequences essential for anatomical definition, coupled with indication-specific additional sequences for either tissue characterization or functional information.

The proposed examination protocols for common pediatric malignancies are described in Table 7.1.

7.3.1 Screening Applications

Cancer Predisposition Syndromes
10% of pediatric cancers may be linked to cancer predisposition syndromes (CPS) [18]. The role of imaging in cancer predisposition syndromes is to be part of tumor surveillance and to allow for detection of tumor recurrence. WB MRI is particularly advantageous due to lack of ionizing radiation and thus can be employed for long-term monitoring in these children. Imaging must be performed from vertex to toes.

Table 7.1 Proposed whole-body MRI protocol for common pediatric malignancies

	T2 (STIR)	T1w	DWI	Additional
Lymphoma *Hodgkin*	✔ Coronal Head to groin	Optional Coronal Head to groin	✔ Axial Head to groin	Axial T2-STIR Axial T1-FS post gad
Non-Hodgkin	✔ Coronal Vertex to toes	Optional Coronal Vertex to toes	✔ Axial Vertex to toes	Axial T2-STIR Axial T1-FS post gad
Neuroblastoma	✔ Coronal Vertex to toes	–	✔ Axial Vertex to toes	Sagittal STIR spine Axial T1-FS post gad
Sarcoma *Soft tissue*	✔ Coronal Vertex to toes Primary tumor in 2 planes	✔ High resolution of primary tumor/single metastases	✔ Axial Vertex to toes	T1-FS post gad primary tumor in 2 planes
Bone sarcoma	✔ Coronal Vertex to toes Primary tumor in 2 planes	✔ High resolution Of primary tumor/single metastases	✔ Axial Vertex to toes	T1-FS post gad primary tumor in 2 planes
Langerhans cell histiocytosis	✔ Coronal Vertex to toes Sagittal spine	✔ Coronal Vertex to toes	–	Axial T2-STIR Axial T1 TSE head

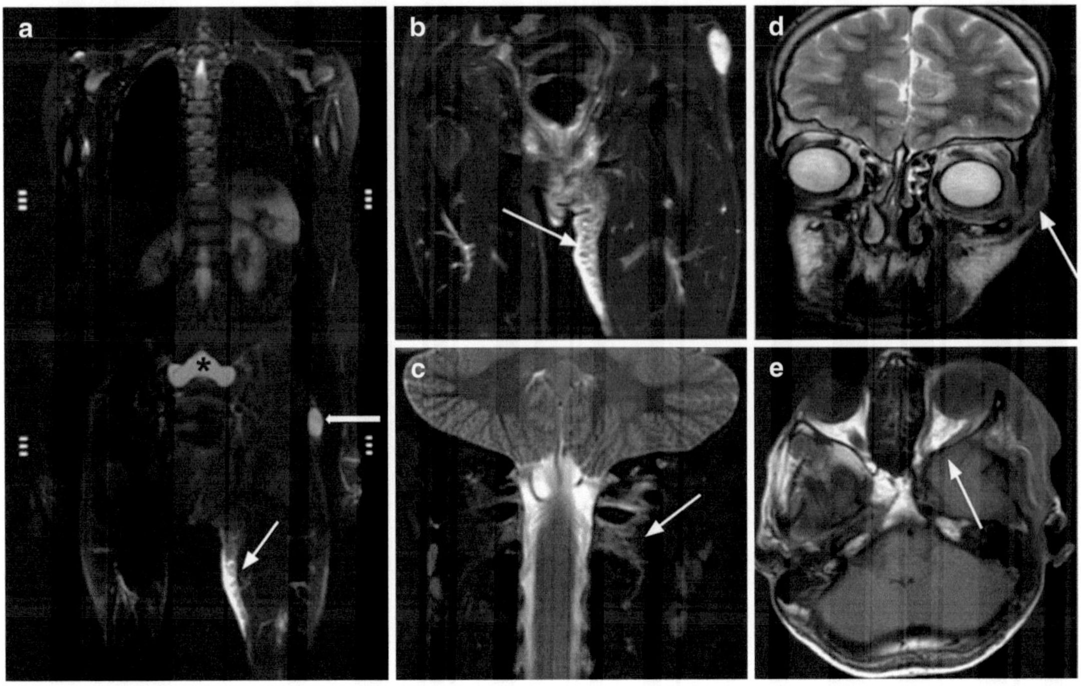

Fig. 7.3 WB MRI in Neurofibromatosis 1. (**a**) Coronal STIR image shows skin thickening along the left medial thigh (arrow), a cutaneous neurofibroma in the left gluteal region (solid arrow), and dural ectasia (*). (**b**) Coronal STIR image of the thigh station shows 'target appearance' in the thigh lesion (arrow) suggesting plexiform neurofibroma. (**c**) Cervical nerve root thickening is also noted (arrow). (**d**, **e**). Coronal T2 (**d**) and axial T1 (**e**) images show another plexiform neurofibroma around left orbit as well as sphenoid wing dysplasia (arrow)

The guidelines for various syndromes are as follows:

1. Li Fraumeni syndrome. Both the National Comprehensive Cancer Network (NCCN) and the American Association for Cancer Research (AACR) recommend annual screening with WB-MRI and brain MRI, with early identification of malignant and premalignant lesions. Notably, due to the risk of sarcomas, the FOV should include the limbs (head-to-toe) [19].
2. Neurofibromatosis: In patients with neurofibromatosis (NF) types 1 and 2, WB-MRI has been shown to be satisfactory for diagnosis and surveillance of tumors, as well as assessment of tumor burden and distribution, with a baseline study recommended between 16 and 20 years of age [20] (Fig. 7.3).
3. Hereditary retinoblastoma: WB MRI to be performed every 12 months from the age of 8 years.

7.4 Imaging Protocols in Screening

Coronal T2-FS/STIR is universally used as the mainstay in all WB MRI protocols. In addition, DWI sequences are recommended, which may be acquired in the axial plane and reconstructed to coronal planes to avoid artifacts when imaging in other planes. The diffusion-weighted imaging with background body signal suppression (DWIBS) sequence has gained popularity for this purpose. The use of gadolinium contrast is not routinely recommended. However, in syndromes where patients are prone to develop tumors of the brain, head, and neck regions, such as Li Fraumeni, hereditary retinoblastoma, neurofibromatosis, contrast evaluation of the brain is recommended. Additional high-resolution images of affected regions may also be acquired, in case any lesions are detected, based on institutional preference.

7.5 Image Interpretation

A step-wise approach to image interpretation in WB MRI is depicted in Fig. 7.4. Few common pitfalls may be encountered in image interpretation [21], these are summarized in Table 7.2. Further, there has been formulation of the Oncologically Relevant Findings Reporting and Data System (ONCO-RADS) for reporting of findings encountered during screening exams in patients with cancer predisposition syndromes [22]. This involves assigning risk categories, along with recommendations, which are summarized in Fig. 7.5. However, the ONCO-RADS risk categories are yet to be validated with actual risk of cancer in prospective studies, and therefore have not found widespread use in reporting of whole-body MRI exams around the globe.

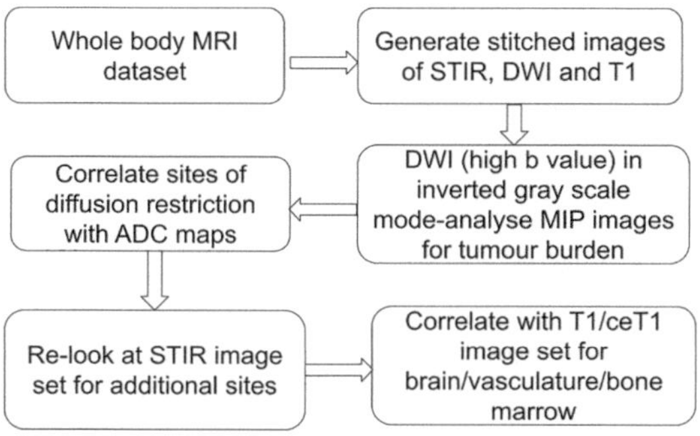

Fig. 7.4 Stepwise approach to image interpretation on WB MRI

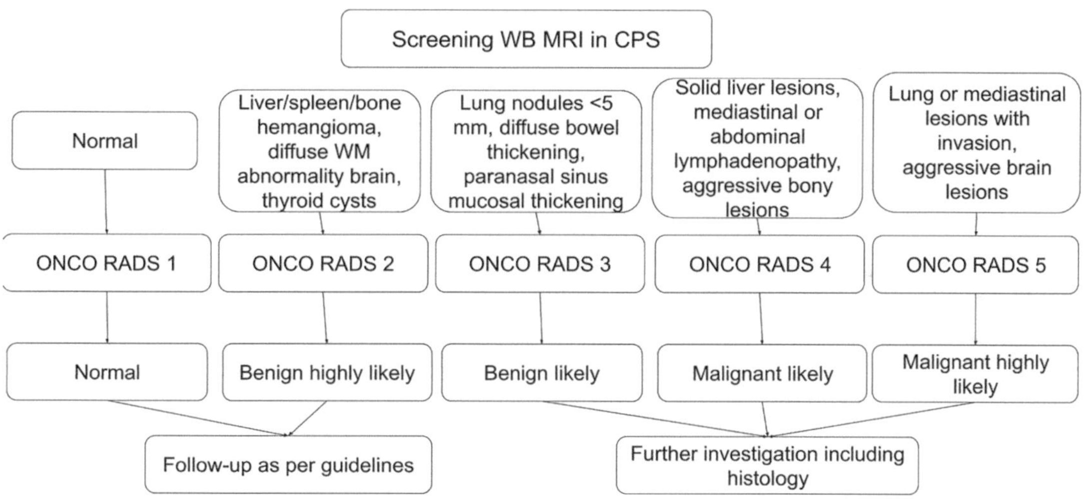

Fig. 7.5 ONCO-RADS risk categories with examples and recommendations based on risk assessment. In children with cancer predisposition syndromes (CPS), ONCO RADS 3 lesions also must be proven benign by further testing

Table 7.2 Pitfalls in WB MRI image interpretation

Pitfalls in WB MRI image interpretation
Subphyseal marrow STIR hyperintensity: physiological in children
Low ADC value in red marrow due to tightly packed cells and bony trabeculae: DIXON sequence may be used to differentiate normal marrow from marrow infiltration [21]
Diffusion restriction in lymph nodes: also seen in normal nodes, cannot be used to differentiate benign from malignant nodes

7.6 Reporting Template

A sample reporting template is shown in Table 7.3. Table 7.4 depicts the imaging appearance of common findings encountered in malignancy/cancer predisposition syndromes in children.

Table 7.3 Structured reporting format for WB MRI in pediatric oncology

Indication for examination	<Diagnostic> <Screening>
Sites	*Assessment*
Head and neck Brain parenchyma	<normal> <focal lesion> <diffuse white/gray matter abnormality>
Calvarium	<normal> <benign lesion> <aggressive lesion>
Orbit	<normal> <intraconal lesion> <extraconal lesion> <optic nerve thickening>
Lymphadenopathy	<present> <absent> Levels involved:
Upper limb Long bones	<normal> <benign lesion> <aggressive lesion> Location: <humerus. <radius> <ulna> <hand bones>
Soft tissue	<normal> <benign lesion> <aggressive lesion>
Thorax Lung	<normal> <solid nodule> <ground glass nodule> <mixed nodule>
Mediastinum	<normal> <thymic hyperplasia> <mass lesion> If mass lesion present, Location: <prevascular> <visceral> <paravertebral> Composition: <solid> <cystic> <mixed>
Lymphadenopathy	<present> <absent> Stations involved:
Ribs	<normal> <benign lesion> <aggressive lesion>
Abdomen Liver Spleen Pancreas Kidney	<normal> <cyst> <benign> <aggressive> <normal> <cyst> <benign> <aggressive> <normal> <cyst> <benign> <aggressive> <normal> <cyst> <benign> <aggressive>
Bowel	<normal> <focal thickening> <diffuse thickening>
Lymphadenopathy	<present> <absent> Sites involved:
Pelvis Ovary Prostate	<normal> <cyst> <benign> <aggressive> <normal> <cyst> <benign> <aggressive>
Lymphadenopathy	<present> <absent> Sites involved:
Lower limb Long bones	<normal> <benign lesion> <aggressive lesion> Location: <femur> <tibia> <fibula> <foot bones>
Soft tissue	<normal> <benign lesion> <aggressive lesion>
Impression	
Recommendation (in case of screening exams)	<no further action> <follow-up> <further testing>

Table 7.4 Summary of common imaging findings on WB MRI

Common pathological findings	T2 signal	T1 signal	Others	Common sites
Lymph nodes	Hyperintense	Iso-hypointense	DWI restriction. Size >10 mm considered positive	Cervical> retroperitoneum> mediastinum >inguinal
Bone metastases	Hyperintense (STIR)	Hypo intense compared to marrow	DWI restriction, convex posterior margin in vertebral collapse	Vertebrae, ribs>calvarium>long bones
Lung	Hyperintense	–	Round morphology, random distribution, lower lobe predominance	Lower lobes>lingula
Abdominal organs				–
Liver	Hyperintense	Hypointense	DWI restriction: Increases sensitivity	
Adrenal	Hyperintense	Hypointense	In-opposed phase (to rule out adenomas)	
Spleen	Hyperintense	Hypointense	Physiological restriction in spleen may mask lesions	
Head and neck				
Orbit	Hyperintense	Hypointense[a]	Enhancement on post gad sequences	
Soft tissue	'Target sign' in plexiform NF	Hypointense	Enhancement on post gad sequences	
Brain	Hyperintense with edema		DWI restriction in malignancy, no restriction/enhancement in NF	Dural surfaces, basifrontal lobes in direct extension from skull base

DWI diffusion-weighted imaging, *NF* Neurofibromatosis, *STIR* short tau inversion recovery
[a]Hyperintensity may be seen in intraocular hemorrhage or retinal detachment due to retinoblastoma

7.7 Limitations

- The most important concern while performing WB MRI is the examination time, especially for the pediatric population. Sedation is usually required in children <6 years old. In these children, distraction techniques or mock examination may sometimes help to reduce the need for anesthesia. In infants <6 months, the 'feed and swaddle' technique can be used for motion limitation.
- The other important limitation is the evaluation of lung nodules, which is of particular importance in evaluation of sarcomas. It has been suggested that nodules >5 mm may be detected, however chest CT remains the standard of care for detection of lung metastases [23].
- WB MRI is unable to perform functional staging for lymph nodes, relying mainly on size criteria. ADC measurements are also limited for distinguishing benign and malignant nodes.

7.8 Recent Advances

- **Positron Emission Tomography Magnetic Resonance Imaging (PET MRI):**
- This is a unique imaging method that allows assessment of both anatomical and functional information. There is an additional advantage

of nearly 80% decrease in radiation compared to PET-CT. The average imaging time is similar to WB MRI.

- The imaging protocol as described by States et al. [7] comprises an initial PET sequence, followed by MRI sequences including a whole-body T1 DIXON and DWI. STIR images may be acquired in case of osseous lesions. PET MRI has shown promise in evaluation of lymphoma, neuroblastoma as well as histiocytosis. It is also helpful in depicting metabolically active areas for biopsy in sarcomas. This modality is particularly useful in post-therapy response assessment as well as evaluation of lymph nodes. There is also a distinct logistics benefit, since PET-MRI serves as a 'one stop shop' and limits the number of visits as well as individual anesthesia exposures for separate PET scans and MRI in children.
- **Ultrasmall Superparamagnetic Iron Oxide (USPIO) Contrast:**
- These agents are taken up by the reticuloendothelial system (RES), with no renal excretion. This is particularly advantageous since there is no risk of nephrogenic systemic fibrosis (NSF) and therefore can be used instead of gadolinium in younger children. It provides long-lasting vessel and tissue enhancement. Due to its RES accumulation, it acts as an excellent contrast for liver, spleen, lymph nodes, and bone marrow. Successful use of a USPIO agent, Ferumoxytol has also been reported for whole body PET-MRI in a study by Muehe et al. [24].

7.9 Conclusion

Whole-body MRI is a promising modality for evaluation of disseminated disease in childhood malignancies, particularly skeletal metastases. Effort must be made to tailor protocols according to specific indications to reduce examination time and increase patient comfort. PET MRI provides a useful alternative for simultaneous functional imaging, important for post-therapy response evaluation.

References

1. Schäfer JF, Granata C, von Kalle T, et al. Whole-body magnetic resonance imaging in pediatric oncology – recommendations by the Oncology Task Force of the ESPR. Pediatr Radiol. 2020;50(8):1162–74. https://doi.org/10.1007/s00247-020-04683-4.
2. Cheson BD, Fisher RI, Barrington SF, et al. Recommendations for initial evaluation, staging, and response assessment of Hodgkin and non-Hodgkin lymphoma: the Lugano classification. J Clin Oncol. 2014;32(27):3059–68. https://doi.org/10.1200/JCO.2013.54.8800.
3. McCarten KM, Nadel HR, Shulkin BL, Cho SY. Imaging for diagnosis, staging and response assessment of Hodgkin lymphoma and non-Hodgkin lymphoma. Pediatr Radiol. 2019;49(11):1545–64. https://doi.org/10.1007/s00247-019-04529-8.
4. Bhalla D, Jana M, Kandasamy D. Diagnostic accuracy of whole-body magnetic resonance imaging versus positron emission tomography-computed tomography for the staging of pediatric lymphoma: a systematic review and meta-analysis. Pediatr Radiol. 2023.; Published online October 10, 2023; https://doi.org/10.1007/s00247-023-05775-7.
5. Wu X, Pertovaara H, Dastidar P, et al. ADC measurements in diffuse large B-cell lymphoma and follicular lymphoma: a DWI and cellularity study. Eur J Radiol. 2013;82(4):e158–64. https://doi.org/10.1016/j.ejrad.2012.11.021.
6. Lin C, Itti E, Luciani A, et al. Whole-body diffusion-weighted imaging with apparent diffusion coefficient mapping for treatment response assessment in patients with diffuse large B-cell lymphoma: pilot study. Investig Radiol. 2011;46(5):341–9. https://doi.org/10.1097/RLI.0b013e3182087b03.
7. States LJ, Reid JR. Whole-body PET/MRI applications in pediatric oncology. Am J Roentgenol. 2020;215(3):713–25. https://doi.org/10.2214/AJR.19.22677.
8. Kembhavi SA, Rangarajan V, Shah S, et al. Prospective observational study on diagnostic accuracy of whole-body MRI in solid small round cell tumours. Clin Radiol. 2014;69(9):900–8. https://doi.org/10.1016/j.crad.2014.04.006.
9. Ishiguchi H, Ito S, Kato K, et al. Diagnostic performance of 18F-FDG PET/CT and whole-body diffusion-weighted imaging with background body suppression (DWIBS) in detection of lymph node and bone metastases from pediatric neuroblastoma. Ann Nucl Med. 2018;32(5):348–62. https://doi.org/10.1007/s12149-018-1254-z.
10. Swift CC, Eklund MJ, Kraveka JM, Alazraki AL. Updates in diagnosis, management, and treatment of neuroblastoma. Radiographics. 2018;38(2):566–80. https://doi.org/10.1148/rg.2018170132.
11. Casali PG, Abecassis N, Aro HT, et al. Soft tissue and visceral sarcomas: ESMO-EURACAN clinical practice guidelines for diagnosis, treatment and follow-up.

Ann Oncol. 2018;29(Suppl 4):iv51–67. https://doi.org/10.1093/annonc/mdy096.
12. Casali PG, Bielack S, Abecassis N, et al. Bone sarcomas: ESMO-PaedCan-EURACAN clinical practice guidelines for diagnosis, treatment and follow-up. Ann Oncol. 2018;29(Suppl 4):iv79–95. https://doi.org/10.1093/annonc/mdy310.
13. Gerrand C, Athanasou N, Brennan B, et al. UK guidelines for the management of bone sarcomas. Clin Sarcoma Res. 2016;6:7. https://doi.org/10.1186/s13569-016-0047-1.
14. Kim JR, Yoon HM, Jung AY, Cho YA, Seo JJ, Lee JS. Comparison of whole-body MRI, bone scan, and radiographic skeletal survey for lesion detection and risk stratification of langerhans cell histiocytosis. Sci Rep. 2019;9(1):317. https://doi.org/10.1038/s41598-018-36501-1.
15. Goo HW, Yang DH, Ra YS, et al. Whole-body MRI of Langerhans cell histiocytosis: comparison with radiography and bone scintigraphy. Pediatr Radiol. 2006;36(10):1019–31. https://doi.org/10.1007/s00247-006-0246-7.
16. Mueller WP, Melzer HI, Schmid I, Coppenrath E, Bartenstein P, Pfluger T. The diagnostic value of 18F-FDG PET and MRI in paediatric histiocytosis. Eur J Nucl Med Mol Imaging. 2013;40(3):356–63. https://doi.org/10.1007/s00259-012-2278-6.
17. Schaefer JF, Kramer U. Whole-body MRI in children and juveniles. ROFO Fortschr Geb Rontgenstr Nuklearmed. 2011;183(1):24–36. https://doi.org/10.1055/s-0029-1245883.
18. Gottumukkala RV, Gee MS, Hampilos PJ, Greer MLC. Current and emerging roles of whole-body MRI in evaluation of pediatric cancer patients. Radiographics. 2019;39(2):516–34. https://doi.org/10.1148/rg.2019180130.
19. Guimarães JB, da Cruz IAN, Ahlawat S, et al. The role of whole-body MRI in pediatric musculoskeletal oncology: current concepts and clinical applications. J Magn Reson Imaging. Published online June 18, 2021. 2021; https://doi.org/10.1002/jmri.27787.
20. Greer MLC, Voss SD, States LJ. Pediatric cancer predisposition imaging: focus on whole-body MRI. Clin Cancer Res. 2017;23(11):e6–e13. https://doi.org/10.1158/1078-0432.CCR-17-0515.
21. van Vucht N, Santiago R, Lottmann B, et al. The Dixon technique for MRI of the bone marrow. Skeletal Radiol. 2019;48(12):1861–74. https://doi.org/10.1007/s00256-019-03271-4.
22. Petralia G, Koh DM, Attariwala R, Busch JJ, Eeles R, Karow D, Lo GG, Messiou C, Sala E, Vargas HA, Zugni F, Padhani AR. Oncologically relevant findings reporting and data system (ONCO-RADS): guidelines for the acquisition, interpretation, and reporting of whole-body MRI for cancer screening. Radiology. 2021;299(3):494–507. https://doi.org/10.1148/radiol.2021201740.
23. Smith EA, Dillman JR. Current role of body MRI in pediatric oncology. Pediatr Radiol. 2016;46(6):873–80. https://doi.org/10.1007/s00247-016-3560-8.
24. Muehe AM, Yerneni K, Theruvath AJ, et al. Ferumoxytol does not impact standardized uptake values on PET/MR scans. Mol Imaging Biol. 2020;22(3):722–9. https://doi.org/10.1007/s11307-019-01409-3.

8 Cancer Predisposition Syndromes

Richa Singh Chauhan and Nihar Kathrani

8.1 Introduction

Majority of the pediatric solid neoplasms are sporadic. However, as the understanding of the human genome has increased, a greater number of childhood malignant tumors associated with germline gene mutations or early somatic mosaicism in cancer predisposing genes and well-known clinical syndromes have been recognized. These neoplasms with genetic predisposition constitute up to 10% of all pediatric neoplasms [1, 2]. Cancer predisposition syndromes (CPS) epitomize a rare section of inherited diseases in which children with a pertinent family history or recognized pathogenic germline gene variant are at greater risk of developing malignant and benign neoplasms during their life span compared with their age-matched peers [3]. In certain instances, clinicians may become cognizant of the related CPS through the distinctive phenotypic presentation or, in other cases there may be a positive family history or positive genetic testing. Nonetheless, majority of CPS patients are recognized with the diagnosis of malignancy as the first sign of the genetic mutation with further detection of CPS-related sequelae [2].

CPS are distinguished by tumorigenesis of pathognomonic tissue types in specific target organs and commonly exhibit an autosomal dominant pattern of inheritance. Although CPS represent a minor fraction of all cancers, their screening, accurate diagnosis, and follow-up might improve mortality and morbidity in this patient group. The diagnosis of these hereditary cancer syndromes is confirmed by detecting causal gene mutation after clinical suspicion [4]. Identifying CPS in children is also imperative to enable surveillance for prompt recognition of second cancers and genetic testing and counselling of relatives [5]. Cross-sectional imaging displays a vital role in the screening, diagnosis, treatment and surveillance of the CPS patients. Early diagnosis guides for prophylactic surgery, which is critical in the management. Thus, for common hereditary CPS, treating physicians ought to be well-versed with the current recommendations and guidelines so as to select proper imaging modality for the diagnosis and decide appropriate time interval for screening and follow-up. Likewise, the radiologists should be pre-informed about the underlying genetic disorder to emphasize on other potential sites of tumors [4, 6].

This chapter offers a brief review of some of the most commonly encountered pediatric hereditary CPS along with their recommended screening/ surveillance guidelines. An overview of imaging modalities, highlighting the importance

R. S. Chauhan (✉) · N. Kathrani
Department of Radiodiagnosis, All India Institute of Medical Sciences (AIIMS), Raipur, Chhattisgarh, India

I. Kumar et al. (eds.), *Practical Approach to Imaging in Pediatric Oncology*,
https://doi.org/10.1007/978-981-96-8158-7_8

of whole-body MRI (WBMRI), for approaching patients with CPS and genetic mutations responsible for CPS will also be discussed.

8.2 When to Suspect CPS?

Individuals with a hereditary CPS may have varied presentations (Box 8.1).

Box 8.1 Clinical Presentations of Individuals with a Hereditary CPS:

1. They may have characteristic neoplasms which are illustrious of a certain CPS (e.g., hemangioblastomas, renal cell carcinomas or pheochromocytomas in VHL syndrome [Fig. 8.1]) (Table 8.1).
2. Patients may also be the members of families with a recognized CPS (e.g., paraganglioma, medullary carcinoma thyroid), especially young-onset neoplasms in several relatives in similar parental descent.
3. They may also have close relatives with a distinct CPS-associated tumor.
4. Patients may report with ≥1 congenital anomalies or key morphological characteristics (Table 8.1) that may raise suspicion or suggest a causal CPS (e.g., cutaneous neurofibromas in NF1).
5. They may have synchronous or metachronous cancers.
6. Bilateral neoplasms or an uncommon neoplasm in an infrequent anatomic site.
7. Finally, individuals may also harbor neoplasms with very early age of onset as compared to the general population (childhood adrenocortical carcinoma in Li-Fraumeni syndrome).

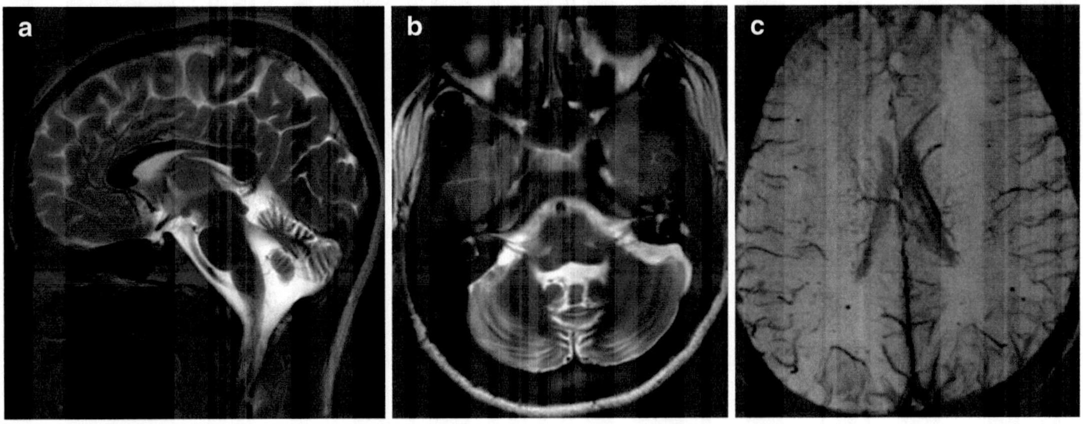

Fig. 8.1 12-year-old child with genetically proven Attaxia Telangiectasia. (**a**, **b**) Sagittal and axial T2w images show marked vermian and cerebellar atrophy. (**c**) Axial SWI image shows multiple microbleeds suggestive of telangiectasias

Table 8.1 Common and uncommon neoplastic and non-neoplastic features associated with CPS

CPS	Gene (s) involved	Inheritance	Associated neoplasms	Non-neoplastic features
Neurofibromatosis (NF) type 1	NF1	Dominant	Neurofibroma, malignant peripheral nerve sheath tumor, optic glioma, Pheochromocytoma, pilocytic astrocytoma, meningiomas, Wilms' tumor, rhabdomyosarcoma, renal angiomyolipoma, carcinoid tumor, leiomyoma, leiomyosarcoma, leukemia, and ganglioglioma	Cutaneous neurofibromas, café-au-lait spots, Lisch nodules (pigmented iris hamartomas)
NF type 2	NF2	Dominant	Vestibular schwannomas, meningiomas, ependymomas	Juvenile cataracts
VHL disease	VHL	Dominant	CNS and retinal hemangioblastomas, renal cell carcinomas, pheochromocytoma, endolymphatic sac tumors, papillary cystadenoma of epididymis and broad ligament, serous cystadenoma, and neuroendocrine tumors of the pancreas	Pancreatic and renal cysts
Tuberous sclerosis	TSC1, TSC2	Dominant	Renal angiomyolipoma, subependymal giant cell astrocytoma (SEGA), cardiac rhabdomyoma	Cortical tubers, white matter abnormalities, subependymal nodules, bone cysts, lymphangioleiomyomatosis, renal cysts
Ataxia telangiectasia (Fig. 8.1)	ATM	Recessive	Leukemia, lymphoma	Progressive cerebellar ataxia, oculocutaneous telangiectasia
Li-Fraumeni syndrome	P53	Dominant	Osteosarcoma and other sarcomas, adrenocortical carcinoma, breast cancer, leukemia, brain tumors (choroid plexus carcinomas and gliomas), neuroblastoma, rhabdomyosarcoma, Wilms' tumor, tumors of the stomach, colon, pancreas, esophagus, or lung; gonadal cell tumors, and early-onset melanoma	–
WAGR (Fig. 8.2)	11p deletion	Dominant	Wilms' tumor, gonadoblastoma	Aniridia, genitourinary anomalies, intellectual disability, pancreatitis, childhood obesity
Beckwith-Wiedemann syndrome	p57, LIT1, H19, CDKN1C, ICR1, NSD1		Wilms' tumor (nephroblastoma), adrenal adenoma/carcinoma, hepatoblastoma, neuroblastoma, leukemia, pancreatoblastoma, and rhabdomyosarcoma	Hemihyperplasia, abdominal wall defects (omphalocele, diastasis recti, umbilical hernia), macroglossia, ear anomalies, capillary malformations, hyperinsulinemic hypoglycemia, nephrourologic malformations, and organomegaly
Cowden syndrome	PTEN	Dominant	Breast cancer, endometrial cancer, thyroid cancer, colorectal cancer, and papillary RCC	Intellectual disability hamartomas, macrocephaly
Peutz-Jeghers syndrome	STK11	Dominant	GI cancers and hamartomas, cervical cancer, ovarian cancer, breast cancer	Hyperpigmented lips

(continued)

Table 8.1 (continued)

CPS	Gene (s) involved	Inheritance	Associated neoplasms	Non-neoplastic features
Multiple endocrine neoplasia type 1 (MEN1)—Wermer syndrome	MEN1	Dominant	Pituitary tumors, pancreas tumors, parathyroid adenomas, well-differentiated endocrine tumors of GI-pancreatic tract, meningioma, angiofibroma, collagenoma, lipoma, foregut carcinoid, adrenocortical tumor	Hypercalcemia, primary hyperparathyroidism, bronchopulmonary and thymic cysts
MEN2a—Sipple syndrome	RET (codon 634)	Dominant	Medullary thyroid carcinoma (MTC), parathyroid tumor, pheochromocytoma	Hyperparathyroidism
MEN2b—Multiple Mucosal neuroma syndrome	RET (codon 918)	Dominant	MTC, mucosal neuromas, pheochromocytoma, intestinal ganglioneuromatosis (secondary megacolon)	Marfanoid habitus, scoliosis, pectus excavatum, ptosis, everted eyelids, thickened lips, high-arched palate, narrow facies, alacrima
MEN4	CDNK1B	Dominant	Parathyroid tumors, pituitary tumors, pheochromocytoma	–
Gorlin syndrome (nevoid basal cell carcinoma syndrome)	PTCH1	Dominant	Basal cell cancers, brain tumors (desmoplastic medulloblastoma), fibromas (ovarian, cardiac), keratocystic odontogenic tumors	Course facies, frontal bossing, macrocephaly, pits on palms and soles, ribs, and vertebral anomalies
Hereditary retinoblastoma syndrome	RB1	Dominant	Retinoblastoma, glioma, melanoma, osteosarcoma, soft-tissue sarcomas, pineoblastoma	–
Rhabdoid tumor predisposition syndrome	SMARCB1/INI1	Dominant	Rhabdoid tumor, choroid plexus tumor, schwannoma, medulloblastoma	–
Hereditary Pheochromocytoma Paraganglioma (HPP) syndrome	SDHx genes	Dominant	Pheochromocytomas, paragangliomas, renal cancers, gastrointestinal stromal tumors, pituitary adenomas	–
DICER1 syndrome	DICER1 gene	Dominant	Familial pleuropulmonary blastoma (PPB), uterine-cervix embryonal rhabdomyosarcoma, cystic nephroma, ovarian Sertoli-Leydig cell tumor, pineoblastoma, pituitary blastoma, intraocular medulloepithelioma, and multinodular goiter	–
Constitutional mismatch repair deficiency syndrome (CMMRDS)	Biallelic: MSH2, MSH6, MLH1, EPCAM, PMS2	Recessive	Brain neoplasms (often anaplastic astrocytoma, glioblastoma, primitive neuroectodermal tumors, medulloblastoma), leukemia, lymphoma, neuroblastoma, Wilms' tumor, lynch syndrome-associated cancers, osteosarcoma, pilomatricoma, rhabdomyosarcoma, neurofibroma, colorectal and small bowel adenomatous polyposis	Hyper–/hypo-pigmented skin lesions including café-au-lait spots, immunodeficiency

Adapted from Refs. [1, 2, 4, 7–11]

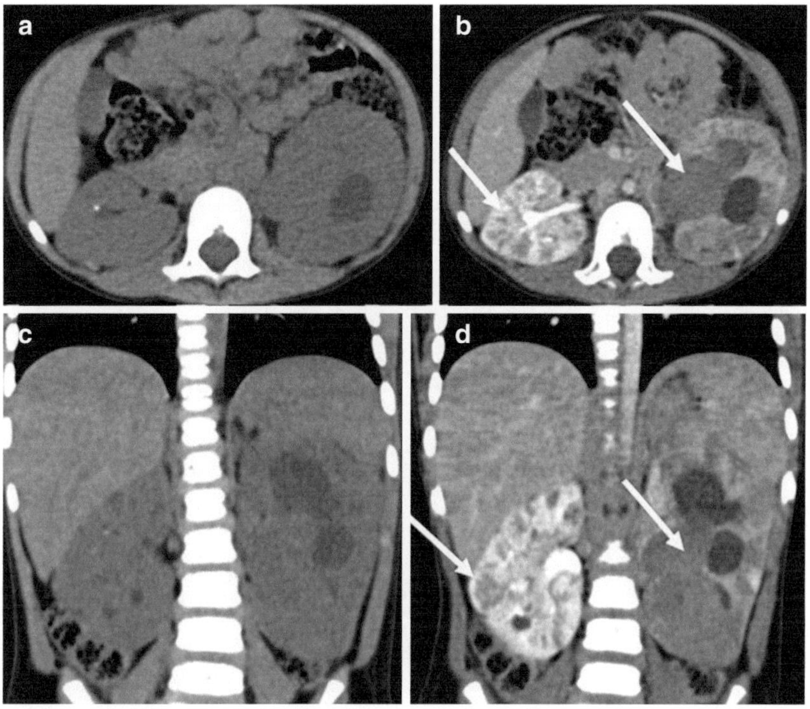

Fig. 8.2 2-year-old child with WAGR syndrome. (**a**, **c**) NCCT and (**b**, **d**) CECT abdomen images show bilateral solid Wilms' tumors (white arrows—biopsy proven)

8.3 Role of Imaging in CPS Diagnosis and Screening

Majority of the familiar CPS have standardized imaging protocols for diagnosis and surveillance. Ultrasound (USG), CT, and MRI are the frequently used imaging modalities. Two recently developed promising imaging techniques viz., WBMRI and functional imaging with FDG-positron emission tomography (PET)/CT have really made the assessment of CPS patients much easier especially for post-treatment surveillance. The WBMRI units use an arrangement of multiple phased-array coils that cover the entire body and aid in the dedicated evaluation of multiple organs with acceptable spatial resolution, soft tissue contrast, and anatomic whole-body coverage [12]. In patients with already diagnosed CPS, screening is aimed at detecting primary tumor recurrence as well as diagnosing any second or subsequently developed pathologically distinct tumors. So, the surveillance is not reduced in these patients after remission or treatment completion as is usually followed in the sporadic cancer survivors. Pediatric CPS patients are at greater risk of developing malignancies, necessitating regular surveillance. Screening guidelines are syndrome-specific and encompass a number of components, imaging being one. Screening in CPS may begin in infancy, childhood, or adolescence. Diagnosis of malignancy in asymptomatic children is promising with regard to upgrading management options and improving survival, however, the risk versus benefit of screening should always be contemplated [3]. Although CT and PET/CT are well-known imaging modalities for tumor imaging, multiple scans could predispose pediatric patients to cancer development because of excessive cumulative radiation exposure. Therefore, USG is the first-line imaging technique for screening, especially for pediatric abdominal imaging, being non-irradiating, non-invasive, and easily available. It allows quick evaluation of solid organ tumors and also guides further targeted cross-sectional imaging [6, 13]. MRI, due to better soft tissue contrast and no risk of ionizing radiation, has also been proved as a beneficial screening tool in this patient group because of young age at diagnosis and the requirement of long-lasting screening. Coronal

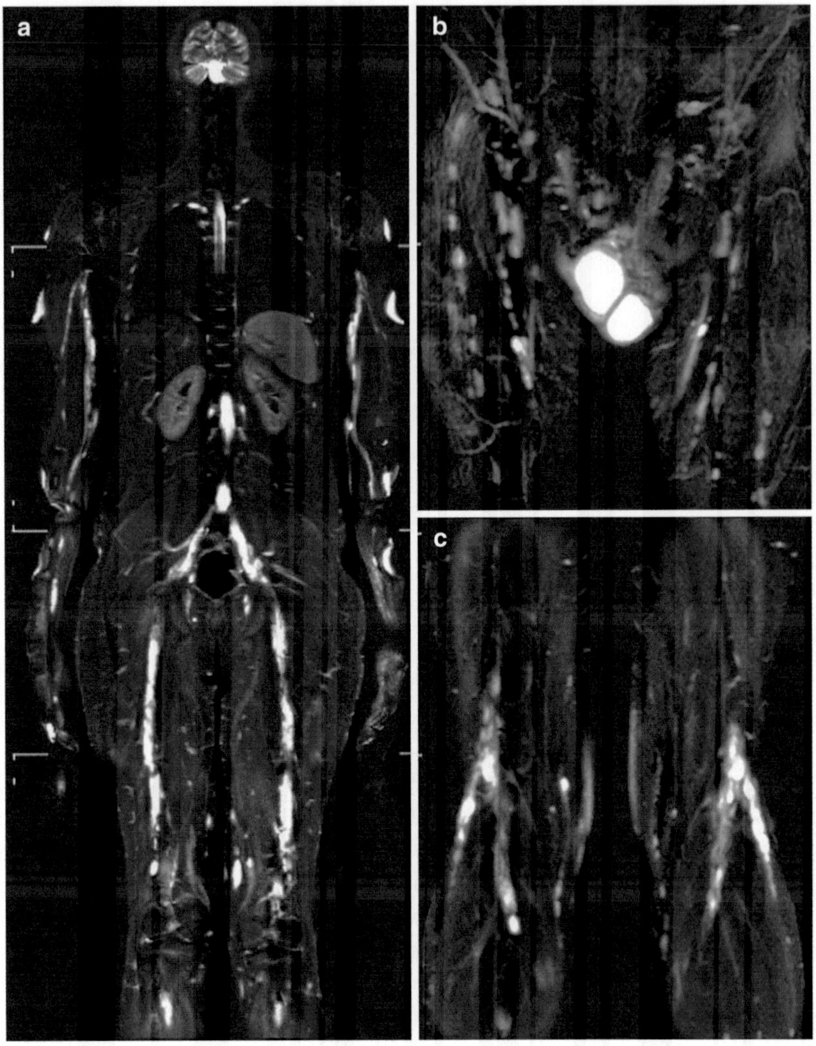

Fig. 8.3 Whole-body coronal STIR MRI in a case of NF1. (**a**) Whole-body pasted image shows multiple neurofibromas along bilateral upper and lower limb nerves. (**b**, **c**) Coronal STIR images acquired at thigh and knee levels showing multiple neurofibromas along the femoral and sciatic nerve and its branches

STIR (short tau inversion recovery) sequence is the basic sequence exploited in WBMRI (Fig. 8.3) because of its greater sensitivity to pick up hyperintense appearing pathologic lesions [14]. 100% sensitivity and 94% specificity of WBMRI have been reported for detection of tumors in children with hereditary CPS [15]. A new evolving sequence, whole-body diffusion-weighted MRI, is being increasingly acquired in WBMRI protocol due to shorter acquisition duration and greater sensitivity to pick bone marrow lesions. This sequence may be used instead of FDG-PET to detect tumors with low FDG uptake, e.g., neuroendocrine tumors and thyroid cancers [16].

Common Cancer Predisposition Syndromes Diagnostic and screening imaging recommendations for some common CPS are deliberated underneath.

8.4 Neurofibromatosis Type 1 (NF1)

NF1 or von Recklinghausen disease is an autosomal dominant hamartomatous neurocutaneous syndrome. It is the commonest phacomatosis triggered due to tumor suppressor NF1 gene mutation (chromosome 17q11.2). De novo mutations are responsible for the onset of the disorder in 50% of patients. The onset is in childhood, with at birth incidence of approximately 1 in 900–2800. There is a variable clinical course with typical features, as per the clinical criteria by the National Institutes of Health (1987), including café-au-lait macules, Lisch nodules, intertriginous freckling, cutaneous and deep plexiform neurofibromas occurring along peripheral nerves, bone dysplasia and optic pathway gliomas (Figs. 8.4 and 8.5) [4, 17, 18] (Box 8.2). About 2–3% of patients can harbor disfiguring plexiform neurofibromas. Some of the neurofibromas may undergo degeneration to malignant peripheral nerve sheath tumors (MPNST) with approximately 8–13% overall lifelong risk. Such lesions usually present with rapid growth and associated pain or neurodeficit [18, 19]. Around 1–2% risk of other neoplasms also exists (Table 8.1) [7, 8]. So, the high-risk anatomical regions warranting careful assessment in NF1 on WBMRI are the brain, orbits, peripheral nerves, skin, and bone marrow; uncommon sites being the adrenals, bowel, urogenital system, and soft tissue/muscle [14]. Patchy multifocal T2/FLAIR hyperintense parenchymal brain lesions known as focal areas of high signal intensity (FASI) may be seen involving the deep grey nuclei, cerebellum, or cerebellar peduncles and brainstem (Figs. 8.4 and 8.5). They are pathognomonic of NF1 and are anticipated to be caused due to aberrant myelination and/or gliosis [20]. CNS gliomas are the major subset of tumors in NF1, especially involving optic pathway (OPG), brainstem, and cerebellum. OPG are WHO grade 1 pilocytic astrocytomas with incidence of around 15% in children with NF1. Symptomatic OPG is most common in children less than 7 years of age [19].

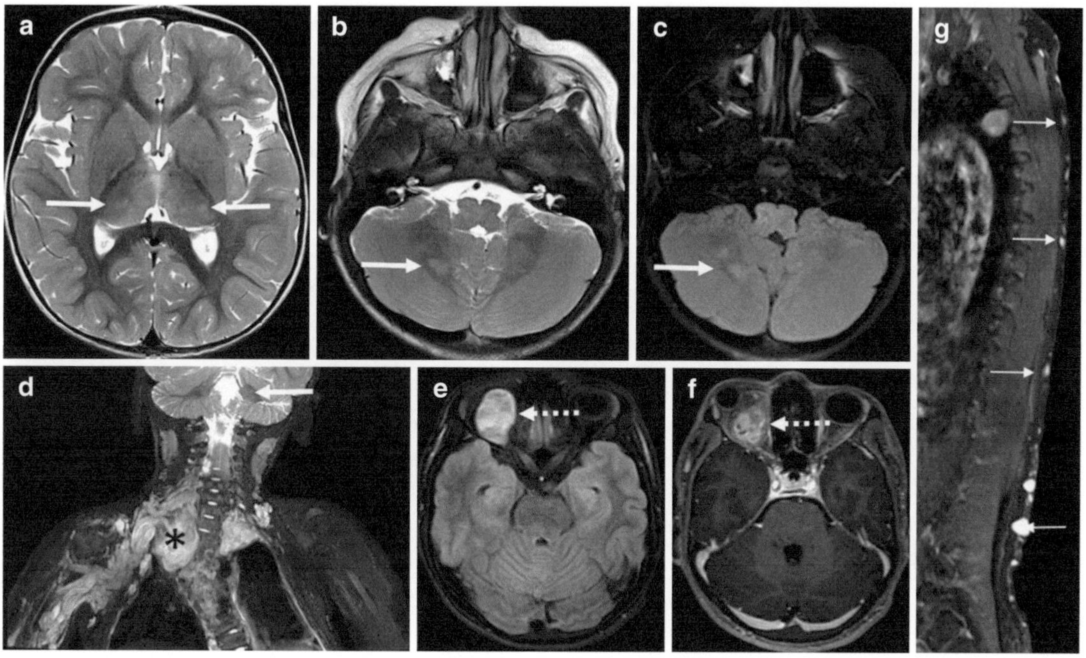

Fig. 8.4 NF1 in an 8-year-old child. (**a–d**) and a 13-year-old child (e-g). (**a, b**) Axial T2w, (**c**) axial FLAIR, and (**d**) coronal T2FS CUBE images show bithalamic and bilateral cerebellar white matter focal areas of high signal intensity (FASI—white arrows). A large right lower cervical-upper dorsal plexiform neurofibroma is also seen (* in **d**) with intraspinal extension. Note the dextroscoliosis. (**e, f**) Axial FLAIR and PCT1w images show right optic nerve glioma. (**g**) sagittal PCT1w image shows multiple cutaneous neurofibromas

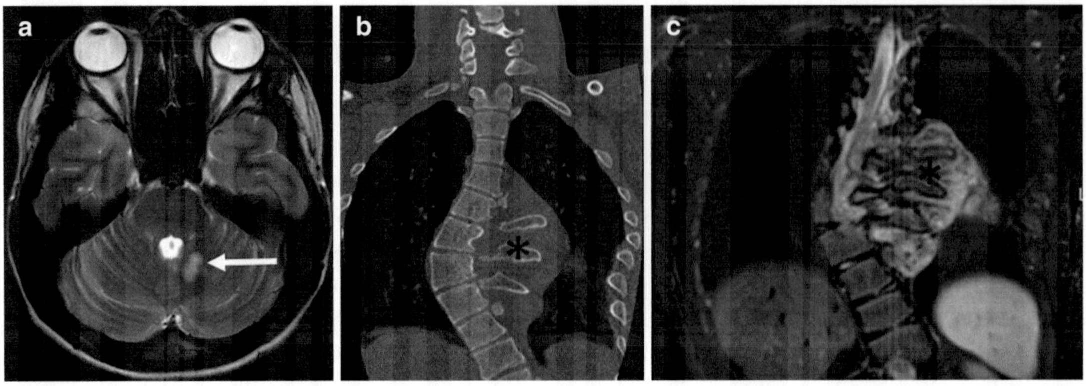

Fig. 8.5 Plexiform neurofibroma in an 11-year-old child with NF1. (**a**) Axial T2w MRI image shows FASI in left cerebellar white matter. (**b**) Coronal NCCT spine in bone window shows a left posterior mediastinal mass with lateral vertebral scalloping and dextroscoliosis. (**c**) Coronal T2-STIR MRI image shows the lesion having intraspinal extension

Box 8.2 (Adapted from Ref. [18])

NF1 Diagnostic criteria (>2 must be there)

1. $\geq$ 6 café-au-lait macules (greatest diameter > 5 mm in prepubertal patients and > 15 mm in postpubertal patients)
2. $\geq$2 neurofibromas of any type, or 1 plexiform neurofibroma
3. Axillary or inguinal freckling.
4. OPG.
5. $\geq$2 Lisch nodules
6. A distinct bony lesion, e.g., pseudarthrosis or sphenoid wing dysplasia.
7. A first degree relative with NF1 consistent with the earlier criteria.

Despite having widespread lesions in NF1, regular MRI surveillance and periodic WBMRI are not done unless the child is symptomatic or has a previously diagnosed tumor, due to low risk of malignancy in childhood. According to the American Association for Cancer Research (AACR) recommendations, a baseline WBMRI before transition to adulthood is recommended to direct long-term monitoring of MPNST (Table 8.2), with clinical and ophthalmic assessment that is done every 6–12 months up to 8 years of age. Female patients transitioning into adulthood should be counselled for increased risk of breast cancer (4–5 times greater than the general population) and for getting screened for the same due to moderate lifetime risk (20%) [14, 18].

Table 8.2 Screening recommendations for imaging in some of the CPS diagnosed in children

Syndrome	Screening
NF 1	Annual MRI, beginning in the teenage years Baseline whole-body MRI: 16–20 years of age
NF 2	Whole-body MRI baseline scan: scheduled on the basis of symptom onset and disease site. Annual brain and spine MRI with and without IV contrast beginning at the age of 10 years (two times annually in the first year to assess the rapid growth). Biennial MRI brain, if baseline scan is negative. MRI of the spine: every 2–3 years (6 monthly, if positive).
Tuberous sclerosis	Renal ultrasound: every 12–36 months. Brain and abdominal MRI or CT: every 12–36 months, until the age of 25 years. CT chest: every 2–3 years if positive for lung cysts; else every 5–10 years. Echocardiography: every 12–36 months from birth in asymptomatic kids; more often, if symptomatic.
Von Hippel-Lindau syndrome	Annual USG abdomen, commencing at the age of 8 years Annual abdominal MRI or CT (>16 years); earlier if biochemical abnormalities are found Brain and spine MRI: every 2 years commencing at 8 years of age and annually after 16 years of age
MEN1	Brain MRI: every 3–5 years, commencing between 5 and 10 years of age Chest and abdominal MRI or CT: every 2–4 years, commencing at 20 years of age Annual chest CT/octreotide or Ga-DOTATATE PET scan for carcinoids/NETs
MEN2	Abdominal MRI or CT: every 4–5 years Annual thyroid USG: beginning at 5 years of age or after thyroidectomy
Hereditary retinoblastoma	WBMRI: every 12 months from 8 to 10 years of age MRI brain: every 6 months to 5 years
HPP syndrome	WBMRI neck-to-pelvis, alternating with WBMRI chest-to-pelvis + dedicated neck MRI Biennially, beginning at the age of 6–8 years
Li-Fraumeni syndrome (birth to age 18 years)	Abdomen and pelvis USG: every 3–4 months for adrenocortical carcinoma Yearly MRI brain (first contrast-enhanced MRI; subsequently non-contrast MRI if the first MRI is negative and there are no new abnormalities) Yearly WBMRI for soft tissue and osseous sarcomas Brain MRI and WBMRI interleaved at 6-month intervals, if no general anesthesia is required
WAGR	USG for Wilms' tumor evaluation: every 3–4 months up to 8 years of age
CMMRD (and lynch) syndrome	WBMRI: Annually from 6 to 8 years age (when general anesthesia not needed) MRI brain: every 6 months after diagnosis USG abdomen and pelvis: every 6 months from the age of 1 year
Peutz-Jeghers syndrome	Yearly testicular examination: birth to teenage years Yearly testicular USG, commencing at teenage years CT or MR enterography, upper gastrointestinal endoscopy, and colonoscopy at 8 years of age; if no polyps, repeat at 18 years age; then every 3 years

Adapted based on the Refs. [1, 2, 4, 6, 9, 10, 18, 21–34]

8.5 Neurofibromatosis Type 2

Neurofibromatosis type 2 is an uncommon autosomal dominant neurocutaneous phakomatosis, caused by a heterogeneous germline NF2 gene mutation (chr 22q12). NF2 gene is responsible for the production of tumor suppressor schwannomin (merlin) protein that is expressed in the Schwann cells, neuronal, and meningeal cells. There is an incidence of nearly 1 in 25,000 live births with virtually 100% penetrance by the late adulthood [4, 21, 35]. It exhibits development of multiple neoplasms of central nervous system like multiple intracranial nerve sheath tumors

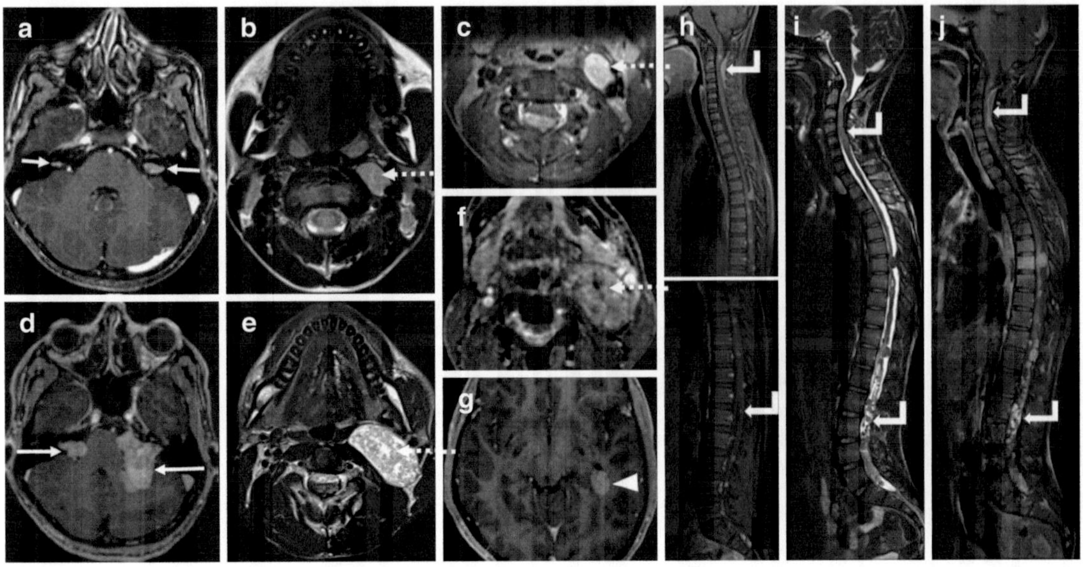

Fig. 8.6 2-year interval MRIs in a 14-year-old child with NF2. (**a**, **c**) Axial T1wPC and (**b**) T2w images show bilateral small intracanalicular vestibular schwannomas (white arrows) and left vagal schwannoma (dotted arrow). (**h**) Sagittal PCT1w image shows multiple small intramedullary and extramedullary-intradural lesions. (**d–g**, **i**, **j**) 2-year follow-up MRI. Note marked increase in the size of bilateral vestibular schwannomas (white arrows in **d**) and left vagal schwannoma (dotted arrows in **e**, **f**), new left atrial meningioma, and marked increase in the size and number of the spinal lesions (curved arrows in **i**, **j**)

(schwannomas), intracranial and spinal meningiomas, and spinal ependymomas (Fig. 8.6, Table 8.1). Neurofibromas can be rarely seen in NF2. The hallmark is simultaneous occurrence of bilateral and often multifocal vestibular nerve schwannomas that cause hearing and balance disturbances. Childhood malignancy is uncommon, with neoplasms usually being benign. Children may also present with a non-cranial schwannoma (Figs. 8.6 and 8.7) or an isolated meningioma [1, 7, 35]. Diagnosis is solely made on the basis of the clinical diagnostic criteria. The detection of NF2 gene mutation is not a requirement for the diagnosis. The Manchester criteria are the most extensively utilized for diagnosing this syndrome (Box 8.3).

Box 8.3: Manchester Criteria for Clinical Diagnosis of NF2 (Adapted from Refs. [35, 36])

Primary finding	Additional findings needed for diagnosis
Bilateral vestibular schwannomas	None
Family history	Unilateral vestibular schwannoma or two NF2-associated lesions (schwannoma, meningioma, glioma, neurofibroma, or cataract)
Unilateral vestibular schwannoma	Two NF2-associated lesions associated with the disorder (schwannoma, meningioma, glioma, neurofibroma, or cataract)
Multiple meningiomas	Unilateral vestibular schwannoma or two other NF2-associated lesions (schwannoma, glioma, neurofibromas, or cataract)

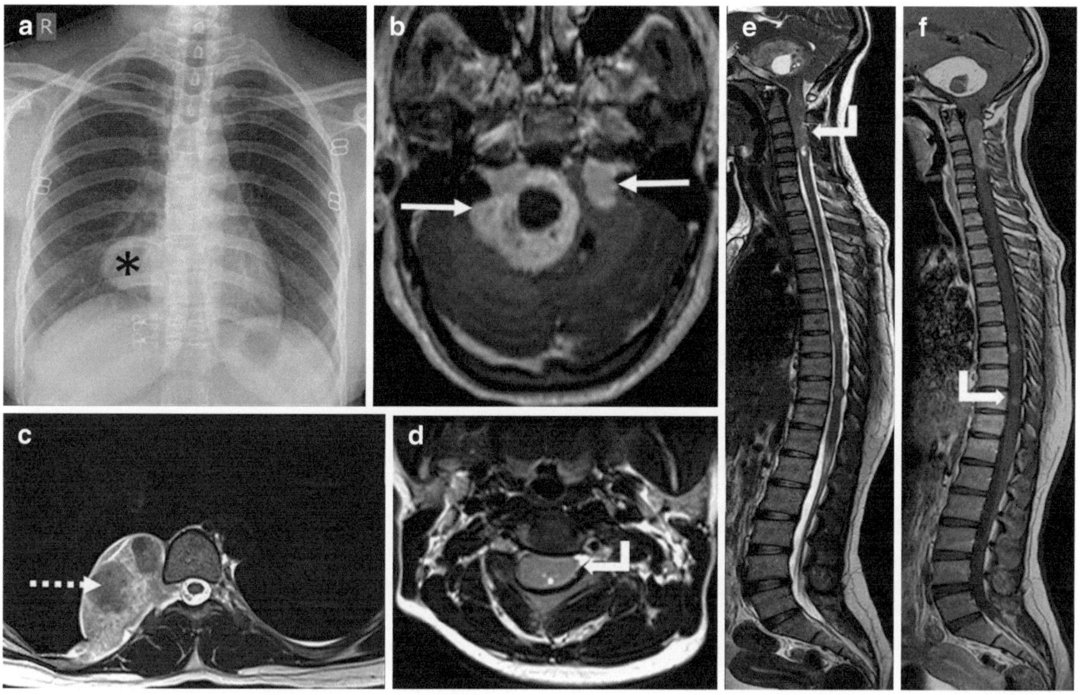

Fig. 8.7 NF2 in a 15-year-old child. (**a**) Chest X-ray PA view shows right posterior mediastinal mass. (**b**) Axial PCT1w image shows bilateral vestibular schwannomas. (**c**) Axial T2w image shows right posterior mediastinal neurogenic tumor with intraspinal extension. (**d**) Axial T2w image at C2 vertebra level shows intramedullary ependymoma. (**e**, **f**) Sagittal T2w and PCT1w images show multiple intramedullary ependymomas

The 2016 AACR Childhood Cancer Predisposition Workshop expert panel advocates MRI brain and spine (with and without intravenous gadolinium contrast) yearly commencing at 10 years of age. Screening may commence earlier in symptomatic children or with high-risk genotypes. Imaging protocol must include high resolution (1–3 mm slice thickness) heavily T2-weighted 3D sequence through the internal auditory meati [1, 21]. If a suggestive lesion is identified, follow-up scan should be performed after 6 months to review the tumor growth. If the baseline imaging does not reveal NF2 features, surveillance frequency may be reduced to biennial MRI brain and spine MRI at 24–36 months interval (Table 8.2). WBMRI may be acquired depending on the symptom onset and known sites of symptoms. As for many other CPSs, the safe time to discontinue the surveillance has not been clearly recognized [9, 21].

8.6 Li–Fraumeni Syndrome (LFS)

LFS is also autosomal dominant and is the most commonly recognized inherited CPS. It predisposes to a greater risk of 6 core cancers including osteosarcomas, soft tissue sarcomas, premenopausal breast carcinoma, CNS tumors, leukemia, and adrenocortical carcinomas as well as of other less common neoplasms (Table 8.1). It results from a loss-of-function germline mutation of TP53 tumor suppressor gene (chromosome 17p13.1) [1, 13]. Carcinoma breast is the most common malignant neoplasm in LFS (30%). A prior history of any of the childhood choroid plexus carcinoma, adrenocortical carcinoma, rhabdomyosarcoma, or multiple childhood cancers is dramatically related to TP53 mutation. Some tumors like childhood adrenocortical carcinoma are so specific for LFS that genetic counseling and TP53 gene testing can be contemplated regardless of positive family history [6, 13]. The lifetime risk for cancer development is 70% for males and ~ 100% for females. There is a risk for radiation-induced second malignancies as well, so radiation therapy is generally avoided and the use of CT and radiography should be minimalized [4, 9]. Surveillance (Table 8.2) should commence as early as a clinical (phenotype suggesting LFS- Box 8.4) or genetic (TP53 mutation) diagnosis has been made.

Box 8.4: Clinical Diagnostic Criteria for LFS (Adapted from Refs. [10, 37])

Classic LFS diagnosis is established when all the following criteria are met in a patient:

1. A sarcoma diagnosed before 45 years of age.
2. A first-degree relative (parent, sibling, or child) with any cancer before 45 years of age.
3. A first-degree or second-degree (grandparent, aunt/uncle, niece/nephew, or grandchild) relative with any cancer before 45 years of age or a sarcoma at any age.

Chompret Criteria for Clinical Diagnosis of LFS. A diagnosis of LFS and carrying out TP53 gene mutation testing is contemplated for someone having a personal and family history that meets 1 of the following 3 criteria:

1. An LFS-spectrum tumor, detected prior to 46 years of age (osteosarcoma, soft-tissue sarcoma, adrenal cortical carcinoma, brain tumor, lung cancer, leukemia, or pre-menopausal breast cancer) **and.**

   At least one first- or second-degree relative harboring an LFS-spectrum tumor, except breast cancer if the person has breast cancer before 56 years of age or with multiple tumors
2. An individual having multiple tumors, except multiple breast tumors, 2 of which belong to the LFS spectrum and first one diagnosed before 46 years of age.
3. An individual having choroid plexus tumor or adrenocortical carcinoma, regardless of positive family history.

8.7 von Hippel-Lindau Syndrome (VHL)

VHL is an inherited autosomal dominant multisystem disorder caused by a germline inactivation mutation in VHL gene (chromosome 3p25.3). VHL is a tumor suppressor gene whose mutation leads to the upregulation of several vascular and somatic growth factors, e.g., vascular endothelial growth factor. This, consequently, results in the development of multiorgan vascular tumors. The prevalence of VHL ranges from 1 in 30,000–50,000. Central nervous system (CNS), kidney, and pancreas are the most frequently involved organs [10, 13, 38]. VHL is associated with various endocrine and non-endocrine, benign and malignant neoplasms (Table 8.1). Children with VHL may stay clinically occult until the symptoms become severe and neoplasms grow sufficiently large, escalating the risks linked to surgical resection [1].

Box 8.5: Clinical Diagnostic Criteria for VHL (Adapted from Ref. [39])

1. Positive family history (first/second degree relative with diagnosis of VHL or ≥ 1 VHL-related tumor) **AND** 1 VHL-related tumor.
2. Patients without a family history: ≥2 HB (CNS/ retinal) **OR** 1 HB and 1 VHL-related manifestation.

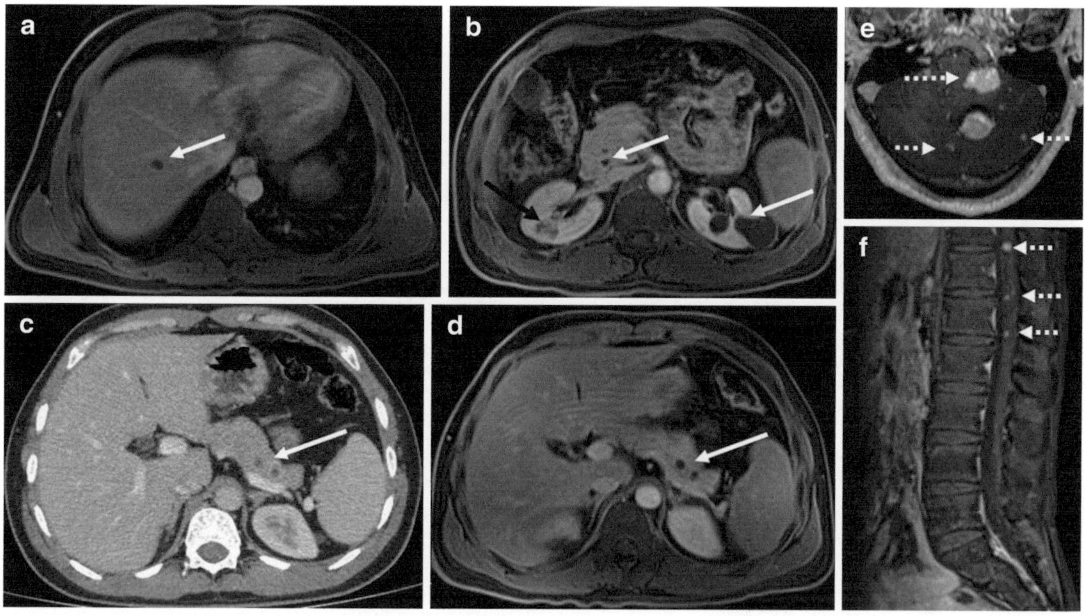

Fig. 8.8 VHL syndrome in a 16-year-old child. (**a**, **b**, and **d**) Axial post-contrast MRI abdomen images show small cysts in liver, pancreas, and left kidney (white arrows). The small right renal heterogeneously enhancing lesion (black arrow in **b**) is biopsy-proven RCC. (**c**) Axial CECT abdomen image shows cysts in pancreatic distal body and tail (white arrow). (**e**) Axial PCT1w MRI brain and (**f**) sagittal PCT1w MRI images show multiple cerebellar and spinal hemangioblastomas (dashed arrows)

CNS hemangioblastomas are the most common tumors in VHL (70% cases) and frequently occur in the retina, cerebellum, and spinal cord. They are usually multiple (Fig. 8.8) with a high recurrence rate and are observed with highest frequency in cerebellum (52%), followed by the cervicothoracic spinal cord (44%), and the brainstem (18%) [4, 10]. MRI demonstrates a cyst with nodule appearance (with intense enhancement of the mural nodule and non-enhancing cyst wall) or a solid enhancing nodular mass. If a cerebellar hemangioblastoma is diagnosed, screening spine MRI for cord hemangioblastomas is compulsory as they generally coexist. Due to the limited role of imaging, the diagnostic workup for retinal lesions comprises ophthalmoscopy and fluorescein angiography. On MRI, a retinal hypervascular nodular lesion and/or retinal detachment may be observed [10].

Renal cell carcinoma (RCC) is another common VHL-associated malignancy (Fig. 8.9) with an average 70% lifetime risk of developing RCC. RCC in VHL are often several in number, predisposed to recurrence, and are the leading cause of mortality. Image-guided radio-frequency or cryo-ablation of RCCs is favored over surgery in VHL, especially for multiple and small-sized (< 3 cm) lesions, because it considerably increases cancer-free survival [6, 10]. Around 20% cases of VHL harbor endolymphatic sac tumors with their bilateral occurrence being a pathognomic feature. MRI brain must include thin section high-resolution T2-weighted images at the level of the internal auditory meati in VHL patients, to evaluate for these lesions. Pancreatic cysts are seen in approximately 75% of patients (Fig. 8.8). on imaging, pancreatic serous cystadenomas display the typical "cluster of cysts" appearance with central scar. They are considered no touch lesions, unless symptomatic. Pancreatic neuroendocrine tumors (NET) harboring a malignant potential can be detected in up to 15% cases; are hypervascular and, on imaging, have early enhancement and washout. There is a significant role of endoscopic ultrasound in the diagnosis, surveillance, and interventional management (tissue sampling and/or

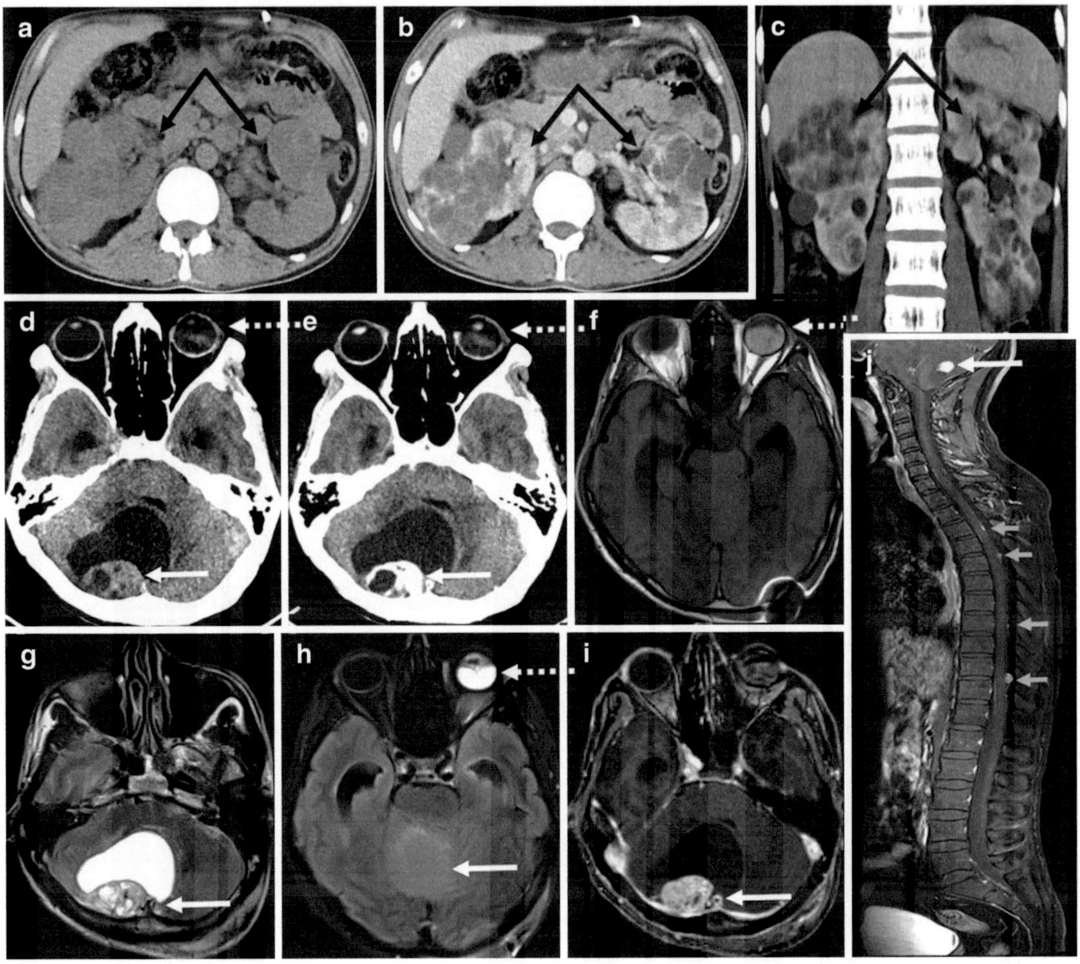

Fig. 8.9 VHL syndrome in a 14-year-old child. (**a**) Axial non-contrast (NCCT), (**b**, **c**) axial and coronal contrast-enhanced CT (CECT) abdomen images show bilateral multiple heterogeneously enhancing RCCs (black arrows). (**d**) Axial NCCT and (**e**) CECT brain showing right cerebellar lesion having 'cyst with avidly enhancing mural nodule' appearance (white arrow). Note the hyperdense left vitreal hemorrhage (dashed arrow). (**f–i**) T1w, T2w, FLAIR and post-contrast (PC) T1w images showing cerebellar hemangioblastoma (white arrows) and the T1 hyperintense left vitreal hemorrhage. (**j**) Sagittal PCT1w MRI of spine shows multiple spinal hemangioblastomas (small grey arrows)

targeted ablation) of NET in VHL. MRI with diffusion-weighted imaging is more sensitive than CT in pancreatic NET detection, comparable to PET/CT [1, 10].

Pheochromocytomas are observed in around 7–18% of VHL patients and do not often present with clinical or biochemical features of catecholamine excess. On imaging, they show early intense arterial phase enhancement with rapid venous phase washout. Calcification, necrotic areas, and hemorrhage can be seen. Meta-iodobenzylguanidine scan can aid in localizing the tumor and to detect occult metastases. WBMRI has been shown to have comparable accuracy to the radionuclide scan for pheochromocytomas [6, 10, 13]. Two subtypes of

VHL have been described based on the low risk (type 1) and high risk (type 2) of pheochromocytoma [40]. Tumor-to-tumor metastasis, a characteristic phenomenon seen in VHL, refers to metastasis from RCC, pheochromocytoma, and NET to existing hemangioblastomas that is suspected when there is abrupt change in hemangioblastoma size [10].

In VHL, lifelong surveillance is recommended and besides physical examination, blood pressure measurement, annual urine, or plasma metanephrine levels, audiology and ophthalmology evaluation, there is a significant role of imaging. By 8 years of age, monitoring for CNS hemangioblastomas should be commenced with biennial brain and spine MRI. Surveillance guidelines for visceral (renal and pancreatic malignancies) manifestations of VHL have recommended annual abdominal MRI starting in teenage years (Table 8.2). Because the sensitivity of biochemical screening is high for detecting pheochromocytomas in VHL, regular surveillance imaging is not advocated [1, 10, 22].

8.8 Tuberous Sclerosis Complex (TSC)

TSC is a neurocutaneous syndrome that follows an autosomal dominant inheritance pattern. Clinically, it presents with the classic triad of epilepsy, mental retardation, and facial angiofibroma/adenoma sebaceum. The triad is, however, observed in only 30–40% cases. The syndrome is triggered due to TSC1 or TSC2 gene mutations (chromosomes 9q34 and 16p13 respectively) and is characterized by multiple hamartomatous lesions involving various organ systems. The estimated prevalence is one in 6000–12,000 and around 2/third cases are sporadic [6, 41]. The updated international TSC diagnostic criteria have 11 major and 7 minor features (Box 8.6).

Box 8.6: Clinical Diagnostic Criteria for TS (Adapted from Ref. [42])

Definite TSC: Either 2 major features **or** 1 major and ≥ 2 minor features
Possible TSC: Either 1 major feature **or** ≥ 2 minor features

Major features	Minor features
Angiofibromas (≥3) or fibrous cephalic plaque	'Confetti' skin lesions
Shagreen patch	Dental enamel pits: ≥3 for the entire dentition
Hypomelanotic macules (≥3, at least 5 mm diameter)	Non-renal hamartomas
Ungual fibromas (≥2)	Intraoral fibromas (≥2)
Multiple cortical tubers and/or cerebral white matter radial migration lines	Multiple renal cysts
Subependymal giant cell astrocytoma (SEGA)	Retinal achromic patch
Subependymal nodule (≥2)	Sclerotic bone lesions
Multiple retinal hamartomas	
Cardiac rhabdomyoma	
Angiomyolipomas (AML) (≥2)[a]	
Lymphangioleiomyomatosis (LAM)[a]	

[a]A combination of the two major features, AML and LAM, without other features does not meet the criteria for a definite diagnosis of TSC.

The commonest intracranial feature of TSC is cortical tubers (~ 95% cases). On CT, they appear as hypodense areas of gyral expansion. MRI exhibits hypointensity on T1-weighted and hyperintensity on T2-weighted images, with the lesions being non-enhancing in greater than 90% cases (Fig. 8.10). Uncommonly, a cyst-like appearance may be observed on MRI. These tubers are linked with more severe epilepsy phenotypes. Seizures are witnessed in up to 90% TSC patients. Tubers associated with medically refractory seizures often necessitate surgery [6, 10]. Presurgical evaluation with ^{18}F FDG-PET/MRI in TSC is an important method to noninvasively identify the tubers responsible for refractory epilepsy [43]. Subependymal nodules appear T1 isointense and T2 iso- to hyperintense and are more predisposed to calcify compared with cortical tubers. Cerebral white matter radial migration lines are the most frequent white matter abnormality recognized in TSC. SEGA, prevalent in approximately 1.7–26% of patients with TSC, are typically the caudothalamic groove lesions at the foramen of Monro showing serial growth (Fig. 8.10). The usual presentation is in the late childhood with acute decompensated obstructive hydrocephalus. On MRI, they are heterogeneous lesions with contrast enhancement. Surgical resection is the customary treatment [44]. LAM is characterized by marked female preponderance with symptom onset in the middle age, and is observed as multiple thin-walled lung cysts on imaging. Association with TSC is seen in ~15% cases of LAM. Around 20% cases of renal AML are seen in TSC patients, and approximately 80% of TSC patients harbor AMLs (Fig. 8.10). Although demonstrable on CT, fat within AML is best appreciated on T1 in- and opposed-phase images on MRI. Multifocal and bilateral AMLs present a surgical challenge, and thus image-

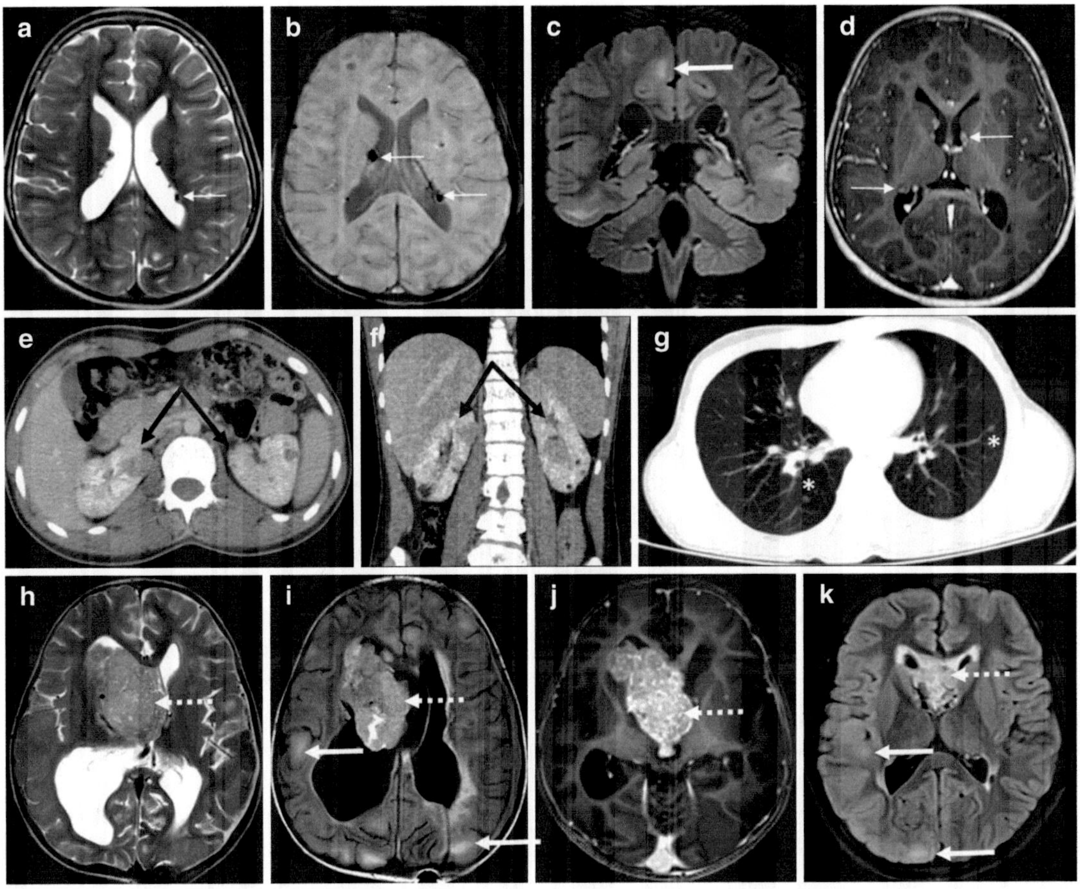

Fig. 8.10 (**a–g**) Tuberous sclerosis complex in a 6-year-old child. (**a**, **b**, and **d**) Axial T2w, SWI and PCT1w show multiple subependymal nodules (thin white arrows), (**c**) coronal FLAIR image showing multiple cortical tubers (thick white arrow), (**e**, **f**) axial and coronal CECT images show bilateral multiple renal angiomyolipomas (black arrows), (**g**) axil CT in lung window shows few bilateral tiny lung nodules (asterisk *). (**h–j**) TSC in a 9-year-old child with subependymal giant cell astrocytoma (SEGA). Axial T2w, FLAIR, and PCT1w images respectively show multiple non-enhancing hyperintense cortical tubers (white arrows) and avidly enhancing SEGA (dashed arrow). (**k**) Axial FLAIR image showing multiple cortical tubers and SEGA in another 6-year-old child with TSC

guided radiofrequency or cryo-ablation techniques are exploited, especially for smaller lesions. The incidence of renal cell carcinoma is slightly high (~4%) [4, 10]. Cardiac rhabdomyomas, detected in approximately 60% of children, are typically asymptomatic and appear as well-defined ventricular septal masses on MRI, which are T1 isointense to myocardium, and T2 hyperintense [10]. The updated International TSC Consensus Group surveillance guidelines published in 2021 have been summarized in Table 8.2.

8.9 Hereditary Retinoblastoma (RB)

RB is the most frequent childhood malignant intraocular neoplasm with an approximate incidence of 1/17,000 live births. Most RB cases are sporadic and only around 10% of RBs are familial. Approximately 10% of unilateral RB and 100% of bilateral RB cases carry a germline RB1 gene (chr 13q14.2) mutation. A de novo occurrence is more common than an autosomal dominant inheritance by the approximate ratio of 4:1. Uncommonly, hereditary RB may be triggered by somatic MYCN amplification mutation [9, 23, 45]. Almost 2/third of RBs are diagnosed before the age of 2 years, and approximately 95% by the age of 5 years. Bilateral tumors (generally hereditary) present at 8 months median age, as compared to the unilateral tumors with 2 years median age of presentation [1, 11]. Hereditary RB also predisposes (3–5% cases) to the development of midline intracranial embryonal tumors and pineoblastomas (trilateral RB) and exaggerate the odds of developing another (often treatment-related) primary tumor; for instance, osteosarcoma, soft tissue sarcoma, brain and nasal tumors, cutaneous, lung, breast, bladder, and uterine neoplasms and other tumors of the orbit. The median age of developing a second primary neoplasm is between 15 and 17 years [1, 9, 46]. Surveillance imaging should be performed along with the intraocular screening and genetic testing. Once the RB mutation is recognized, a routine brain MRI every 6 months until 5 years of age is suggested. There are no distinguished imaging guidelines for the assessment of RB survivors for second malignancies. Although there is no consensus for WBMRI, yet because of an enhanced risk of sarcoma development, a few authors have also suggested it annually after 8–10 years of age [1, 23]. The main anatomical locations for review on the WBMRI are brain, orbits, soft tissue, and bones. The AACR WBMRI screening recommendations are mentioned in Table 8.2 [14].

8.10 Multiple Endocrine Neoplasia Syndrome (MEN)

MEN group of disorders are autosomal dominant syndromes characterized by concurrent tumors in ≥2 endocrine organs. Two major types have been classified: MEN1 (Wermer's syndrome) and MEN2 (Sipple's syndrome). MEN1 affects males and females equally irrespective of age with an estimated prevalence of 2 in 100,000. MEN2 is more prevalent (1 in 200,000 live births) [10, 47, 48]. MEN4 is a newly designated type comprising patients having risk of development of pituitary and parathyroid tumors [1].

8.11 MEN1

MEN 1 predisposes to the tumors of parathyroid and pituitary glands, and pancreas. Germline mutations in tumor suppressor gene MEN1 (chromosome 11q13) lead to its development. Primary hyperparathyroidism is the commonest abnormality (90–100%), caused due to single or several parathyroid adenomas. Nuclear medicine scans for parathyroid adenomas utilize technetium^{99m} (^{99m}Tc) sestamibi where there is asymmetric uptake and longer retention of the tracer in parathyroid adenomas compared with the thyroid gland. On multiphase neck CECT, there is early arterial phase enhancement and venous washout with a > 90% sensitivity of parathyroid adenoma detection [6, 49]. CT is, however, inferior to dynamic MRI to demonstrate the hypervascularity of parathyroid adenomas. Quantitative assessment of perfusion parameters of the adenomas is possible with contrast-time curve that demonstrates a greater peak enhancement, rapid time-to-peak, and quicker wash-in and wash-out in comparison to thyroid/cervical lymph nodes [50]. Entero-pancreatic NET (30–70%), mostly, are functional in MEN1 with low risk of malignancy and are a major cause of morbidity and mortality. Endoscopic ultrasound exhibits a higher sensitivity (100%) and specificity (95%) than transabdominal USG. On cross-sectional imaging, they are seen as a well-defined mass with avid arterial enhancement [51]. Anterior pituitary tumors (30–40%) are generally microadenomas (~66%) with prolactinoma being the commonest one, and are best visualized on dynamic sellar MRI. ^{68}Ga-DOTATATE PET/CT can distinguish functioning and nonfunctioning tumors and may also detect residual normal pituitary tissue post-surgery and recurrence of functioning adenomas [52]. Surveillance protocol for MEN1 is mentioned in Table 8.2.

8.12 MEN2

Germline RET proto-oncogene mutations (10q11) are responsible for MEN2 syndrome [53]. MEN2 is subclassified into MEN2A, MEN2B, and familial MTC. The common feature is MTC, observed in 90–95% cases. MEN2-associated MTC present earlier are multicentric as compared to the sporadic MTC. MEN2B is less frequent than MEN2A but more aggressive. USG should be done for initial assessment in all MTC patients where it is seen as large solid strikingly hypoechoic mass with/without microcalcifications, showing marked vascularity [6]. Evaluation should be done for local invasion, nodal (cervical and mediastinal), hepatic, and lung metastases. American Thyroid Association (2015) has recommended CECT neck and chest, hepatic triple-phase CECT, MRI abdomen, and bone scintigraphy in patients with high serum calcitonin (>500 pg/dL) or widespread neck disease to exclude remote metastasis [10, 54]. European Association of Nuclear Medicine guidelines (2020) have recommended the use of ^{18}F-FDOPA-PET/CT in persistent MTC. Use of ^{18}F-FDG-PET/CT is restricted to aggressive MTC variants [55]. Benign or malignant pheochromocytomas (usually bilateral) may be associated with MEN2; so it is mandatory to exclude pheochromocytoma on confirmation of RET mutation and the screening (biochemical or imaging) should commence in the childhood (5 years age). ^{123}I-MIBG, due to high sensitivity (87–90%), is recommended if cross-sectional imaging is inconclusive or shows unilateral disease. Prophylactic thyroidectomy is recommended for patients having the mutated gene. When MTC and pheochromocytoma are diagnosed synchronously, pheochromocytoma should be managed first. Parathyroid tumors in MEN2A need to be investigated similar to MEN1. MEN2B does not predispose to parathyroid tumors so screening for those is not needed [10, 24]. Surveillance protocol for MEN2 is mentioned in Table 8.2.

8.13 Hereditary Paraganglioma Pheochromocytoma Syndromes (HPP)

HPP are also autosomal dominant syndromes, characterized by multiple, generally benign neural crest neoplasms that are symmetrically dispersed from the skull base to pelvis along the paravertebral axis [56]. They are caused due to germline pathogenic SDHx gene mutations (multiple genes encoding the succinate dehydrogenase enzyme) or mutations in certain non-SDHx genes like MAX gene, with near 90% penetrance [6, 9]. Moreover, syndromic patients can also develop gastrointestinal stromal tumors (GIST), renal cancers, and pituitary adenomas [22]. There are four types of HPP syndromes (types 1, 2, 3, and 4) depending upon the mutated genes, of which types 1 and 4 are more common. HPP1 is characterized by multiple head and neck PGs (60–79% of patients). The risk of pheochromocytoma and extra-adrenal PGs is comparatively lower (~16–21%). These are usually benign tumors with lower malignant potential. The common tumors detected in HPP4 patients are extraadrenal PGs (~52–84%) and pheochromocytomas (~18–28%) with low risk of head and neck PGs. HPP4 is characterized by an increased risk of malignancy (20–41%) [57, 58]. A family history of PGs, bilateral and multiple PGs, and earlier age of onset of PGs and pheochromocytomas are suggestive of HPP syndromes. Detected from the age of 6 years, these tumors may manifest by hormonal effect (catecholamine secreting tumors) or by mass effect. The common sites of head and neck PGs are carotid bifurcation (carotid body tumor), along the vagus nerve (glomus vagale), jugular foramen (glomus jugulare), and middle ear cavity (glomus tympanicum). On CT, they appear as avidly enhancing tumors with local bony erosions, typically observed with glomus jugulare at jugular foramen. MRI shows a characteristic salt-and-pepper appearance on T1-weighted images (hypointensities due to flow voids and hyperintensities due to hemorrhage) and marked contrast enhancement. Whole-body screening can be accomplished by nuclear imaging with ^{123}I-MIBG or ^{111}In-octreotide [6]. Imaging surveillance should commence by the age of 6–8 years with biennial WBMRI and optional dedicated neck MRI. The main anatomical locations for review on WBMRI are the adrenals, paravertebral sympathetic trunk, aortocaval region, organ of Zukerkandl, carotid body, vas deferens, kidneys, and bowel. Routine screening for GIST is not recommended, however, a CECT/FDG-PET CT should be acquired in symptomatic patients with anemia or gastric bleeding [15, 22, 25]. AACR WBMRI screening recommendations are stated in Table 8.2.

8.14 Conclusion

In this chapter, we discussed the vital role of imaging in the diagnosis and screening of children with CPS. Early detection of cancers is crucial to improve the outcomes in this population. Imaging recommendations are being amended with more and more understanding of the genetic components of these disorders. It is imperative to have a standardized image interpretation approach and communication with the multidisciplinary oncology team so that the best possible care can be offered to the affected children and their families.

Acknowledgments Dr. Jitender Saini, MD, DM; Professor, Dept. of Neuroimaging and Interventional Radiology (NIIR), NIMHANS, Bangalore.

References

1. Anupindi SA, Smith EA, Chauvin NA. Imaging of children with cancer predisposition syndromes. In: Voss SD, McHugh K, editors. Imaging in pediatric oncology. Cham: Springer; 2019. p. 369–86. (Pediatric Oncology). Available from: http://link.springer.com/10.1007/978-3-030-03777-2_20.
2. Grant CN, Rhee D, Tracy ET, Aldrink JH, Baertschiger RM, Lautz TB, et al. Pediatric solid tumors and associated cancer predisposition syndromes: Workup, management, and surveillance. A summary from the APSA Cancer Committee. J Pediatr Surg. 2022;57(3):430–42. https://doi.org/10.1016/j.jpedsurg.2021.08.008. PMID: 34503817.
3. Al-Sarhani H, Gottumukkala RV, Grasparil ADS 2nd, Tung EL, Gee MS, Greer MLC. Screening of cancer predisposition syndromes. Pediatr Radiol. 2022;52(2):401–17. https://doi.org/10.1007/s00247-021-05023-w. PMID: 33791839.
4. Kahraman G, Çeltikçi P, Karasu Ş. Radiological screening for hereditary cancer predisposition syndromes. In: Dilek ON, Uranues S, Latifi R, editors. Prophylactic surgery. Cham: Springer; 2021. p. 497–512. Available from: https://link.springer.com/10.1007/978-3-030-66853-2_42.
5. Bakhuizen JJ, Hopman SMJ, Bosscha MI, Dommering CJ, Van Den Heuvel-Eibrink MM, Hol JA, et al. Assessment of cancer predisposition syndromes in a national cohort of children with a neoplasm. JAMA Netw Open. 2023;6(2):e2254157. https://doi.org/10.1001/jamanetworkopen.2022.54157. PMID: 36735256.
6. Tiwari R, Singh AK, Somwaru AS, Menias CO, Prasad SR, Katabathina VS. Radiologist's primer on imaging of common hereditary cancer syndromes. Radiographics. 2019;39(3):759–78. https://doi.org/10.1148/rg.2019180171. PMID: 31059391.
7. Ahlawat S, Fayad LM, Khan MS, Bredella MA, Harris GJ, Evans DG, et al. Current whole-body MRI applications in the neurofibromatoses: NF1, NF2, and schwannomatosis. Neurology. 2016;87(7 Suppl 1):S31–9. https://doi.org/10.1212/WNL.0000000000002929. PMID: 27527647; PMCID: PMC5578359.

8. Boyd KP, Korf BR, Theos A. Neurofibromatosis type 1. J Am Acad Dermatol. 2009;61(1):1-14; quiz 15–6. https://doi.org/10.1016/j.jaad.2008.12.051. PMID: 19539839.
9. Greer MLC. Imaging of cancer predisposition syndromes. Pediatr Radiol. 2018;48(9):1364–75. https://doi.org/10.1007/s00247-018-4113-0. PMID: 30078044.
10. Majithia J, Mahajan A, Vaish R, Prakash G, Patwardhan S, Sarin R. Imaging recommendations for diagnosis, staging, and management of hereditary malignancies. Indian J Med Paediatr Oncol. 2023;44(03):287–301. https://doi.org/10.1055/s-0042-1760325.
11. Garber JE, Offit K. Hereditary cancer predisposition syndromes. J Clin Oncol. 2005;23(2):276–92. https://doi.org/10.1200/JCO.2005.10.042. PMID: 15637391.
12. Schmidt GP, Haug AR, Schoenberg SO, Reiser MF. Whole-body MRI and PET-CT in the management of cancer patients. Eur Radiol. 2006;16(6):1216–25.
13. Monsalve J, Kapur J, Malkin D, Babyn PS. Imaging of cancer predisposition syndromes in children. Radiographics. 2011;31(1):263–80. https://doi.org/10.1148/rg.311105099. Erratum in: Radiographics. 2011;31(2):624. PMID: 21257945.
14. Greer MLC, Voss SD, States LJ. Pediatric Cancer predisposition imaging: focus on whole-body MRI. Clin Cancer Res. 2017;23(11):e6–e13. https://doi.org/10.1158/1078-0432.CCR-17-0515. PMID: 28572262.
15. Anupindi SA, Bedoya MA, Lindell RB, Rambhatla SJ, Zelley K, Nichols KE, et al. Diagnostic performance of whole-body MRI as a tool for cancer screening in children with genetic cancer-predisposing conditions. AJR Am J Roentgenol. 2015;205(2):400–8.
16. Kwee TC, Takahara T, Ochiai R, Koh DM, Ohno Y, Nakanishi K, et al. Complementary roles of whole-body diffusion-weighted MRI and 18F-FDG PET: the state of the art and potential applications. J Nucl Med Off Publ Soc Nucl Med. 2010;51(10):1549–58.
17. De Bella K, Szudek J, Friedman JM. Use of the National Institutes of Health Criteria for Diagnosis of Neurofibromatosis 1 in Children. Pediatrics. 2000;105(3):608–14. https://doi.org/10.1542/peds.105.3.608. PMID: 10699117.
18. Evans DGR, Salvador H, Chang VY, Erez A, Voss SD, Schneider KW, et al. Cancer and central nervous system tumor surveillance in pediatric neurofibromatosis 1. Clin Cancer Res. 2017;23(12):e46–e53. https://doi.org/10.1158/1078-0432.CCR-17-0589. PMID: 28620004.
19. Ferner RE, Huson SM, Thomas N, Moss C, Willshaw H, Evans DG, et al. Guidelines for the diagnosis and management of individuals with neurofibromatosis 1. J Med Genet. 20067;44(2):81–8. https://doi.org/10.1136/jmg.2006.045906. PMID: 17105749.
20. Calvez S, Levy R, Calvez R, Roux CJ, Grévent D, Purcell Y, et al. Focal Areas of High Signal Intensity in Children with Neurofibromatosis Type 1: Expected Evolution on MRI. AJNR Am J Neuroradiol. 2020;41(9):1733–39. https://doi.org/10.3174/ajnr.A6740. PMID: 32816766.
21. Evans DGR, Salvador H, Chang VY, Erez A, Voss SD, Druker H, et al. Cancer and central nervous system tumor surveillance in pediatric neurofibromatosis 2 and related disorders. Clin Cancer Res. 2017;23(12):e54–e61. https://doi.org/10.1158/1078-0432.CCR-17-0590. PMID: 28620005.
22. Rednam SP, Erez A, Druker H, Janeway KA, Kamihara J, Kohlmann WK, et al. Von Hippel–Lindau and hereditary pheochromocytoma/paraganglioma syndromes: clinical features, genetics, and surveillance recommendations in childhood. Clin Cancer Res. 2017;23(12):e68–e75. https://doi.org/10.1158/1078-0432.CCR-17-0547. PMID: 28620007.
23. Kamihara J, Bourdeaut F, Foulkes WD, Molenaar JJ, Mossé YP, Nakagawara A, et al. Retinoblastoma and neuroblastoma predisposition and surveillance. Clin Cancer Res. 2017;23(13):e98–e106. https://doi.org/10.1158/1078-0432.CCR-17-0652. PMID: 28674118.
24. Brandi ML, Gagel RF, Angeli A, Bilezikian JP, Beck-Peccoz P, Bordi C, et al. Guidelines for diagnosis and therapy of MEN type 1 and type 2. J Clin Endocrinol Metab. 2001;86(12):5658–71.
25. Jasperson KW, Kohlmann W, Gammon A, Slack H, Buchmann L, Hunt J, et al. Role of rapid sequence whole-body MRI screening in SDH-associated hereditary paraganglioma families. Fam Cancer. 2014;13(2):257–65. https://doi.org/10.1007/s10689-013-9639-6. PMID: 23934599.
26. Kratz CP, Achatz MI, Brugières L, Frebourg T, Garber JE, Greer MLC, et al. Cancer screening recommendations for individuals with li-fraumeni syndrome. Clin Cancer Res. 2017;23(11):e38–e45. https://doi.org/10.1158/1078-0432.CCR-17-0408. PMID: 28572266.
27. Villani A, Tabori U, Schiffman J, Shlien A, Beyene J, Druker H, et al. Biochemical and imaging surveillance in germline TP53 mutation carriers with Li-Fraumeni syndrome: a prospective observational study. Lancet Oncol. 2011;12(6):559–67. https://doi.org/10.1016/S1470-2045(11)70119-X. PMID: 21601526.
28. Villani A, Shore A, Wasserman JD, Stephens D, Kim RH, Druker H, et al. Biochemical and imaging surveillance in germline TP53 mutation carriers with Li-Fraumeni syndrome: 11 year follow-up of a prospective observational study. Lancet Oncol. 2016;17(9):1295–305. https://doi.org/10.1016/S1470-2045(16)30249-2. PMID: 27501770.
29. Tabori U, Hansford JR, Achatz MI, Kratz CP, Plon SE, Frebourg T, et al. Clinical management and tumor surveillance recommendations of inherited mismatch repair deficiency in childhood. Clin Cancer Res.

2017;23(11):e32–e37. https://doi.org/10.1158/1078-0432.CCR-17-0574. PMID: 28572265.
30. Krueger DA, Northrup H; International Tuberous Sclerosis Complex Consensus Group. Tuberous sclerosis complex surveillance and management: recommendations of the 2012 International tuberous sclerosis complex consensus conference. Pediatr neurol. 2013;49(4):255–65. https://doi.org/10.1016/j.pediatrneurol.2013.08.002. PMID: 24053983.
31. Thakker RV, Newey PJ, Walls GV, Bilezikian J, Dralle H, Ebeling PR, et al. Clinical practice guidelines for multiple endocrine neoplasia type 1 (MEN1). J Clin Endocrinol Metab. 2012;97(9):2990–3011.
32. Coury SA, Schneider KA, Schienda J, Tan WH. Recognizing and managing children with a pediatric cancer predisposition syndrome: A Guide for the Pediatrician. Pediatr Ann. 2018;47(5):e204–e216. https://doi.org/10.3928/19382359-20180424-02. PMID: 29750288.
33. Kim JY, Byeon JS. Genetic counseling and surveillance focused on lynch syndrome. J Anus Rectum Colon. 2019;3(2):60–68. https://doi.org/10.23922/jarc.2019-002. PMID: 31559369.
34. Villani A, Greer MLC, Kalish JM, Nakagawara A, Nathanson KL, Pajtler KW, et al. Recommendations for cancer surveillance in individuals with rasopathies and other rare genetic conditions with increased cancer risk. Clin Cancer Res. 2017;23(12):e83–e90. https://doi.org/10.1158/1078-0432.CCR-17-0631. PMID: 28620009
35. Asthagiri AR, Parry DM, Butman JA, Kim HJ, Tsilou ET, Zhuang Z, et al. Neurofibromatosis type 2. Lancet Lond Engl. 2009;373(9679):1974–86.
36. Evans DGR, Baser ME, O'Reilly B, Rowe J, Gleeson M, Saeed S, et al. Management of the patient and family with neurofibromatosis 2: a consensus conference statement. Br J Neurosurg. 2005;19(1):5–12.
37. Criteria for LFS [Internet]. Li-Fraumeni syndrome association. Available from: https://www.lfsassociation.org/what-is-lfs/lfscritieria/
38. Kaelin WG. Von Hippel-Lindau disease. Annu Rev Pathol. 2007;2:145–73.
39. Shuin T, Yamasaki I, Tamura K, Okuda H, Furihata M, Ashida S. Von Hippel-Lindau disease: molecular pathological basis, clinical criteria, genetic testing, clinical features of tumors and treatment. Jpn J Clin Oncol. 2006;36(6):337–43.
40. van Leeuwaarde RS, Ahmad S, van Nesselrooij B, et al. Von Hippel-lindau syndrome. 2000. In: Adam MP, Feldman J, Mirzaa GM, et al., editors. GeneReviews®. Seattle(WA): University of Washington, Seattle; 1993. Available from: http://www.ncbi.nlm.nih.gov/books/NBK1463/
41. Umeoka S, Koyama T, Miki Y, Akai M, Tsutsui K, Togashi K. Pictorial review of tuberous sclerosis in various organs. Radiogr Rev Publ Radiol Soc N Am Inc. 2008;28(7):e32.
42. Northrup H, Aronow ME, Bebin EM, Bissler J, Darling TN, de Vries PJ, et al; International Tuberous Sclerosis Complex Consensus Group. Updated International Tuberous Sclerosis Complex Diagnostic Criteria and Surveillance and Management Recommendations. Pediatr Neurol;123:50-66. https://doi.org/10.1016/j.pediatrneurol.2021.07.011. PMID: 34399110.
43. Liu S, Cai Y, Rong R, Hu P, Chen S, Wang X, et al. Tuberous sclerosis complex (TSC) with epilepsy on 18F-FDG simultaneous PET/MR. Eur J Nucl Med Mol Imaging. 2020;47(10):2471–2.
44. Roth J, Roach ES, Bartels U, Jóźwiak S, Koenig MK, Weiner HL, et al. Subependymal giant cell astrocytoma: diagnosis, screening, and treatment. Recommendations from the international tuberous sclerosis complex consensus conference 2012. Pediatr Neurol. 2013;49(6):439–44.
45. Rothschild PR, Lévy D, Savignoni A, Lumbroso-Le Rouic L, Aerts I, Gauthier-Villars M, et al. Familial retinoblastoma: fundus screening schedule impact and guideline proposal. A retrospective study. Eye Lond Engl. 2011;25(12):1555–61.
46. Fabius AWM, van Hoefen Wijsard M, van Leeuwen FE, Moll AC. Subsequent malignant neoplasms in retinoblastoma survivors. Cancers (Basel). 2021;13(6):1200. https://doi.org/10.3390/cancers13061200. PMID: 33801943.
47. Kamilaris CDC, Stratakis CA. Multiple Endocrine Neoplasia Type 1 (MEN1): An Update and the significance of early genetic and clinical diagnosis. Front Endocrinol (Lausanne). 2019;10:339. https://doi.org/10.3389/fendo.2019.00339. PMID: 31263451.
48. Moline J, Eng C. Multiple endocrine neoplasia type 2: an overview. Genet Med Off J Am Coll Med Genet. 2011;13(9):755–64.
49. Chazen JL, Gupta A, Dunning A, Phillips CD. Diagnostic accuracy of 4D-CT for parathyroid adenomas and hyperplasia. AJNR Am J Neuroradiol. 2012;33(3):429–33. https://doi.org/10.3174/ajnr.A2805. PMID: 22135127.
50. Nael K, Hur J, Bauer A, Khan R, Sepahdari A, Inampudi R, et al. Dynamic 4D MRI for characterization of parathyroid adenomas: multiparametric analysis. AJNR Am J Neuroradiol. 2015;36(11):2147–52.
51. Singh Ospina N, Donegan D, Rodriguez-Gutierrez R, Al-Hilli Z, Young WF. Assessing for multiple endocrine neoplasia type 1 in patients evaluated for Zollinger-Ellison syndrome-clues to a safer diagnostic process. Am J Med. 2017;130(5):603–5.
52. Iglesias P, Cardona J, Díez JJ. The pituitary in nuclear medicine imaging. Eur J Intern Med. 2019;68:6–12.
53. Mulligan LM, Kwok JB, Healey CS, Elsdon MJ, Eng C, Gardner E, et al. Germ-line mutations of the RET proto-oncogene in multiple endocrine neoplasia type 2A. Nature. 1993;363(6428):458–60.
54. Wells SA, Asa SL, Dralle H, Elisei R, Evans DB, Gagel RF, et al. Revised American Thyroid

Association guidelines for the management of medullary thyroid carcinoma. Thyroid Off J Am Thyroid Assoc. 2015;25(6):567–610.
55. Castinetti F, Taïeb D. Positron emission tomography imaging in medullary thyroid carcinoma: time for reappraisal? Thyroid Off J Am Thyroid Assoc. 2021;31(2):151–5.
56. Santos P, Pimenta T, Taveira-Gomes A. Hereditary Pheochromocytoma. Int J Surg Pathol. 2014;22(5): 393–400.
57. Pasini B, Stratakis CA. SDH mutations in tumorigenesis and inherited endocrine tumours: lesson from the phaeochromocytoma-paraganglioma syndromes. J Intern Med. 2009;266(1):19–42.
58. Neumann HPH, Erlic Z, Boedeker CC, Rybicki LA, Robledo M, Hermsen M, et al. Clinical predictors for germline mutations in head and neck paraganglioma patients: cost reduction strategy in genetic diagnostic process as fall-out. Cancer Res. 2009;69(8):3650–6.

Non-oncological Diseases Affecting the Children with Cancers

9

Richa Singh Chauhan and Nihar Kathrani

9.1 Introduction

Recent advances in cancer treatment and a better insight into the molecular pathways regulating tumorigenesis and metastasis have dramatically enhanced overall survival rates of several childhood cancers with consequent greater life expectancy. Therefore, there is an increasing number of pediatric patients formerly treated for cancers [1]. The acute and chronic consequences of cancer, caused not only by the cancer itself but also by the treatment methods employed, are impacting the life of many children. Cancers can trigger an immune response that could damage various components of the organ systems not primarily involved by the cancer. Radiation therapy (RT), chemotherapy, hematopoietic stem-cell transplantation (HSCT), and surgery are the mainstays of treatment of pediatric solid tumors as well as hemato-lymphoid malignancies. All of these treatment methods can instigate acute life-threatening complications, as well as the late consequences like chronic organ dysfunction or secondary cancers. Even though there have been advancements in decreasing toxicity from cancer therapy, several complications stay unavoidable [2]. Additionally, the evolution of new treatment regimes inevitably leads to the development of novel complications. According to present estimations, greater than 75% childhood cancer survivors will suffer nonetheless 1 late effect post treatment [3]. Early detection of treatment-related complications (TRCs) and their management have become pivotal for better patient outcomes. TRCs can be early or late. Early complications present during treatment or arise in a few months after treatment, whereas late complications usually take months to years to develop after treatment and could cause long-lasting morbidity [4]. Understanding of these potential aftereffects makes the clinicians more vigilant for the signs and symptoms guiding the further management of pediatric cancer patients. Early in the treatment course (i.e., within 1 year), the complications are usually due to infections or treatment toxicity, whether chemotherapy-related or toxic effects resulting from radiation therapy. Secondary cancers that develop due to treatment complications most often involve the bone marrow, brain, thyroid, and breast [4, 5].

Radiologists play critical role in multidisciplinary teams taking care of pediatric cancer patients and often aid in diagnosing cancer-induced or therapy-related complications and distinguishing them from conditions like tumor recurrence or secondary cancers. This chapter reviews the indirect consequences of pediatric cancers and their treatment-related toxicities

R. S. Chauhan (✉) · N. Kathrani
Department of Radiodiagnosis, All India Institute of Medical Sciences (AIIMS),
Raipur, Chhattisgarh, India

I. Kumar et al. (eds.), *Practical Approach to Imaging in Pediatric Oncology*,
https://doi.org/10.1007/978-981-96-8158-7_9

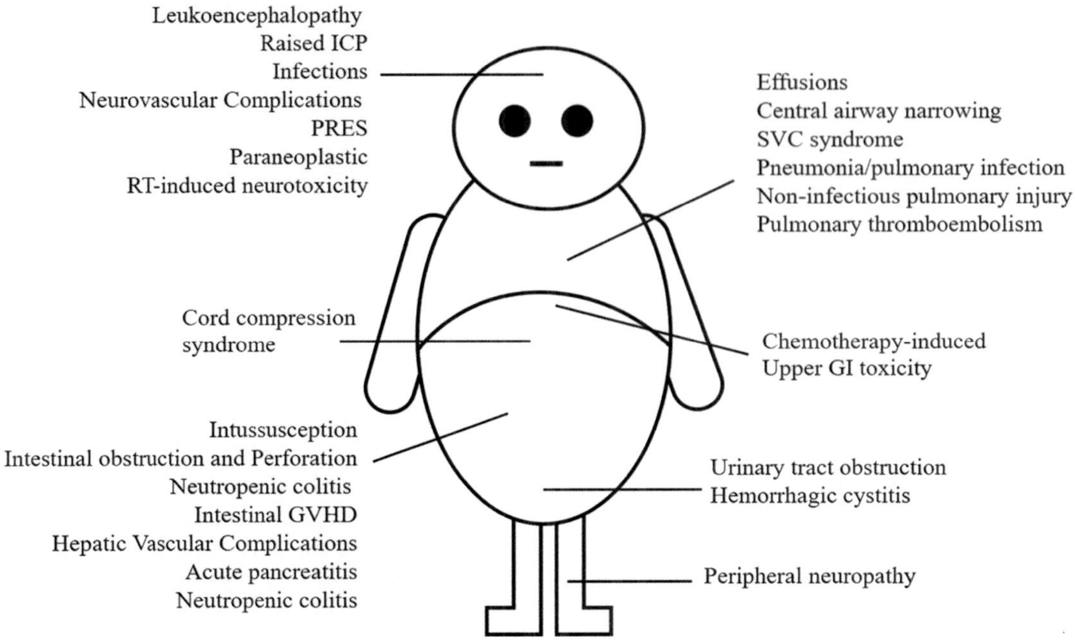

Fig. 9.1 Illustration of various cancers and their therapy-related diseases in children. *ICP* intracranial pressure, *PRES* posterior reversible encephalopathy syndrome, *RT* radiotherapy, *GVHD* graft versus host disease, *SVC* superior vena cava, *GI* gastrointestinal

(Fig. 9.1) on various organ systems with a brief description of the imaging findings. Because of a longer lifespan of pediatric cancer survivors compared with their adult counterparts this becomes particularly important to recognize the imaging features of these conditions.

9.2 Treatment-Related Febrile Neutropenia and Infections: Imaging Recommendations

Cancer treatment-related bone marrow as well as immune system suppression render patients at risk to systemic infections (Fig. 9.2). In fact, the infections are the chief source of treatment-related morbidity and mortality and lead to frequent hospitalization. Severe neutropenia (absolute neutrophil count <500/mm^3) is the most significant risk factor. Although just 20–30% of cancer patients with febrile neutropenia exhibit blood culture positivity [6]. Mortality rate, due to infections, may range between 1% and 3% during febrile neutropenia after relapse or progression [7]. About 70% bloodstream infections are triggered by gram-positive (staphylococci, streptococci, enterococci, etc.) and ~ 23% by gram-negative (E.coli, pseudomonas, klebsiella, proteus, etc.) bacteria, and ~7% by viruses or fungi (candida, cryptococcus, pneumocystis jirovecii, aspergillus, cytomegalovirus, adenovirus). Severe and long-standing neutropenia usually leads to invasive fungal infections (Figs. 9.3, 9.4, 9.5 and 9.6), which are more frequent in patients with hematologic cancers compared with those having solid tumors. An indwelling central venous catheter and corticosteroid treatment further predispose to multisystemic fungal infections [8]. Chest radiographs can be normal in children with FN and pulmonary infection due to a feeble inflammatory response. When positive, the radiographic abnormalities are usually non-specific which increases the risk of a delay in diagnosis and treatment [7, 9]. Further, the incidence of pneumonia in asymptomatic children is <3%, so chest X-ray is recom-

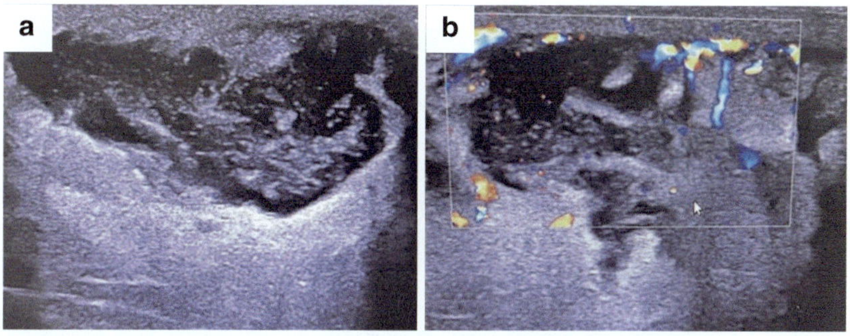

Fig. 9.2 Left axillary abscess in a neutropenic child on chemotherapy (**a**, grey scale and **b**, color Doppler image)

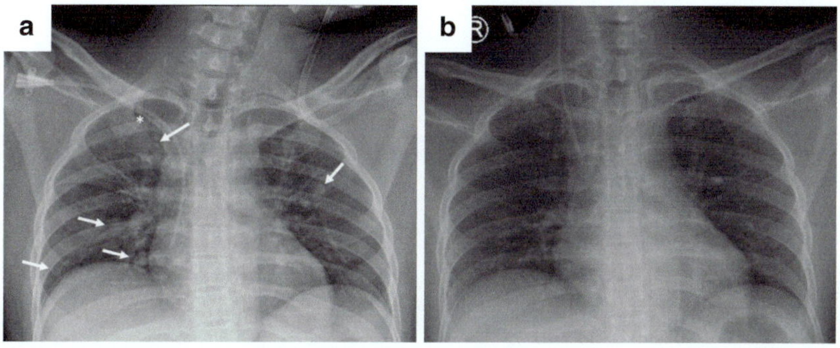

Fig. 9.3 Disseminated invasive Aspergillosis in a 14-year-old boy with acute myeloid leukemia (AML) post hematopoietic cell transplant. (**a**) Pre and (**b**) Post treatment chest radiographs. (**a**) Multiple nodules (white arrows) are seen in bilateral lung fields (right > left) with right upper lobe interstitial markings (asterisk). Repeat radiograph after 1 month (**b**) shows resolution of most of the radiographic abnormalities

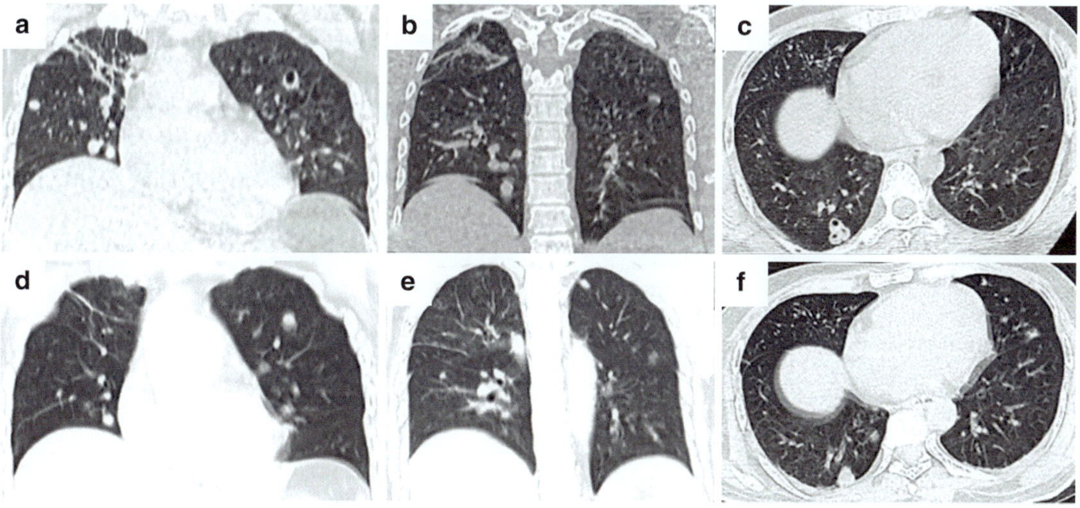

Fig. 9.4 Disseminated invasive Aspergillosis (same child as above). (**a–c**) Pre and (**d–f**) Post treatment chest CT. (**a–c**) Multiple nodules are seen in bilateral lung fields (right > left) with few of them showing cavitation. Atelectatic bands and septal thickening are seen in the right upper lobe. Repeat CT 3 weeks after starting antifungal treatment (**d–f**) shows resolution of majority of the nodules as well as right upper lobe interstitial changes. The cavitatory nodules in the apicoposterior segment of the left upper lobe and posterior basal segment of the right lower lobe are showing decrease in size with loss of cavitation

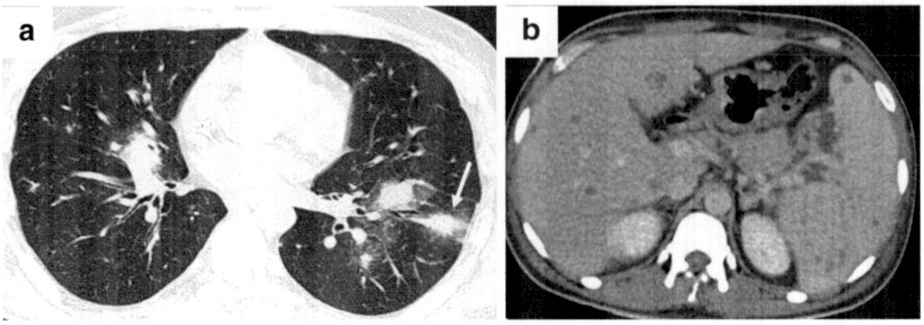

Fig. 9.5 Disseminated invasive Aspergillosis (same child as above). (**a**) Axial CT chest in lung window shows 'Halo sign' of invasive pulmonary Aspergillosis (white arrow). (**b**) Axial CECT abdomen shows splenomegaly with multiple hypo-enhancing hepato-splenic granulomas

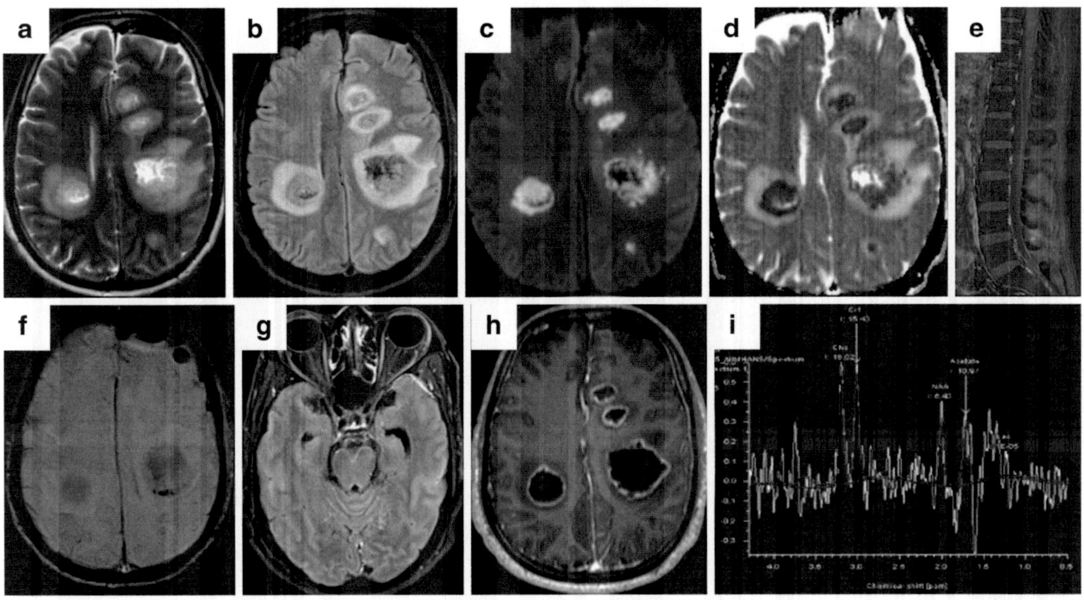

Fig. 9.6 Disseminated invasive Aspergillosis (same child as above). (**a** to **i**—axial T2W, FLAIR, diffusion weighted trace and ADC maps, sagittal T1 PC spine, axial SWI, PC FLAIR, PC T1 MPRAGE and MRS (at intermediate TE) images respectively) Multiple T2 hyperintense lesions partially inverting on FLAIR, showing predominantly peripheral diffusion restriction and ring enhancement are seen in bilateral cerebral hemispheres. The largest lesion in left centrum semiovale is showing blooming foci of hemorrhage along dorsal aspect of its wall. PC FLAIR (**g**) and sag PCT1 spine images show meningitis. MRS (**i**) from the wall of the largest lesion shows reduced NAA, elevated lipid-lactate and a trehalose peak at 3.6–3.8 ppm. *PC* post-contrast

mended only in children showing positive respiratory symptoms or signs [9, 10]. In the guideline for the management of fever and neutropenia in pediatric patients with cancer and HSCT recipients: 2023 update, the imaging recommendations formulated in the 2017 update remain unchanged. Imaging to evaluate prolonged (≥96 hours) febrile neutropenia (FN) in high-risk invasive fungal disease patients includes chest CT and abdominal ultrasound (strong recommendation, low quality evidence). CT of paranasal sinuses is not routinely recommended as it often turns out to be positive in prolonged FN and does not necessarily discriminate fungal infections from other causes [11, 12]. Chest CT possesses greater sensitivity for detecting lung infections, however, its utility is limited by the radiation exposure. A few studies have reported the technical feasibility of lung MRI in pediatric FN patients showing high correlation with HRCT and comparable specificity and sensitivity [13, 14]. However, further research is desirable to establish pulmonary MRI as a preferred diagnostic tool in such patients. Furthermore, whole-body MRI may be performed in these patients due to the systemic involvement by the fungal infection (paranasal sinuses, lungs, liver, spleen, muscles, and kidneys) [7].

9.3 CNS Complications

9.3.1 Infections

CNS infections in children with cancer may be due to malignancy- or treatment-related immunosuppression, surgical complications, or indwelling devices like external ventricular drain or ventriculostomy catheters. Hematologic malignancy is a chief predisposing factor for invasive opportunistic fungal infections in children [15]. The incidence of treatment-related CNS infections has been reported to be 2–14%. They occur most commonly in patients undergoing HSCT or neurosurgical procedures [7]. The chief clinical features can be either meningoencephalitic features or focal neurological deficits due to mass lesions. Imaging aids in diagnosing the infection, detecting complications, and monitoring the treatment response. Imaging features depend on the type of infection and the causative organism. CNS infections may appear as invasive sinusitis, encephalitis, meningitis, focal lesion, demyelination, or infarct. CT is often nonspecific showing areas of hypodensity with or without enhancement or mass effect [16]. Thus, children with cancer suspected to harbor a CNS infection should undergo MRI instead of CT. Simultaneous lung infection is observed in about 90% of patients with CNS fungal infection [17]. Cerebral and spinal abscesses are commonly caused by the organisms that spread via hematogenous route, or via direct extension from adjoining infected tissues (sinuses or vertebrae), or along a shunt [18].

Fungal abscesses are common in immunocompromised children compared with bacterial abscesses in immunocompetent children. Aspergillus most commonly causes CNS fungal infections in this patient group. The main clinical symptom is headache. Imaging reveals hypodense lesions with little or no mass effect on CT without significant enhancement. The lesions are hyperintense on T2W images with perilesional edema and rim enhancement (Fig. 9.6). Nonetheless, angioinvasive aspergillus lesions are frequently non-enhancing in severe immunocompromised patients [16, 19]. Sometimes, a hemorrhagic component may be seen secondary to vascular occlusion by hyphae, finally leading to infarction. Susceptibility artefacts can also be seen due to paramagnetic effect of the fungal hyphae. Focal lesions are frequently more noticeable on DWI than on conventional sequences. Fungal cerebral abscesses in immunocompromised children may frequently show central diffusion restriction like that of bacterial abscesses, may be because of highly proteinaceous content and cellular infiltration. However, the diffusion restriction may be absent or of a different pattern with different organisms. Aspergillus or mucor often leads to invasive fungal sinusitis; so if there is sinus disease along with cerebral involvement, aspergillus infection should be sought after [7].

CNS viral infection may present variedly in the form of encephalitis (herpes, EBV, CMV, enteroviruses, influenza), vasculitic infarcts (herpes zoster virus), and/or progressive multifocal leukoencephalopathy (PML; JC virus) [20]. In PML, there is progressive and long-lasting injury to the subcortical white matter. Varicella zoster virus may also lead to myelitis if it spreads to the spinal cord [18]. CNS infection with human-herpesvirus (HHV), particularly HHV-6, is rare in immunocompetent children, but reactivation may occur in 50% of patients 2–4 weeks after bone marrow transplantation, and may be followed by encephalopathy in a few patients. CT is less sensitive for viral encephalitis changes. On T2/FLAIR images, uni- or bilateral hyperintensity is seen in the amygdala, hippocampi, or parahippocampal gyri, often without diffusion restriction. This hyperintensity is followed by volume loss in the medial temporal lobes [17].

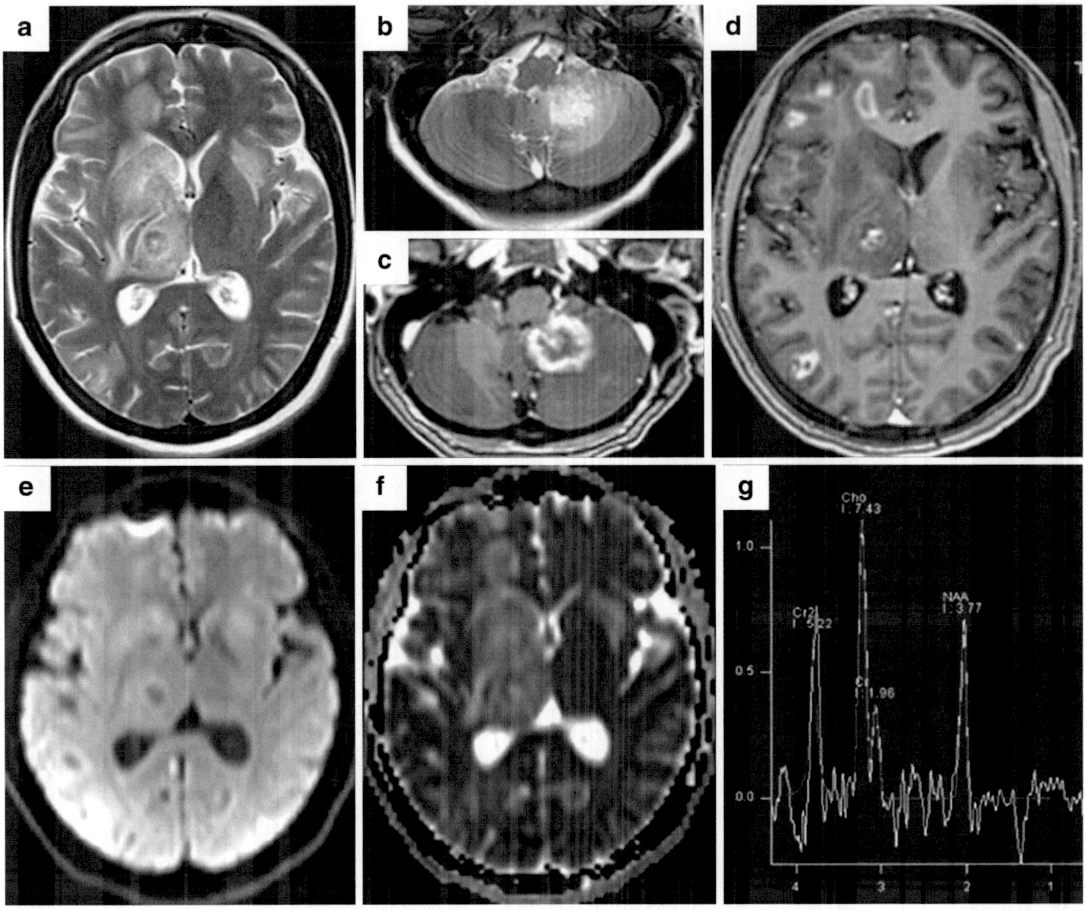

Fig. 9.7 CNS toxoplasmosis in a 14-year-old child receiving chemotherapy for non-Hodgkin lymphoma. Axial T2W (**a**, **b**) and PCT1 MPRAGE (**c**, **d**) show T2 hyperintense right frontal, thalamic, occipital, bilateral gangliocapsular, and right cerebellar lesions with marked edema, post contrast rim enhancement and typical 'eccentric target sign' sign in right thalamic and cerebellar lesions. Diffusion-weighted trace (**e**) and ADC (**f**) maps show patchy peripheral diffusion restriction, and MRS (**g**) from the cerebellar lesion depicts reduced NAA and inverted lactate peak at intermediate TE (144 ms)

CNS toxoplasmosis is caused due to reactivation of the latent infection, and presents with fever, seizures, focal neurological deficits, and altered mental status. Patients are vulnerable to the infection in the second phase after HSCT. On imaging, multiple ring-enhancing lesions or abscesses are seen in bilateral cerebral hemispheres and basal ganglia (Fig. 9.7) [18].

9.3.2 Raised Intracranial Pressure

Raised intracranial pressure (ICP) in children with intracranial neoplasms can be due to acute hydrocephalus, massive peritumoral edema, or tumoral hemorrhage [21]. Both low and high grade intracranial neoplasms may cause hydrocephalus from extrinsic compression (Fig. 9.8a–c) on the ventricular outflow, intraventricular tumor extension, or CSF overproduction (Fig. 9.8d). Non-obstructive hydrocephalus may also be seen in patients with diffuse leptomeningeal carcinomatosis that impedes CSF reabsorption by blocking the arachnoid granulations [22]. In case of acute presentation, the role of imaging is directed to the localization of the mass, identifying the complications (hydrocephalus or bleed), and aiding the clinicians to plan subsequent interventions

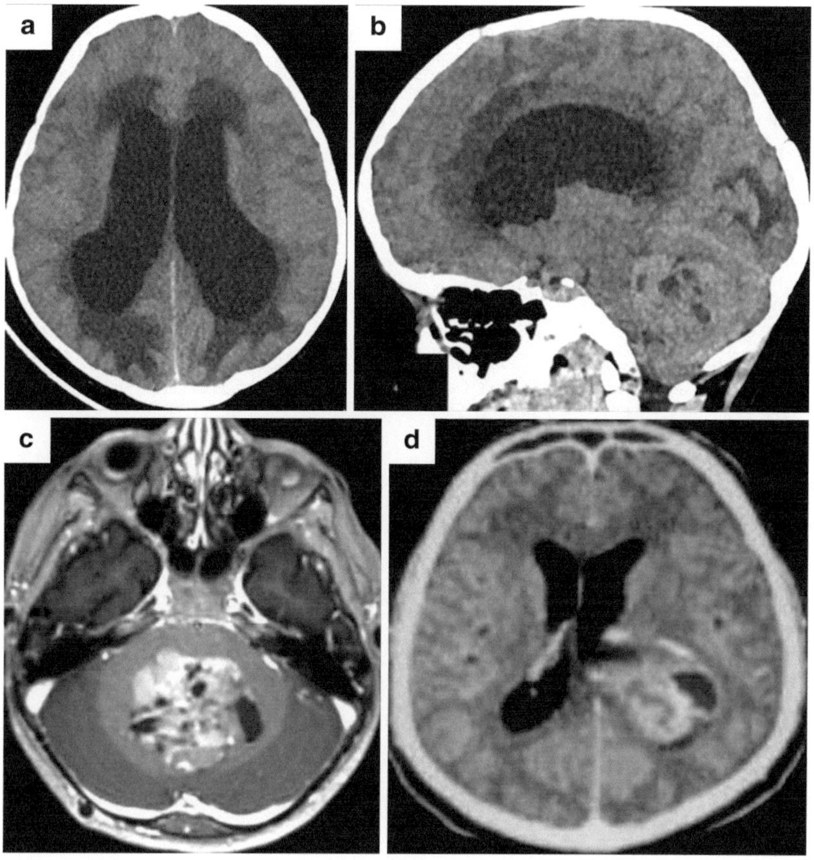

Fig. 9.8 Raised intracranial pressure due to hydrocephalus. (**a**–**c**) Acute decompensated intraventricular obstructive hydrocephalus secondary to WNT-activated medulloblastoma in a 2-year-old child. (**d**) Overproduction hydrocephalus in another 2-year-old child with left atrial choroid plexus papilloma

which may include insertion of an extra-ventricular drain (EVD) [23]. Clinical signs of a raised ICP may be Cushing's triad (bradycardia, decreased respiratory rate, systolic hypertension) as well as seizures. Focal neurological deficits and stroke-like symptoms can also be seen due to tumor bleed or venous sinus thrombosis causing venous infarction [24]. Cranial USG is a quick screening tool in infants with patent fontanelles for findings such as dilated ventricles, focal cerebral mass lesion, and hemorrhage. Superior sagittal sinus thrombosis can also be detected with Doppler examination. In the emergency setting, NCCT detects hemorrhage, midline shift, hydrocephalus, parenchymal herniations, and edema readily, and CECT can demonstrate venous sinus thrombosis. MRI may be employed further for lesion characterization and as a complementary modality in cases where CT shows no identifiable cause [22, 23].

9.3.3 Leukoencephalopathy

Methotrexate MTX is well-known for its neurotoxic effects in the form of leukoencephalopathy. The predisposing factors can be intrathecal exposure, high dosage, or simultaneous intracranial irradiation. The pathophysiology of MTX-related leukoencephalopathy is not well-comprehended and is reported to be due to altered folate metabolism causing demyelination and white matter damage [15, 25]. Patients may be asymptomatic or may report with seizure, confusion, headache, or hemiparesis that develop within 2 weeks of administration. Characteristic MRI findings of acute MTX toxicity are T2/FLAIR hyperintensities in bilateral centrum semiovale and periventricular white matter, with diffusion restriction. The restricted diffusion generally resolves with improvement in symptoms, however T2 signal changes can persist (Fig. 9.9) [26]. In chronic

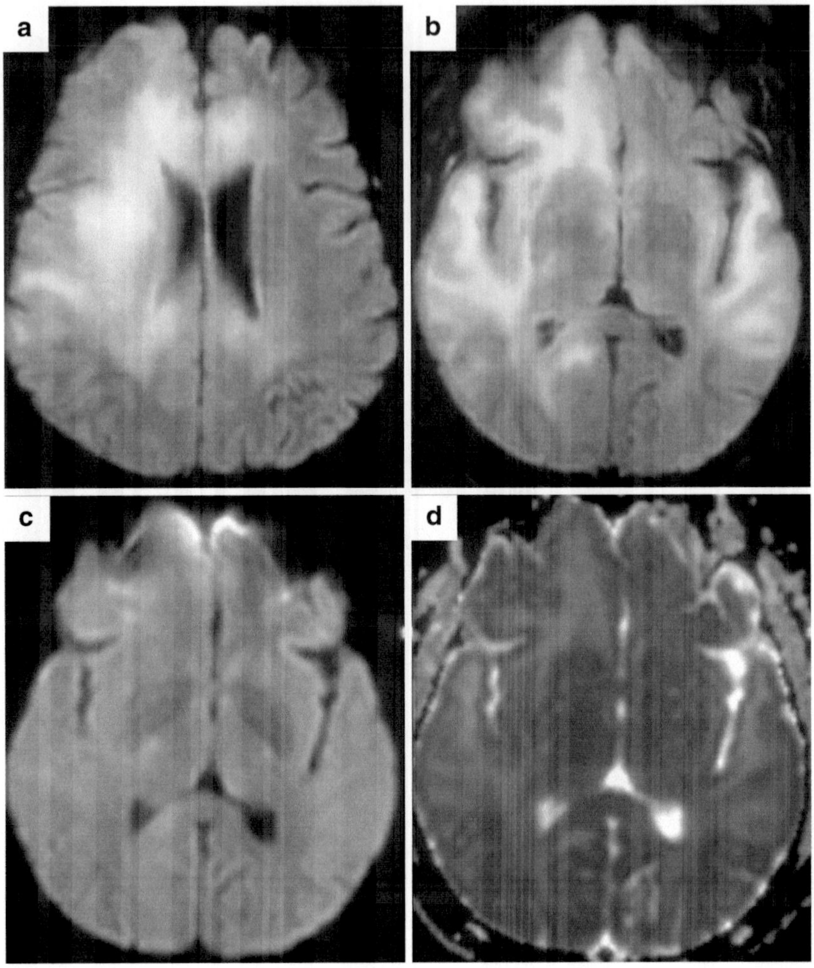

Fig. 9.9 Subacute methotrexate toxicity. A 15-year-old child taking methotrexate for NHL. Axial FLAIR (**a** and **b**) and diffusion-weighted trace (**c**) and ADC (**d**) maps depict extensive signal changes in bilateral subcortical and deep white matter (right > left) with facilitated diffusion. Note, the diffusion restriction is seen only in the acute phase of methotrexate toxicity. *NHL* Non-Hodgkin lymphoma

toxicity, white matter signal changes may persist, and non-resolving changes on diffusion-tensor imaging have been reported to correlate with neurocognitive impairment [27]. An infrequent, however, potentially lethal complication of intrathecal MTX when administered alone or with intracranial radiation is disseminated necrotizing leukoencephalopathy that follows a rapidly progressive course. MRI depicts widespread white matter edema with areas of T2 hypointensity, restricted diffusion, and enhancement (typically labelled as "soap bubble-like" or "Swiss cheese-like"), due to necrosis and hemorrhage [15].

Several other chemotherapeutic drugs like carboplatin, cytarabine, vincristine, and fludarabine; bone marrow transplantation and few antimicrobial agents can cause similar leukoencephalopathy [15].

9.3.4 Posterior Reversible Encephalopathy Syndrome

Posterior reversible encephalopathy syndrome (PRES) is a clinico-radiological syndrome that can ensue in children on cancer treatment, commonly those with hematologic malignancies, or allogeneic hematopoietic cell transplant [28]. Some anticancer medications can also be associated with PRES including methotrexate (MTX), vincristine, L-asparaginase, cisplatin, and immunosuppressive agents [29]. PRES patients are usually hypertensive. Clinical symptoms include headache, seizures, and/or altered mental status [28]. The distinctive imaging finding is bilateral but asymmetric subcortical patchy T2 hyperintensities, commonly involving the posterior brain

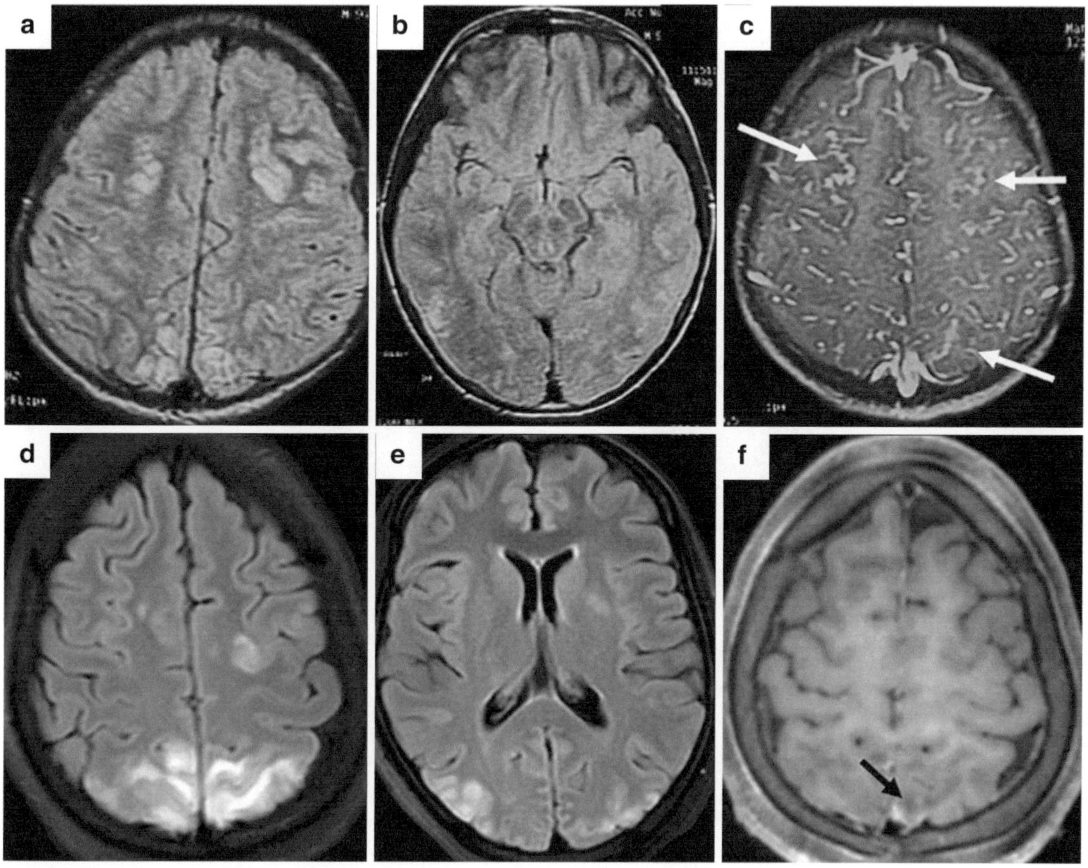

Fig. 9.10 (**a**–**c**) PRES in a 3-year-old child with altered mental status, on chemotherapy for ALL. Axial FLAIR (**a** and **b**) images show bilateral cortical and subcortical hyperintensities along the frontal, parietal, and occipital lobes. (**c**) Axial PCT1 image shows enhancement in the same regions (arrows). (**d**–**f**) Another 9-year-old child on chemotherapy for ALL shows similar pattern of bilateral cerebral involvement with subtle enhancement along the left parietal lesion. Pediatric PRES may show atypical features like frontal, cerebellar, or spinal involvement and post-contrast enhancement. *ALL* acute lymphoblastic leukemia, *PRES* posterior reversible encephalopathy syndrome

areas, i.e., posterior parietal, posterior temporal, and occipital lobes. In children, PRES may have atypical imaging appearances, involving the anterior brain areas (frontal lobe) (Fig. 9.10), deep grey nuclei, brainstem, cerebellum, or cord. Rarely, there can be isolated cerebellar involvement, parenchymal or subarachnoid hemorrhage, patchy restricted diffusion, or patchy parenchymal and leptomeningeal enhancement [28, 30, 31]. Microbleeds are best depicted on susceptibility-weighted imaging (SWI). PRES can be treated with conservative management, antiepileptics, antihypertensives, and stopping the offending drug, wherever feasible [28].

9.3.5 RT-Induced Neurotoxicity

Cranial irradiation is required for treating certain CNS neoplasms and hematologic malignancies regardless of recognized neurological adverse effects. In children, post-radiation somnolence syndrome (PRSS) occurs 3–12 weeks post-RT and presents with fever, anorexia, somnolence, cerebellar ataxia, nausea, vomiting, and EEG slowing. PRSS typically spontaneously resolves within 3–14 days [32].

Stroke-like migraine attacks after radiation therapy (SMART) syndrome is also a late complication of cranial RT, ensuing after

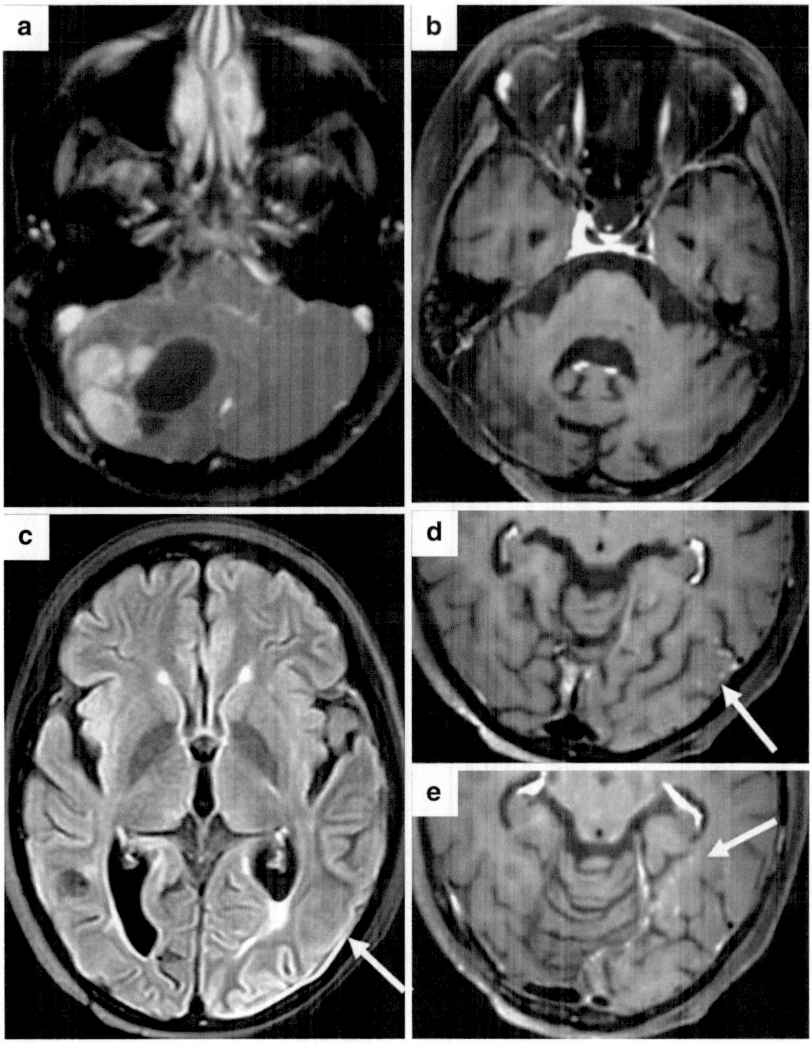

Fig. 9.11 SMART syndrome in a child with recurrent right cerebellar medulloblastoma post-radiotherapy. (**a**, **b**, **d**, and **e**) Axial post contrast T1 MPRAGE and (**c**) axial FLAIR images. (**a**) Enhancing solid-cystic recurrent right cerebellar medulloblastoma and (**b**) post-resection MRI image of the same. Note the right occipital craniectomy defect. Signal abnormalities in left posterior temporal and occipital regions on FLAIR (**c**) with patchy dot-like enhancement (**d** and **e**) suggestive of post-radiation changes

2–10 years. Symptoms include recurrent migrainous headaches, seizures, and/or focal neurological deficits. EEG commonly reveals subclinical seizures and imaging may depict cerebrovascular abnormalities with hemispheric hypoperfusion. Distinctive MRI findings include unilateral cortical T2 hyperintensity with gyriform postcontrast enhancement (Fig. 9.11) [15, 32, 33].

Myelopathy may occur after spinal irradiation. Early-onset myelopathy is usually reversible while late-onset is generally progressive [34].

Another late effect of cranial RT is cognitive dysfunction, usually noted years after treatment. Young age at the time of RT is a predisposing factor for its development [32].

9.3.6 Neurovascular Complications of Cancer

Approximately 1% of children with cancer can suffer from stroke, caused either by the cancer itself, or its therapy. Both ischemic and hemorrhagic strokes can occur. L-asparaginase that is often used for treating hematologic malignancies is a well-known inciting factor for cerebral venous sinus thrombosis (CVST) and venous hemorrhage [35, 36]. CVST is a serious

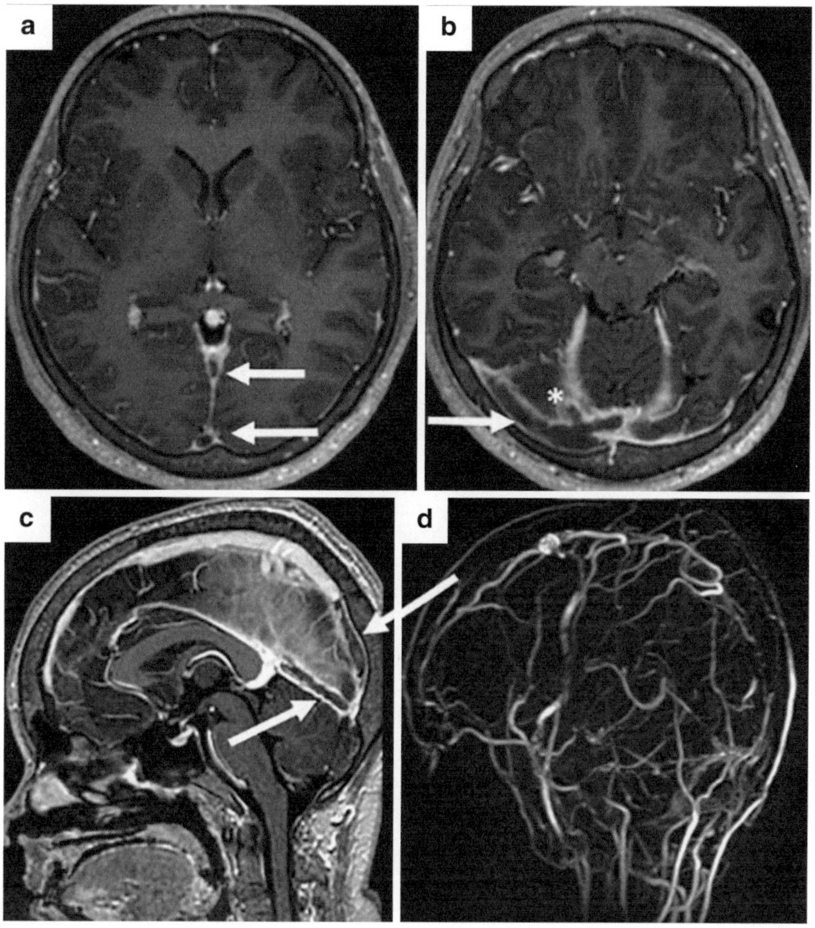

Fig. 9.12 Cortical venous sinus thrombosis in an 11-year-oolld child with ALL. Superficial as well as deep sinus thrombosis seen as filling defects (arrows) on PCT1 images (**a**–**c**). Note the thrombus extension into one of the cortical veins (* in **b**). (**d**) Phase contrast magnetic resonance venography image depicts lack of filling of almost all the major venous sinuses

complication seen in children with hematologic malignancies. The predisposing factors are leukemia-induced increased thrombin production, L-asparaginase administration, corticosteroids, and infections. It usually occurs within 3–4 weeks of therapy. Symptoms can be variable, from just headache to seizures, multifocal neurologic deficits, or coma [7]. NCCT may detect acute CVST, seen as hyperattenuating deep and cortical veins and venous sinuses. When the attenuation of thrombus decreases, it is seen as a filling defect in the venous sinuses on CECT (Fig. 9.12). MRI with MR venography is now the method of choice for diagnosis. The subacute thrombus is easily recognizable, however, in the acute phase it can be erroneously considered as flowing blood, but MR venography will demonstrate the absence of flow (Fig. 9.12d) [17].

Post-RT arteriopathy, a type of moyamoya syndrome, is a late complication of cranial RT that is characterized by steno-occlusive disease of supraclinoid internal carotid and proximal anterior and middle cerebral arteries, increasing the risk of stroke. The greatest at-risk patients are the children receiving RT close to the circle of Willis [26]. MRI may show acute infarcts, and/or areas of gliosis and volume loss. MR angiography can demonstrate the vascular stenosis (Fig. 9.13) and associated collaterals, although catheter angiography remains the gold standard for assessment [15].

Vascular malformations can also occur as a late effect of cranial RT, especially cerebral cavernous malformations (CCM), with reported cumulative incidence of 3–4% at 10 years post-RT. Medulloblastoma and ALL are most often

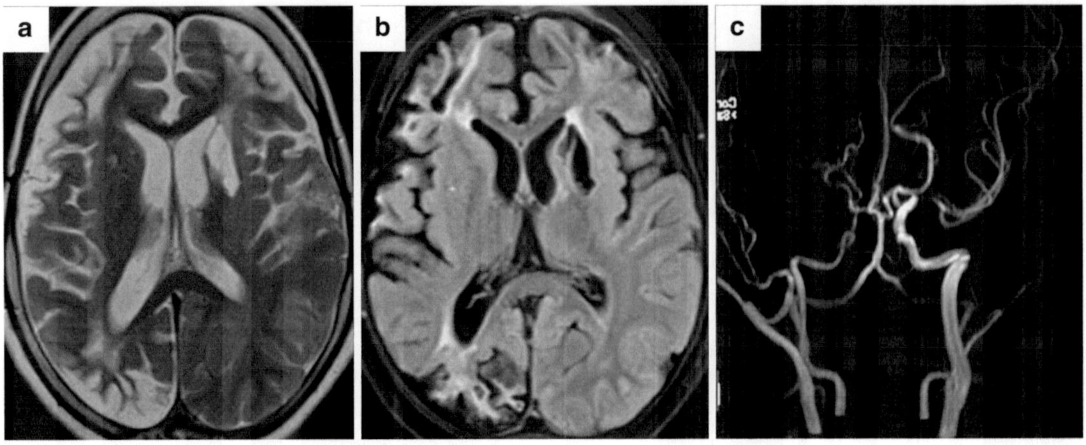

Fig. 9.13 Post-RT arteriopathy. A 15-year-old child post resection and intracranial radiation for craniopharyngioma presenting with recurrent strokes. Axial T2 (**a**) and FLAIR (**b**) images show gliosis and cystic encephalomalacic changes in the right cerebral hemisphere and left frontal and striatal regions. TOF MRA image (**c**) shows marked steno-occlusive involvement of right distal ICA, MCA, and ACA. On the left side, there is comparatively less severe involvement of the terminal ICA and proximal part of M1 MCA. *TOF* time-of-flight, *MRA* magnetic resonance angiography

reported to be associated with the development of CCM, although they can arise after cranial RT for any disease. Patients present with bleed or seizures approximately 8–12 years after RT [15, 32]. Rarely, cerebral aneurysms may be seen [37].

9.3.7 Paraneoplastic Neurologic Syndromes

Paraneoplastic syndromes are the remote systemic effects of cancer not caused by metastases or treatment and are mediated by hormonal or immunologic mechanisms [32]. Many paraneoplastic syndromes affect the CNS and peripheral nerves. Limbic encephalitis is the most well-known paraneoplastic neurologic syndrome. Others are paraneoplastic brain stem encephalitis, cranial neuropathy, paraneoplastic cerebellar degeneration, myelitis, myasthenia gravis, stiff-person syndrome, opsoclonus myoclonus syndrome, Lambert-Eaton myasthenic syndrome, retinopathy, enteric nervous system dysfunction, and polyneuropathy. They are often associated with CSF or serum positivity of onconeuronal antibodies in cancer patients [38]. The criteria for diagnosis of paraneoplastic syndrome in children are similar to that of adults. Although an amendment to reduce the interval between symptom presentation and tumor diagnosis has been suggested, since the common tumor types in children (neuroblastoma, lymphoma, etc.) present earlier than common tumor types in adults [39]. There are certain other differences in the adult and childhood paraneoplastic syndromes: (i) the specificity and sensitivity of antibody panel are not yet established in children, (ii) the similar clinical syndromes can exist with non-paraneoplastic autoimmune antibodies, (iii) certain paraneoplastic antibodies like anti-Hu, VGKC antibodies can occur without tumors in children [32].

CSF antibody analysis, which is more sensitive than serum analysis, is done to assess limbic encephalitis. CSF features that may support the diagnosis include moderate lymphocyte-predominant CSF pleocytosis (80% cases), oligoclonal bands (50–60% cases), elevated protein (30% cases), or positive IgG index. Other features include EEG showing slowing or epileptiform activity, and MRI FLAIR signal changes or contrast enhancement in limbic areas (Fig. 9.14), deep gray structures, cortex, brainstem, or cerebellum. There may not be any positive findings early in the course of the disease [32].

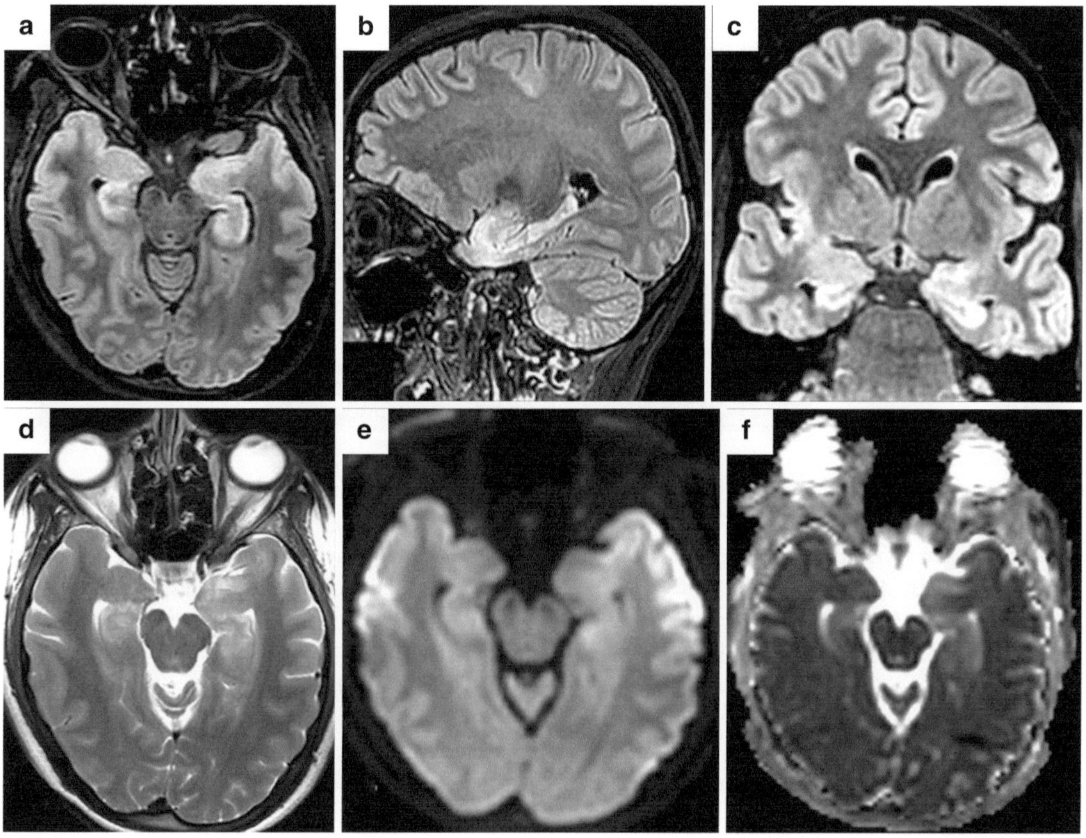

Fig. 9.14 Anti-N-methyl-D-aspartate (NMDA) receptor encephalitis in a 10-year-old child with immature ovarian teratoma and strongly positive cerebrospinal fluid anti-NMDAR antibody. (**a–c**) FLAI and (**d**) T2W images show bilateral (left > right) medial temporal hyperintensity involving hippocampi and parahippocampal gyri. Diffusion-weighted trace (**e**) and ADC (**f**) maps show facilitated diffusion

Opsoclonus myoclonus ataxia syndrome is rare, and is caused due to autoantibodies against cerebellar cells. Up to 50% children with the syndrome harbor a neuroblastoma whereas only 2–3% of children with neuroblastoma will have the syndrome. Three of the four characteristic features are needed for the diagnosis, which are opsoclonus (abnormal eye movements), ataxia and/or myoclonic jerks, behavioral or sleep changes (drooling, speech changes, hypotonia, emotional lability, etc.), and underlying neuroblastoma [40, 41].

9.3.8 Cord Compression Syndrome

Acute spinal cord compression occurs in 2.5–6% of all cancer patients and in 3–5% of children with cancer [22, 23], commonly from compression by an extradural paravertebral tumor (Fig. 9.15), frequently reported with backache. Prompt diagnosis is imperative to prevent neurological sequelae like paraplegia and loss of bowel/bladder control, as longstanding compression may progress to irreversible neurological damage [42]. Potential contributory neoplastic lesions include neuroblastomas, soft tissue sarcomas, lymphoma, primary spinal cord tumors (like astrocytomas, ependymomas), and intraspinal leukemic deposits [23]. The non-neoplastic pathologies causing cord compression in cancer patients may include traumatic spinal fractures and abscesses [43]. Plain spine radiographs are usually not beneficial except in patients with fractures. MRI is the modality of choice and must include the whole neuraxis

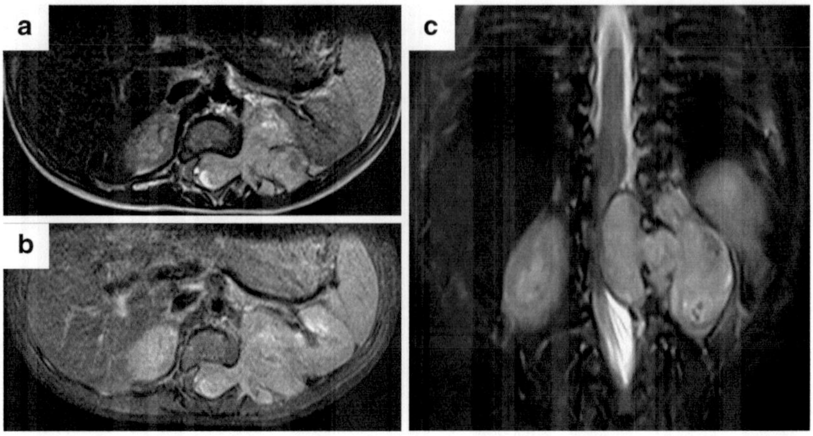

Fig. 9.15 Cord compression syndrome. Axial T2W (**a**), T1PC (**b**) and coronal T2W (**c**) images depict left-sided neuroblastoma having transforaminal intraspinal extension with cord compression, displacement, and signal changes

(brain and cord) imaged in the same sitting. MRI enables evaluation of the extent of the compression and aids in treatment planning. Dorsal spine is the most commonly affected region (70% cases) [44]. The malignant spinal tumors are generally seen as T1 hypointense and T2 hyperintense lesions with patchy to solid contrast enhancement. The extradural metastatic lesions may cause cortical erosions and displace and compress the spinal cord. There can be resultant cord edema, seen as T2 hyperintense signal (Fig. 9.15c). In case MRI is unavailable or contraindicated, CT with myelography is indicated.

9.3.9 Peripheral Neuropathy

Chemotherapy-induced peripheral neuropathy (CIPN) can be caused by taxanes, vinca alkaloids, platins, thalidomide, and bortezomib. RT, paraneoplastic syndromes, antibiotics like voriconazole and malnutrition-associated vitamin B12 deficiency may also trigger neuropathy. CIPN typically instigates weakness and distal sensory loss, severity of which is dependent on the dose and treatment duration [45]. Weak reflexes are the presenting sign followed by paresthesias in the feet and hands. There may be motor weakness or loss of vibration sense and proprioception. CIPN may improve when the inciting drug is stopped or the dose is reduced, however, the neuropathic symptoms may continue irrespective of intervention [46].

9.4 Cardiopulmonary Complications

9.4.1 Mediastinal Tumor Causing Central Airway Narrowing and Superior Vena Cava Syndrome

Anterior mediastinal masses (commonly germ cell tumors, leukemia, and lymphoma) pose a greater risk of airway narrowing (Fig. 9.16a, b) in children owing to more compressibility and lesser caliber of trachea. The other complication of these neoplasms is vascular compression causing SVC syndrome (Fig. 9.16c). Children usually present with cough, dyspnea, and stridor secondary to airway compression or with cardiogenic shock due to decreased venous return secondary to SVC compression [23]. In 97% cases, chest radiographs can detect mediastinal mass and the tracheal narrowing. CT scan or MRI can be done to confirm and further evaluate the lesion. CECT/MRI can depict the site and extent of narrowing and facilitates to distinguish extrinsic compression by the tumor from the direct airway invasion or vascular thrombosis. Additionally, cross-sectional imaging can also demonstrate the tumor characteristics and the relation of the

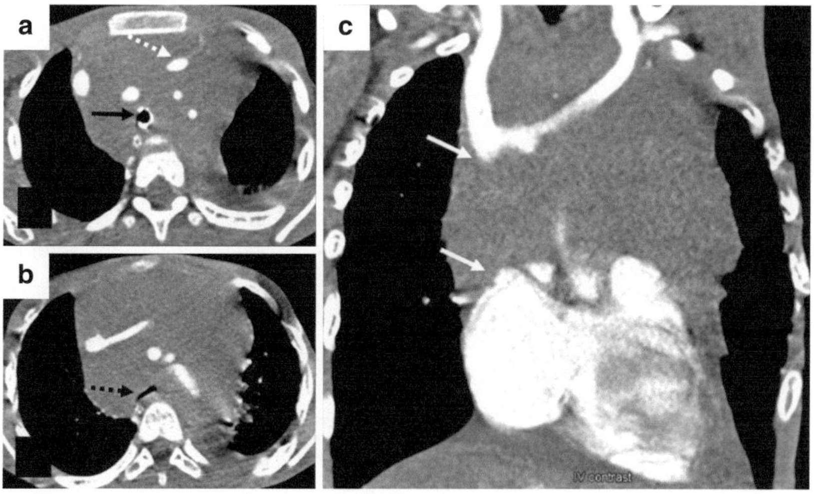

Fig. 9.16 Central airway compression and superior vena cava (SVC) syndrome in a 5-year-old child with superior mediastinal lymphoma. Axial (**a** and **b**) and coronal (**c**) CECT chest images show a homogeneously enhancing superior mediastinal mass encasing the great vessels of the medisastinum and the trachea. Note marked tracheal compromise (dashed black arrow in **b**), endotracheal tube in situ (black arrow in **a**), left brachiocephalic vein luminal narrowing (dashed white arrow in **a**) and non-visualization/opacification of entire length of SVC (white arrows in **c**)

tumor to other mediastinal structures aiding in the treatment planning [22, 47].

9.4.2 Infection

Chemotherapy-induced bone marrow aplasia, a central venous catheter, and treatment with steroids and calcineurin inhibitors are the important predisposing factors for chest infection in pediatric cancer patients [48]. The type of immune dysfunction and duration post-HSCT in children are important factors to predict potential infectious organisms. In the pre-engraftment period (<30 days) there is neutropenia and compromised mucosal immunity due to preparative chemotherapy; in the early post-engraftment period, there is impaired cell-mediated immunity; and in the late post-engraftment period there is impaired humoral- as well as cell-mediated immunity [49].

Bacterial pneumonia mostly ensues following chemotherapy-induced severe neutropenia and in the pre-engraftment phase after HSCT. Common causative microorganisms are Staphylococcus aureus, S. epidermidis, Streptococcus spp., Klebsiella spp., and Pseudomonas aeruginosa. On radiographs, there will be lung (focal, segmental, or lobar) opacities [50]. Lymphopenia predisposes to viral infections. Frequently encountered respiratory viruses in these children are parainfluenza, influenza A and B, rhino, respiratory syncytial (RSV), and coronaviruses. Viral infections may have normal imaging appearances or may depict all or a combination of the ground-glass opacities, nodules, and consolidation [51, 52].

CT imaging of invasive pulmonary aspergillosis (Figs. 9.3 and 9.4) can reveal variable-sized nodules, consolidation areas, masses, cavities, ground-glass and/or tree-in-bud opacities, and effusion [20] which can be observed in other infections as well. As per the European Organization for Research and Treatment of Cancer and the Mycoses Study Group Education and Research Consortium (EORTC/MSGERC) criteria, at least one of the four of air crescent sign; dense, well-circumscribed lesion(s) with or without halo sign (Fig. 9.5); cavity; or wedge-shaped and segmental or lobar consolidation, should be observed on CT to diagnose fun-

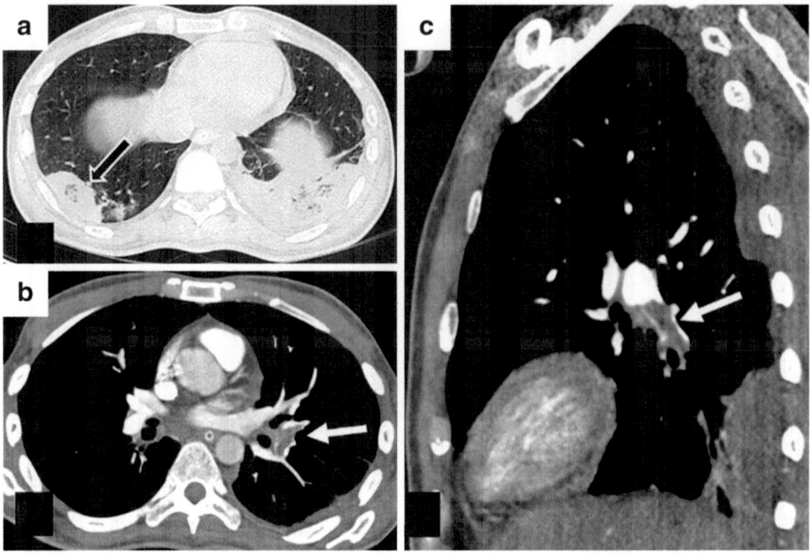

Fig. 9.17 'Reverse-Halo sign' (black arrow in **a**) and pulmonary thromboembolism (white arrows in **b** and **c**) in a child with neutropenic fever and invasive pulmonary aspergillosis

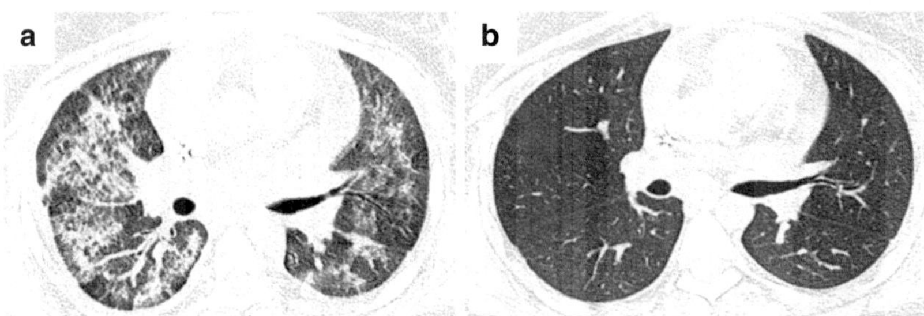

Fig. 9.18 Broncho-alveolar lavage (BAL)-confirmed Pneumocystis jiroveci pneumonia (**a**) in a 16-year-old female child with acute lymphocytic leukemia (ALL) on therapy with prolonged febrile neutropenia. Axial CT image shows predominantly central ground glass opacification. (**b**) Post-antibiotic resolution of the CT findings. *BAL* Bronchoalveolar lavage

gal aspergillosis. For fungal infection other than aspergillus, reversed halo sign (Fig. 9.17a) is also added to the criteria [53]. A nodular or consolidation area surrounded by ground-glass opacity indicates halo sign, which comes early in FN patients, i.e., within 5 days from fever onset. In 50% cases, after 2–3 weeks of recovery of neutropenia, the air crescent sign appears [7]. Clinico-radiological features of pulmonary fungal infections in children may be non-specific and considerably differ from adult features, especially the air crescent sign, halo sign, or cavitation are infrequent in children for undetermined reasons [54]. Pneumocystis jirovecii pneumonia presents with fever, dry cough, and dyspnea. Chest radiographs classically demonstrate bilateral perihilar gradually coalescing interstitial infiltrates (Fig. 9.18). However, imaging may be nonspecific with unilateral infiltrates; nodules, consolidations, or cavities [48]. Rarely, Candida spp. can infect the lungs secondary to hematogenous spread from other organs. Invasive candidiasis occurs more frequently in neonates than the older children. CT features are nonspecific with bilateral nodules and consolidation [7, 54].

9.4.3 Non-infectious Pulmonary Injury

Non-infectious pulmonary injury usually occurs in an anticipated period post-HSCT and leads to acute respiratory failure. It includes idiopathic pneumonia syndrome (IPS) or idiopathic interstitial pneumonitis (IIP) that occurs within 120 days of HSCT with approximate incidence of 10%. IPS may cause injury to alveoli, airway epithelium, or vascular endothelium with radiographs showing diffuse bilateral pulmonary infiltrates. Broncho-alveolar lavage (BAL) is mostly culture-negative. IPS carries a mortality rate of 50–75% [55, 56].

Other subsets of IPS are periengraftment respiratory distress syndrome (PRDS; within 5–7 days), diffuse alveolar hemorrhage (DAH; within 100 days), cryptogenic organizing pneumonia (COP; within 2–12 months) and bronchiolitis obliterans syndrome (BOS; late-onset; within 3–24 months) with fever, cough, dyspnea, and hypoxia being the most prominent symptoms. PRDS signifies an inflammatory condition that happens during post-HSCT neutrophil recovery and leads to noncardiogenic pulmonary edema [52]. Pulmonary injury may be accompanied by hepatorenal failure in up to 25% cases with encephalopathy in a minor subset [56].

On radiographs, PRDS and DAH appear as diffuse bilateral pulmonary infiltrates (Fig. 9.19) while patchy infiltrates are observed in COP. On HRCT, ground glass infiltrates can be seen in DAH and COP which are diffuse and dense in DAH with predominant perihilar distribution (Fig. 9.20), and patchy with accompanying air space consolidation and nodules in COP. To establish the diagnosis of DAH bronchoscopy is done that reveals increasingly bloody BAL [52, 56]. Chest x-ray in BOS can be normal or may show hyperinflated lung fields. On CT, there may be centrilobular nodules and areas of air trapping, mosaic attenuation, or bronchiectasis. BOS diagnosis is confirmed by an obstructive pulmonary function test [57].

Early recognition and management of these complications is obligatory as children who suffer from acute post-HSCT respiratory failure carry a high mortality rate of up to 60% [58].

9.4.4 Pulmonary Embolism

Children with cancer are highly predisposed to pulmonary thromboembolism (PTE). Venous thromboembolism (VTE) risk, including DVT and PTE, is 4–7 times greater in cancer patients compared with general population [59]. According to a study, one-fourth of children with VTE harbor a neoplasm [60]. Another study stated that approximately 2% of children with cancer showed PTE in their routine chest CT [61]. It warrants urgent reporting and initiation of treatment as it is usually accompanied by the occurrence of other thromboembolic events and DVT. Factors predisposing to PTE development in pediatric cancer patients may include tumor- or therapy-related (e.g., L-asparaginase) coagulopathy, a central venous catheter, parenteral hyperalimentation, post-transfusion platelet microaggregates, tumor thrombi, and tumor lysis [47]. Chest X-ray findings are often non-specific and classical signs of PTE are rarely observed.

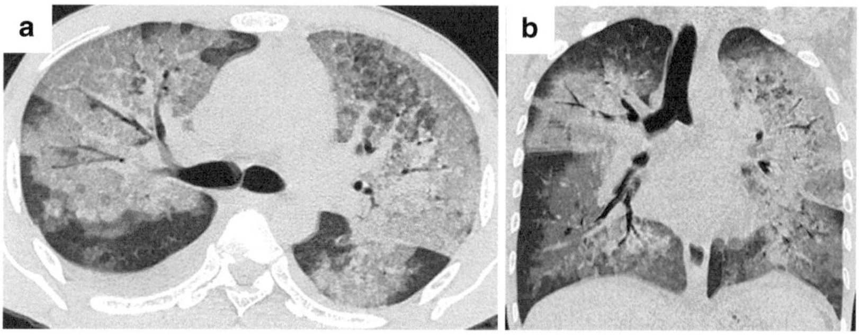

Fig. 9.19 Periengraftment respiratory distress syndrome (PRDS) in a 13-year-old child with AML on day 14 after allogenic bone marrow transplant. Axial (**a**) and coronal (**b**) CT images show diffuse bilateral pulmonary ground-glass opacities and consolidation areas

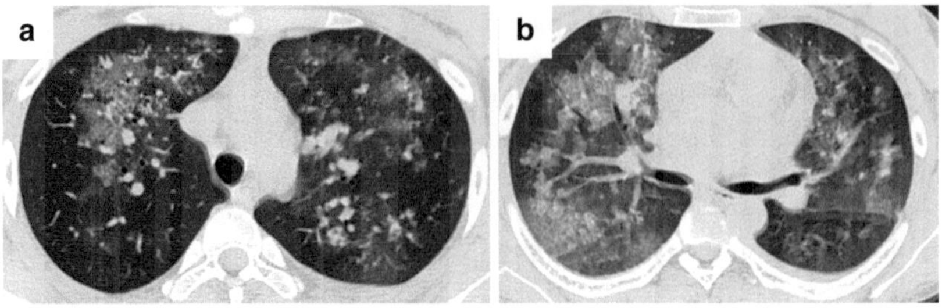

Fig. 9.20 BAL-proven diffuse alveolar hemorrhage (DAH) in a 14-year-old child with AML post allogenic stem cell transplant. (**a**, **b**) Axial CT images show bilateral, central, diffuse ground-glass opacities (GGO) and a 'crazy paving' pattern due to the GGO with septal thickening

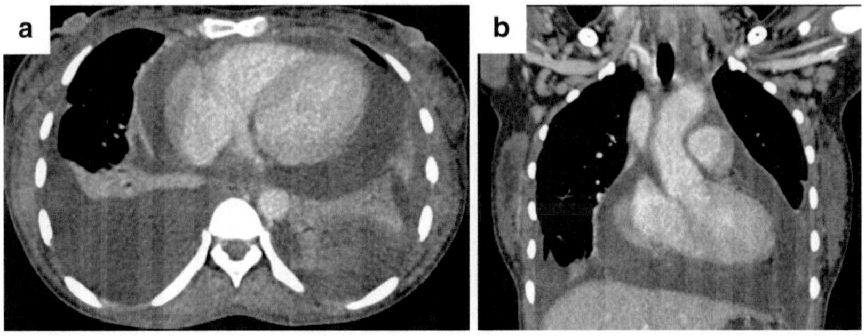

Fig. 9.21 Moderate to gross tubercular pericardial and pleural effusions in a 12-year-old child on chemotherapy for lymphoma. Axial (**a**) and coronal (**b**) CECT images showing the effusions. Note the bilateral axillary round, homogeneous and discrete lymph nodes in image (**b**)

For diagnosing PTE, CT pulmonary angiography is the current technique of choice that depicts intraarterial filling defects (Fig. 9.17) and the extent of vascular involvement. There may be wedge-shaped peripheral pulmonary consolidation areas [22]. Not many clinical studies are there to depict the role of MR angiography in diagnosing PTE in children. Further, nuclear scans are also rarely performed in pediatric patients with suspected PTE [47].

9.4.5 Effusions

Pericardial effusion, when rapid and massive, can lead to cardiac tamponade due to marked cardiac compression and diminished venous return and cardiac output. Direct tumor invasion (leukemia/lymphoma/metastasis), opportunistic infections, or radiation fibrosis are the common causes. Pericardial teratoma and cardiac hemangioma may lead to neonatal pericardial effusion. Echocardiography is the imaging technique of choice to confirm pericardial effusion, assess its hemodynamics, and to guide fluid drainage [22]. Chest radiographs and CT may incidentally detect pericardial effusion where increased cardiothoracic ratio will be observed on chest x-rays with globular cardio-mediastinal outline. CT will show pericardial fluid accumulation with or without pericardial thickening (Fig. 9.21), nodularity, hemorrhage, or features of cardiac failure like contrast reflux into IVC, azygous and hepatic veins, and congested liver. MRI can characterize effusions to be serous or hemorrhagic, however, it is rarely performed to diagnose pericardial effusion [47].

Pleural effusions in children with cancer can be benign or malignant. Large pleural fluid collections can lead to respiratory compromise by causing passive lung compression (Fig. 9.21). Infectious/inflammatory causes, reduced lymphatic drainage, or reduced oncotic pressure usually cause benign effusions while malignant effusions are typically caused by the primary disease. Lymphoma is a common cause in the pediatric age group. The diagnosis can be established by chest radiograph or USG. USG can aid in guiding therapeutic drainage, whenever needed. CT can assess the severity and cause of effusion, pulmonary parenchyma, as well as the underlying malignancy. The evidence of thickened nodular pleura suggests malignancy [22].

9.5 Abdominal Complications

9.5.1 Chemotherapy-Induced Upper GI Toxicity

Esophageal toxicity may be acute, occurring during or closely after thoracic irradiation, or late, occurring months or years after thoracic irradiation. The acute toxicity displays impaired peristalsis on fluoroscopy and usually resolves within 12 weeks. Late radiation toxicity results in slowly progressive dysphagia secondary to fibrotic stenosis/stricture that can be seen as long, smooth narrowed segment with tapered margins. The median onset is typically 6 months from RT. Uncommonly, intermittent esophageal spasms, chronic ulcerations, fistulation, bleeding, or perforation may occur. On CT, circumferential esophageal wall thickening can be realized in both early and late toxicities [62, 63]. Similar to the esophagus, stomach and duodenum may be affected post RT. Gastric and duodenal ulcerations, impaired peristalsis, luminal narrowing, nonspecific gastric wall thickening with perigastric fat stranding may be observed on CT [64].

9.5.2 Intussusception/ Intestinal Obstruction and Perforation

Intussusception may be caused by primary bowel neoplasms (polyps, lipoma, neurofibroma, leiomyoma, gastrointestinal stromal tumor (GIST), lymphoma, and carcinoid) or metastases [22, 47]. It is the presenting feature in about 17–25% of patients with abdominal Burkitt's lymphoma. Underlying pathological lead point should be strongly suspected when children >2 years of age present with intussusception [23, 65]. Abdominal radiograph may suggest intestinal obstruction. Ultrasound (USG) and CT show bowel within bowel (target/concentric ring sign) with or without accompanying mesenteric fat and vessels (Fig. 9.22). Long length >3.5 cm, an identifiable lead point, and an evidence of bowel

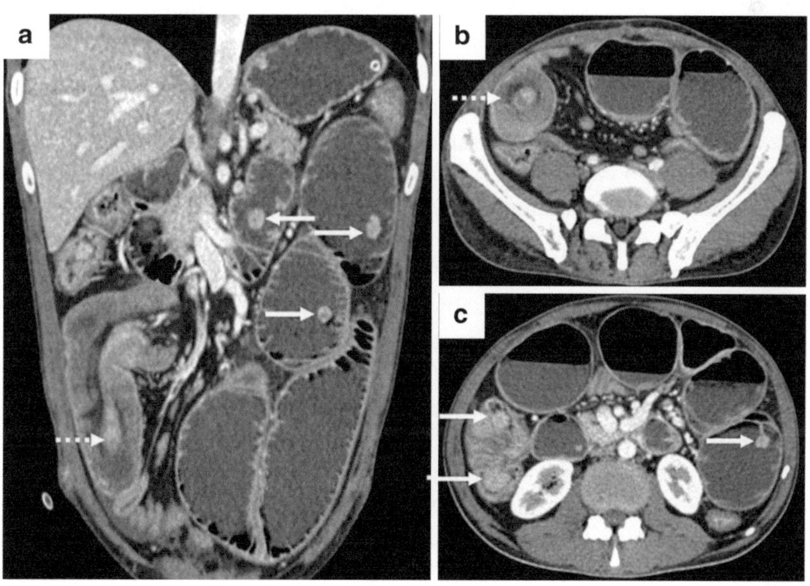

Fig. 9.22 Intussusception in a 7-year-old child with Peutz-Jegher syndrome. Coronal (**a**) and axial (**b**, **c**) CECT images depict multiple gastric and jejuno-ileal polyps (arrows) with one of the lesions as the lead point of the intussusception (dashed arrow in **a** and **b**). Note the grossly dilated proximal small bowel loops

obstruction suggest pathological intussusception on USG [66].

Other causes of bowel obstruction in children with cancer can be benign like postoperative adhesions following abdomino-pelvic surgery, inflammatory or post-infectious strictures, and nonobstructive adynamic ileus secondary to certain drugs like vinca alkaloids group, or the obstruction can be malignancy-associated [22, 47]. Malignant small bowel obstruction is caused more frequently by metastatic tumors while colonic obstruction is generally caused by the primary malignancy [22]. Erect abdominal radiograph typically displays dilated bowel loops with multiple air-fluid levels and lack of fecal matter and gas in the distal bowel. In paralytic ileus, uniform dilatation of the entire bowel is observed without abrupt transition point. Contrast-enhanced CT is the imaging modality of choice as it demonstrates both the site and the cause of obstruction [47].

Bowel perforation, an infrequent presentation, may result due to bowel obstruction, tumor infiltration (e.g., in Burkitt's lymphoma), gastritis/peptic ulcers, or after rigorous chemotherapy or radiation. An erect chest or abdominal radiograph may demonstrate pneumoperitoneum and CECT may reveal the free air as well as the site of perforation [23, 67].

9.5.3 Neutropenic Colitis

Neutropenic colitis/typhlitis, a potentially life-threatening ailment, is transmural necrotizing bowel inflammation affecting profoundly neutropenic children post chemotherapy for hematologic cancers. The exact incidence in children is unknown, but it occurs infrequently in pediatric patients than in adults. It usually involves the cecum, terminal ileum, appendix, and ascending colon although rest of the bowel can also be involved [47, 68]. Due to similar symptomatology, it is clinically difficult to differentiate typhlitis from acute appendicitis in neutropenic children. So, imaging, usually USG or CT, is often obligatory for diagnosis. Imaging characteristically shows bowel wall thickening (Fig. 9.23), pericolic/pericecal mesenteric inflammation, ascites, mucosal enhancement, and less commonly, pneumatosis intestinalis [15, 69]. The bowel wall thickness may be striking (>8 mm; as compared to aGVHD where wall thickening is generally moderate) [70]. Neutropenic colitis can be complicated by bowel perforation. Other differential diagnoses include postinfectious enterocolitis like pseudomembranous colitis, and intestinal GVHD.

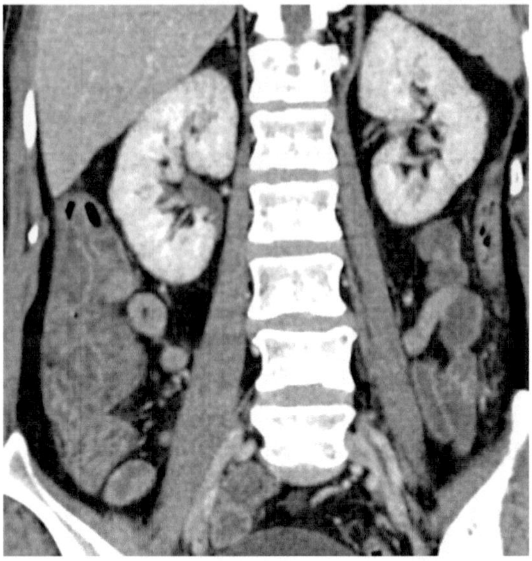

Fig. 9.23 Neutropenic typhlitis in a severely neutropenic child with ALL

9.5.4 Intestinal Graft-Versus-Host Disease

Graft-versus-host disease (GVHD) is a severe complication of hematopoietic cell transplantation (HCT). It ensues when donor T cells cross-react with the host tissues in the skin, liver, or GI tract [71]. Acute GVHD typically occurs within 100 days post-transplantation. Patients with intestinal GVHD commonly present with nausea, vomiting, crampy abdominal pain, and copious diarrhea. Pathologically, acute intestinal GVHD triggers destruction of intestinal crypts and results in focal or diffuse mucosal ulceration. Small bowel is typically more severely involved.

Abdominal radiograph shows ileus with separation of bowel loops, and air–fluid levels [47]. USG reveals dilated fluid-filled bowel loops with wall thickening (>3 mm) while CECT shows marked mucosal enhancement. Further, there is characteristic "target sign" seen due to hyperenhancing mucosal and serosal surfaces with a hypoenhancing intervening layer signifying intramural/submucosal edema [72]. Pneumatosis intestinalis, mesenteric vascular engorgement, and ascites can also be seen [47].

9.5.5 Acute Pancreatitis

Many chemotherapeutic drugs may induce pancreatitis in pediatric patients, especially those used in the treatment of ALL (acute lymphoblastic leukemia) or lymphoma, e.g., l-asparaginase, vincristine, doxorubicin, and corticosteroids [73]. L-asparaginase commonly causes necrotizing pancreatitis and affects about 5–18% of patients being treated with this drug. Pancreatitis may occur as an early or late complication [6, 74]. Re-treatment with L-asparaginase after an attack of mild pancreatitis predisposes to the risk of recurrent pancreatitis, the risk and severity of which are unrelated to the severity of the first attack. On imaging, typical features of acute pancreatitis like diffuse pancreatic enlargement, decreased enhancement, peripancreatic fat streaking, fluid collections, and/or pancreatic necrosis/pseudocysts can be seen (Fig. 9.24). Pseudocysts are the commonest complication and are seen in 18–30% of patients [7, 73].

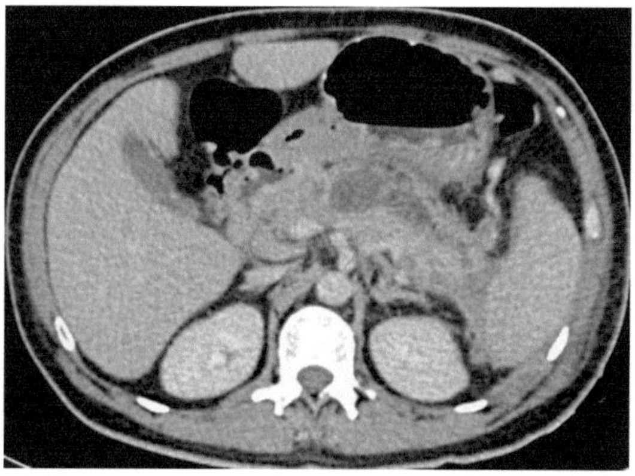

Fig. 9.24 L-asparaginase-induced acute pancreatitis in a 10-year-old child with ALL. Axial CECT abdomen shows pancreatic enlargement with intra- and peri-pancreatic necrosis and peri-pancreatic inflammation

9.5.6 Hepatic Vascular Complications

Hepatic sinusoidal obstruction syndrome (HSOS) is a critical, life-threatening complication of high-dose chemotherapeutic treatment, especially with HSCT. The incidence in pediatric patients is 10–20% [75]. Infrequently, conventional chemotherapy may incite milder form of HSOS that generally resolves spontaneously [7, 76]. The pathophysiology behind HSOS involves hepatic venous microvasculature damage causing decreased liver outflow and, thereby, portal hypertension [15]. Imaging features are nonspecific including hepatosplenomegaly, ascites, periportal edema, edematous gallbladder wall, decreased velocity (<10 cm/s) or reversed portal vein flow, narrowed but patent hepatic veins with loss of phasicity, and raised hepatic artery resistive index >0.75 [77]. Additionally, increase in hepatic artery peak systolic velocity and in liver stiffness on transient elastography might represent early imaging features of HSOS in children [7].

Another infrequent abdominal vascular complication is portal vein thrombosis in children on intensive chemotherapy with HSCT, having an incidence of 0.7%. The diagnosis is imaging-based; ultrasound being highly sensitive and specific for diagnosis. In the majority of patients, HSOS is followed by portal venous thrombosis [78].

9.5.7 Hemorrhagic Cystitis

Chemoradiation, infections, and HSCT may cause transitional epithelial injury as well as injury to the urinary tract blood vessels leading to diffuse mucosal hemorrhage from any part of the urothelium, urinary bladder (UB) being the most vulnerable organ [6, 79]. Cyclophosphamide

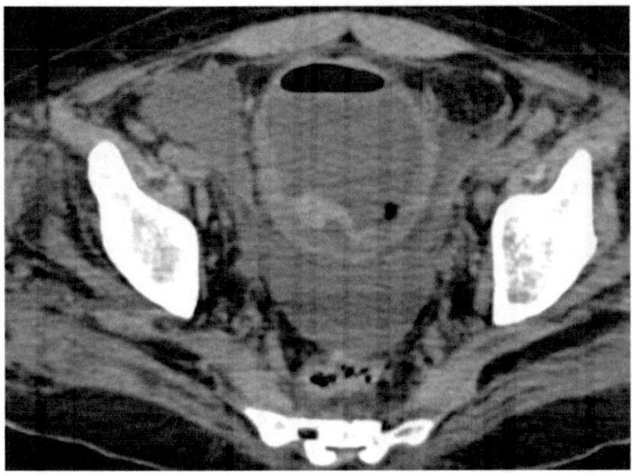

Fig. 9.25 Cyclophosphamide-induced hemorrhagic cystitis in a 14-year-old child with germ cell tumor post-HSCT. Axial CECT pelvis image showing diffuse bladder wall thickening with echogenic blood clot. Note the air within the bladder secondary to catheterization

is a common cause of hemorrhagic cystitis (HC). HC has been reported to be seen in approximately 6% of the pediatric patients with cancer with the incidence being greater in post HSCT patients (up to 25%). It can occur as an early or a late effect of the therapy. Severe cystitis poses the risk of complications like reflux or obstructive hydronephrosis, bladder perforation, and renal damage. The imaging method of choice is USG that may reveal focal or diffuse UB wall thickening (>3 mm in distended and > 5 mm in non-distended UB) with hypervascularity and intraluminal blood clots (Fig. 9.25) [79, 80]. Recurrent/chronic HC may ultimately lead to UB fibrosis with small appearing contracted UB on imaging. Fibrosis results in a reduced UB capacity, causing reflux, hydroureteronephrosis, and renal damage over time [15].

9.6 Conclusion

In this chapter, we reviewed various indirectly cancer-related as well as cancer therapy-related diseases and complications in the pediatric age group with brief discussion of their imaging features. These conditions may present any time in the course of cancer management, i.e., at the time of diagnosis, while on treatment, in remission phase, or during end-of-life care and may pose a substantial diagnostic challenge. Imaging plays a crucial role in ruling out or diagnosing majority of these conditions, thereby aiding in improvement of overall outcomes in pediatric cancers. So a collaborative multidisciplinary approach and interpretation of the imaging findings with reference to the clinical symptomatology as well as treatment details (type and phasing) is essential to provide the most efficient care to the affected children without delay.

Acknowledgements
1. Dr. Jitender Saini, Professor, Department of NeuroImaging and Interventional Radiology, NIMHANS, Bangalore, Karnataka.
2. Dr. Yashwant Kashyap, Senior, Consultant, Department of Medical Oncology, Balco Medical Center, Raipur, Chhattisgarh.

References

1. Siegel RL, Miller KD, Fuchs HE, Jemal A. Cancer statistics, 2021. CA Cancer J Clin. 2021;71(1):7–33.
2. Butler E, Ludwig K, Pacenta HL, Klesse LJ, Watt TC, Laetsch TW. Recent progress in the treatment of cancer in children. CA Cancer J Clin. 2021 Jul;71(4):315–32.
3. Hudson MM, Ness KK, Gurney JG, Mulrooney DA, Chemaitilly W, Krull KR, et al. Clinical ascertainment of health outcomes among adults treated for childhood cancer. JAMA. 2013;309(22):2371–81.
4. Cheung C, Fung KFK, Ng CWK, Chan PKJ, Wong KC, Lam KSG, et al. Treatment-related complications in children with cancer. Radiographics. 2024;44(4):e230072.
5. Shelmerdine SC, Chavhan GB, Babyn PS, Nathan PC, Kaste SC. Imaging of late complications of cancer therapy in children. Pediatr Radiol. 2017;47(3):254–66.
6. Chavhan GB, Babyn PS, Nathan PC, Kaste SC. Imaging of acute and subacute toxicities of cancer therapy in children. Pediatr Radiol. 2016;46(1):9–20. quiz 6–8
7. Voss SD, McHugh K, editors. Imaging in pediatric oncology [internet]. Cham: Springer; 2019. (Pediatric Oncology). Available from: http://link.springer.com/10.1007/978-3-030-03777-2
8. Mor M, Gilad G, Kornreich L, Fisher S, Yaniv I, Levy I. Invasive fungal infections in pediatric oncology. Pediatr Blood Cancer. 2011;56(7):1092–7.
9. Roberts SD, Wells GM, Gandhi NM, York NR, Maron G, Razzouk B, et al. Diagnostic value of routine chest radiography in febrile, neutropenic children for early detection of pneumonia and mould infections.

Support Care Cancer Off J Multinatl Assoc Support Care Cancer. 2012;20(10):2589–94.
10. Phillips RS, Lehrnbecher T, Alexander S, Sung L. Updated systematic review and meta-analysis of the performance of risk prediction rules in children and young people with febrile neutropenia. PLoS One. 2012;7(5):e38300.
11. Lehrnbecher T, Robinson PD, Ammann RA, Fisher B, Patel P, Phillips R, et al. Guideline for the management of fever and neutropenia in pediatric patients with cancer and hematopoietic cell transplantation recipients: 2023 update. J Clin Oncol. 2023;41(9):1774–85.
12. Lehrnbecher T, Robinson P, Fisher B, Alexander S, Ammann RA, Beauchemin M, et al. Guideline for the management of fever and neutropenia in children with cancer and hematopoietic stem-cell transplantation recipients: 2017 update. J Clin Oncol Off J Am Soc Clin Oncol. 2017;35(18):2082–94.
13. Peltola V, Ruuskanen O, Svedström E. Magnetic resonance imaging of lung infections in children. Pediatr Radiol. 2008;38(11):1225–31.
14. Sodhi KS, Khandelwal N, Saxena AK, Bhatia A, Bansal D, Trehan A, et al. Rapid lung MRI – paradigm shift in evaluation of febrile neutropenia in children with leukemia: a pilot study. Leuk Lymphoma. 2016;57(1):70–5.
15. Snyder EJ, Sarma A, Poussaint TY, Krishnasarma R, Pruthi S. Complications of cancer therapy in children: a comprehensive review of neuroimaging findings. J Comput Assist Tomogr. 2023;47(5):820–32.
16. Chu WCW, Lee V, Howard RG, Roebuck DJ, Chik KW, Li CK. Imaging findings of paediatric oncology patients presenting with acute neurological symptoms. Clin Radiol. 2003;58(8):589–603.
17. Vázquez E, Delgado I, Sánchez-Montañez A, Barber I, Sánchez-Toledo J, Enríquez G. Side effects of oncologic therapies in the pediatric central nervous system: update on neuroimaging findings. Radiogr Rev Publ Radiol Soc N Am Inc. 2011;31(4):1123–39.
18. Weaver L, Samkari A. Neurological complications of childhood cancer. Semin Pediatr Neurol. 2017;24(1):60–9.
19. Nickerson JP, Richner B, Santy K, Lequin MH, Poretti A, Filippi CG, et al. Neuroimaging of pediatric intracranial infection--part 2: TORCH, viral, fungal, and parasitic infections. J Neuroimaging Off J Am Soc Neuroimaging. 2012;22(2):e52–63.
20. Zerizer I, Humphries PD. Imaging 'the lost tribe': a review of adolescent cancer imaging. Part 2: imaging of complications of cancer treatment. Cancer Imaging. 2009;9(1):82–8.
21. Prabhu SP, Young-Poussaint T. Pediatric central nervous system emergencies. Neuroimaging Clin N Am. 2010;20(4):663–83.
22. Guimaraes MD, Bitencourt AG, Marchiori E, Chojniak R, Gross JL, Kundra V. Imaging acute complications in cancer patients: what should be evaluated in the emergency setting? Cancer Imaging. 2014;14(1):18.
23. Gaunt T, D'Arco F, Smets AM, McHugh K, Shelmerdine SC. Emergency imaging in paediatric oncology: a pictorial review. Insights Imaging. 2019;10(1):120.
24. Okabe T, Nozaki T, Aida N, Starkey J, Enokizono M, Niwa T, et al. MR imaging findings in some rare neurological complications of paediatric cancer. Insights Imaging. 2018;9(3):313–24.
25. Bhojwani D, Sabin ND, Pei D, Yang JJ, Khan RB, Panetta JC, et al. Methotrexate-induced neurotoxicity and leukoencephalopathy in childhood acute lymphoblastic leukemia. J Clin Oncol. 2014;32(9):949–59.
26. Sun LR, Cooper S. Neurological complications of the treatment of pediatric neoplastic disorders. Pediatr Neurol. 2018;85:33–42.
27. Sabin ND, Cheung YT, Reddick WE, Bhojwani D, Liu W, Glass JO, et al. The impact of persistent leukoencephalopathy on brain white matter microstructure in long-term survivors of acute lymphoblastic leukemia treated with chemotherapy only. AJNR Am J Neuroradiol. 2018;39(10):1919–25.
28. Sommers KR, Skiles J, Leland B, Rowan CM. Posterior reversible encephalopathy syndrome: incidence and clinical characteristics in children with cancer. J Pediatr Hematol Oncol. 2022;44(2):54–9.
29. Musioł K, Waz S, Boroń M, Kwiatek M, Machnikowska-Sokołowska M, Gruszczyńska K, et al. PRES in the course of hemato-oncological treatment in children. Childs Nerv Syst. 2018;34(4):691–9.
30. Donmez FY, Guleryuz P, Agildere M. MRI findings in childhood PRES: what is different than the adults? Clin Neuroradiol. 2016;26(2):209–13.
31. Khan RB, Sadighi ZS, Zabrowski J, Gajjar A, Jeha S. Imaging patterns and outcome of posterior reversible encephalopathy syndrome during childhood cancer treatment. Pediatr Blood Cancer. 2016;63(3):523–6.
32. Armstrong C, Sun LR. Neurological complications of pediatric cancer. Cancer Metastasis Rev. 2020;39(1):3–23.
33. Fan EP, Heiber G, Gerard EE, Schuele S. Stroke-like migraine attacks after radiation therapy: a misnomer? Epilepsia. 2018;59(1):259–68.
34. Stubblefield MD. Neuromuscular complications of radiation therapy. Muscle Nerve. 2017;56(6):1031–40.
35. Noje C, Cohen K, Jordan LC. Hemorrhagic and ischemic stroke in children with cancer. Pediatr Neurol. 2013;49(4):237–42.
36. Fullerton HJ, Stratton K, Mueller S, Leisenring WW, Armstrong GT, Weathers RE, et al. Recurrent stroke in childhood cancer survivors. Neurology. 2015;85(12):1056–64.
37. Sciubba DM, Gallia GL, Recinos P, Garonzik IM, Clatterbuck RE. Intracranial aneurysm following radiation therapy during childhood for a brain tumor. Case report and review of the literature. J Neurosurg. 2006;105(2 Suppl):134–9.
38. Madhavan AA, Carr CM, Morris PP, Flanagan EP, Kotsenas AL, Hunt CH, et al. Imaging review of

paraneoplastic neurologic syndromes. AJNR Am J Neuroradiol. 2020;41(12):2176–87.
39. Wells EM, Dalmau J. Paraneoplastic neurologic disorders in children. Curr Neurol Neurosci Rep. 2011;11(2):187–94.
40. Hsu M, Tejani I, Shah N, Olaosebikan R, Kumar A, Naik S. Review of Opsoclonus-myoclonus ataxia syndrome in pediatric patients. Children. 2024;11(3):367.
41. Ma GM, Chow JS, Taylor GA. Review of paraneoplastic syndromes in children. Pediatr Radiol. 2019;49(4):534–50.
42. Traylor KS, Kralik SF, Radhakrishnan R. Pediatric spine emergencies. Semin Ultrasound CT MR. 2018;39(6):605–17.
43. Tantawy AAG, Ebeid FSE, Mahmoud MA, Shepl OE. Spinal cord compression in childhood pediatric malignancies: multicenter egyptian study. J Pediatr Hematol Oncol. 2013;35(3):232–6.
44. Schiff D. Spinal cord compression. Neurol Clin. 2003;21(1):67–86. viii. https://doi.org/10.1016/s0733-8619(02)00033-6. PMID: 12690645.
45. Neil EC, Hanmantgad S, Khakoo Y. Neurological complications of pediatric cancer. J Child Neurol. 2016;31(12):1412–20.
46. Lee EQ, Arrillaga-Romany IC, Wen PY. Neurologic complications of cancer drug therapies. Contin Minneap Minn. 2012;18(2):355–65.
47. Handa A, Nozaki T, Makidono A, Okabe T, Morita Y, Fujita K, et al. Pediatric oncologic emergencies: clinical and imaging review for pediatricians. Pediatr Int. 2019;61(2):122–39.
48. Toma P, Bertaina A, Castagnola E, Colafati GS, D'Andrea ML, Finocchi A, et al. Fungal infections of the lung in children. Pediatr Radiol. 2016;46(13):1856–65.
49. Wingard JR, Hsu J, Hiemenz JW. Hematopoietic stem cell transplantation: an overview of infection risks and epidemiology. Infect Dis Clin N Am. 2010;24(2):257–72.
50. Gertz SJ, McArthur J, Hsing DD, Nitu ME, Smith LS, Loomis A, et al. Respiratory pathogens associated with intubated pediatric patients following hematopoietic cell transplant. Transpl Infect Dis Off J Transplant Soc. 2020;22(4):e13297.
51. Fisher BT, Danziger-Isakov L, Sweet LR, Munoz FM, Maron G, Tuomanen E, et al. A multicenter consortium to define the epidemiology and outcomes of inpatient respiratory viral infections in pediatric hematopoietic stem cell transplant recipients. J Pediatr Infect Dis Soc. 2018;7(4):275–82.
52. Morin CE, McBee MP, Elbahlawan L, Griffin LM, Maron GM, Nguyen HN, et al. Early pulmonary complications related to cancer treatment in children. Pediatr Radiol. 2022;52(10):2017–28.
53. Alexander BD, Lamoth F, Heussel CP, Prokop CS, Desai SR, Morrissey CO, et al. Guidance on imaging for invasive pulmonary aspergillosis and mucormycosis: from the imaging working group for the revision and update of the consensus definitions of fungal disease from the EORTC/MSGERC. Clin Infect Dis Off Publ Infect Dis Soc Am. 2021;72(Suppl 2):S79–88.
54. Donnelly JP, Chen SC, Kauffman CA, Steinbach WJ, Baddley JW, Verweij PE, et al. Revision and update of the consensus definitions of invasive fungal disease from the European Organization for Research and Treatment of Cancer and the Mycoses Study Group Education and Research Consortium. Clin Infect Dis Off Publ Infect Dis Soc Am. 2020;71(6):1367–76.
55. Nishio N, Yagasaki H, Takahashi Y, Hama A, Muramatsu H, Tanaka M, et al. Engraftment syndrome following allogeneic hematopoietic stem cell transplantation in children. Pediatr Transplant. 2009;13(7):831–7.
56. Elbahlawan L, Galdo AM, Ribeiro RC. Pulmonary manifestations of hematologic and oncologic diseases in children. Pediatr Clin N Am. 2021;68(1):61–80.
57. Glanville AR, Benden C, Bergeron A, Cheng GS, Gottlieb J, Lease ED, et al. Bronchiolitis obliterans syndrome after lung or haematopoietic stem cell transplantation: current management and future directions. ERJ Open Res. 2022;8(3):00185–2022.
58. Yanik GA, Grupp SA, Pulsipher MA, Levine JE, Schultz KR, Wall DA, et al. TNF-receptor inhibitor therapy for the treatment of children with idiopathic pneumonia syndrome. A joint pediatric blood and marrow transplant consortium and children's oncology group study (ASCT0521). Biol Blood Marrow Transplant J Am Soc Blood Marrow Transplant. 2015;21(1):67–73.
59. Stein PD, Beemath A, Meyers FA, Skaf E, Sanchez J, Olson RE. Incidence of venous thromboembolism in patients hospitalized with cancer. Am J Med. 2006 Jan;119(1):60–8.
60. Monagle P, Adams M, Mahoney M, Ali K, Barnard D, Bernstein M, et al. Outcome of pediatric thromboembolic disease: a report from the Canadian childhood thrombophilia registry. Pediatr Res. 2000 Jun;47(6):763–6.
61. Lee EY, Kritsaneepaiboon S, Arellano CMR, Grace RF, Zurakowski D, Boiselle PM. Unsuspected pulmonary emboli in pediatric oncology patients: detection with MDCT. AJR Am J Roentgenol. 2010;194(5):1216–22.
62. Benveniste MF, Gomez D, Carter BW, Betancourt Cuellar SL, Shroff GS, Benveniste APA, et al. Recognizing radiation therapy-related complications in the chest. Radiogr Rev Publ Radiol Soc N Am Inc. 2019;39(2):344–66.
63. Benveniste MF, Gomez D, Carter BW, Betancourt Cuellar SL, De Groot PM, Marom EM. Radiation effects in the mediastinum and surroundings: imaging findings and complications. Semin Ultrasound CT MR. 2016;37(3):268–80.
64. Albano D, Benenati M, Bruno A, Bruno F, Calandri M, Caruso D, et al. Imaging side effects and complications of chemotherapy and radiation therapy: a pictorial review from head to toe. Insights Imaging. 2021;12(1):76.

65. Gupta H, Davidoff AM, Pui CH, Shochat SJ, Sandlund JT. Clinical implications and surgical management of intussusception in pediatric patients with Burkitt lymphoma. J Pediatr Surg. 2007;42(6):998–1001. discussion 1001
66. Munden MM, Bruzzi JF, Coley BD, Munden RF. Sonography of pediatric small-bowel intussusception: differentiating surgical from nonsurgical cases. AJR Am J Roentgenol. 2007;188(1):275–9.
67. Fallon SC, Redell MS, El-Bietar J, Lopez ME, Vasudevan SA, Brandt ML. Intestinal perforation after treatment of Burkitt's lymphoma: case report and review of the literature. J Pediatr Surg. 2013;48(2):436–40.
68. Fike FB, Mortellaro V, Juang D, St Peter SD, Andrews WS, Snyder CL. Neutropenic colitis in children. J Surg Res. 2011;170(1):73–6.
69. McCarville MB, Adelman CS, Li C, Xiong X, Furman WL, Razzouk BI, et al. Typhlitis in childhood cancer. Cancer. 2005;104(2):380–7.
70. Mahgerefteh SY, Sosna J, Bogot N, Shapira MY, Pappo O, Bloom AI. Radiologic imaging and intervention for gastrointestinal and hepatic complications of hematopoietic stem cell transplantation. Radiology. 2011;258(3):660–71.
71. Jacobsohn DA. Acute graft-versus-host disease in children. Bone Marrow Transplant. 2008;41(2):215–21.
72. Lubner MG, Menias CO, Agrons M, Alhalabi K, Katabathina VS, Elsayes KM, et al. Imaging of abdominal and pelvic manifestations of graft-versus-host disease after hematopoietic stem cell transplant. AJR Am J Roentgenol. 2017;209(1):33–45.
73. Wolthers BO, Frandsen TL, Baruchel A, Attarbaschi A, Barzilai S, Colombini A, et al. Asparaginase-associated pancreatitis in childhood acute lymphoblastic leukaemia: an observational Ponte di Legno toxicity working group study. Lancet Oncol. 2017;18(9):1238–48.
74. Flores-Calderón J, Exiga-Gonzaléz E, Morán-Villota S, Martín-Trejo J, Yamamoto-Nagano A. Acute pancreatitis in children with acute lymphoblastic leukemia treated with L-asparaginase. J Pediatr Hematol Oncol. 2009;31(10):790–3.
75. Corbacioglu S, Carreras E, Ansari M, Balduzzi A, Cesaro S, Dalle JH, et al. Diagnosis and severity criteria for sinusoidal obstruction syndrome/veno-occlusive disease in pediatric patients: a new classification from the European society for blood and marrow transplantation. Bone Marrow Transplant. 2018;53(2):138–45.
76. Mohty M, Malard F, Abecassis M, Aerts E, Alaskar AS, Aljurf M, et al. Sinusoidal obstruction syndrome/veno-occlusive disease: current situation and perspectives-a position statement from the European Society for Blood and Marrow Transplantation (EBMT). Bone Marrow Transplant. 2015;50(6):781–9.
77. Chung H, Im SA, Kim SK. Ultrasound in Hepatic Veno-occlusive Disease (HVOD) after Pediatric Hematopoietic Stem Cell Transplantation (HSCT): comparison of diagnostic criteria including the pediatric criteria of European Society for Blood and Marrow Transplantation (EBMT). Pediatr Hematol Oncol. 2020;37(4):275–87.
78. Brisse H, Orbach D, Lassau N, Servois V, Doz F, Debray D, et al. Portal vein thrombosis during antineoplastic chemotherapy in children: report of five cases and review of the literature. Eur J Cancer Oxf Engl 1990. 2004;40(18):2659–66.
79. Johnston D, Schurtz E, Tourville E, Jones T, Boemer A, Giel D. Risk factors associated with severity and outcomes in pediatric patients with hemorrhagic cystitis. J Urol. 2016;195(4 Pt 2):1312–7.
80. McCarville MB, Hoffer FA, Gingrich JR, Jenkins JJ. Imaging findings of hemorrhagic cystitis in pediatric oncology patients. Pediatr Radiol. 2000;30(3):131–8.

Part II

Neuro and Head and Neck

Supratentorial Pediatric Brain Tumors

10

Arpita Sahu, Aishvarya Shri Rajasimman, Nihaal Reddy, Karuna Shekdar, Tejas Kapadia, and Kshitij Mankad

10.1 Introduction

Brain tumors are the most prevalent solid neoplasms in the pediatric age group and account for around 20% of all childhood cancers [1].

Pilocytic astrocytomas and embryonal tumors are the commonest CNS tumors under 10 years of age and gliomas are more common in older children and adults [2]. Other tumors in children include glioneuronal tumors, ependymal tumors, choroid plexus tumors, and germ cell tumors.

More than one-third of the pediatric brain neoplasms are supratentorial. The supratentorial neoplasms belong to a wide variety of histological origin ranging from glial & glioneuronal cells, neuroectodermal origin, choroid plexus, pineal gland, etc. Supratentorial brain tumors of higher grade (WHO category 3 and 4) are commonly seen in infants and younger children and behave more aggressively than the infratentorial tumors.

Over several decades, there has been tremendous progress in understanding the biology and molecular characteristics of these tumors. Molecular and genomic testing with next-generation sequencing (NGS) has changed the landscape of the pediatric brain tumors with many changes and newer additions in the recent fifth edition of WHO classification of brain tumors (Table 10.1) [3].

The main role of imaging is to differentiate between high-grade and low-grade tumors, study the extent to guide surgical outcome, and to evaluate other associated features like metastasis.

The aim of this chapter is to provide an overview of the imaging characteristics of the supratentorial pediatric brain tumors with a special focus on newly added entities.

All authors have reviewed and approved the final manuscript.

A. Sahu (✉) · A. S. Rajasimman
Department of Radiodiagnosis, Tata Memorial Centre & Homi Bhabha National Institute, Mumbai, Maharashtra, India

N. Reddy
Rainbow Children's Hospital, Hyderabad, Telangana, India

K. Shekdar
Perelman School of Medicine, The Children's Hospital of Philadelphia, Department of Radiology, Neuro-radiology Division, University of Pennsylvania, Philadelphia, PA, USA

T. Kapadia
Royal Manchester Children's Hospital, Manchester, UK

K. Mankad
Great Ormand Street Hospital, London, UK

I. Kumar et al. (eds.), *Practical Approach to Imaging in Pediatric Oncology*,
https://doi.org/10.1007/978-981-96-8158-7_10

Table 10.1 Classification of pediatric brain tumors based and adapted from 5th edition WHO classification (2021)

Pediatric-type diffuse low-grade gliomas	Diffuse astrocytoma MYB- or MYBL1 altered* Angiocentric glioma Polymorphous low-grade neuroepithelial tumor of the young* Diffuse low-grade glioma, MAPK pathway altered*
Pediatric-type diffuse high-grade gliomas	Diffuse midline glioma H3 K-27 altered ** Diffuse hemispheric glioma H3 G34 mutant* Diffuse pediatric type diffuse high-grade glioma, H3 & IDH- wildtype* Infant-type hemispheric glioma*
Circumscribed astrocytic glioma	Pilocytic astrocytoma Pleomorphic xanthoastrocytoma Subependymal giant cell astrocytoma Chordoid glioma Astroblastoma MN1-altered
Glioneuronal and neuronal tumors	Ganglioglioma Gangliocytoma Desmoplastic infantile ganglioglioma Desmoplastic infantile astrocytoma Dysembryoplastic neuroepithelial tumor (DNET) Diffuse glioneuronal tumor with oligodendroglioma-like features and nuclear clusters* Papillary glioneuronal tumor Rosette-forming glioneuronal tumor Myxoid glioneuronal tumor * Diffuse leptomeningeal glioneuronal tumor** Multinodular and vacuolating neuronal tumor** Central neurocytoma
Embryonal tumors	Medulloblastoma Atypical teratoid/rhabdoid tumor Embryonal tumor with multilayered rosettes** Cribriform neuroepithelial tumor* CNS neuroblastoma, FOXR2-activated* CNS tumor with BCOR internal tandem duplication* CNS embryonal tumor NEC/NOS
Ependymal tumors	Supratentorial ependymoma, ZFTA fusion positive Supratentorial ependymoma, YAP1 fusion positive * Supratentorial ependymoma NOS Posterior fossa ependymoma, NOS Posterior fossa group A (PFA) ependymoma Posterior fossa group B (PFB) ependymoma Spinal ependymoma, NOS Spinal ependymoma, MYCN-amplified Myxopapillary ependymoma Subependymoma
Choroid plexus tumors	Choroid plexus papilloma Atypical choroid papilloma Choroid plexus carcinoma
Pineal tumors	Pineoblastoma Pineocytoma Pineal parenchymal tumor of intermediate differentiation Papillary tumor of the pineal region Desmoplastic myxoid tumor, SMARCB1-mutant*
Mesenchymal non-meningothelial tumors involving the CNS	Solitary fibrous tumor Rhabdomyosarcoma Intracranial mesenchymal tumor, FET::CREB fusion positive* CIC-rearranged sarcoma* Primary intracranial sarcoma, DICER1-mutant* Ewing sarcoma

(continued)

Table 10.1 (continued)

Tumors of the sellar region	Adamantinomatous craniopharyngioma Pituitary adenoma, pituitary neuroendocrine tumor Pituitary blastoma*
Hematolymphoid tumors involving the CNS	Primary diffuse large B-cell lymphoma of the CNS Immunodeficiency-associated CNS lymphomas Lymphomatoid granulomatosis Miscellaneous rare lymphomas of the CNS Secondary CNS lymphomas Langerhans cell histiocytosis Rare histiocytic tumors
Germ cell tumors	Germinoma and non-germinomatous germ cell tumors

Newly added tumors in 2021 classification are marked with * and those were added in 2016 classification are marked with **

10.2 Clinical Presentation

The common presenting features of pediatric brain tumors are headache, nausea, and papilledema associated with raised intracranial pressure [4]. The mass effect could also lead to various herniation syndromes that could result in brainstem compression and related symptoms like vomiting, diplopia, facial weakness, and gagging. One of the frequent symptoms in patients with brain tumors is seizure which has a variable incidence of 30–100% among brain tumor patients [5]. The neuronal and neuroglial neoplasms are the ones to commonly present with seizures as they tend to co-exist with cortical dysplasia.

Apart from these there are localizing signs and symptoms. Frontal lobe tumors present with personality changes and cognitive disturbances while the temporal lobe lesions present with seizures. Visual symptoms are usually seen with the occipital lobe lesions and sometimes with temporal lobe lesions (when the optic radiation is involved).

Pineal region tumors can be associated with Parinaud syndrome secondary to the compression of the tectum. Parinaud syndrome is a triad of upward gaze palsy, light-near dissociation of pupillary reflex, and nystagmus [6].

10.3 Diagnostic Workup

MRI is the primary investigation of choice for suspected intracranial space-occupying lesion, owing to its superior resolution and non-ionizing nature. CT is helpful in ruling out other causes of neurological symptoms like infarct, hemorrhage, or meningitis. If a lesion is seen characterization is limited to look at the location, extent of the lesion, associated mass effect, and intralesional calcifications/hemorrhage. Owing to the excellent bony structure visualization, CT is helpful to evaluate lesions close to the skull-base [5].

MRI with gadolinium-enhanced protocols forms the workhorse of brain tumor assessment. With the advent of many newer sequences, MRI could help narrowing to a diagnosis in most of the cases. Conventional MR sequences comprising T1, T2, and FLAIR (fluid attenuated inversion recovery) are the primary sequences acquired in a suspected case of brain tumor. These sequences give basic details of the lesion like its size, location, heterogeneity, and fluid content.

Additional sequences like diffusion-weighted imaging (DWI) and susceptibility weighted imaging (SWI) have become the standard of care. Diffusion-weighted imaging and apparent diffusion coefficient (ADC) values indicate the cellularity of the lesion, with lower ADC values associated with higher cell density. Susceptibility-weighted imaging (SWI) can detect calcifications and hemorrhage in lesions, the differentiation between them being done using phase information. In lesions with ambiguous phase, phase information at its cranial or caudal margin can be used to reliably determine calcifications versus hemorrhage [7].

Proton MR spectroscopy provides information on the biochemical and metabolic profile within the tumor. Contrast sequence can be supplemented by perfusion which is generally a non-contrast perfusion technique like arterial spin labelling (ASL) [8, 9].

Post contrast T2-weighted FLAIR sequence is more sensitive in detecting leptomeningeal metastases and is recommended in CNS tumors with known metastatic potential [9]. Spine imaging is also recommended in tumors with CSF spread; to detect drop metastases and lately it has become a norm to include post-contrast spinal imaging as part of the pediatric brain tumor MRI protocol. The recommended standard of care MRI protocol tailored for brain tumors is discussed in the next section.

10.4 Consensus/Guidelines

A standardized imaging protocol is essential to maintain the uniformity of oncologic evaluation across various institutions to ensure quality imaging and compatibility. Hence in 2022, the Onco-imaging committee of the Society of Pediatric Radiology (SPR) and the Children's Oncology Group (COG) under International Society of Pediatric Oncology (SIOP) and American Society of Pediatric Hematology/Oncology formed a committee and published a white paper on imaging recommendations for pediatric brain tumors.

(i) Imaging Modality

In a child with a suspicious brain lesion, MRI is the recommended modality. However, if the child is unstable or if the facility does not have an available MRI, CT is recommended for initial assessment (Grade A, very strong recommendation) [10].

MRI of brain is the recommended modality for diagnosing and following-up of brain tumors (Grade A, very strong recommendation). It helps in characterizing and assessing the extent and dissemination of the disease. A 3-Tesla MRI is preferred over 1.5-Tesla in all cases except in cases where a metallic implant is present since the former has better spatial resolution and the latter is associated with lesser susceptibility artifacts (Grade B, strong recommendation). Spine screening is advised in high-grade pediatric tumors with risk of leptomeningeal dissemination and recommended by RAPNO to be done immediately after brain MRI, with a postcontrast T1-weighted series acquired first, followed by a steady-state acquisition (either, constructive interference steady-state or fast imaging employing steady-state acquisition) sequence in the sagittal plane [11].

(ii) Use of Contrast and Sedation

Unless an immediate surgical intervention is planned that requires or warrants a contrast examination, a contrast-enhanced CT is not essential and further characterization should be proceeded with an MRI. Contrast-enhanced MRI is recommended both at initial and follow-up imaging while macrocyclic contrasts are preferred over linear gadolinium agents [10].

Sedation or general anesthesia is needed in children less than 6 years of age, however when anesthesia could be avoided through the usage of video goggles, it should be tried.

(iii) MRI Protocol

An institutional MRI protocol for brain tumors has to be followed based on the recommended protocols. The minimum recommended sequences as per the recent white paper are given in Table 10.2.

(iv) Grading of Tumors

WHO has given grading for brain tumors that act as a scale for malignancy and disease prognosis based on pathology (Table 10.3).

Table 10.2 Minimum recommended MRI brain tumor protocol

Sequence	Plane of acquisition	Slice thickness
3D T1 TSE	Axial or sagittal	1–1.5
DWI with ADC (B value of 0 and 1000)	Axial	≤4
SWI or GRE	Axial	≤4
T2 TSE/FSE	Axial or coronal	≤4
Post contrast 3D T1 IR GRE	Axial or sagittal	1–1.5
Post contrast T1 TSE	Axial or coronal	1
Post contrast T2 FLAIR TSE/ FSE	Axial	≤4
Other optional sequences	Perfusion (DCE/DSC/ASL)	
	MR spectroscopy (TE short/long)	
	DTI (for surgical guidance)	
Spine screening	Sagittal spine screening on post-contrast sequences (pre-contrast sagittal images are optional)	

Adapted from COG diagnostic imaging committee white paper [9]
Abbreviations: *TSE* turbo spin echo, *DWI* diffusion-weighted imaging, *ADC* apparent diffusion coefficient, *SWI* susceptibility weighted imaging, *GRE* gradient echo, *FSE* fast spin echo, *IR* inversion recovery, *FLAIR* fluid attenuated inversion recovery, *DCE* dynamic contrast enhanced, *DSC* dynamic susceptibility contrast, *ASL* arterial spin labelling, *TE* time to echo, *DTI* diffusion tensor imaging

Table 10.3 Grading of brain tumors [5]

Grade	Tumoral pathology	Prognosis
Grade I	Low proliferative potential	Cure after surgical resection possible
Grade II	Infiltrative pattern of growth	Has potential to recur or progress to higher grade
Grade III	Pathologically malignant	Worse than III, better than IV
Grade IV	Pathologically malignant with more areas of necrosis	Rapid disease progression with fatal outcomes

10.5 Structured Reporting Template

MRI is the investigation of choice for detection and characterization of these masses. Systematically approaching these tumors on imaging for their typical imaging characteristics can help narrow down the diagnosis. In this section, a systematic and structured reporting format for supratentorial pediatric brain tumors is given in Table 10.4.

Table 10.4 Structured reporting template for supratentorial brain tumors

Age of the patient		
Number of lesions		
Compartment	Intra-axial/extra-axial/indeterminate	
Supratentorial/infratentorial		
Location		
Eloquent areas involved?	Yes/no, if yes please mention	
Size in cm		
Lesion characteristics		
T1 appearance		
T2/FLAIR appearance		
Uniformity	<homogeneous> < heterogeneous>	
If heterogeneous,		
Cyst	Yes/no	If not distinguishable, mentioned as cystoid component
Necrosis	Yes/no	
Bleed	Yes/no	Sometimes cannot be differentiated, may be mentioned as blooming on GRE
Calcification	Yes/no	
Diffusion restriction in solid areas	Yes/no	
Advanced sequences		
Perfusion relative to normal brain parenchyma	Hypo/iso/hyperperfused	
rCBV value		
Spectroscopy		
Choline/NAA ratio	≤2.5/ >2.5	
Choline/creatinine ratio	≤2/ >2	
Peri lesional and rim characteristics		
Margin definition	Circumscribed/non-circumscribed	
Peritumoral edema	Maximum distance in cm	
Any characteristic rim present?	Mention if different from lesion	
Peri-tumoral cyst	Present/absent	
Extent (mention as applicable)		
Nerve involvement	Yes/no/not applicable	
Vessel involvement	Yes/no	
Bone (calvarium/skull base)	Yes/no/not applicable	
Mass effect		
Sulcal effacement	Yes/no	
Any compression of brain matter	Yes/no	
Any compression of ventricle	Yes/no	
Any herniation	Yes/no, if yes please mention	
Post contrast findings		
Intralesional enhancement	Homogeneous/heterogeneous	
Margin of lesion		
Extralesional enhancement	Present/absent	
Additional findings		
Leptomeningeal spread	Present/absent	
Bone involvement/changes	Present/absent, if present describe	
Spinal cord changes/drop metastasis	Present/absent	
Other findings if any mention		
Impression		
Findings suggestive of	High or low-grade tumor	

10.6 Imaging Features

The brain tumor classification is broad and covering every tumor is beyond the scope of this chapter. So, the imaging features of newer and important supratentorial tumors shall be discussed in this section.

10.6.1 Pediatric-Type Diffuse Low-Grade Gliomas

10.6.1.1 Diffuse Astrocytoma MYB- or MYBL1-Altered

This is a rare WHO grade 1 pediatric glioma that has non-specific histological and imaging characteristics and needs molecular markers for diagnosis. These are characterized by fusion, amplification, or rearrangement of transcriptional regulators like MYB or MYBL1 [12]. Commonly involved locations include cerebral hemispheric cortex followed by supratentorial white matter and deep grey nuclei. On imaging, these are T2/FLAIR hyperintense lesion lacking post-contrast enhancement or diffusion restriction (Fig. 10.1). Though infiltrative, the lesion is usually well defined, preserving the brain structure. Hemorrhage, calcification, and necrosis are rare and the lesions show increased Cho/NAA ratio on spectroscopy [8]. More than half of the cases can show T2-FLAIR mismatch, this is more common in MYBL1-altered diffuse astrocytomas [13].

10.6.1.2 Angiocentric Glioma

Angiocentric gliomas are cortical-based low-grade (WHO grade 1) tumors associated with epilepsy. The median age of presentation is 13 years [8]. Predominantly occurs in frontal or temporal lobes appearing T2/FLAIR hyperintense without enhancement or diffusion restriction (Fig. 10.2). More than 50% of angiocentric gliomas show T1 hyperintense areas. A stalk-like structure could be seen from the tumor to the adjacent ventricular lining and is a frequent feature along with surrounding brain atrophy [14].

10.6.1.3 Polymorphous Low-Grade Neuroepithelial Tumor of the Young (PLNTY)

This is also a WHO grade 1 tumor that is cortical or subcortical in location. These occur in the second and third decades with a median age of 15 years. Temporal lobe is the common location and thus refractory seizure being the presenting complaint. These are usually a well-circumscribed tumor presenting with peripheral cysts interspersed with calcifications [15]. They appear T2/FLAIR hyperintense without enhancement or diffusion restriction (Fig. 10.3) [12]. Since the tumor contains oligodendroma-like components, dense and prominent calcifications are typically seen. These tumors are CD34 immunopositivity with mitogen-activated protein kinase (MAPK) alterations including FGFR or BRAF [16].

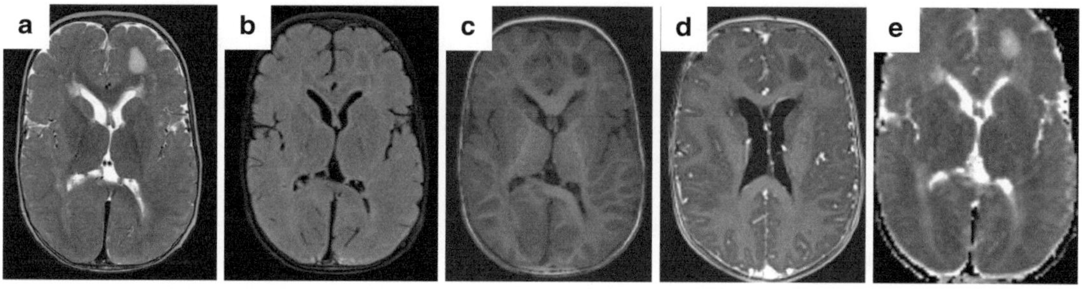

Fig. 10.1 A 1-year-old boy with a history of generic overgrowth syndrome with PIK3CA mutation. (**a**, **b**) MRI shows a well-defined T2 hyperintense lesion with T2-FLAIR mismatch. (**c**, **d**) It appears T1 hypointense without contrast enhancement or diffusion restriction (**e**). Note is also made on polymicrogyria. HPR – Diffuse Astrocytoma MYB-MYBL1 altered

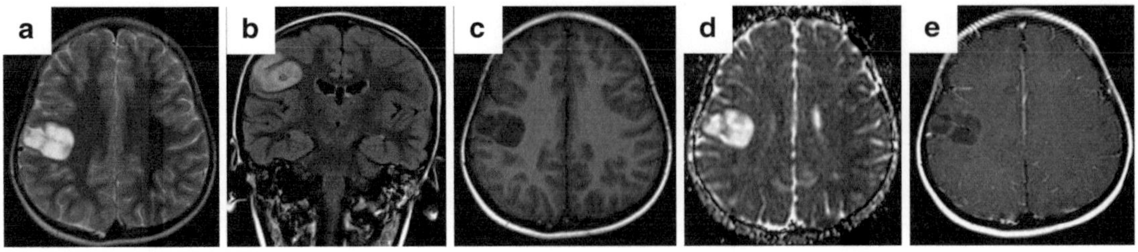

Fig. 10.2 A 14-year-old presented with left facial or brachial seizures. (**a**, **b**) MRI shows a well-defined T2W/FLAIR hyperintense lesion in the right parietal lobe. (**c**) It is hypointense on T1W. (**d**, **e**) No diffusion restriction or enhancement is seen. HPR – Angiocentric glioma

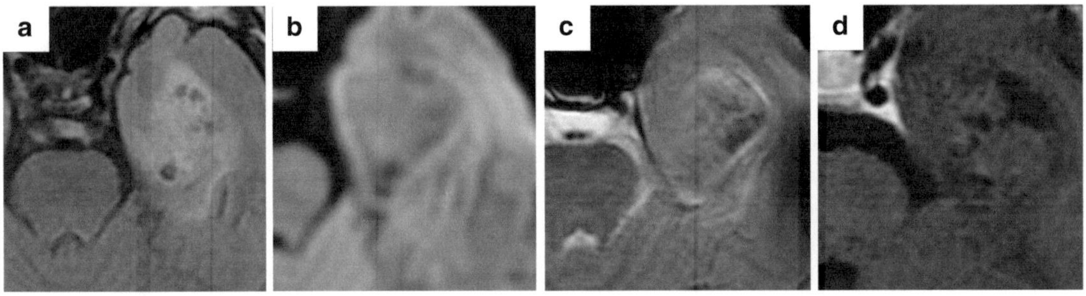

Fig. 10.3 A 15-year-old boy presented with episodes of seizures. (**a**, **b**) A well-defined FLAIR hyperintense lesion is seen in the left temporal lobe showing no diffusion restriction. (**c**, **d**) Few focal areas of blooming are seen without perilesional edema or enhancement is noted. HPR - Polymorphous low-grade neuroepithelial tumor of the young (PLNTY)

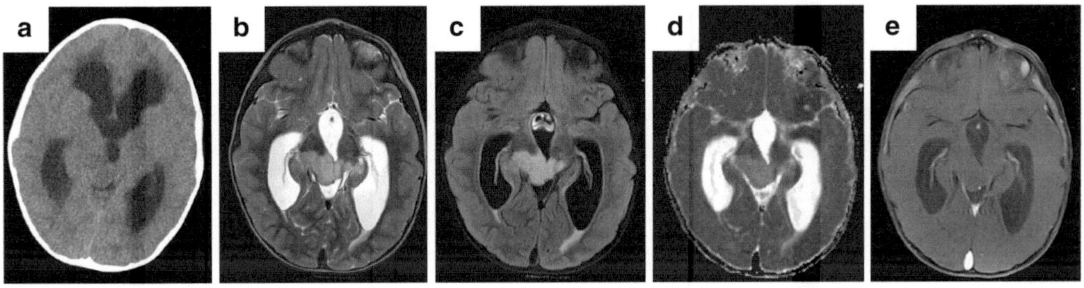

Fig. 10.4 A 8-year-old female presented with focal seizures. (**a**, **b**, **c**) CT shows an isodense lesion that appears hyperintense on T2/FLAIR involving the tectum, thalamus and brainstem on right. (**d**, **e**) No diffusion restriction or enhancement is seen. HPR - Diffuse low grade glioma MAPK pathway-altered

10.6.1.4 Diffuse Low-Grade Glioma, MAPK Pathway-Altered

These are low-grade gliomas with molecular alterations involving the MAPK pathway like FGFR and BRAF. IDH and H3F3 mutations must be absent. It has 3 molecular subtypes, diffuse low-grade glioma FGFR1 tyrosine kinase domain-duplicated, diffuse low-grade glioma FGFR1-mutant, and diffuse low-grade glioma BRAF V600E mutant [12]. The most common location is the temporal lobe. Literature on MRI findings of this rare tumor is very limited. They appear T2/FLAIR hyperintense and T1 hypointense. Enhancement may or may not be seen (Fig. 10.4).

10.6.2 Pediatric-Type Diffuse High-Grade Gliomas

These are grade 4 tumors with morphological features discussed below.

10.6.2.1 Diffuse Hemispheric Glioma H3G34-Mutant

This tumor involves the cerebral hemisphere, mostly parietal and temporal lobes. It has a male predilection and is more common in adolescents with median age of diagnosis being 15–19 years. The defining feature of this tumor is the missense mutation involving H3G34 [8]. The imaging features are similar to high-grade gliomas. These tumors are T2/FLAIR hyperintense, T1 hypointense with variable post-contrast enhancement and diffusion restriction (Fig. 10.5). They show increased perfusion with raised Cho/NAA ratio and Lip/Lac peaks on spectroscopy. Hemorrhage, calcification, and necrosis may be present [12, 17].

10.6.2.2 Diffuse Pediatric-Type High-Grade Glioma H3-Wildtype, IDH-Wildtype

It is a malignant high-grade glioma occurring in children which is wildtype for both IDH and H3. These were earlier classified as pediatric glioblastomas. Median age of involvement is 8 years [12]. Commonly, these are supratentorial but can also involve brainstem. These are aggressive neoplasms that appear heterogenous on T1, T2, and FLAIR with areas of hemorrhage and necrosis. It appears hyperintense on T2/FLAIR with inhomogeneous post-contrast enhancement and diffusion restriction (Fig. 10.6). As with any high-grade tumor, this entity also shows increased perfusion with elevated Cho/NAA ratio [8, 18].

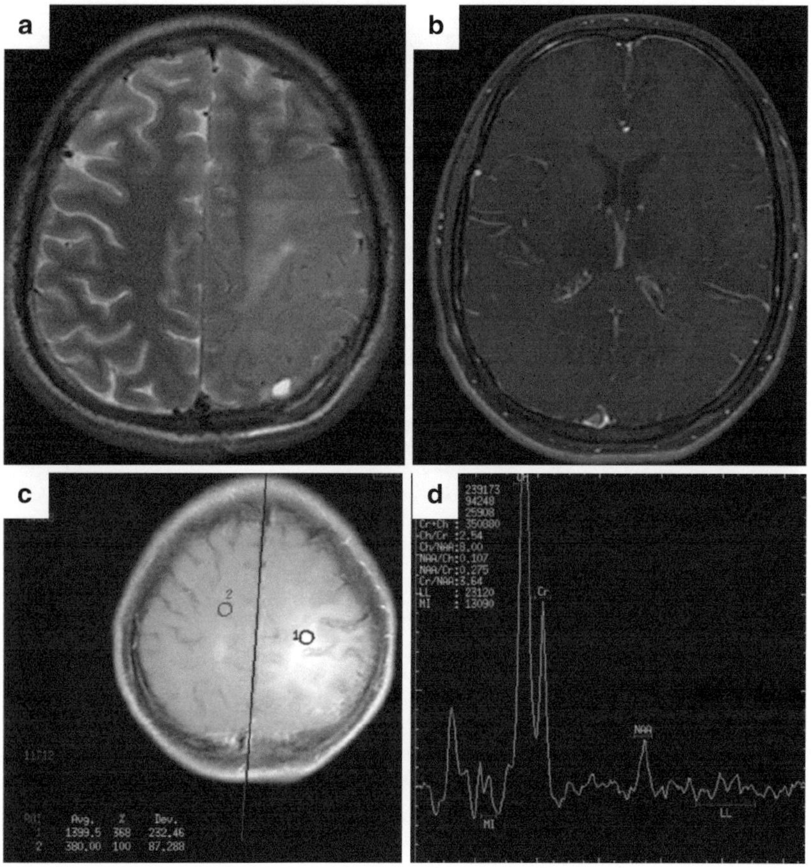

Fig. 10.5 A 15-year-old boy presented with hemiparesis for past 6 months with decreased speech and memory disturbances for 2 weeks. (**a**) T2 shows an ill-defined hyperintense lesion involving the left cerebral hemisphere. (**c**, **d**) The lesion is hyperperfused with elevated choline peak

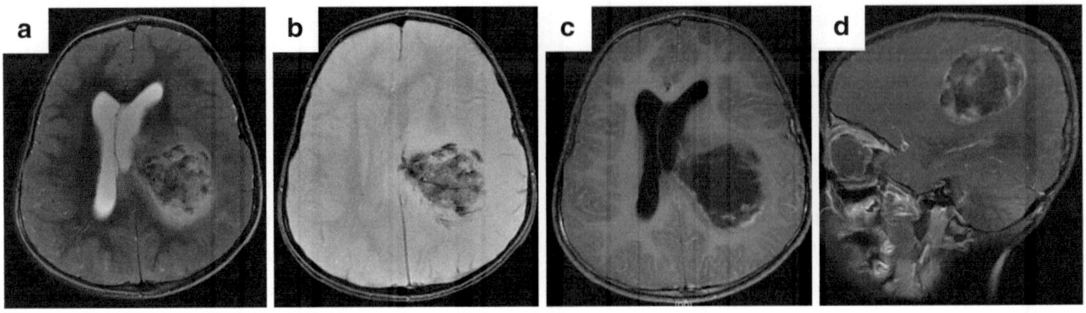

Fig. 10.6 A 6-year-old boy with headache, vomiting and right sided weakness for 15 days. Examination revealed Cafe au lait spots and family history of Cafe au lait spots. (**a**, **b**) MRI brain shows a T2 heterogenous lesion in the left parietal lobe with areas of blooming. (**c**, **d**) Note the lesion is necrotic with peripheral enhancement. HPR -Diffuse pediatric type diffuse high grade glioma, H3 & IDH- wildtype

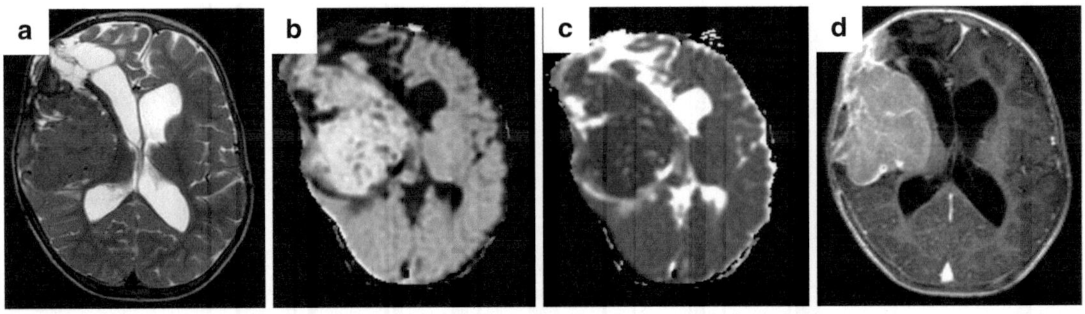

Fig. 10.7 A 11-month-old boy presented with projectile vomiting and GTCS. (**a**) MRI brain shows a large ill-defined heterogenous solid-cystic lesion involving the right fronto-temporal lobes and the adjacent meninges. (**b–d**) Note the diffusion restriction and avid contrast enhancement. HPR - Infant-type hemispheric glioma

10.6.2.3 Infant-Type Hemispheric Glioma

Infant-type hemispheric glioma is a high-grade tumor that shows tyrosine receptor kinase fusion (like ALK, MET, NTRK family, ROS1) [8]. These are large cortical-based supratentorial lesions occurring in infants with median age of 2–3 months. It carries a worse prognosis. These are large lesions involving one or two lobes or an entire hemisphere showing solid-cystic appearance and extensive areas of intralesional hemorrhage. They show avid heterogeneous enhancement (Fig. 10.7) [19].

10.6.3 Circumscribed Gliomas

10.6.3.1 Pleomorphic Xanthoastrocytoma (PXA)

These are WHO grade 2 astrocytic glial tumors that are common between 10 and 30 years, usually supratentorial in location. Characteristically, these are superficial tumors involving the cerebral cortex in the temporal lobe, presenting with seizures. They can be BRAF V600E mutated or wild type. On imaging these appear as T2/FLAIR hyperintense solid-cystic lesion with infiltrative appearance and vivid enhancement of the solid component near the pial surface. Usually, there is no diffusion restriction or perilesional edema (Fig. 10.8). PXA can be associated with adjacent meningeal enhancement or scalloping of the bone (one of the distinctive features) [4, 8].

10.6.3.2 Subependymal Giant Cell Astrocytoma (SEGA)

SEGA is a tumor of periventricular region that is associated with tuberous sclerosis (TS), arising in 5–15% of patients with TS. It classically arises in the subependymal region near the foramen of Monro. A SEGA can be defined as any caudothalamic lesion of size >1 cm or any subependymal

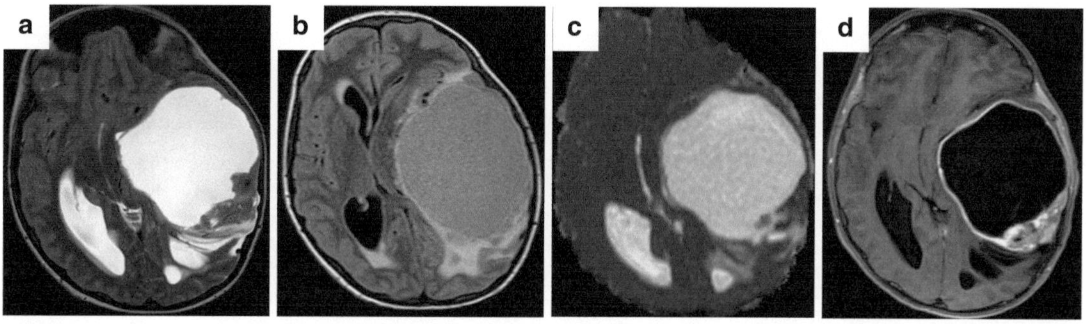

Fig. 10.8 A 12-year-old presented with severe headache, vomiting and visual distrubances. (**a, b**) T2W and FLAIR images show a large hyperintense lesion involving the left temporo-parietal cortex. The lesion shows thin peripheral enhancement with an eccentric enhancing component (**d**) without significant diffusion restriction (**c**). HPR – Pleomorphic Xanthoastrocytoma

lesion showing rapid growth in size [20]. It presents as a well-defined lesion in the foramen of Monro with calcifications, cystic areas, and avid enhancement. They are usually associated with hydrocephalus [21].

10.6.3.3 Astroblastoma MN1-Altered

Astroblastoma is a supratentorial glial neoplasm occurring in adolescents and young adults. This tumor doesn't have any assigned tumor grading. Previously, no particular molecular biomarker was associated with this tumor; but the 2021 classification has assigned MN1-alteration as a defining feature of astroblastoma. These are solid-cystic tumors that are T2/FLAIR iso-hyperintense, peripherally located, showing heterogeneous contrast enhancement, diffusion restriction in solid component. These are characterized by the multicystic or bubbly appearance (Fig. 10.9). Areas of hemorrhage and calcifications within have also been observed [4, 22].

Pilocytic astrocytoma comprises an important tumor of this classification category. Since predominant cases of pilocytic astrocytoma are infratentorial, it will be discussed in the next section.

10.6.4 Glioneuronal and Neuronal Tumors

This category comprises of many tumors, only the supratentorial tumors in children are being discussed here.

10.6.4.1 Ganglioglioma

These are slow-growing WHO grade 1 supratentorial tumors that are predominantly seen in temporal lobes. It is a tumor of adolescents and young adults occurring in the first 2 decades of life. They might show BRAF V600E mutation. On imaging, these are well-circumscribed lesions that present as a cyst with a mural nodule or as a solid-cystic lesion [9]. The solid component shows variable enhancement but is not restricted on diffusion-weighted imaging. Associated perilesional edema and scalloping of adjacent calvarial bone may be seen. When imaging shows an infiltrative lesion, it is associated with a higher grade of the tumor [4].

10.6.4.2 Dysembryoplastic Neuroepithelial Tumor (DNET)

DNETs are low-grade gliomas that are predominantly seen in children and adolescents. They commonly present with epilepsy. DNETs are cortical in location and are common in temporal lobe. Sometimes, these tumors are surrounded by a rim of dysplastic cortex [23]. On imaging, these are cortical tumors that appear bubble-like or pop-corn-like. These are hyperintense on T2 and FLAIR and are hypointense on T1. The lesion shows minimal to poor enhancement and shows no diffusion restriction (Fig. 10.10) [24].

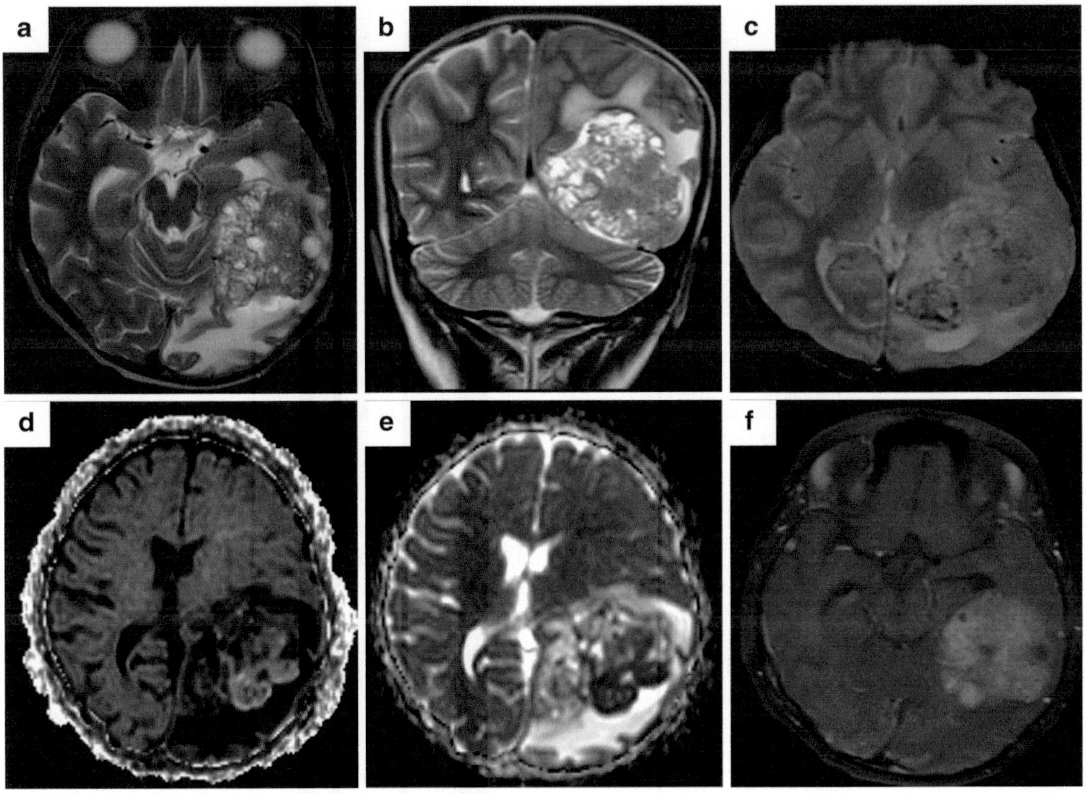

Fig. 10.9 An 8-year-old girl presented with vomiting, headache and giddiness. (**a**, **b**) MRI brain shows a T2/FLAIR hyperintense solid-cystic lesion with bubby appearance. (**c**) Small hemorrhagic foci are seen within. (**d**–**f**) Note the diffusion restriction and heterogeneous enhancement. HPR- Astroblastoma MN-1 altered

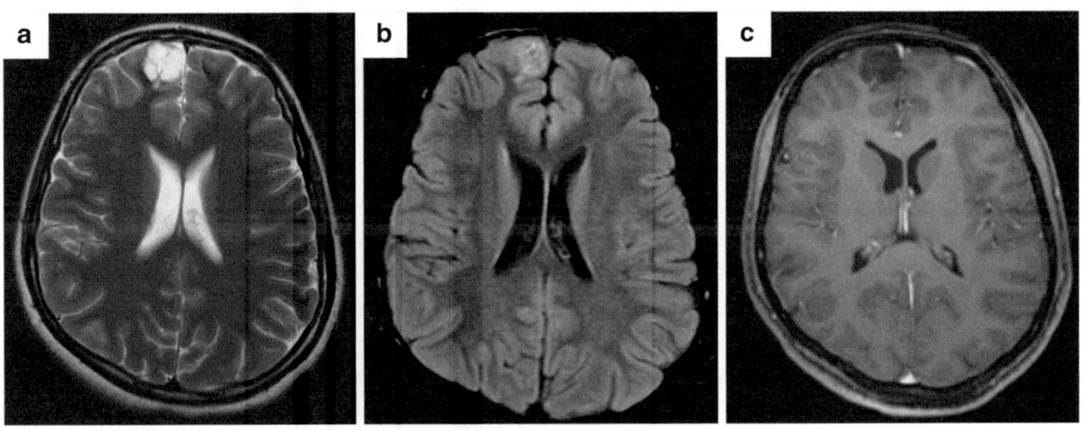

Fig. 10.10 (**a**) MRI brain of a 14-year-old boy with GTCS for 6 months shows a T2W hyperintense bubbly superficial lesion. (**b**, **c**) Note the FLAIR hyperintense rim and absence of contrast enhancement. HPR-Dysembryoplastic neuroepithelial tumor (DNET)

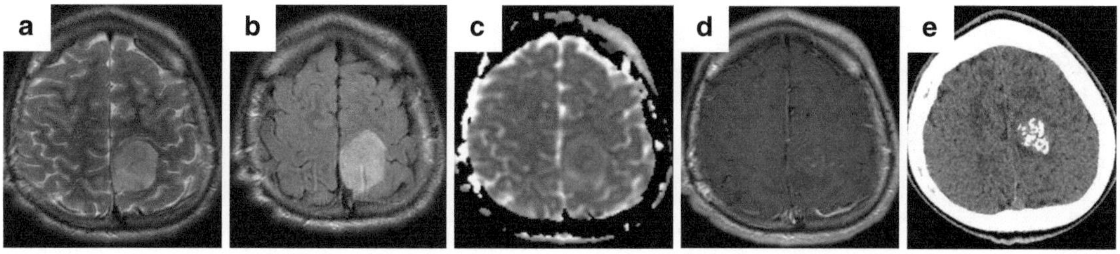

Fig. 10.11 A 7-year-old girl presented with headache and seizures. (**a**, **b**) MRI brain shows a well-defined T2/FLAIR hyperintense lesion in the left fronto-parietal lobe. (**c**, **d**) The lesion shows no diffusion restriction with minimal contrast enhancement. (**e**) Note the coarse calcification on the CT image. HPR-Diffuse glioneuronal tumor with oligodendroma-like features and nuclear clusters (DGONC)

10.6.4.3 Diffuse Glioneuronal Tumor with Oligodendroma-Like Features and Nuclear Clusters (DGONC)

This is a newly added provisional entity that belongs to neuroepithelial tumors showing a unique methylation profile and monosomy of chromosome 14. These are supratentorial tumors that are common in temporal lobes. Among the few cases reported, the median age of involvement was 9 years [25]. On MRI, this tumor appears hyperintense on T2/FLAIR with no perilesional edema. They show minimal to nil contrast enhancement with variable to nil diffusion restriction [26] (Fig. 10.11). Calcification has also been observed [12].

10.6.4.4 Papillary Glioneuronal Tumor (PGNT)

These are grade 1 tumors seen in young adults and sometimes in adolescents. Initially introduced as 'pseudopapillary glioneurocytoma', these tumors have been revised as PGNTs in 2021 classification. PRKCA gene fusion is their molecular marker [8]. PGNTs are supratentorial tumors that are common in the temporal lobe [27]. These tumors are commonly cystic with solid components. Rarely may also present as cyst with a mural nodule or a complete cystic lesion. The solid component whenever present, shows post-contrast enhancement and is not diffusion-restricting. The presence of calcifications and hemorrhage is common. 'T2-FLAIR mismatch' has been observed in the complete cystic variants of PGNT [28]. Perilesional edema is usually absent or minimal.

10.6.4.5 Myxoid Glioneuronal Tumor (MGNT)

MGNT is a low-grade glioneuronal tumor characterized by PDGFRA mutation. These tumors occur in adolescents and young adults. MGNT has very typical locations like septum pellucidum, foramen of Monro, corpus callosum, and periventricular region. As the name suggests, the myxoid tumors are T2/FLAIR hyperintense. MGNT are well-circumscribed solid tumors that are T1 hypointense without contrast enhancement or diffusion restriction [29]. Calcification and hemorrhage are also very rare.

10.6.4.6 Diffuse Leptomeningeal Glioneuronal Tumor (DLGNT)

Diffuse leptomeningeal glioneuronal tumor is a glioneuronal tumor comprising of both neuronal and glial cells. They are positive for OLIG1, MAP2, and S100. Based on the molecular characteristics, this tumor has been subtyped into DLGNT with 1q gain, with methylation class 1 and with methylation class 2 [30]. It is a rare pediatric tumor with a median of 4 years of age. On MRI, this characteristically shows diffuse nodular leptomeningeal thickening and enhancement in the intracranial and intraspinal compartment. Multiple T2 hyperintense cysts are seen along the subpial aspect of brain, along CSF spaces and spinal cord (Fig. 10.12). These cysts are non-enhancing usually. Sometimes, an associated spinal cord mass can also be seen. An important imaging differential is meningitis and other less common differential is racemose neurocysticercosis. Thus, clinical presentation and associated findings should be reviewed together for raising the suspicion of DLGNT [31, 32].

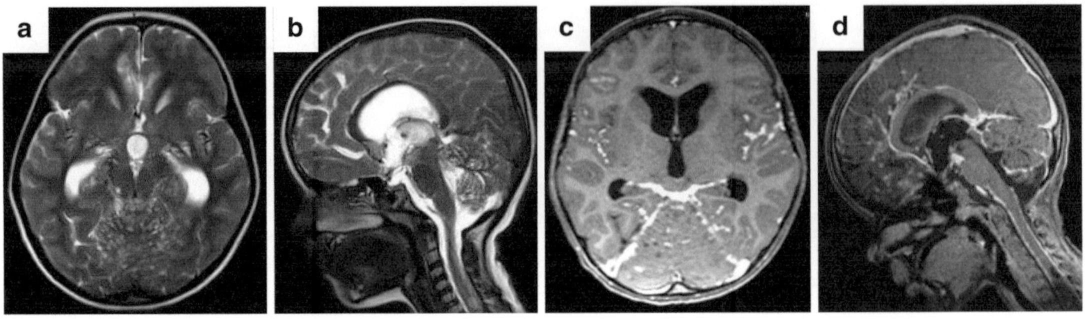

Fig. 10.12 A 4-yar-old girl had presented with drowsiness, drooling of saliva and lower limb weakness. (**a**, **b**) MRI shows ill-defined T2 hyperintense cysts along the subpial and periventricular aspect. (**c**) Note the characteristic diffuse nodular leptomeningeal enhancement along the sulcal and cisternal spaces. (**d**) Similar meningeal enhancement is also seen along the spinal cord. HPR-Diffuse leptomeningeal glioneuronal tumor (DLGNT)

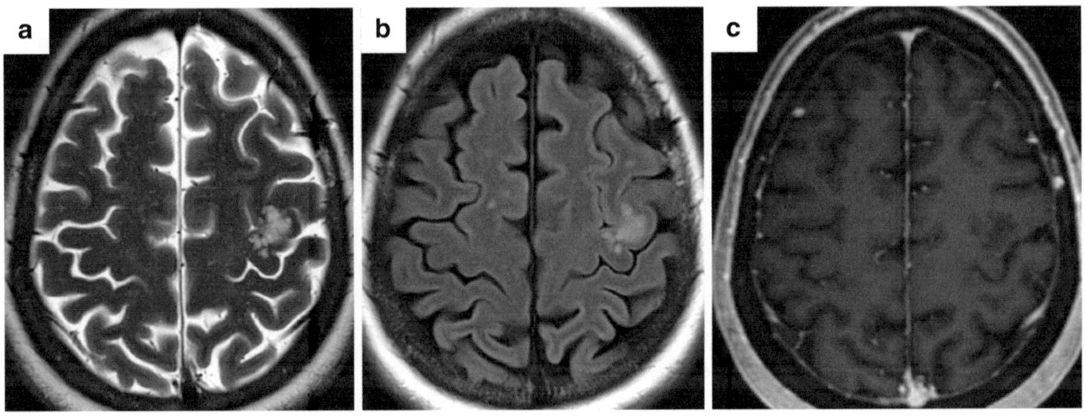

Fig. 10.13 A 17-year-old male with known Neurofibromatosis came for screening MRI. (**a**, **b**) T2/FLAIR shows clustered hyperintense nodules in the subcortical aspect of left frontal lobe. (**c**) No perilesional edema or enhancement is seen. HPR - Multinodular Vacuolating Neuronal Tumor (MVNT)

10.6.4.7 Multinodular Vacuolating Neuronal Tumor (MVNT)

These are rare WHO grade 1 tumors that occur both in adults and children. These are composed of immature neuronal cells showing vacuolization changes in the matrix and associated with MAP2K1 mutation [12]. It involves the subcortical ribbon and subcortical white matter. On imaging, MVNT has a characteristic appearance of variable-sized T2/FLAIR hyperintense discrete nodules without surrounding edema. These nodules occur along the gyral contour (Fig. 10.13). This lesion does not show enhancement, diffusion restriction, calcification, or mass effect and are generally asymptomatic [33].

10.6.5 Embryonal Tumors

All embryonal tumors are grade 4 tumors.

10.6.5.1 Atypical Teratoid/Rhabdoid Tumor (AT/RT)

AT/RT is characterized by activation of SMARCB1 or SMARCA4 genes. They occur in both supratentorial and infratentorial locations

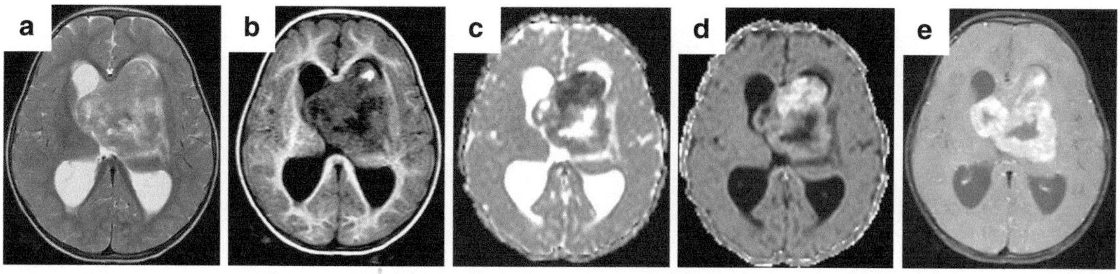

Fig. 10.14 A 20-months-old boy presented with right sided weakness and difficulty in walking. (**a**, **b**) MRI shows a large T2/FLAIR heterogeneously hyperintense lesion along the left lateral ventricle with few cystic areas. Note diffusion restriction (**c**, **d**) and homogeneous enhancement (**e**) of solid component. HPR - Atypical teratoid/rhabdoid tumor

predominantly in children less than 4 years [8]. While supratentorial, these tumors are along the ventricles and cisterns occurring as a large heterogeneous lesion with peripheral cystic areas. The lesion shows diffusion restriction and variable enhancement of the solid component and rarely non-enhancing (Fig. 10.14). A characteristic wavy thick enhancement of the cyst wall could be seen. Calcifications and hemorrhage are also seen [34]. A variable amount of perilesional edema can be observed. ATRT can present as a diffuse leptomeningeal plaque-like disease without a parenchymal mass lesion and can rapidly progress. Infratentorial AT/RT are not usually associated with cysts and are briefed in the next chapter.

10.6.5.2 Embryonal Tumor with Multilayered Rosettes (ETMR)

ETMR is characterized by amplification of 19q13.42 chromosome [35]. It predominantly occurs in children especially those below 4 years of age more in supratentorial than infratentorial location. ETMR are large heterogeneous tumors showing areas of calcification, hemorrhage, and necrosis with irregular post-contrast enhancement [8]. They are restricted on DWI and show hyperperfusion. There is no distinguishing imaging feature specific for ETMR.

10.6.5.3 Cribriform Neuroepithelial Tumors

This is a new entity under provisional type defined by heterozygous deletion of SMARCB1. This tumor is positive for tyrosinase, EMA, vimentin, and synaptophysin. These are intraventricular or occur adjacent to ventricles and common in children between 0 and 10 years. From the limited available literature, imaging features are non-specific showing a large heterogenous tumor that is T2/FLAIR hyperintense with heterogeneous enhancement and diffusion restriction [12, 36].

10.6.5.4 CNS Neuroblastoma, FOXR2-Activated

It is an aggressive supratentorial neoplasm occurring in children (median age of 4.5 years). They are defined by the activation and overexpression of FOXR2 transcription factor. On imaging, these are large exclusively supratentorial tumors involving the white matter and cortex of the cerebral hemisphere, commonly frontal lobe [8]. They often show cystic/necrotic changes with moderate enhancement and diffusion restriction. Calcifications and hemorrhage are common (Fig. 10.15). When the tumor is large, cortical remodeling, a feature of slow-growing neoplasm has also been observed [37].

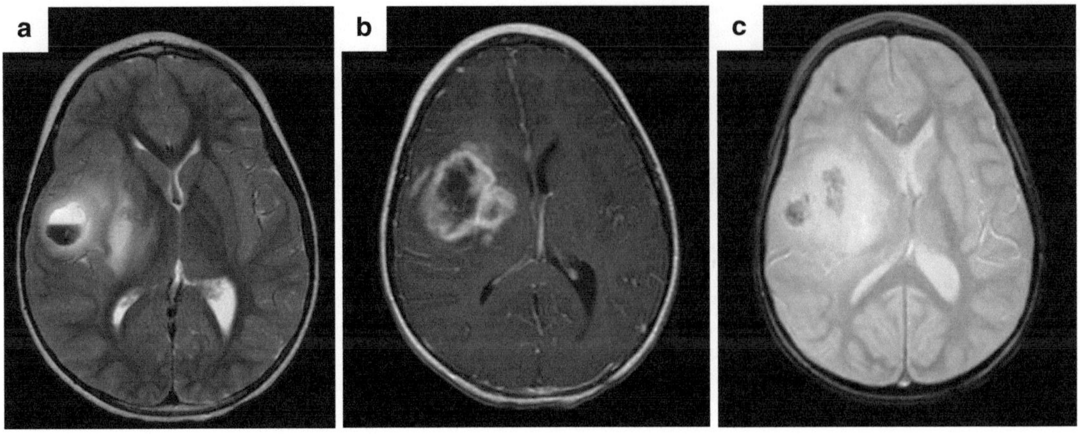

Fig. 10.15 A 9-year-old girl came with chronic headache. (**a**) MRI brain shows a heterogeneously T2 hyperintense lesion in the right temporal lobe. (**b**, **c**) The lesion is necrotic with peripheral enhancement with areas of hemorrhage within. HPR- CNS neuroblastoma FOXR2

10.6.5.5 CNS Tumor with BCOR Internal Tandem Duplication

These are rare tumors seen in children between 1 and 7 years of age. It can be both supra- or infratentorial. Characteristically, these are positive for BCOR, OLIG2, NeuN while S100 and GFAP are negative [8]. The tumors are large and T2 hyperintense with necrotic areas showing enhancement and diffusion restriction (Fig. 10.16). Dural abutment of the tumor is usually present. Sometimes, large intratumoral vessels can be seen. Perilesional edema is usually not seen, if seen it is minimal [38].

10.6.5.6 CNS Embryonal Tumor, NEC/ NOS

These are rare tumors of neuroepithelial origin. They lack any molecular feature to be classified into one of the embryonal tumors. These have features overlapping with those tumors that were previously called primitive neuroectodermal tumor (PNET). The imaging is non-specific similar to any high-grade tumor. They commonly have cystic areas within the tumor with calcification and minimal peritumoral edema [39].

Embryonal tumors also comprise of medulloblastoma which is a tumor of infratentorial compartment and shall be discussed in the following chapter.

10.6.6 Ependymal Tumors

10.6.6.1 Supratentorial Ependymoma

Supratentorial ependymomas are tumors with rosettes or pseudo-rosettes of uniform small cells surrounded by a matrix. The RELA-fusion positive ependymoma of 2016 classification shows C11orf95 mutation (now ZFTA) has been updated now into the 'supratentorial tumors ZFTA-fusion positive' category [8]. These are WHO grade 2 or 3 tumors common in children. Supratentorial ependymomas occur either within the ventricles or adjacent to them. YAP1 fusion-positive tumors have better prognosis than ZFTA-fusion-positive. These are heterogenous circumscribed tumors with cystic components, areas of hemorrhage, and calcifications. They are iso to hyperintense on T2/ FLAIR showing diffusion restriction in the solid component and heterogeneous enhancement [40]. YAP1 subtypes have larger cystic component associated than the ZFTA subtypes (Fig. 10.17). However, in many instances the subtypes appear similar on imaging, and it is almost impossible to differentiate solely on imaging [41].

The other ependymal tumors are predominantly infratentorial and spinal and shall be discussed in corresponding chapters.

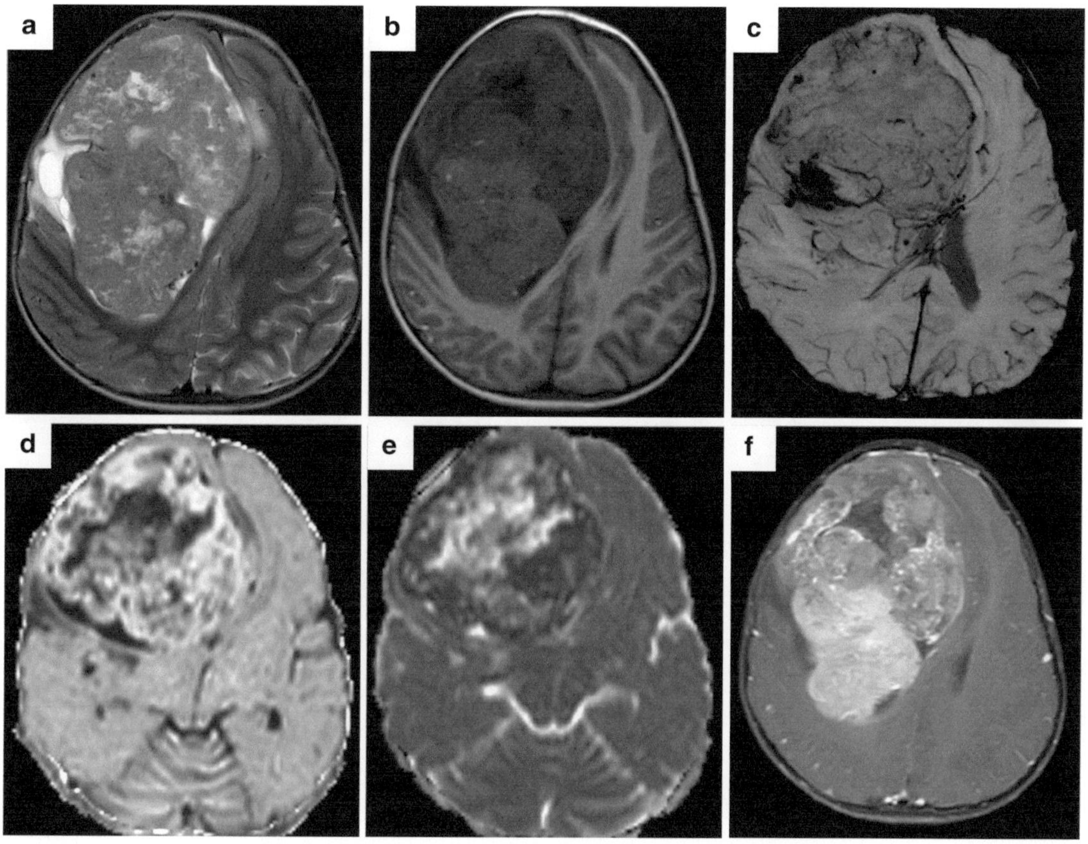

Fig. 10.16 A 7-year-old girl came with scalp swelling for 2 months with forehead bossing and left sided weakness since 1 month. (**a**, **b**) A large heterogeneous T1 hypointense and T2 hyperintense large lesion is seen involving the right fronto-temporal lobes. (**c**–**e**) Note the tumoral hemorrhage and diffusion restriction within. f) The lesion shows heterogeneously enhancing. HPR - CNS tumor with BCOR internal tandem duplication

10.6.7 Choroid Plexus Tumors

The tumors of choroid plexus are childhood tumors that are commonly supratentorial but can occur infratentorial as well. It consists of choroid plexus papilloma (WHO grade 1), atypical choroid plexus papilloma (WHO grade 2), and choroid plexus carcinoma (WHO grade 3 tumor). It affects infants and young children from birth to 4 years [9]. Choroid plexus papilloma and the atypical papilloma are indistinguishable from each other on imaging. They appear as a solid-cystic lesion within the ventricle or sometimes as asymmetrically large choroid plexus with vivid enhancement of the solid component. Diffusion restriction is usually absent. They have a predilection for trigone [8]. Whereas, choroid plexus carcinoma presents as a large lesion, more heterogeneous than papilloma with areas of necrosis and calcifications. These show diffusion restriction, elevated lactate, and choline peak. Sometimes, choroid plexus carcinoma may invade the adjacent parenchyma with associated edema [4]. All these tumors can show CSF dissemination and a neuraxis screening has to be performed.

10.6.8 Pineal Tumors

Almost all pineal tumors except pineoblastoma are adulthood tumors and thus are not included in our discussion. Germinomas also occur in pineal region but are described separately later.

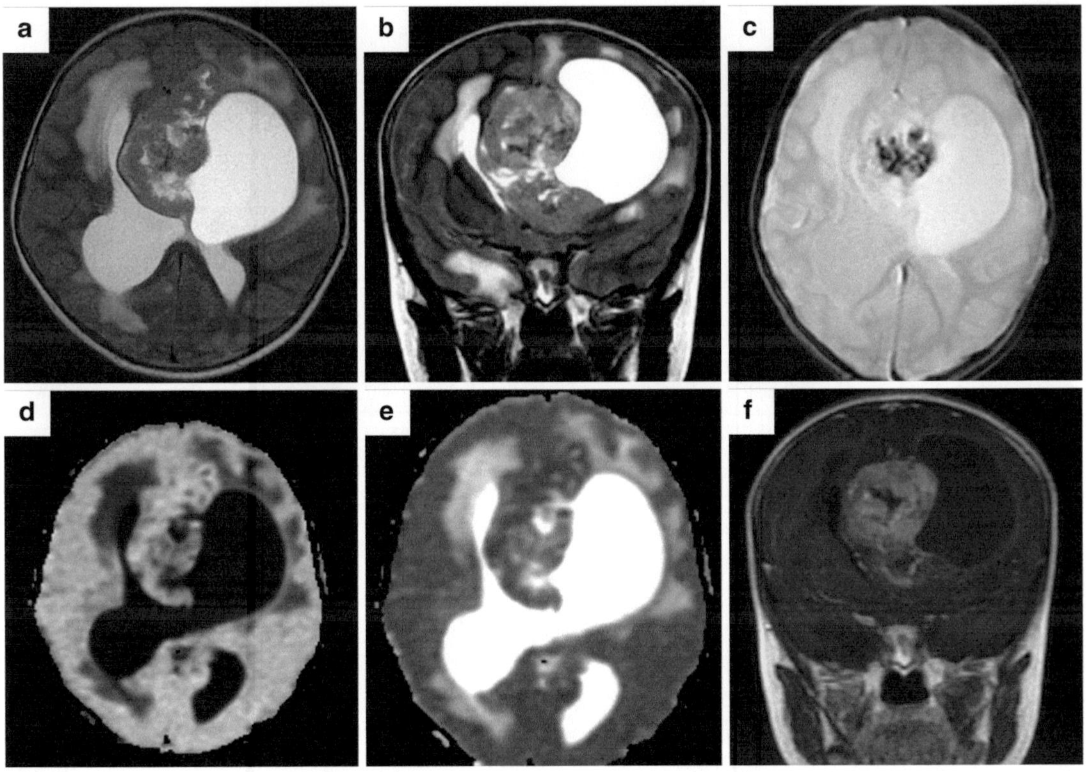

Fig. 10.17 A 8-year-old girl presented with headache and vomiting. (**a**) MRI brain shows a heterogeneous solid-cystic T2 hyperintense intraventricular lesion epicentered in the septum pellucidum. (**b**, **c**) It is associated with large cystic component and areas of hemorrhage. (**c**–**f**) The lesion shows associated peritumoral edema with diffusion restriction and heterogenous contrast enhancement. HPR – Supratentorial ependymoma YAP1 positive

10.6.8.1 Pineoblastoma

Pineoblastoma is WHO grade 4 poorly differentiated tumor originating from the pineal gland. It is a tumor of childhood and the common differential being germ cell tumors of pineal region. These can be seen associated with DICER1 syndrome, with hereditary retinoblastoma or with MYC amplification [8]. It is a large heterogenous lesion of pineal gland often seen invading the adjacent structures. It shows cystic changes, hemorrhage, calcifications, and necrosis. Diffusion restriction and inhomogeneous contrast enhancement is often seen. The calcifications on CT have been termed 'exploding' helping it differentiate from germ cell tumors. Diffuse craniospinal metastases are frequently seen and hence always a neuraxial screening must be performed [9].

10.6.9 Mesenchymal Non-meningothelial Tumors Involving the CNS

10.6.9.1 Intracranial Mesenchymal Tumor, FET-CREB Fusion Positive

These tumors are of mesenchymal origin. Intracranial angiomatoid fibrous histiocytoma and intracranial myxoid mesenchymal tumor have now been brought under this entity which is characterized by fusion of FET (a RNA binding protein) with CREB (transcription factor) [12]. These are predominantly extra-axial tumors that are common along the cerebral convexities in the supratentorial component. On imaging, they appear heterogeneous with post-contrast enhancement and areas of hemorrhage. They are usually associated with significant perilesional edema and sometimes a dural tail or calvarial involvement can be seen [42].

10.6.9.2 Primary Intracranial Sarcoma, DICER1-Mutant

This is a rare intracranial sarcoma defined by DICER1 mutation. It can be seen associated with familial DICER1 syndrome or neurofibromatosis 1. Usually these are extra-axial tumors, if intra-axial these commonly involve the supratentorial location. Due to its rarity, the data on imaging is limited. Imaging shows a complex heterogeneously enhancing lesion with hemorrhage and meningeal involvement [12, 43].

10.6.10 Tumors of Sellar Region

Around 10% of supratentorial tumors occur in the sellar region. This includes craniopharyngioma, germinoma, and pituitary tumors. However, the pituitary tumors are less common in childhood [44].

10.6.10.1 Adamantinomatous Craniopharyngioma

Adamantinomatous craniopharyngioma accounts for 5–11% of pediatric intracranial tumors whereas papillary craniopharyngioma is a tumor of adults. It is a tumor originating from squamous cells characterized by activation of CTNNB1 [8]. They present as a heterogeneous solid-cystic suprasellar mass with variable amounts of calcifications. The cyst is usually T1 hyperintense or may follow CSF signal intensity. The solid component almost always enhances while the cyst wall enhancement is variable. When large they exhibit mass effect on the optic chiasma resulting in visual symptoms. Diffusion restriction is usually absent or difficult to evaluate because of coarse calcifications [45].

10.6.11 Germ Cell Tumors

GCTs can be divided into germinoma and non-germinomatous germ cell tumors (NGGCT) and are seen in children. Sometimes, GCTs have also been reported in the fetus. They occur in pineal and suprasellar regions. NGGCT occurs in infants and younger children, while germinomas are common among older children and adolescents [4]. Germinomas are homogenous mass that are hyperdense on CT and iso-hyperintense on T2/FLAIR showing diffusion restriction and contrast enhancement. Whereas, NGGCT are heterogeneous tumors. GCTs show calcifications and hemorrhage. The calcifications in GCT are termed as 'engulfing' calcifications on CT. Neuraxial screening must be performed owing to known dissemination [9].

10.7 Low-Grade Developmental and Epilepsy-Associated Tumors (LEAT)

These are a group of tumors that are associated with epilepsy in children, usually the drug-resistant ones. LEAT includes pediatric-type diffuse low-grade gliomas, circumscribed astrocytic gliomas, glioneuronal tumors, and developmental disorders like focal cortical dysplasia. LEAT had been earlier described as "Long-term epilepsy associated tumors", but owing to the inclusion of neurodevelopmental causes, the name has been aptly revised [46]. LEAT constitutes the second common surgical cause of epilepsy in children and young adults. The recent 2021 WHO classification insists on understanding the molecular or genetic basis of the tumor; however, owing to the poor inter-observer agreement between the histopathologists in arriving at a specific diagnosis among these tumors, these tumors were grouped into LEAT tumors. Roughly, LEAT tumors can be classified into astrocyte predominant tumors with BRAF mutations and oligodendrocyte predominant tumors with FGFR-1 alterations [47]. Seizures caused by LEAT group of tumors can be treated by surgery.

10.8 Response Assessment and Surveillance Imaging

Post-treatment imaging of brain tumors is a challenging task by itself. Identifying treatment changes, residual, pseudo progression, and recurrence is vital, and imaging plays a crucial role in the management. Standard adult criteria cannot be used in children and hence the Response Assessment in Pediatric Neurooncology (RAPNO) working group has published criteria for assessing post-treatment response in children. Different set of criteria are available separately for pediatric high-grade gliomas (HGGs), low-grade gliomas (LGGs), craniopharyngiomas, medulloblastomas, and leptomeningeal seeding tumors [10]. These criteria focus on two-dimensional measurements of tumor on T2/FLAIR or contrast sequences for assessment. Certain cases like LGGs cysts are also taken into consideration [48, 49]. A dedicated description of these criteria is beyond the scope of our chapter. The readers are advised to refer to these criteria for a detailed reading.

Surveillance imaging is used to follow-up patients after treatment to look for response and to detect asymptomatic recurrences earlier. RAPNO suggests MRI once in 3 months for the first year and then slowly increasing the interval between MRI in cases without relapses or progression for HGGs [49]. In LGGs, a presurgical MRI and another MRI after 24–72 hours of surgery are recommended. If post-treatment changes are obscuring the evaluation of a residual tumor, RAPNO recommends a repeat MRI after 2–3 weeks. During trials or treatment MRI once in 3 months is recommended. A spine screening is also added wherever indicated [48]. Whereas in pediatric craniopharyngioma MRI taken within 2 weeks of surgery should be considered as baseline for further assessment. Adjuvant therapy is recommended to be started within 4–6 weeks of post-surgical MRI with surveillance imaging done every 3 months during the treatment period [50].

10.9 Recent Updates and Advances in Imaging

Research and advances in neuroimaging have improved dramatically in the past decade. These include advances in imaging sequences and artificial intelligence.

MRI Perfusion

Understanding the tumoral perfusion by assessing the cerebral blood volume (CBV) and cerebral blood flow (CBF) helps not only in diagnosing and grading the tumors, but also in guiding biopsies and post-treatment evaluation. The more aggressive the tumor, higher is the grade of neovascularization, leading to increased relative CBV (rCBV) and CBF. A cut-off of 1.75 rCBV has been highly sensitive in differentiating high-grade tumors [51]. The techniques employed in perfusion imaging includes dynamic contrast enhancement (DCE) based on T1 acquisition, dynamic susceptibility contrast enhancement (DSC) with T2* acquisition, and arterial spin labelling (ASL). ASL is based on magnetically labelling the blood and it does not use intravenous contrast administration. Perfusion imaging is a vital tool especially in follow-up post-treatment imaging in neuro-oncology [52].

MR Spectroscopy

MR spectroscopy is a metabolic imaging based on hydrogen proton signals. It provides chemical information of brain parenchyma. MRS can be acquired with varying TE and thus classified into short (20–40 ms), intermediate (135–144 ms), and long (270–280 ms) [53]. The long TE gives fewer metabolites than short TE. The important metabolites of MRS include

1. N-acetyl cysteine (NAA), a neuronal marker.
2. Choline (Cho), indicates membrane turnover.
3. Creatinine (Cr), an energy metabolite.
4. Lactate (Lac), seen in anerobic glycolysis, indicates necrosis in tumors.
5. Myoinositol (MI), a marker of glial cell.

Typically, all tumors have an elevated Cho peak and decreased NAA peak. A high Cho/Cr ratio indicates a higher tumor grade. A Cho/Cr ratio greater than 2 is considered as cut-off for high-grade tumors [54]. Elevated MI is seen in low-grade tumors like astrocytoma and ependymoma. A recent study has shown that the myo-inositol/contralateral creatinine (MI/c-Cr) helps in evaluating treatment response in high-grade tumors [51].

Diffusion Tensor Imaging (DTI)

DTI studies the white matter tract based on water diffusion properties. DTI can provide color-coded anisotropy maps based on the degree and direction of the diffusion. Additional fiber tractography could also be processed. These help in understanding the relationship between the tumors and the white matter tracts like corticospinal tract, etc., it is essential especially in supratentorial and brainstem tumors. Based on the FA values and the direction of the tracts, displacement, edema, and infiltration of the tract by the tumor can be made out [52, 55].

Functional MRI (fMRI)

Functional MRI is based on the blood oxygen level-dependent (BOLD) signals of the brain parenchyma that acts as a tool to assess the eloquent areas of brain for tumor involvement [52]. The commonly performed is task-based fMRI like finger tapping where the task and rest period are alternated in the paradigm. During the task, for example finger-tapping, the motor cortex gets activated and utilizes more oxygen and thereby more blood flow with alterations in the oxyhemoglobin levels which is reflected as MR signals. fMRI can also be used to determine the language dominance based on the laterality score [53]. Recently resting state-fMRI (rs-fMRI) has been studied in pediatric supratentorial tumors to assess the resting state networks like sensory motor network, language network, medial visual, and lateral visual networks. Localization of these networks and their involvement by the tumor can help surgeons in planning the preoperative extent of resection. This approach can minimize the risk of losing critical or specialized function secondary to resection [56, 57].

Radiomics and Artificial Intelligence

The current incline toward artificial intelligence has not spared brain tumors as well. Radiomics which is a method to extract tumor-related information from CT and MRI images has been incorporated along with machine learning and artificial intelligence models to predict a wide range of information ranging from diagnosis, characterizing biomarkers, and predicting the prognosis and survival [58]. Similar concept with inclusion of genetic and molecular characteristics of the tumors from radiological images is radiogenomics. Recently, radiogenomic models were able to predict the mutation status in both high- and low-grade gliomas like IDH mutation, etc., however, owing to difficulties in generalizability and reproducibility, the clinical application of such research is still lacking [51].

Magnetic Resonance Fingerprinting (MRF)

Magnetic resonance fingerprinting (MRF) is a method of quantifying the tissue property from T1 and T2 values. This can aid in accurate margin delineation and in differentiating high- from low-grade gliomas. The applications of MRF in pediatric brain tumors are being explored [51]. MRF has potential in aiding tumor diagnosis, molecular subtyping and grading, etc.

Magnetic Resonance Elastography (MRE)

MRE measures the mechanical properties of the tissues and tumors. The normal brain cells, tumor, and extracellular matrix all show varied stiffness that can be measured. These mechanical properties can help identify the grade of the tumor. When MRE is combined with genetic or molecular information of the tumor to predict the mutation status, etc., it has been termed as 'mechanogenomics' [51]. These techniques are still under research.

The continuing advancement in the field of neuroimaging has improved the quality of imaging, the accuracy of diagnosis, and evaluation of treatment responses.

10.10 Conclusion

Supratentorial tumors in children are a vast group of tumors that are classified based on molecular characteristics. They have varied imaging features making it a challenge for the radiologist. By understanding imaging features, diagnosis can be made to a certain extent. A fair understanding of these tumors could enable radiologists in guiding the management by differentiating high-grade from low-grade tumors, identifying associated acute/emergency findings and in evaluating tumor response.

Acknowledgement None.

Disclosures The authors have no conflict of interest to disclose.

Financial Interests The authors declare they have no financial interests.

Funding The authors did not receive funding from any organization for the submitted work.

References

1. Ostrom QT, Price M, Neff C, et al. CBTRUS statistical report: primary brain and other central nervous system tumors diagnosed in the United States in 2016—2020. Neuro-Oncology. 2023;25:iv1–iv99. https://doi.org/10.1093/neuonc/noad149.
2. Newton HB, Malkin MG. Overview of brain tumor epidemiology. In: Handbook of neuro-oncology neuroimaging. Elsevier; 2008. p. 3–8.
3. Louis DN, Perry A, Wesseling P, et al. The 2021 WHO classification of tumors of the central nervous system: a summary. Neuro-Oncology. 2021;23:1231–51. https://doi.org/10.1093/NEUONC/NOAB106.
4. Resende LL, Alves CAPF. Imaging of brain tumors in children: the basics – a narrative review. Transl Pediatr. 2021;10:1138–68.
5. Triulzi FM. General overview. In: Triulzi FM, editor. Neuroradiology of brain tumors: practical guide based on the 5th edition of WHO classification. Cham: Springer International Publishing; 2023. p. 1–32.
6. Sciacca S, Lynch J, Davagnanam I, Barker R. Midbrain, pons, and medulla: anatomy and syndromes. Radiographics. 2019;39:1110–25. https://doi.org/10.1148/RG.2019180126.
7. Tay KL, Leason SR, Dawes LC, et al. Haemorrhage and calcification on susceptibility-weighted imaging: a quick and reliable qualitative technique for differentiating lesions with ambiguous phase. Clin Neuroradiol. 2022;32:705–15. https://doi.org/10.1007/S00062-021-01094-2.
8. Triulzi FM. Neuroradiology of brain tumors practical guide based on the 5th edition of WHO classification. Springer Nature; 2023.
9. Jaju A, Yeom KW, Ryan ME. MR imaging of pediatric brain tumors. Diagnostics. 2022;12
10. Jaju A, Li Y, Dahmoush H, et al. Imaging of pediatric brain tumors: a COG diagnostic imaging committee/SPR oncology committee/ASPNR white paper. Pediatr Blood Cancer. 2023;70:e30147. https://doi.org/10.1002/pbc.30147.
11. Erker C, Tamrazi B, Poussaint TY, et al. Response assessment in paediatric high-grade glioma: recommendations from the response assessment in pediatric neuro-oncology (RAPNO) working group. Lancet Oncol. 2020;21:e317–29. https://doi.org/10.1016/S1470-2045(20)30173-X.
12. Rigsby RK, Brahmbhatt P, Desai AB, et al. Newly recognized CNS tumors in the 2021 World Health Organization classification: imaging overview with histopathologic and genetic correlation. Am J Neuroradiol. 2023;44:367–80.
13. van Maren EA, Dankbaar JW, Wesseling P, et al. T2-FLAIR mismatch: an imaging biomarker for children's *MYB/MYBL1* –altered diffuse astrocytoma or Angiocentric glioma. Am J Neuroradiol. 2024;45:747. https://doi.org/10.3174/ajnr.A8203.
14. Kurokawa R, Baba A, Emile P, et al. Neuroimaging features of angiocentric glioma: a case series and systematic review. J Neuroimaging. 2022;32:389–99. https://doi.org/10.1111/jon.12983.
15. Johnson DR, Giannini C, Vaubel RA, et al. A radiologist's guide to the 2021 WHO central nervous system tumor classification: part I – key concepts and the Spectrum of diffuse gliomas. Radiology. 2022;304:494–508. https://doi.org/10.1148/radiol.213063.
16. Golub D, Lynch DG, Pan PC, et al. Polymorphous low-grade neuroepithelial tumor of the young with FGFR3-TACC3 fusion mimicking high-grade glioma: case report and series of high-grade correlates. Front Oncol. 2023;13 https://doi.org/10.3389/fonc.2023.1307591.
17. Kurokawa R, Baba A, Kurokawa M, et al. Neuroimaging features of diffuse hemispheric glioma, H3 G34-mutant: a case series and systematic review. J Neuroimaging. 2022;32:17–27. https://doi.org/10.1111/jon.12939.
18. Tauziède-Espariat A, Debily M-A, Castel D, et al. The pediatric supratentorial MYCN-amplified high-grade gliomas methylation class presents the same radiological, histopathological and molecular features as their pontine counterparts. Acta Neuropathol Commun. 2020;8:104. https://doi.org/10.1186/s40478-020-00974-x.
19. Bader A, Heran M, Dunham C, Steinbok P. Radiological features of infantile glioblastoma and

desmoplastic infantile tumors: British Columbia's children's hospital experience. J Neurosurg Pediatr. 2015;16:119–25. https://doi.org/10.3171/2014.10.PEDS13634.
20. Elousrouti LT, Lamchahab M, Bougtoub N, et al. Subependymal giant cell astrocytoma (SEGA): a case report and review of the literature. J Med Case Rep. 2016;10:35.
21. Stein JR, Reidman DA. Imaging manifestations of a subependymal Giant cell astrocytoma in tuberous sclerosis. Case Rep Radiol. 2016;2016:1–5. https://doi.org/10.1155/2016/3750450.
22. Mhatre R, Sugur HS, Nandeesh BN, et al. MN1 rearrangement in astroblastoma: study of eight cases and review of literature. Brain Tumor Pathol. 2019;36:112–20. https://doi.org/10.1007/s10014-019-00346-x.
23. Phi JH, Kim SH. Dysembryoplastic Neuroepithelial tumor: a benign but complex tumor of the cerebral cortex. Brain Tumor Res Treat. 2022;10:144. https://doi.org/10.14791/btrt.2022.0015.
24. Liao D, Zheng X, Feng Q, Xia T. Association of CT and MRI manifestations with pathology in Dysembryoplastic Neuroepithelial tumors. J Belg Soc Radiol. 2022;106:135. https://doi.org/10.5334/jbsr.2940.
25. Deng MY, Sill M, Sturm D, et al. Diffuse glioneuronal tumour with oligodendroglioma-like features and nuclear clusters (DGONC) – a molecularly defined glioneuronal CNS tumour class displaying recurrent monosomy 14. Neuropathol Appl Neurobiol. 2020;46:422–30. https://doi.org/10.1111/nan.12590.
26. Benesch M, Perwein T, Apfaltrer G, et al. MR imaging and clinical characteristics of diffuse Glioneuronal tumor with Oligodendroglioma-like features and nuclear clusters. Am J Neuroradiol. 2022;43:1523–9. https://doi.org/10.3174/ajnr.A7647.
27. Li D, Wang JM, Li GL, et al. Clinical, radiological, and pathological features of 16 papillary glioneuronal tumors. Acta Neurochir. 2014;156:627–39. https://doi.org/10.1007/s00701-014-2023-y.
28. Du X, He Y, Li F, et al. Imaging manifestations of papillary glioneuronal tumors. Neurosurg Rev. 2024;47:179. https://doi.org/10.1007/s10143-024-02393-1.
29. Caporalini C, Scagnet M, Giunti L, et al. Myxoid glioneuronal tumor: histopathologic, neuroradiologic, and molecular features in a single center series. Neoplasia (United States). 2023;37 https://doi.org/10.1016/j.neo.2023.100885.
30. Patankar AP, Vaghela P, Nasit J, Gohil R. Diffuse leptomeningeal Glioneuronal tumor: a rare case report with review of literature. Asian J Neurosurg. 2022;17:532–5. https://doi.org/10.1055/s-0042-1756637.
31. Lakhani DA, Mankad K, Chhabda S, et al. Diffuse leptomeningeal glioneuronal tumor of childhood. Am J Neuroradiol. 2020;41:2155–9.
32. Nandi D, Sahu A. Know the less known: diffuse leptomeningeal glioneuronal tumour. Indian J Med Res. 2020;152:148. https://doi.org/10.4103/ijmr.IJMR_2233_19.
33. Turan A, Gunes Tatar I, Hekimoglu A, et al. Advanced magnetic resonance imaging findings of multinodular and vacuolating neuronal tumor. Turk Neurosurg. 2021;31:725. https://doi.org/10.5137/1019-5149.JTN.32215-20.3.
34. Calandrelli R, Massimi L, Pilato F, et al. Atypical Teratoid Rhabdoid tumor: proposal of a diagnostic pathway based on clinical features and neuroimaging findings. Diagnostics. 2023;13
35. Meliti A, Gasim W, Al-Maghrabi H, Mokhtar G. Embryonal tumor with multilayered rosettes; rare pediatric CNS tumor. A case report and review of literature. Int J Pediatr Adolesc Med. 2022;9:174–8. https://doi.org/10.1016/j.ijpam.2021.11.002.
36. Tauziède-Espariat A, Guerrini-Rousseau L, Puget S, et al. A novel case of cribriform neuroepithelial tumor: a potential diagnostic pitfall in the ventricular system. Pediatr Blood Cancer. 2021;68:e29037. https://doi.org/10.1002/pbc.29037.
37. Tietze A, Mankad K, Lequin MH, et al. Imaging characteristics of CNS neuroblastoma- *FOXR2*: a retrospective and multi-institutional description of 25 cases. Am J Neuroradiol. 2022;43:1476–80. https://doi.org/10.3174/ajnr.A7644.
38. Cardoen L, Tauziède-Espariat A, Dangouloff-Ros V, et al. Imaging features with histopathologic correlation of CNS high-grade Neuroepithelial tumors with a *BCOR* internal tandem duplication. Am J Neuroradiol. 2022;43:151–6. https://doi.org/10.3174/ajnr.A7367.
39. Gojo J, Kjaersgaard M, Zezschwitz B, et al. Rare embryonal and sarcomatous central nervous system tumours: state-of-the art and future directions. Eur J Med Genet. 2023;66:104660. https://doi.org/10.1016/j.ejmg.2022.104660.
40. Sahu A, Venkatesh A, Snehil A, et al. Imaging of supratentorial ependymomas with radio-pathological correlation. Explor Target Antitumor Ther. 2024;5:766–79. https://doi.org/10.37349/etat.2024.00245.
41. Jabeen S, Konar SK, Prasad C, et al. Conventional and advanced magnetic resonance imaging features of Supratentorial Extraventricular Ependymomas. J Comput Assist Tomogr. 2020;44:692–8. https://doi.org/10.1097/RCT.0000000000001080.
42. Sloan EA, Chiang J, Villanueva-Meyer JE, et al. Intracranial mesenchymal tumor with FET-CREB fusion—a unifying diagnosis for the spectrum of intracranial myxoid mesenchymal tumors and angiomatoid fibrous histiocytoma-like neoplasms. Brain Pathol. 2021;31:e12918. https://doi.org/10.1111/bpa.12918.
43. Kamihara J, Paulson V, Breen MA, et al. DICER1-associated central nervous system sarcoma in children: comprehensive clinicopathologic and genetic analysis of a newly described rare tumor. Mod

Pathol. 2020;33:1910–21. https://doi.org/10.1038/s41379-020-0516-1.
44. Sepulveda F, Scotto Opipari R, Coppola F, et al. Approaches to supratentorial brain tumours in children. Neuroradiology. 2024;66:1495–512. https://doi.org/10.1007/s00234-024-03398-9.
45. Lee IH, Zan E, Bell WR, et al. Craniopharyngiomas : radiological differentiation of two types. J Korean Neurosurg Soc. 2016;59:466. https://doi.org/10.3340/jkns.2016.59.5.466.
46. Xie M, Wang X, Duan Z, Luan G. Low-grade epilepsy-associated neuroepithelial tumors: tumor spectrum and diagnosis based on genetic alterations. Front Neurosci. 2023;16 https://doi.org/10.3389/fnins.2022.1071314.
47. Park YW, Vollmuth P, Foltyn-Dumitru M, et al. The 2021 WHO classification for gliomas and implications on imaging diagnosis: part 2 – summary of imaging findings on pediatric-type diffuse high-grade gliomas, pediatric-type diffuse low-grade gliomas, and circumscribed astrocytic gliomas. J Magn Reson Imaging. 2023;58:690–708. https://doi.org/10.1002/jmri.28740.
48. Fangusaro J, Neuroradiology P, Kadom N, et al (2020) Imaging Guidelines for Paediatric Brain Tumours 1 Response assessment in paediatric low-grade glioma: recommendations from the Response Assessment in Pediatric Neuro-Oncology (RAPNO) working group.
49. Mata-Mbemba D, Mueller S, Erker C et al. Imaging Guidelines for paediatric brain tumours 2 response assessment in paediatric high-grade glioma: recommendations from the Response Assessment in Pediatric Neuro-Oncology (RAPNO) working group. 2020
50. Hoffman LM, Jaimes C, Mankad K, et al. Response assessment in pediatric craniopharyngioma: recommendations from the response assessment in pediatric neuro-oncology (RAPNO) working group. Neuro-Oncology. 2023;25:224–33.
51. Sabeghi P, Zarand P, Zargham S, et al. Advances in neuro-oncological imaging: an update on diagnostic approach to brain tumors. Cancers (Basel). 2024;16
52. Goo HW, Ra Y-S. Advanced MRI for pediatric brain tumors with emphasis on clinical benefits. Korean J Radiol. 2017;18:194. https://doi.org/10.3348/kjr.2017.18.1.194.
53. Nikam RM, Yue X, Kaur G, et al. Advanced neuroimaging approaches to pediatric brain tumors. Cancers (Basel). 2022;14:14.
54. Rafique Z, Awan MW, Iqbal S, et al. Diagnostic accuracy of magnetic resonance spectroscopy in predicting the grade of glioma keeping histopathology as the gold standard. Cureus. 2022;14:e22056. https://doi.org/10.7759/cureus.22056.
55. Poussaint TY, Rodriguez D. Advanced neuroimaging of pediatric brain tumors: MR diffusion, MR perfusion, and MR spectroscopy. Neuroimaging Clin N Am. 2006;16:169–92. https://doi.org/10.1016/j.nic.2005.11.005.
56. Anwar A, Radwan A, Zaky I, et al. Resting state fMRI brain mapping in pediatric supratentorial brain tumors. Egypt J Radiol Nucl Med. 2022;53 https://doi.org/10.1186/s43055-022-00713-3.
57. Sparacia G, Parla G, Mamone G, et al. Resting-state functional magnetic resonance imaging for surgical neuro-oncology planning: towards a standardization in clinical settings. Brain Sci. 2021;11:1613. https://doi.org/10.3390/brainsci11121613.
58. Kaifi R. A review of recent advances in brain tumor diagnosis based on AI-based classification. Diagnostics (Basel). 2023;13(18):3007. https://doi.org/10.3390/diagnostics13183007.

Infratentorial Pediatric Brain Tumors

11

Priscilla Joshi, Aditi Dongre, Shriyash Pinglikar, Somashree Manna, and Isha Shah

11.1 Introduction

Infratentorial or posterior fossa tumors predominate in children after the age of 3–4 years, and account for more than 50% of brain tumors. The most common presentation in children is symptomatic elevated intracranial pressure (ICP) like headache secondary to obstructive hydrocephalus. Symptoms also depend on age of presentation. Infants may present with macrocrania, drowsiness, nausea, and vomiting. Truncal and gait ataxia, tinnitus is seen more often in older children. Common intra-axial posterior fossa tumors include medulloblastoma, pilocytic astrocytoma, ependymoma, atypical teratoid-rhabdoid tumor (ATRT), brainstem glioma, and rarely teratoma. Cerebellar hemangioblastoma may be seen in the context of Von Hippel-Lindau (VHL) disease but otherwise it is rare. Extra-axial tumors are infrequently encountered, and include dermoid, epidermoid, enterogenous cyst, teratoma, schwannoma, meningioma, and skull base tumors.

P. Joshi (✉)
Department of Radiodiagnosis, Bharati Vidyapeeth University Medical College, Pune, Maharashtra, India

Department of Radiodiagnosis, Bharati Vidyapeeth (DU) Medical College and Hospital, Pune, Maharashtra, India

A. Dongre · S. Pinglikar · I. Shah
Department of Radiodiagnosis, Bharati Vidyapeeth University Medical College, Pune, Maharashtra, India

S. Manna
Department of Radiodiagnosis and Imaging, Institute of Medical Sciences, Banaras Hindu University, Varanasi, Uttar Pradesh, India

11.2 Imaging Recommendations

- Brain malignancies are the most common solid tumor malignancies in children. It is important to standardize their imaging protocols to ensure quality and uniformity in tumor evaluation, facilitate research, and compare post-treatment outcomes [1–3].
- Head computed tomography (CT)—may be the initial imaging modality in suspected intracranial tumor, when patient is unstable, or when MRI is not available. Post-contrast CT may be done if urgent surgical intervention is needed, otherwise it is not routinely recommended. CT dose should always be optimized and kept as low as reasonably achievable (ALARA). The effective pediatric dose range is 0.3–3 mSv in non-contrast head CT and 3–10 mSv in contrast head CT.
- Brain MRI with contrast is the modality of choice for diagnosis and follow-up of brain tumors. Macrocyclic gadolinium-based contrast agents (GBCAs) are preferred over linear agents due to better safety profile, however their judicious use is recommended. Sedation is usually needed for children less than 6 years, but may differ on a case-by-case basis. For infants up to 3 months of age, 'feed and bundle' method may be used instead of sedation.

I. Kumar et al. (eds.), *Practical Approach to Imaging in Pediatric Oncology*,
https://doi.org/10.1007/978-981-96-8158-7_11

- Minimum recommended standard MRI sequences for tumor diagnosis and follow-up include pre- and post-contrast T1-weighted, T2-weighted, T2-FLAIR, and diffusion-weighted imaging (DWI).

Pre- and post-contrast T1	3D isotropic sequences are preferred over 2D due to better spatial resolution and sensitivity to small lesions IR-prepped sequences are used more commonly; 3D TSE/FSE sequences can also be used, they provide improved detection of leptomeningeal disease Ideally acquired after 5 min of contrast administration in the plateau phase, using slice thickness of 1–1.5 mm
An additional post contrast 2D T1-SE/TSE/FLAIR is recommended for comparing true enhancement versus artifact	
T2-weighted sequence	Contiguous 2D TSE axial sections with ≤4 mm slice thickness is recommended T2 sequence is recommended for lesion measurement in partial or non-enhancing tumors, and is often more reliable for response assessment due to variability in post-contrast enhancement
T2-FLAIR	It helps in detection of edema, and post-treatment changes, and along with T2, may be used for tumor size measurement Delayed post-contrast T2-FLAIR improves sensitivity of detection of leptomeningeal disease. It should be timed to acquire after acquiring post-contrast T1 images
Diffusion-weighted imaging (DWI)	Contiguous axial sections with ≤4 mm slice thickness is recommended Restricted diffusion helps differentiate recurrent high-grade tumor from post-treatment change It improves detection of recurrent and metastatic medulloblastomas which may show variable enhancement, but always demonstrates restricted diffusivity
Susceptibility-weighted imaging (SWI)	Recommended for detection of calcification and hemorrhage Also helps in evaluation of post-surgical and post-radiation changes like post-radiation cavernomas T2*GRE may be used instead, but is less sensitive

Optional Sequences

Other optional sequences that may further assist in tumor characterization and surgical planning and navigation include:

3D T2 TSE/FSE and 3D bSSFP sequences like CISS/ FIESTA-C—for detecting small lesions. CISS is also useful in planning endoscopic third ventriculostomy in patients, e.g., with tectal glioma.

MRI DTI and tractography—Help in delineation of tumor with respect to adjacent white matter tracts, and improve surgical outcome.

Functional MRI—Helps in delineation of tumor with respect to eloquent areas of brain like motor, sensory, visual, speech areas, and improve surgical outcome.

MR perfusion imaging—Post-contrast perfusion techniques like dynamic susceptibility (DSC), and dynamic contrast-enhanced (DCE) perfusion are recommended. Applications include grading of tumors, differentiate pseudo-progression from recurrence on follow-up, differentiate residual or recurrent disease from post-radiation changes. Utility of non-contrast arterial spin labelling (ASL) remains unclear.

MR spectroscopy (MRS)—Single voxel proton MRS at short TE (35 msec) is recommended, as it can detect many tumor-specific biochemical metabolites. Multivoxel MRS performs better in infiltrative and heterogeneous tumors.

Spine imaging—Imaging of spine is recommended for evaluation of drop metastases in spinal canal, based on suspected tumor histology. Contrast is typically needed for evaluation. Additional sequences like 3D steady-state T2-weighted images and DWI play an important role in non-enhancing lesions. Preoperative spine imaging is strongly recommended for initial staging in a newly diagnosed posterior fossa tumors. If not done preoperatively, it should be done at least 2 weeks after the posterior fossa surgery to avoid misinterpretation.

11.3 Post-treatment Imaging and Surveillance

The Response Assessment in Paediatric Neuro-Oncology (RAPNO) working group has six publications till date, laying down consensus recommendations for response assessment in pediatric brain tumors including medulloblastoma and other leptomeningeal seeding tumors, diffuse intrinsic pontine glioma, ependymoma, pediatric low-grade glioma, pediatric high-grade glioma, and craniopharyngioma. Recommendations pertaining to the former four groups of tumors, which are frequently encountered in the posterior fossa are further elaborated under respective headings [4–7].

11.4 Structured Reporting Template for Posterior Fossa Brain Tumors

A structured reporting template (Table 11.1) can improve quality, clarity, and completeness of reporting, standardize use of terminology, and ensure uniformity in long-term follow-up. A prototype reporting template is discussed below:

11.4.1 Age of Patient

Certain tumors like teratoma are frequently congenital or encountered in infants <1 year of age. High-grade gliomas and embryonal tumors are other common tumors in infancy. Amongst embryonal tumors, atypical teratoid-rhabdoid tumor is more common in children below 2–3 years of age [8].

11.4.2 Number of Lesions

Brain tumors are usually single. Occasionally, multifocal synchronous lesions of same histological subtype may be encountered. Multifocal lesions have been reported in anaplastic gliomas. Synchronous brain tumors of diverse subtype, like coexistence of pilocytic astrocytoma with medulloblastoma or choroid plexus carcinoma have also been reported, but these are extremely

Table 11.1 structured reporting template

Age of patient	
Tumor focality	<unifocal> < multifocal—Mention number of lesion>
Size	< > x < > x < > cm
Anatomical location:	Ex: < right/ left cerebellar hemisphere> < fourth ventricle> < midbrain/pons/medulla> <cerebellopontine angle> <others>
Lesion characteristics	
Matrix	< T1, T2, FLAIR signal characteristics>
Uniformity	<homogeneous/ heterogeneous> <cyst* > necrosis* > <hemorrhage> <calcification> *If not distinguishable, mentioned as cystoid component*
Diffusion restriction in solid areas	<restricted> <facilitated> < ADC value>
Peri-lesional and rim characteristics	< Margin: Circumscribed/non-circumscribed> < Peritumoral edema/white matter infiltration: Maximum distance in cm > <Peri-tumoral cyst>
Extent	Compartment: <intraaxial> <extraaxial > <indeterminate> Nerve involvement: <displaced> <involved> Vessel involvement: <displaced> <encased> <thrombosed> Bone (calvarium/skull base)
Mass effect	< Cerebellar folial effacement> < Any compression of brain matter> < Any compression of ventricle> < Any herniation>
Enhancement characteristics	<intra lesional> <Margin of lesion> <Extra lesional> < Leptomeningeal enhancement> <Craniospinal spread>
Advanced imaging	< Perfusion characteristics> <Magnetic resonance spectroscopy>
Additional findings:	
Impression:	Findings suggestive of: <benign> <indeterminate> <malignant> Diagnosis suggestive of:

rare. Theories to explain this phenomenon include the carcinogenic stimulus theory, Cohnheim theory of embryonic remnant as origin for all primary brain tumors, genetic susceptibility, and the common origin of all gliomas from a single stem cell [9–12].

11.4.3 Anatomical Location

It is important to determine the intra- or extra-axial location of mass. Features like broad dural base, presence of CSF cleft and pial vessels at the tumor-brain interface, buckling of gray matter are associated with extra-axial lesions, while intra-axial lesions expand the brain parenchyma. Precise anatomical localization of brain tumors helps to narrow down the differentials and predict molecular subtype in few lesions. The most common tumors in each location are enlisted below:

- Cerebellum—Medulloblastoma, pilocytic astrocytoma, ATRT, Diffuse low grade glioma, Hemangioblastoma; rare—Pilomyxoid astrocytoma, dysplastic cerebellar gangliocytoma.
- Fourth Ventricle—Medulloblastoma, ependymoma, pilocytic astrocytoma, choroid plexus papilloma.
- Brainstem—Diffuse midline glioma, Diffuse low-grade glioma, Pilocytic astrocytoma, rare—Pilomyxoid astrocytoma.
- Cerebellopontine angle—Ependymoma, Choroid plexus papilloma, Astrocytoma.
- Diffuse leptomeningeal glioneuronal tumors—tend to involve the basal cisterns, posterior fossa and spinal cord, and present as leptomeningeal thickening and subpial microcysts.

11.4.4 Size of Lesion

The size of brain tumors is usually measured in two or three planes. Post-contrast 3D sequences are preferred for volumetric analysis, which may be done by manual tracing or automation, and assist in both surgical planning as well as response assessment. The most reproducible way to obtain bidimensional measurements consists of the longest measurement (width) of the tumor and the longest measurement perpendicular to the width. The most reproducible way to determine measurements for three perpendicular planes consists of determining the maximum diameters in the standard anterior–posterior, transverse, and caudo-cranial dimensions obtained on multiplanar imaging [13].

T2/ FLAIR sequence is considered to be the best measure of tumor size in non-enhancing tumors like pediatric low-grade gliomas and diffuse intrinsic pontine glioma [4, 13]. For high-grade gliomas, Response Assessment in Pediatric Neuro-Oncology (RAPNO) recommends the sequence most representative of the tumor be used to determine response assessment, whether this sequence is T1-weighted for contrast-enhancing disease or T2-FLAIR in tumors with minimal or no enhancement on baseline MRI. The sequence selected for measurable disease at baseline should be used thereafter in follow-up [14]. In few cases, determining the margins of non-enhancing tumors for measurement is challenging because of difficulty in distinguishing the tumor from vasogenic oedema. In these cases, concurrent involvement of T2-FLAIR signal within grey matter structures or the presence of diffusion restriction supports tumor involvement over oedema, and might help to determine the tumor margin.

Similarly for other tumors, the sequence most representative of the lesion with appreciable margins—either T2/FLAIR or contrast-enhanced T1 should be chosen for size measurement.

In a solid-cystic tumor morphology, the cystic component is considered measurable only if it is integrated within the solid component (soap bubble appearance), is not readily separable from the solid component, or has thick wall enhancement, or both; or there is a cluster of small microcysts within a tumor. However, reactive cyst at the interface of the solid component of the tumor and healthy brain, or cysts intermingled with the resection cavity, or predominantly cystic tumors with non-enhancing wall with solid enhancing mural nodule are not included in the measurement for response assessment. *This is further elaborated under cerebellar pilocytic astrocytomas* [13].

11.4.5 Lesion Characteristics

11.4.5.1 Internal Matrix on Basic Sequences

Basic MR sequences throw light on cell composition and relative water content of the tumor. Brain tumors are usually iso to hypointense to grey matter on T1, and hyperintense to gray matter on T2-FLAIR sequence. Tumors that show CT hyper-density and T2 hypo-intensity often have high nucleus-cytoplasm ratios with decreased relative water content, and is suggestive of densely cellular lesion like small round blue cell tumors, lymphoma, medulloblastoma, and other embryonal tumors [15]. T1 hyperintensity may represent hemorrhage (methemoglobin), melanin (in metastatic melanomas), fat, calcification, or slow vascular flow. T2 hypointensity may also represent hemorrhage (hemosiderin), calcification, proteinaceous material, or flow voids.

11.4.5.2 Cystoid Component

Brain tumors may be entirely solid or have a more variegated appearance comprising non-solid areas. These areas may be designated as cyst or necrosis, but sometimes cannot be distinguished. Cysts are round structures with fluid signal intensity which may have thin, smooth, regular, slightly enhancing, or non-enhancing walls. The biological mechanism of cyst formation is different for each tumor, and still unclear. Necrosis is identified on post-contrast axial images as regions of tumor having low signal intensity on T1, high signal intensity on T2 and an irregular enhancing border. Necrosis is seen frequently in high-grade lesions, and occurs due to rapid cell proliferation leading to nutritional imbalance, hypoxia, and cell death. It heralds poor prognosis [16].

Low-grade gliomas are usually solid or have a mixed solid-cystic appearance. High-grade gliomas have a more ominous appearance with solid and hallmark necrotic areas. Although classically described as cyst with nodule, pilocytic astrocytoma may also appear as entirely solid, or partly solid, partly cystic or complex cyst with septations. Diencephalic lesions are often entirely solid. The variable appearance of cystic component on FLAIR is due to proteinaceous content [17].

The presence of a thick, wavy/irregular rim of enhancing tissue partially or completely surrounding central cystic-necrotic areas is considered to be highly specific (95%) and sensitive (83%) for ATRT [18]. Cystic changes are present in up to 40–50% of medulloblastomas, and are typically small. These are frequently encountered in ependymomas as well, and appear larger than in medulloblastomas [2].

11.4.5.3 Hemorrhage and Calcification

Intra-tumoral bleed is multifactorial and can be attributed to abnormal tumor vascularization, invasion into parenchymal vessels, and tumor necrosis. It can occur in both benign and malignant lesions. High-grade gliomas appear heterogeneous due to the presence of necrosis and hemorrhage. Diffuse midline gliomas usually do not have significant hemorrhage but small internal hemorrhagic foci are detected on SWI sequence in up to half the cases [19]. Pilocytic astrocytoma may also show some bleed. [20]

Calcifications are detected better on CT. They are seen in up to 50% of ependymomas [21]. Calcifications are relatively rare in medulloblastomas, seen in 10–40% [22, 23]. Atypical teratoid rhabdoid tumors often have cysts, calcification and hemorrhage, and the presence of eccentric cysts can be used to differentiate these from medulloblastoma in posterior fossa [24].

11.4.6 Diffusion Patterns

The T2 and post-contrast T1-weighted images are utilized to exclude cystoid areas, calcifications/ hemorrhage, edema, and select the axial sections containing solid areas. The diffusion pattern and quantitative measure of apparent diffusion coefficient are obtained for these solid areas. ADC map is a quantitative scanner software-generated sequence, and has been shown to be reproducible across different scanners and field strengths [25, 26].

Low-grade gliomas usually do not show diffusion restriction. In contrast, high-grade gliomas may show localized or marked diffusion restriction. Diffusion restriction in densely cellular lesions like embryonal tumors is characteristic, and can be used to distinguish medulloblastomas from other tumors in the posterior fossa. Pavlisa et al. reported ADC values greater than 120×10^{-5} mm^2/s indicative of pilocytic astrocytoma, while an ADC between 80 and 120×10^{-5} mm^2/s is characteristic of ependymoma, and strong diffusion restriction, with ADC less than 80×10^{-5} mm^2/s is typically encountered in medulloblastoma [27].

11.4.7 Margin Definition

Tumor margins are usually described as well-defined or infiltrative. Diffuse gliomas usually show infiltrative margins, however occasionally, may have well-defined margins on imaging. The differentiation between low- and high-grade glioma is usually based on lack of diffusion restriction and contrast enhancement in the former [28]. Tumor margin is not a predictor of tumor grade, and merely suggests the containment zone of lesions. Infiltrative margins point toward involvement of adjacent apparently normal appearing parenchyma, and needs caution in surgical planning. Advanced imaging techniques like diffusion tensor imaging to identify infiltration of white matter tracts, magnetic resonance spectroscopy to detect biochemical changes in the peritumoral edema, and perfusion imaging that depicts increased rCBV in involved areas can help to delineate the areas of invasion in infiltrative lesions [29].

Pilocytic astrocytoma shows variable margin features based on their location, with purely expansive lesions with well-circumscribed margins more common in cerebral and cerebellar hemisphere. Infiltrative lesions are more common in the optic-diencephalic region and brainstem with variable degree of extension [30].

11.4.8 Perilesional Vasogenic Edema

The bright T2-weighted signal region surrounding the tumor should be defined as peritumoral edema, and is estimated based on the maximum distance from the tumor margin to the outer edge of the edema. It is usually graded as minor, if <10 mm, and major or marked if >10 mm [16, 31]. According to the method reported by Hartmann et al. [17], the morphological classification of peri-tumoral edema was performed on the basis of the T2-weighted images. Rapidly growing and invasive brain lesions produce more vasogenic edema compared to slow-growing lesions. In some cases, the peritumoral altered signal intensity is produced by both vasogenic edema and tumor cell infiltration. MRS of the peritumoral white matter will reflect biochemical changes like increased choline and reduced NAA in cases of tumoral infiltration in contrast to that in vasogenic edema which will retain normal biochemical composition of white matter [32].

Diffuse high-grade lesions usually have significant edema and mass effect. However, occasionally, they may show relatively mild edema; and size of edema does not correlate with their grade [33–35].

11.4.9 Pattern of Contrast Enhancement

Contrast enhancement merely suggests the breakdown of blood-brain barrier and does not correlate with the grade of tumor. Benign lesions like pilocytic astrocytoma may show avid enhancement of its solid component, due to rich vascularity or focal breakdown of blood-brain barrier, and does not correlate with tumor grade [17]. Choroid plexus papilloma also shows strong homogeneous enhancement. High-grade gliomas show variable enhancement, which does not correlate with tumor grade or prognosis.

The enhancement patterns may be described as absent or mild diffuse or patchy in low-grade gliomas. High-grade gliomas owing to their heterogeneous matrix frequently show a complex variable pattern of enhancement. Centrally necrotic tumors with a thick irregular rind of enhancement are seen in embryonal tumors, ATRT, and high-grade gliomas.

11.4.10 Imaging Findings in Common Infratentorial Tumors

11.4.10.1 Medulloblastoma

Classified under embryonal tumors, they are the most common malignant pediatric brain tumor and most common infratentorial, accounting for 40% posterior fossa tumors. Patients usually present with signs of raised intracranial hypertension like headache, vomiting, and ataxia.

They are highly malignant WHO grade 4 tumors. The 2021 WHO classification groups them into WNT activated, Sonic Hedgehog (SHH) activated TP53—wild type, Sonic Hedgehog (SHH) activated TP53-mutant, and non-WNT/non-SHH medulloblastoma—*comprises group 3 and group 4 tumors.*

The previously mentioned histological subtypes in 2016 classification, namely classic, desmoplastic/nodular, medulloblastoma with extensive nodularity (MBEN), and large cell/anaplastic, have now been combined under a single designation, *Medulloblastoma, histologically defined.* [36]

Histologically Defined Medulloblastoma Subgroups

The histological or morphological categories of medulloblastoma are intended to be reported in a layered manner with the molecular subgroups.

Classic morphology is the most common, characterized by classic 'small round blue cell' appearance, and rarely well-defined Homer Wright rosettes.

Desmoplastic/nodular (D/N) medulloblastomas are characterized by nodular zones of cellular tumor, surrounded by dense cellularity and intercellular reticulin, giving it a packeted appearance. Reticulin staining is an important diagnostic indicator in this subgroup.

Medulloblastomas with extensive nodularity (MBEN) are variants of D/N medulloblastoma, which presents with larger nodules containing more differentiated tumor cells, and are more midline in location. These are the rarest histological subtype, accounting for <5% of medulloblastoma. Both D/N and MBEN are common in younger patients less than 3 years of age, have excellent prognosis in early childhood, and are largely associated with SHH-activated molecular pathway.

Medulloblastomas with large cell/anaplastic (LC/A) morphology are characterized by anaplastic cellular appearance, and are associated with worse prognosis, metastasis, recurrence, cerebrospinal fluid dissemination [37, 38].

Imaging Appearance

Typical medulloblastomas are sharply defined midline mass in 75–90% of patients, arising from the inferior medullary velum, and growing into and distending the fourth ventricle, with associated hydrocephalus. In 15% of cases, they may extend into cerebellopontine angle via foramen of Luschka [23]. The characteristic hyperdense appearance on NCCT is attributed to increased cellularity and nuclear-cytoplasmic ratio (N:C), and has been reported in 62–97% cases.

On MRI, they appear as circumscribed mass, usually hypointense on T1 and hypo-iso-minimally hyperintense or heterogeneous on T2. Cystic component is common, seen in 50–95% of cases. Calcification is seen in 10–40%, and intratumoral hemorrhage is rare, seen in 5–15% of cases.

Contrast enhancement is variable and can be subtle/minimal (<5% enhancing component), heterogeneous or intense (>90% enhancement). Meningeal enhancement at contact point may be seen. Diffusion restriction is characteristic; however, desmoplastic variant may have minimal or absent restriction.

On MR spectroscopy, Group 3 and 4 tumors exhibit high taurine peak at 3.4 ppm, and elevated creatine. SHH activated tumors show low to negligible taurine and low creatine values [39] (Fig. 11.1).

The new WHO classification (Table 11.2) emphasizes on molecular subtyping, due to its vital role in prognosis and precise, and tailored therapeutic interventions. While genomic profiling provides accurate molecular identification, the need for tissue sample makes it an

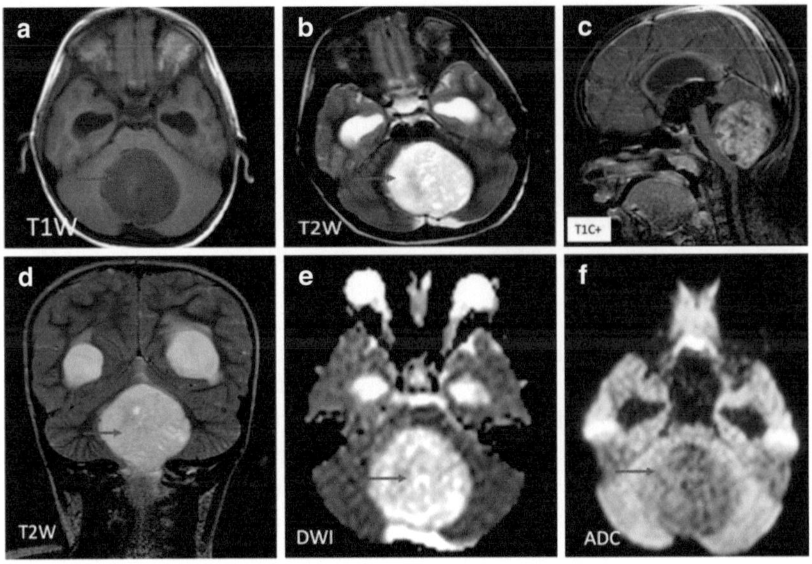

Fig. 11.1 5-year-old child with headache and vomiting. Well-defined large mass is seen in the midline in the posterior fossa. It has a low T1 signal intensity (**a**) and a high T2 signal intensity (**b** and **d**) with heterogeneous contrast enhancement (**c**). On corresponding DWI restricted diffusion is seen (**e** and **f**) No normal vermis can be identified and the mass is likely to arise from it, completely effacing the fourth ventricle and abutting the dorsal aspect of the brainstem without evidence of extension into the pons. As a result of the mass effect on the fourth ventricle, significant obstructive hydrocephalus has developed. Diagnosis: Medulloblastoma

Table 11.2 The new WHO classification

	WNT	SHH	Group 3	Group 4
Prevalence	Rarest (10%)	30%	25%	Most common (35%)
Key mutation pathways	*CTNNB1, APC*	*TP53, PTCH1, SUFU, SMO, MYCN, GLI2 (methylome)*	*MYC, MYCN, PRDM6, KDM6A (methylome)*	
Histology	*Classic*	*Most common desmoplastic/nodular, classic*	*Classic, large cell/anaplastic*	
Demographics	Older children and teens, M:F = 1:1	Bimodal; infants and teens/adults	Infants and young children (M:F = 2:1)	Infants, children, adults Peaks at 10 years (M: F = 3:1)
Imaging features:				
Tumor location (horizontal axis)	Midline, but commonly extends to CP/CPA cistern (approx. 75% tumors in CPA cistern)	Lateralized location involving cerebellar hemisphere, but midline common in infants/young children	Predominantly midline location involving the vermis or fourth ventricle	
Tumor location (vertical axis)	Central, but can extend inferiorly sometimes	Superior location highly specific (it often reaches or abuts the tentorium)	Central in location, but can extend inferiorly also	Inferior in location, with dilatation of superior recess of IVth ventricle
Relation with dorsal brainstem	Often infiltrating the dorsal brainstem	Over 50% tumors away from dorsal brainstem	Closely related to and abuts the dorsal brainstem	

(continued)

Table 11.2 (continued)

	WNT	SHH	Group 3	Group 4
Characteristics on T2-weighted sequence	Mostly isointense and homogeneous	Mostly isointense and heterogeneous	Mostly hypointense and homogeneous	Hyperintense/ isointense and homogeneous
Peri-tumoral edema	Mild or absent	Significant edema, often >1.5 cm beyond the tumor	Absent or mild	Absent or mild
Intra-tumoral hemorrhage	Can be present	Absent	Absent	Absent
Cyst (size and location)	Microcysts; intra-tumoral	Microcysts and macro-cysts; Intra-tumoral and peri-tumoral	Macro-cyst; peri-tumoral	Micro-cysts; Intra-tumoral
Enhancement pattern	Homogeneous bright enhancement involving majority of tumor	Variable pattern with moderate enhancement	Heterogeneous "fluffy" enhancement	Heterogeneous "patchy" enhancement
Associated hydrocephalus	Generally absent (mild-moderate if present)	Seldom (mild-moderate if present)	Moderate to severe	Moderate to severe
Potential metastases	Rare	Variable incidence, Spinal and posterior fossa, Possible multi-centricity	Highest incidence, Spinal metastases, Laminar metastases	Moderate incidence, Supra-sellar and infundibular, Nodular metastases
Prognosis (5-year survival rate)	Good prognosis (95%)	Intermediate prognosis (75%) (mutations in MYCN or TP53 oncogenes worsen prognosis)	Worst prognosis (50%)	Intermediate prognosis (75%) (MYCN amplification do not worsen prognosis)
Syndromic association		Gorlin syndrome, Fanconi anemia	Neurocutaneous syndromes like tuberous sclerosis	

Adapted from Dasgupta et al. [40]

invasive investigation. MRI imaging has been explored as a non-invasive alternative modality for prediction of molecular marker. Present literature shows that anatomical location and contrast enhancement patterns correlate well with their molecular expression [41]. The distinguishing characteristics of different molecular subgroups of medulloblastoma are summarized below:

Treatment of medulloblastomas entails a combination of surgery and chemoradiation. In current understanding, therapeutic approach of these tumors may be guided by their molecular phenotype. For example: opting for less invasive or low risk surgery in WNT phenotype, and neoadjuvant chemoradiation in group 4 tumors, and high grade SHH-α subtypes. Radio-genomic studies have been conducted which involves using machine learning models to extract quantitative biomarkers from conventional MRI sequences, and use these to predict the molecular subgroup. So far, it shows promising results [41, 42] (Fig. 11.2).

Imaging Consideration and Post-treatment Surveillance

The consensus recommendations given by The Response Assessment in Paediatric Neuro-Oncology group (RAPNO) are applicable for medulloblastoma as well as other leptomeningeal seeding tumors (include germ cell subtypes, choroid plexus tumors, and embryonal tumors such

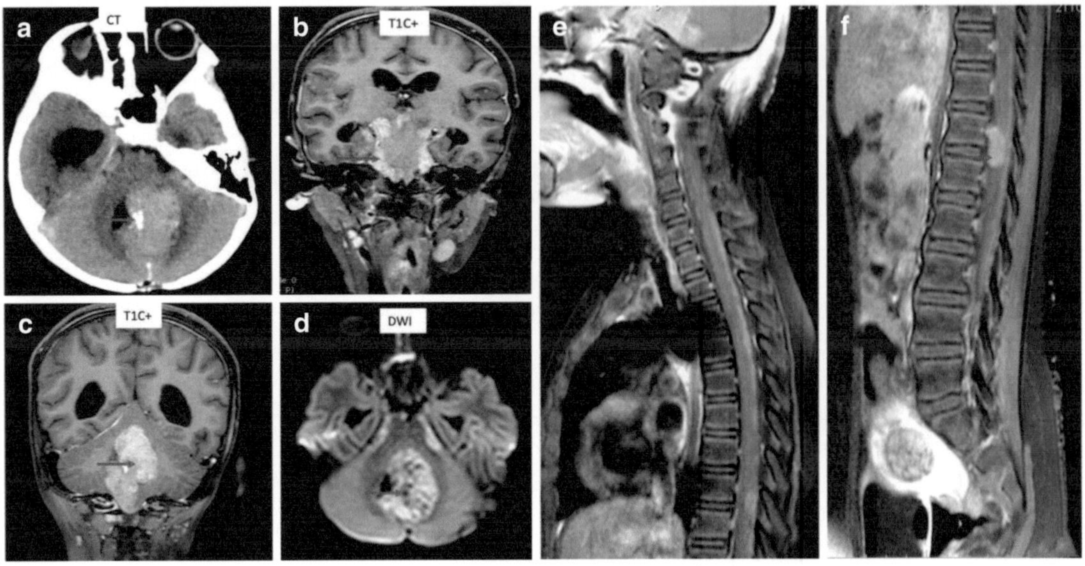

Fig. 11.2 A large ill-defined mass is seen in the midline in the posterior fossa. It appears isodense on CT with areas of calcification within (**a**). On post contrast T1WI it shows heterogeneous contrast enhancement (**b** and **c**). Areas of restricted diffusion are seen within the lesion (**d**). No normal vermis can be identified and the mass is likely to arise from it, completely effacing the fourth ventricle. As a result of the mass effect on the fourth ventricle, significant obstructive hydrocephalus has developed (**b**). Sagittal images of the spine show well-defined hyperintense lesions in the spinal cord (arrow), indicative of "drop metastasis" (**e** and **f**). Diagnosis: Medulloblastoma with drop metastasis

as pinealoblastoma, and atypical teratoid rhabdoid tumor).

- Treatment is usually surgical resection of the primary mass, followed by craniospinal radiation therapy and chemotherapy.
- Brain imaging recommendations are same as discussed previously. Fast turbo spin echo (FSE) sequences are recommended over spoiled gradient recalled acquisitions (SPGR) for post-contrast T1 due to less vascular artifact. Vascular flow compensation and fat saturation pulses are discouraged. Diffusion-weighted sequences are recommended for both primary tumor and sites of metastasis. Post contrast T2-FLAIR is recommended for leptomeningeal disease. Spine imaging is recommended with post-contrast T1 and 3D myelographic T2-weighted images.
- Postoperative MRI for residual disease is recommended within 72 hours of surgery. If the images are not clear, a repeat MRI is recommended 2–3 weeks after surgery. During the course of adjuvant chemotherapy, follow-up MRI imaging is recommended every 2 cycles of chemotherapy, and not less frequent than at 3-month interval.
- Leptomeningeal disease assessment should be done using both MRI and CSF cytology.
- FOR RESPONSE ASSESSMENT: Measurable lesion should be seen on at least two slices. In multifocal lesions, up to 4 target lesions should be chosen for response assessment. Standard bidimensional measurement (i.e., largest diameter and its largest perpendicular diameter) should be used unless specified otherwise (Table 11.3).
- Summary of response definitions:

11.4.10.2 Cerebellar Pilocytic Astrocytoma

They are WHO grade I circumscribed astrocytic gliomas, accounting for 20–30% of all pediatric tumors, and typically occur in the first two decades of life. In the posterior fossa, they are

Table 11.3 response to treatment

	Complete response (CR)	Partial response (PR)	Stable disease	Progressive disease (PD)
Fulfilled criteria	All	All	All	Any
MRI brain	Complete disappearance of all disease for at least 4 weeks	≥ 50% decrease (compared to baseline) in sum of products of perpendicular diameters of up to 4 measurable lesions for at least 4 weeks No progression of non-measurable disease	Does not meet criteria for CR, PR, PD	≥25% increase (compared to any time point) in the sum of the products of perpendicular diameters of all measurable lesions; Significant progression of non-measurable disease (not therapy related) any new tumor (not treatment related)
MRI spine	Complete disappearance of all disease for at least 4 weeks	≥ 50% decrease (compared to baseline) in sum of products of perpendicular diameters of up to 4 measurable lesions for at least 4 weeks No progression of non-measurable disease	Does not meet criteria for CR, PR, PD	≥25% increase (compared to any time point) in the sum of the products of perpendicular diameters of all measurable lesions; Significant progression of non-measurable disease (not therapy related) any new tumor (not treatment related)
CSF cytology	Negative on two samples 2 weeks apart	Absent/present	Absent/present	Newly positive
Neurologic exam	Stable/improving	Stable/improving	Stable/improving	Deterioration
Steroid use	Off steroid	Stable/less than baseline dose	Stable/less than baseline dose	
Extra-CNS disease	Absent	No new site	No new site	New site
Serum markers (in germ cell tumors)	Normal			New positive

most common in the cerebellum followed by the brainstem. They usually arise from alteration in *KIAA1549-BRAF*, *BRAF*, and *NF1* genes. Neurofibromatosis type 1 (NF1) syndrome-associated pilocytic astrocytoma frequently involves the optic pathway, and have better prognosis. Other syndromic associations include Turcot syndrome, PHACE(S) syndrome, and Ollier's disease. Supratentorial location is more common in adults.

11.4.11 Imaging Appearance

50% of cerebellar lesions are cystic with an enhancing solid mural nodule. Cyst walls may be enhancing or non-enhancing. Other presentations include solid with central non-enhancing necrotic component, and rarely pure solid lesion. The solid component is T1 iso to hypointense and T2/FLAIR hyperintense and shows variable post-contrast enhancement. The cyst content is usually

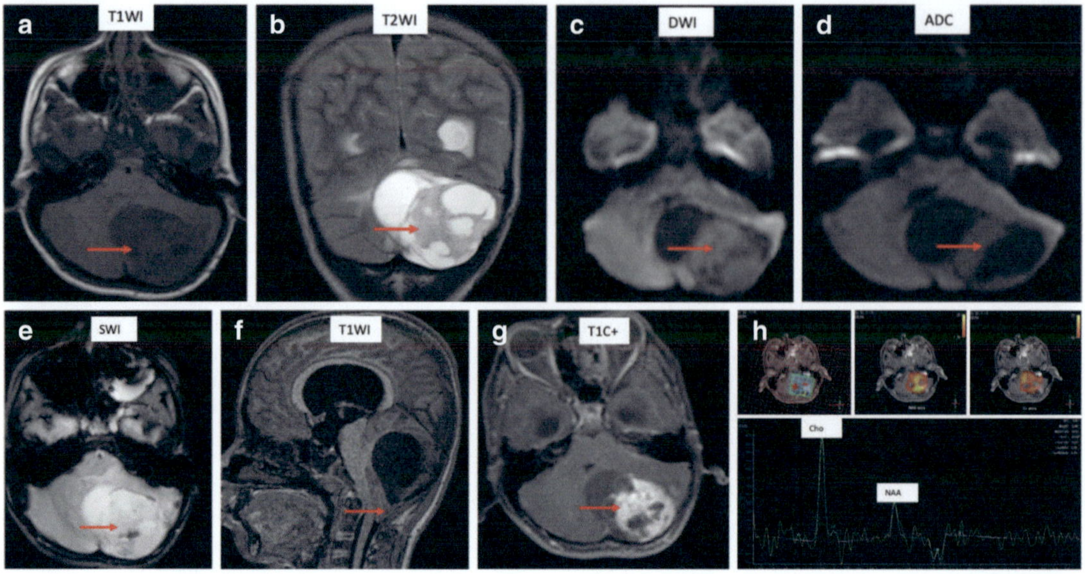

Fig. 11.3 Thirteen years male with fever, multiple episodes of vomiting and headache. MRI Brain (with contrast) (**a**): Axial T1WI, (**b**): Coronal T2WI (**c**) and (**d**): Axial DWI, (**e**): axial SWI (**f**): sagittal TWI (**g**)T1C+ Axial image: Well-defined solid-cystic left cerebellar hemisphere mass with secondary moderate obstructive hydrocephalus, tonsillar and ascending transtentorial herniation. Areas of restricted diffusion are seen and patchy post contrast enhancement. (**f**): axial Gradient images showing a focus of blooming indicative of calcification/hemorrhage and (**h**)MR spectroscopy (MRS) images showing a raised choline peak. Diagnosis: Astrocytoma

T2 and FLAIR hyperintense compared to CSF. Intra-lesional bleed has been rarely reported in pilocytic astrocytoma, and are usually not massive. Diffusion-weighted imaging shows high ADC (> 120 x 10 $^{-5}$ mm^2/s by Pavlisa et al), reflecting the low cellular density of the tumor [43]. MRS shows high choline level, high lactate level, low N-acetyl aspartate (NAA) levels, features that are usually associated with high-grade tumors. MR perfusion shows low perfusion with decreased rCBV of the enhancing component (Fig. 11.3).

11.4.11.1 Imaging Consideration and Post-treatment Surveillance

Pediatric low-grade gliomas comprise ~40–50% of all pediatric brain tumor, with pilocytic astrocytoma being the most common. The following RAPNO surveillance guidelines are relevant to all WHO grade I and II tumors of glial origin.

- A combination of clinical, imaging, and functional evaluation is recommended to assess treatment response.
- Brain imaging recommendations are the same as discussed previously. Contrast sequences, although used routinely and required under protocol, are not reliable due to variable enhancement patterns. Many patients receive molecular targeted therapy like MEK inhibitors and BRAF inhibitors, which reduce tumoral enhancement. Hence, changes in enhancement pattern should not be considered as a treatment response. T2 and FLAIR sequences should be considered for standard bidimensional measurement of lesion.
- 3D post contrast T1 and post contrast T2-FLAIR are optional sequences unlike elsewhere.
- Postoperative MRI for residual disease is recommended within 24–72 hours of surgery. If not clear, a repeat MRI is recommended

2–3 weeks after surgery. Spine imaging is recommended when there is a concern for metastatic disease in specific high-risk pathology (such as pleomorphic xantho-astrocytoma) or in clinically symptomatic cases.

- For cystic tumors, it is important to distinguish tumoral cyst from non-tumor cyst. Only tumoral cysts are measured and included under response assessment. Tumor cysts include those which are integrated within the solid component (like soap bubble appearance), are not readily separable from the solid component, show thick wall enhancement, or appear as a cluster of small microcysts within the tumor.
- The cysts to be excluded from measurement and response assessment include.

  - Reactive cyst at the interface of solid component of the tumor and healthy brain.
  - Resection cavity or cyst intermingled with the resection cavity.
  - Cystic component of a predominantly cystic tumor with a solid enhancing mural nodule but without substantial cyst wall enhancement.

Although tumor cysts are included in size measurements, imaging features indicating progression differ for cystic versus solid portions of the tumor.

11.4.11.2 Brainstem Gliomas

They account for up to 12% of all pediatric intracranial tumors in children. Mean age of presentation is 7 years.

They can be further classified into diffuse brainstem tumors, and non-diffuse or focal brainstem tumors.

11.4.12 Diffuse Midline Glioma, H3 K27 Altered

These lesions were previously grouped as H3K27 mutant in the old WHO classification. Their new nomenclature in the recent 2021 classification reflects the multiple mechanisms of tumorigenesis, which can involve H3 K27, TP 53, ACVR1, PDGFRA, EGFR, EZHIP pathways. They typically involve midline structures with a predilection for pons (32%), followed by thalamus (27%), fourth ventricle/cerebellum (15%), and spinal cord (6%). They are highly aggressive lesions with median age of survival less than 1 year (Fig. 11.4).

11.4.12.1 Imaging Appearance

The imaging appearance is highly variable. Classically these are described as expansile masses involving at least 50% of pons, without enhancement or necrosis, and with large areas of surrounding infiltrative growth. Pontine lesions tend to involve the ventral aspect of pons, and encase the basilar artery without causing associated vascular narrowing. These tumors often extend beyond their site of origin into adjacent structures like mid brain and cerebellum [34, 35]. They can also present as peripherally enhancing masses with central necrosis and significant surrounding mass effect but, with little surrounding T2/FLAIR hyperintensity. Most tumors do not show diffusion restriction. Occasionally, mild restriction may be seen, and apparent diffusion coefficient (ADC) values are characteristically higher than medulloblastomas (Fig. 11.5).

11.4.12.2 Imaging Consideration and Pre- and Post-treatment Surveillance

- The mainstay of treatment in diffuse midline glioma is steroids and anti-angiogenic agents like bevacizumab. These often produce a phenomenon called pseudo-progression, seen in up to 21–44% of DIPG patients, which is characterized by worsening of clinical symptoms and/or imaging appearance. This phenomenon can lead to confounding appearance of the primary tumor on follow-up MRI, and should be kept in mind.
- RAPNO recommends pre- and post-contrast T1, T2, and FLAIR sequence, acquired with ≤ 4 mm slice thickness. DWI is not recommended due to variability in diffusion characteristics.

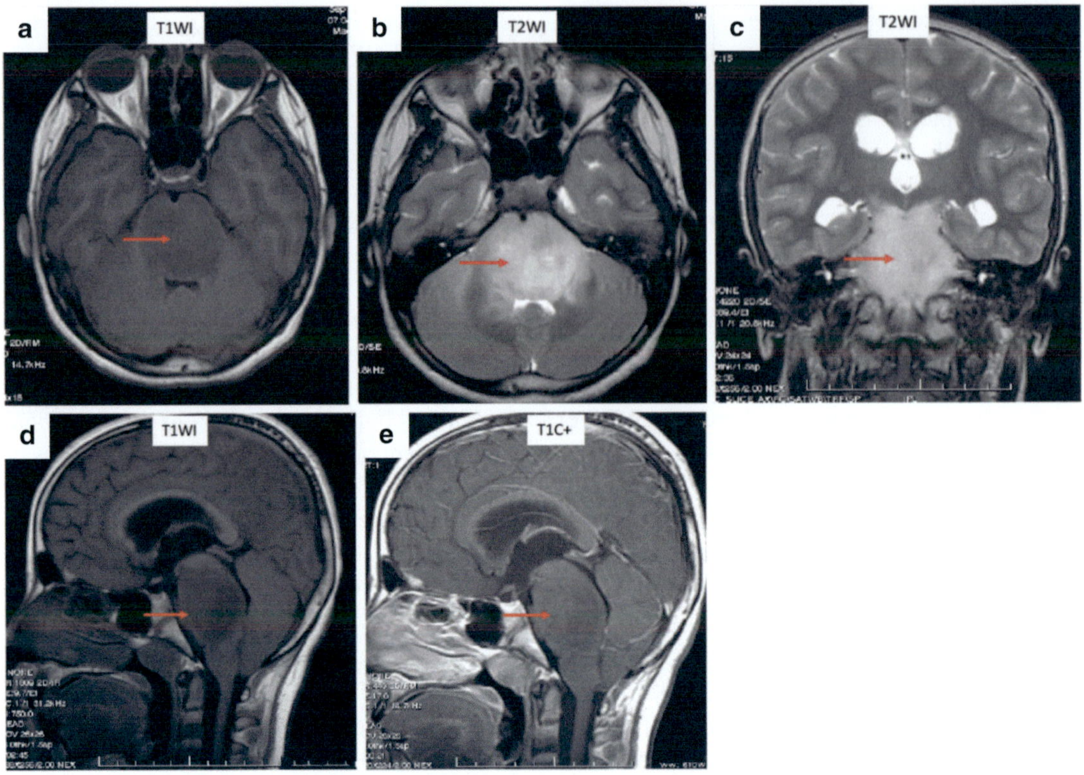

Fig. 11.4 12-year-old female. A fairly well-defined intra-axial intrapontine mass lesion is seen causing pontine enlargement. It appears hypointense on T1WI (**a**) and (**d**) and hyperintense on T2WI (**b**) and (**c**). The lateral ventricles and the third ventricle appear dilated due to the obstruction by the lesion. It shows mild enhancement on post-contrast images (**e**). Diagnosis: Brainstem glioma

- In patients on chemotherapy, the baseline MRI scan for response assessment is recommended within 4 weeks from entry into the clinical trial, or 4–6 weeks after radiotherapy has been completed. For all trials, follow-up MRI should be done every 2 cycles.
- FOR RESPONSE ASSESSMENT: Either T2 or FLAIR sequence is used to measure the lesion. For multifocal disease, 3 target lesions are chosen. Standard bidimensional measurement is used. Measurable disease should be at least 1 cm or two times slice thickness plus interslice gap.

11.4.13 Other Brainstem Gliomas

Other brainstem gliomas include focal gliomas like pilocytic astrocytoma, ganglioglioma, and diffuse low-grade gliomas. Imaging considerations and post-treatment surveillance discussed previously under cerebellar pilocytic astrocytoma is also applicable to these brainstem gliomas (Figs. 11.6 and 11.7).

Most tectal gliomas fit histologically and genetically into either pilocytic astrocytoma with BRAF alterations and NRAS mutations or diffuse low-grade glioma, MAPK pathway–altered, and are not considered as separate entities in the classification.

The other common low-grade brainstem gliomas are discussed below.

11.4.13.1 Pilocytic Astrocytoma

Brainstem pilocytic astrocytoma are usually focal circumscribed expansile lesions, and typically present with exophytic growth (more often arising from dorsal brainstem). They may have

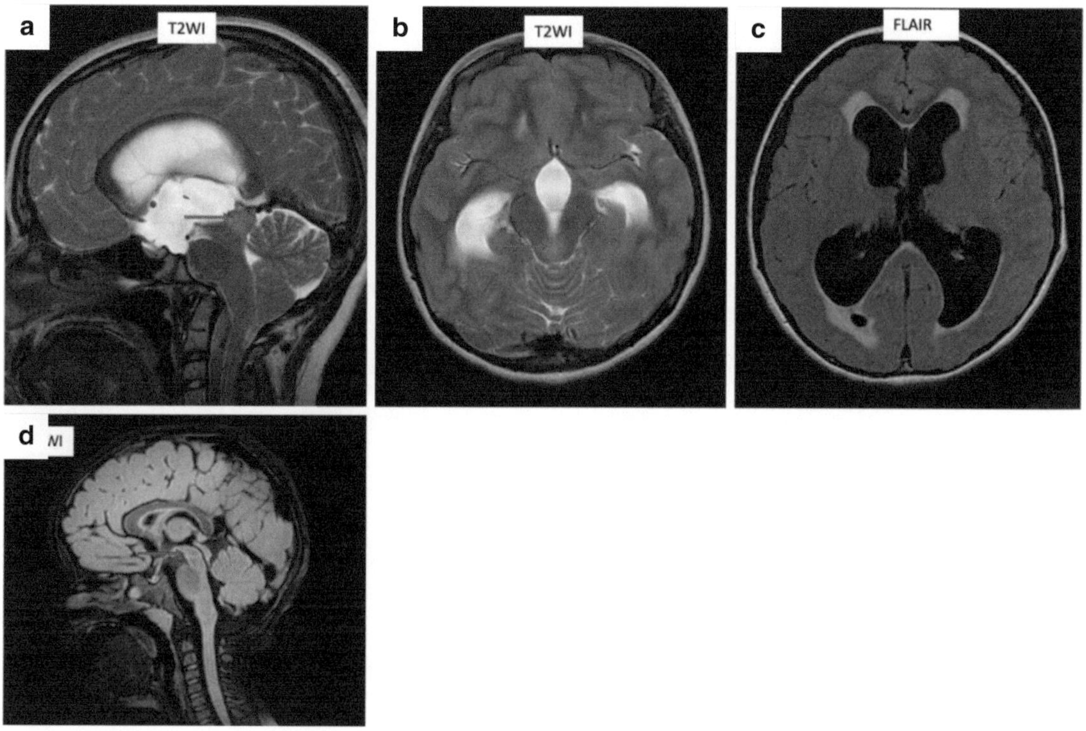

Fig. 11.5 A 7-year-old girl presented with headaches with early morning worsening, projectile vomiting and squintA subtle ill defined T2 hyperintense mass lesion is noted in the tectum (arrow) with tectal enlargement, causing obstructive hydrocephalus (**a**) and (**b**). Periventricular ooze is seen on FLAIR images (**c**). Normal tectum for comparison (**d**). Diagnosis: Tectal glioma

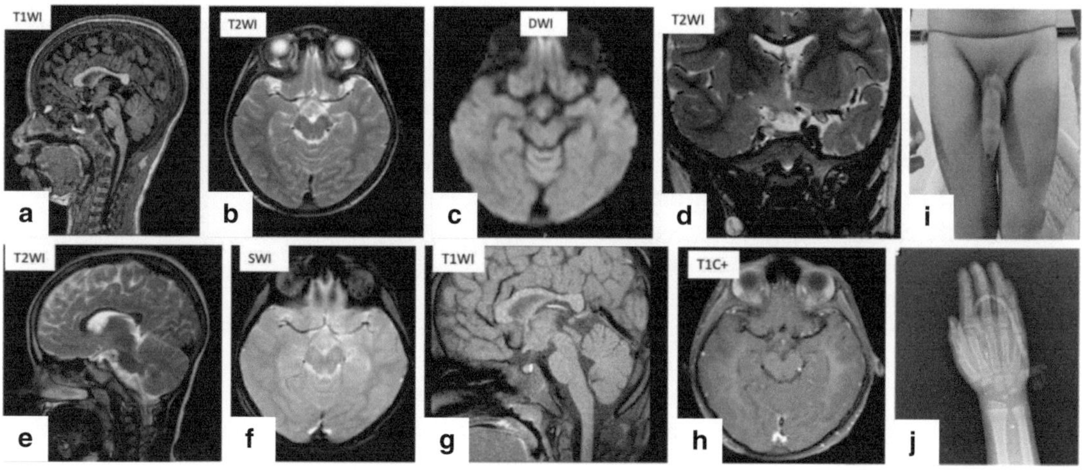

Fig. 11.6 A 2 years 9 months male child, first and only issue of a NCM was brought with concerns of: Development of excessive pubic hair 2 months Increase in size of phallus. (**a**): sagittal TWI, (**b**): axial T2WI, (**c**): Axial DWI, (**d**) coronal T2WI, (**e**) sagittal T2WI, (**f**) Axial SWI, (**g**) TIWI, (**h**) Post contrast TIWI (**i**)Bone age is 7–8 years (**j**). A soft tissue mass between the right optic tract and mammillary bodies involving the right half of tuber cinereum. Causing indentation on prechiasmatic optic nerve. It is extending superiorly along the lateral wall of third ventricle and infiltrating the optic tract and right medial temporal lobe laterally (**a**, **b**, **d**).T1WI: hypointense (**a**). T2WI: mildly hyperintense (**b**). No diffusion restriction (**c**) SWI: No blooming (**f**) T1C+: Post-contrast enhancement (**h**). Diagnosis: Low-grade glioma

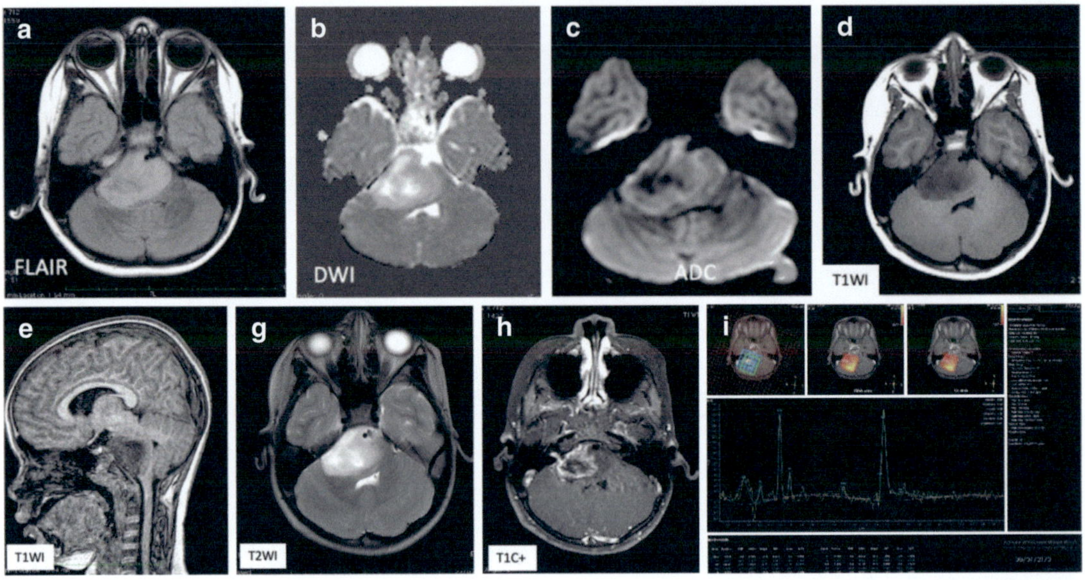

Fig. 11.7 A 7-year-old boy progressive left sided weakness (**a**): Axial FLAIR, (**b**) axial diffusion and (**c**) axial ADC, (**d** and **e**) Axial and sagittal TIWI, (**g**) axial T2WI, (**h**) axial post contrast TIWI, (**i**) MRS. A large ill-defined mass is seen with epicentre in the right CP angle cistern which appears to be an exophytic brainstem mass arising from the pons. It appears hypointense on T1WI and hyperintense on T2WI. Incomplete suppression is seen on FLAIR images (**a**) (T2/FLAIR mismatch).It shows central restricted diffusion (**b** and **c**) .Peripheral enhancement is seen on post-contrast images (**h**). On MR spectroscopy a choline peak and a lipid lactate peak is seen (**i**)

cystic areas. The dorsally exophytic tumors have been observed to push the fourth ventricle upward. Solid component is usually T2 hyperintense, and shows homogeneous or heterogeneous enhancement. Tectal plate lesions present with obstruction of Aqueduct of Sylvius, and frequently do not enhance after contrast administration [44].

11.4.13.2 Diffuse Low-Grade Glioma

9% of all diffuse low-grade gliomas occur in the brainstem. They appear as infiltrative lesion with heterogeneous enhancement and with no obvious diffusion restriction.

Posterior Fossa Ependymoma

They constitute around 8–15% of pediatric posterior fossa tumors and are graded 2 or 3 based on histopathology. Posterior fossa (PF) ependymoma is now described as a separate entity in the latest WHO classification (Table 11.4), and is further sub-classified into two groups—PFA and PFB based on DNA-methylation and transcriptional profiling.

Table 11.4 Types of posterior fossa ependymoma

Posterior fossa group A (PFA) ependymomas	Posterior fossa group B (PFB) ependymomas
Seen in younger patients (median age 2.5 years)	Seen in older age group (median age 20 years)
More likely to arise laterally in the cerebellopontine angles	More likely to arise in the spinal cord or midline cerebellum
Lateral type tumors that cause lateral brainstem displacement without obex involvement	Mid-floor type tumors that tend to displace the brainstem anteriorly and infiltrate obex,
Worse prognosis and associated with greater recurrence	Relatively better prognosis

Imaging Appearance

Infratentorial/posterior fossa ependymomas arise from the ependymal lining of fourth ventricle or foramen of Luschka, and frequently show 'plastic nature'—extension through the foramina of Luschka into the cerebellopontine angle (15%) and/or inferiorly through the foramen of Magendie (60%) onto the posterior aspect of the upper cervical cord. [21] The foraminal exten-

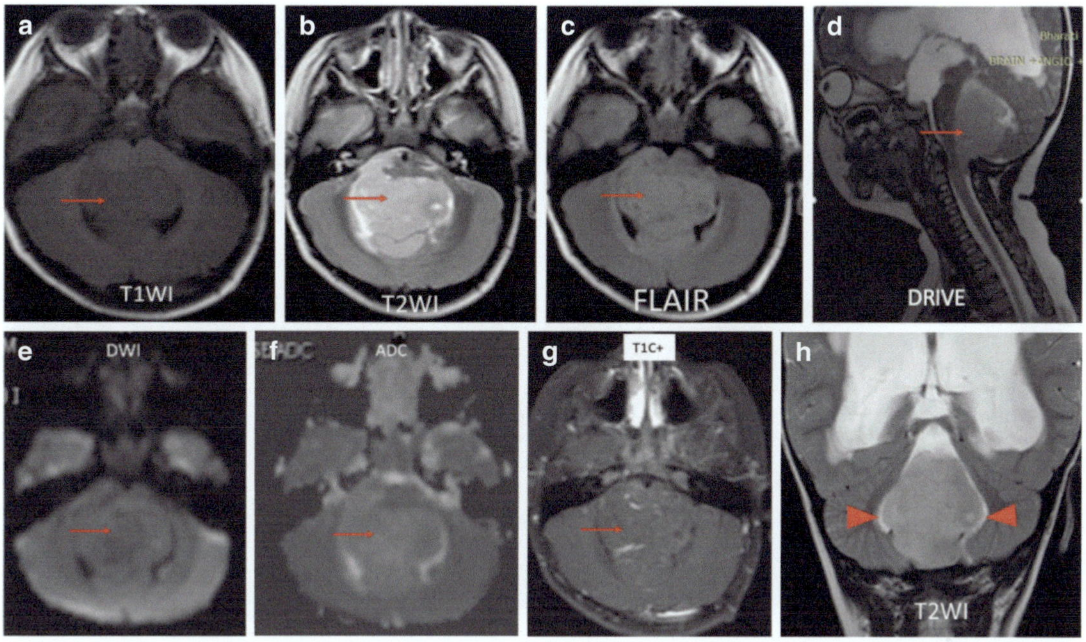

Fig. 11.8 2-year-old female child, with fever, vomiting, and difficulty in walking since 2 days. History of child having head tilt toward one side with restriction of movement of neck to the left side (**a**) Axial TIWI, (**b** and **h**) axial and coronal T2WI, (**c**) axial FLAIR, (**d**) CSF DRIVE sagittal, (**e** and **f**) axial DWI and ADC, (**g**) post-contrast TIWI. Large well-defined heterogeneous mass in the posterior fossa with epicentre in the fourth ventricle, extending into the foramina of Luschka (arrow heads) and pre pontine cistern. It is isointense on T1WI (**a**), hyperintense on T2 (**b**) with areas of higher signal, suggestive of cystic change. The mass shows no restricted diffusion (**e** and **f**). On post-contrast images heterogeneous contrast enhancement is seen (**g**). Mass effect and fourth ventricular obstruction is seen with hydrocephalus and periventricular ooze (**d** and **h**). Diagnosis: Ependymoma

sions tend to be slender unlike mass like bulbous extensions in medulloblastoma, that may aid in differentiation [45].

They are typically heterogeneous on CT and MRI with necrosis, calcifications, hemorrhage, and cysts. They demonstrate low T1, high T2, and intermediate-to-high FLAIR signal intensity relative to both grey and white matter, likely due to intracellular myxoid accumulation and cyst formation. They are typically slow-growing lesions and frequently insinuate between and encase vessels and cranial nerves. Diffusion restriction is intermediate (ADC between 80 and 120× 10^{-5} mm^2/s by Pavlisa et al) (Fig. 11.8).

Imaging Consideration and Post-treatment Surveillance

- Brain MRI sequences should include pre and post-contrast T1, T2, post-contrast T2 FLAIR for leptomeningeal disease, and DWI.
- Surgery is the treatment of choice. Gross total resection is defined by RAPNO as no measurable disease. Near total resection is measurable disease ≤5 mm. Subtotal resection is measurable disease ≥5 mm.
- Postoperative MRI is recommended within 2 weeks, and if not clear, a repeat MRI should be done 2-3 weeks later.
- Measurable disease may be either enhancing or non-enhancing; The size of the lesion to qualify as measurable should be at least 1 cm or two times slice thickness plus interslice gap.

11.4.13.3 Atypical Teratoid Rhabdoid Tumor

Classified under embryonal tumors, they are highly malignant grade 4 tumors and most commonly present in <2–3 years of age. They are relatively rare, and constitute 1–2% of all pediatric tumors. Imaging features resemble medulloblastoma, and definitive diagnosis requires molecular detection of inactivated SMARCB1 (INI1) or SMARCA4 (BRG1) gene.

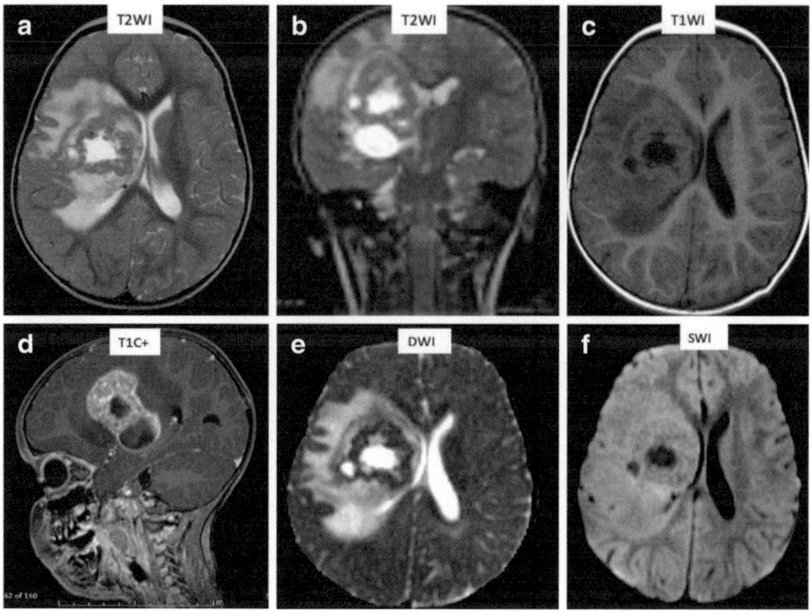

Fig. 11.9 Large intra axial ill-defined, heterohenous, mass right basal ganglia. It appears hypointense on T1WI (**c**) and hyperintense on T2WI (**a**) and (**b**). Right lateral ventricular compression is seen with heterogenous contrast enhancement (**d**). Central non enhancing area is consistent with necrosis. Diagnosis: Supratentorial ATRT

Imaging Appearance

They typically present as large heterogeneous mass in cerebellum or fourth ventricle with necrosis, calcifications, and hemorrhage. Nearly all tumors show diffusion restriction, and cranial nerve involvement may already be present at the onset. Contrast enhancement is heterogeneous. MRS shows an aggressive metabolite pattern. However, myoinositol and taurine peaks are typically absent.

A younger patient age at presentation and a relatively more heterogeneous appearance of the lesion favors preoperative diagnosis of ATRT. Presently, machine learning-based radiomic studies have shown promising result in distinguishing ATRT from medulloblastoma [46]. MRI imaging sequence recommendations and post-treatment surveillance are the same as medulloblastoma (Fig. 11.9).

11.4.13.4 Hemangioblastoma

These are extremely rare in children, with an incidence of <1 case per million, and are commonly associated with Von Hippel-Lindau (VHL) syndrome. Typical hemangioblastomas are solid-cystic, the solid component being T1 hypo- to isointense and T2 hyperintense relative to grey matter with enhancement of the mural nodule. The cyst wall most commonly does not enhance unless lined by neoplasm. They can mimic pleomorphic xanthoastrocytoma and pilocytic astrocytoma, and are differentiated by high rCBV values on perfusion MRI.

11.5 Post-treatment Changes and Secondary Tumors

Brain tumors require a combined therapeutic approach of surgery and chemoradiation. The relevant imaging protocols, as mentioned under RAPNO guidelines, have been discussed for individual tumors.

As far as post-surgical imaging is concerned, MRI should be done early within 24–72 hours of surgery to reduce the artifactual effect of surgical scar. But, in case of extensive edema or hemorrhage obscuring the operative site, MRI is recommended 2–3 weeks after surgery.

11.5.1 Radiation Effects

Acute radiation effects include presence of vasogenic oedema and new contrast enhancement, but these are usually confined around the radiation area.

Pseudo-progression is an important subacute/early delayed effect seen within 3–6 months of radiotherapy, and is characterized by new or enlarging areas of contrast enhancement in the absence of true tumor growth. Sequences used to differentiate this entity from recurrent lesion include perfusion MRI which shows reduced rCBV, diffusion-weighted imaging which demonstrates high diffusivity, MR spectroscopy which displays variable decrease in NAA, and lack of pronounced increase in choline level.

In patients receiving high-dose radiation therapy, *radiation necrosis* is an important late complication. It usually presents at 1–2 years post radiation therapy. It is usually seen as a heterogeneously enhancing mass lesion with central necrosis and reactive oedema. Its enhancement pattern is often described as "spreading wavefront," or "soap bubble–like" or "Swiss cheese–like," or cut green pepper appearance. It may be multifocal, but always develops in the radiation field. With time, it can lead to marked shrinkage of the white matter and cortex and result in focal brain atrophy. Demonstration of decreased rCBV on perfusion and elevated lipid/lactate peaks on 1H MRS differentiates this entity from recurrent tumor.

Other lesions observed in the late stage include *vascular proliferative lesion*s like capillary telangiectasia and cavernous malformations (cavernomas). Radiation-induced neoplasms are another delayed effect. Criteria for diagnosis of radiation-induced neoplasms include location in the irradiated field, sufficient latent period, and histopathology different from the original neoplasm. Examples include meningioma, glioma, and sarcoma.

11.6 Chemotherapy Effects

Effects of chemotherapy are usually acute and include posterior reversible encephalopathy syndrome (PRES) and acute leukoencephalopathy. Of note, tumors treated with antiangiogenic agents like bevacizumab (in gliomas as mentioned earlier) may show reduced enhancement, perfusion, oedema, and mass effect soon after initiation of therapy, despite the persistence of the biological tumor. This phenomenon is known as pseudo-response. In such cases, T2-FLAIR sequence which identifies the tumor as persistent hyperintense signal, is used for response assessment.

11.7 Recent Developments

11.7.1 Diffusion Tensor Imaging

It uses at least 6 diffusion-sensitizing gradients to detect anisotropic diffusion and generate fractional anisotropy maps and tractography maps. The spatial relationship of brain tumor with respect to adjacent white matter tracts in terms of displacement versus infiltration is demonstrated well on these maps, which further aid in surgical planning. In addition, it also plays a role in the detection of radiation-induced white matter injury, which demonstrates lower fractional anisotropy (FA) values than the normal white matter [47].

11.7.2 Application of Artificial Intelligence in Brain Tumor Imaging

Radiomics refers to the extraction of quantifiable biometric parameters from radiographic images and relies heavily on artificial intelligence. A subset of radiomics Radio-genomics—applies to correlation of imaging lesion phenotypes with their genotypes. Machine learning is another branch of artificial intelligence which provides automated recognition of data patterns [48]. Artificial intelligence, radiomics, machine learning, and deep learning models are being studied currently for preoperative segmentation and molecular subtyping of brain tumors, and distinction between diverse tumor groups.

11.7.3 Sodium MRI

Few studies conducted with sodium (^{23}Na) MRI on brain gliomas show increased sodium concentration in the pathological areas, and these areas are substitute markers of tumor proliferation. Their study in pediatric patients is limited. One pediatric study shows increased total sodium concentration (TSC) in pathological areas in diffuse brainstem gliomas treated with radiation therapy and supratentorial gliomas, compared to uninvolved normal brain parenchyma [49].

Other novel MRI techniques which are under clinical investigation in adult brain tumors include chemical exchange saturation transfer (CEST) imaging [47].

Acknowledgments We would like to thank Dr. Isha Shah for her help with the images.

References

1. Jaju A, Li Y, Dahmoush H, Gottardo NG, Laughlin S, Mirsky D, et al. Imaging of pediatric brain tumors: a COG diagnostic imaging committee/SPR oncology committee/ASPNR white paper. Pediatr Blood Cancer. 2023;70(S4):e30147.
2. Jaju A, Yeom KW, Ryan ME. MR imaging of pediatric brain tumors. Diagnostics (Basel). 2022;12(4):961.
3. Jung AY. Basics for pediatric brain tumor imaging: techniques and protocol recommendations. Brain Tumor Res Treat. 2024;12(1):1–13.
4. Cooney TM, Cohen KJ, Guimaraes CV, Dhall G, Leach J, Massimino M, et al. Response assessment in diffuse intrinsic pontine glioma: recommendations from the response assessment in pediatric neuro-oncology (RAPNO) working group. Lancet Oncol. 2020;21(6):e330–6.
5. Warren KE, Vezina G, Poussaint TY, Warmuth-Metz M, Chamberlain MC, Packer RJ, et al. Response assessment in medulloblastoma and leptomeningeal seeding tumors: recommendations from the response assessment in pediatric neuro-oncology committee. Neuro-Oncology. 2018;20(1):13–23.
6. Lindsay HB, Massimino M, Avula S, Stivaros S, Grundy R, Metrock K, et al. Response assessment in paediatric intracranial ependymoma: recommendations from the response assessment in pediatric neuro-oncology (RAPNO) working group. Lancet Oncol. 2022;23(8):e393–401.
7. Bhatia A, Sabin ND, Fisher MJ, Poussaint TY. Review of imaging recommendations from response assessment in pediatric neuro-oncology (RAPNO). Pediatr Radiol. 2023;53(13):2723–41.
8. Shih RY, Koeller KK. Embryonal tumors of the central nervous system: from the radiologic pathology archives. Radiographics. 2018;38(2):525–41.
9. Tunthanathip T, Kanjanapradit K, Ratanalert S, Phuenpathom N, Oearsakul T, Kaewborisutsakul A. Multiple, primary brain tumors with diverse origins and different localizations: case series and review of the literature. J Neurosci Rural Pract. 2018;9(4):593–607.
10. Kim BS, Jung TY, Jang WY, Baek HJ, Kim SK, Lee KH. Multiple craniospinal tumors in a pediatric patient with neurofibromatosis type 2: a case report. Childs Nerv Syst. 2022;38(11):2205–9.
11. Yan J, Cheng J, Liu F, Liu X. Pleomorphic xanthoastrocytomas of adults: MRI features, molecular markers, and clinical outcomes. Sci Rep. 2018;8(1):14275.
12. Taha M, Issawi W, Al-Umran S, Shamdine O, Abdulkader M, Housaawi Y. Synchronous Primary Brain Tumor in pediatric age group. Report on two cases and review of the literature. 2019.
13. Fangusaro J, Witt O, Hernáiz Driever P, Bag AK, de Blank P, Kadom N, et al. Response assessment in paediatric low-grade glioma: recommendations from the response assessment in pediatric neuro-oncology (RAPNO) working group. Lancet Oncol. 2020;21(6):e305–16.
14. Erker C, Tamrazi B, Poussaint TY, Mueller S, Mata-Mbemba D, Franceschi E, et al. Response assessment in paediatric high-grade glioma: recommendations from the response assessment in pediatric neuro-oncology (RAPNO) working group. Lancet Oncol. 2020;21(6):e317–29.
15. Young RJ, Knopp EA. Brain MRI: tumor evaluation. J Magn Reson Imaging. 2006;24(4):709–24.
16. Wu CX, Lin GS, Lin ZX, Zhang JD, Chen L, Liu SY, et al. Peritumoral edema on magnetic resonance imaging predicts a poor clinical outcome in malignant glioma. Oncol Lett. 2015;10(5):2769–76.
17. NCBI. Manifestations of pilocytic astrocytoma: a pictorial review – PubMed. 2023. Available from: https://pubmed.ncbi.nlm.nih.gov/24789122/
18. Au Yong KJ, Jaremko JL, Jans L, Bhargava R, Coleman LT, Mehta V, et al. How specific is the MRI appearance of supratentorial atypical teratoid rhabdoid tumors? Pediatr Radiol. 2013;43(3):347–54.
19. Leach JL, Roebker J, Schafer A, Baugh J, Chaney B, Fuller C, et al. MR imaging features of diffuse intrinsic pontine glioma and relationship to overall survival: report from the international DIPG registry. Neuro-Oncology. 2020;22(11):1647–57.
20. Ostrowski RP, He Z, Pucko EB, Matyja E. Hemorrhage in brain tumor – an unresolved issue. Brain Hemorrhages. 2022;3(2):98–102.
21. Yuh EL, Barkovich AJ, Gupta N. Imaging of ependymomas: MRI and CT. Childs Nerv Syst. 2009;25(10):1203.

22. Plaza MJ, Borja MJ, Altman N, Saigal G. Conventional and advanced MRI features of pediatric intracranial tumors: posterior fossa and Suprasellar tumors. Am J Roentgenol. 2013;200(5):1115–24.
23. Dangouloff-Ros V, Varlet P, Levy R, Beccaria K, Puget S, Dufour C, et al. Imaging features of medulloblastoma: conventional imaging, diffusion-weighted imaging, perfusion-weighted imaging, and spectroscopy: from general features to subtypes and characteristics. Neurochirurgie. 2021;67(1):6–13.
24. Arslanoglu A, Aygun N, Tekhtani D, Aronson L, Cohen K, Burger PC, et al. Imaging findings of CNS atypical teratoid/rhabdoid tumors. AJNR Am J Neuroradiol. 2004;25(3):476–80.
25. Novak J, Zarinabad N, Rose H, Arvanitis T, MacPherson L, Pinkey B, et al. Classification of paediatric brain tumours by diffusion weighted imaging and machine learning. Sci Rep. 2021;11(1):2987.
26. Gauvain KM, McKinstry RC, Mukherjee P, Perry A, Neil JJ, Kaufman BA, et al. Evaluating pediatric brain tumor cellularity with diffusion-tensor imaging. Am J Roentgenol. 2001;177(2):449–54.
27. Pavlisa G, Pavlisa G, Rados M. Diffusion differences between pilocytic astrocytomas and grade II ependymomas. Radiol Oncol. 2011;45(2):97–101.
28. Chiang J, Harreld JH, Tinkle CL, Moreira DC, Li X, Acharya S, et al. A single-center study of the clinicopathologic correlates of gliomas with a MYB or MYBL1 alteration. Acta Neuropathol. 2019;138(6):1091–2.
29. Price SJ, Gillard JH. Imaging biomarkers of brain tumour margin and tumour invasion. Br J Radiol. 2011;84(Spec Iss 2):S159–67.
30. Gaudino S, Martucci M, Russo R, Visconti E, Gangemi E, D'Argento F, et al. MR imaging of brain pilocytic astrocytoma: beyond the stereotype of benign astrocytoma. Childs Nerv Syst. 2017;33(1):35–54.
31. Moore W, Mathis D, Gargan L, Bowers DC, Klesse LJ, Margraf L, et al. Pleomorphic Xanthoastrocytoma of childhood: MR imaging and diffusion MR imaging features. AJNR Am J Neuroradiol. 2014;35(11):2192–6.
32. Panigrahy A, Blüml S. Neuroimaging of pediatric brain tumors: from basic to advanced magnetic resonance imaging (MRI). J Child Neurol. 2009;24(11):1343–65.
33. Gonçalves FG, Viaene AN, Vossough A. Advanced magnetic resonance imaging in pediatric glioblastomas. Front Neurol. 2021;12 https://doi.org/10.3389/fneur.2021.733323.
34. Aboian MS, Solomon DA, Felton E, Mabray MC, Villanueva-Meyer JE, Mueller S, et al. Imaging characteristics of pediatric diffuse midline gliomas with histone H3 K27M mutation. AJNR Am J Neuroradiol. 2017;38(4):795–800.
35. Rao S, Sahay A, Epari S. Paediatric type diffuse high grade gliomas in the WHO CNS5 classification: what the pathologist needs to know? Indian J Pathol Microbiol. 2022;65(Supplement):S50–8.
36. Louis DN, Perry A, Wesseling P, Brat DJ, Cree IA, Figarella-Branger D, et al. The 2021 WHO classification of tumors of the central nervous system: a summary. Neuro-Oncology. 2021;23(8):1231–51.
37. Orr BA. Pathology, diagnostics, and classification of medulloblastoma. Brain Pathol. 2020;30(3):664–78.
38. Cotter JA, Hawkins C. Medulloblastoma: WHO 2021 and beyond. Pediatr Dev Pathol. 2022;25(1):23–33.
39. Blüml S, Margol AS, Sposto R, Kennedy RJ, Robison NJ, Vali M, et al. Molecular subgroups of medulloblastoma identification using noninvasive magnetic resonance spectroscopy. Neuro-Oncology. 2016;18(1):126–31.
40. Dasgupta A, Gupta T. Radiogenomics of medulloblastoma: imaging surrogates of molecular biology. J Transl Genet Genom. 2018;2
41. Colafati GS, Voicu IP, Carducci C, Miele E, Carai A, Di Loreto S, et al. MRI features as a helpful tool to predict the molecular subgroups of medulloblastoma: state of the art. Ther Adv Neurol Disord. 2018;11:1756286418775375.
42. Zhang M, Wong SW, Wright JN, Wagner MW, Toescu S, Han M, et al. MRI Radiogenomics of pediatric Medulloblastoma: a multicenter study. Radiology. 2022;304(2):406–16.
43. Chourmouzi D, Papadopoulou E, Konstantinidis M, Syrris V, Kouskouras K, Haritanti A, et al. Manifestations of pilocytic astrocytoma: a pictorial review. Insights Imaging. 2014;5(3):387.
44. Coley BD. Caffey's pediatric diagnostic imaging: Caffey's pediatric diagnostic imaging E-book. Elsevier Health Sciences; 2018. p. 2745.
45. Barkovich AJ. Pediatric neuroimaging. Lippincott Williams & Wilkins; 2005. p. 995.
46. Zhang M, Wong SW, Lummus S, Han M, Radmanesh A, Ahmadian SS, et al. Radiomic phenotypes distinguish atypical Teratoid/Rhabdoid tumors from Medulloblastoma. AJNR Am J Neuroradiol. 2021;42(9):1702–8.
47. Goo HW, Ra YS. Advanced MRI for pediatric brain tumors with emphasis on clinical benefits. Korean J Radiol. 2017;18(1):194–207.
48. Cè M, Irmici G, Foschini C, Danesini GM, Falsitta LV, Serio ML, et al. Artificial intelligence in brain tumor imaging: a step toward personalized medicine. Curr Oncol. 2023;30(3):2673–701.
49. Bhatia A, Lee VK, Qian Y, Paldino MJ, Ceschin R, Hect J, et al. Quantitative sodium (23Na) MRI in pediatric gliomas: initial experience. Diagnostics (Basel). 2022;12(5):1223.

Imaging of Paediatric Spine and Cord Lesions

12

Bernice Thamarai Selvi and Anitha Jasper

12.1 Introduction

Primary spinal tumours account for 10% of all central nervous system (CNS) tumours in children, half intramedullary and the other half extramedullary [1]. Extramedullary tumours include intradural extramedullary and extradural tumours. Extradural tumours include osseous lesions of the spine and paraspinal soft tissue lesions. Spinal osseous tumours can be primary osseous or metastatic from non-CNS primary neoplasms (Table 12.1).

Table 12.1 List of few common paediatric spinal lesions and their locations

Intramedullary lesion	IDEM lesion	Extradural lesion	Vertebral lesion
Astrocytoma Ependymoma Ganglioglioma Hemangioblastoma ATRT (rarely in cord)	Drop metastases (MB) Myxopapillary ependymoma Nerve sheath tumours Dermoid/epidermoid Meningioma Paraganglioma Neuroenteric cyst Arachnoid cyst	Lymphoma Leukaemia Neuroblastoma Germ cell tumours Rhabdomyosarcoma	Hemangioma Osteoid osteoma Osteoblastoma LCH ABC Sacrococcygeal teratoma

B. T. Selvi · A. Jasper (✉)
CMC, Vellore, India

I. Kumar et al. (eds.), *Practical Approach to Imaging in Pediatric Oncology*,
https://doi.org/10.1007/978-981-96-8158-7_12

12.2 Imaging Aspects

The clinical presentation of spinal masses is usually relatively non-specific, so they are often initially imaged with conventional radiographs. Intradural extramedullary and intramedullary tumours may cause spinal canal widening and vertebral scalloping; however, these are not early indicators of disease. On the contrary, extradural lesions may cause bone changes in the early stages. Magnetic resonance imaging (MRI) is the modality of choice for evaluating paediatric spinal tumours because it allows the evaluation of the entire neuraxis, provides anatomical details, and best characterises the tumour. MRI is also the mainstay for follow-up imaging of children with suspected cord/spinal lesions or to look for metastases. Older children may cooperate for an MRI, while young children may require sedation or general anaesthesia [2]. Specific paediatric spine MRI protocols should be followed for imaging. CT is rarely needed in some cases to delineate the osseous component and for surgical planning [2].

12.2.1 Imaging Techniques

- Appropriate technique to minimise CSF flow-related and pulsation artefacts from the heart and great vessels.
- Select proper 2D or 3D techniques, minimum possible slice thickness, and minimum or nil slice gap to detect small dural lesions.
- Reduce scan time to minimise the duration of general anaesthesia. Brain and spine imaging should be done concurrently.
- Diffusion-weighted imaging (DWI) can be performed to detect small meningeal deposits in cellular tumours.

12.2.2 Recommended Imaging Protocol

- T2W sequence in the sagittal plane and a T2-based high-resolution sequence like DRIVE in the axial plane of the whole spine.

Table 12.2 Recommended MRI parameters in evaluating primary spinal lesions and for metastatic work-up

MRI sequence	Slice thickness/gap	Plane of imaging
Spine imaging for primary spinal tumour		
T2W SE/TSE	ST 3 mm/SG 0.5 mm	Sagittal whole spine
T2W SE/TSE	ST 4–5 mm/No SG	Axial at the level of the lesion
Heavily T2W	High resolution	Sagittal whole spine
T1W SE/TSE	ST 3 mm/SG 0.5 mm pre and post contrast	Sagittal whole spine
T1W 3D volume	ST 3 mm/no SG. Post contrast	Axial whole spine
Metastatic workup—spine imaging for brain tumours		
T1W SE/TSE with contrast	ST 3 mm/SG 0.5 mm	Sagittal whole spine
T1W SE/TSE with contrast	ST 4–5 mm/No SG	Axial whole spine

- T1W pre- and post-contrast 3D volume sequences with fat suppression of the entire spine in sagittal, axial and coronal (optional) planes.
- DWI and STIR sequences wherever applicable.
- Axial plane can be tailored down through the extent of the lesion.
- Cranio-caudal coverage on sagittal can be done in a single stack or two stacks, depending upon the age/height of the child and the type of scanner (Table 12.2).

12.2.3 Recommendations for Follow-Up or Surveillance MRI Scans

As per the SIOPE (European Society of Pediatric Oncology) and RAPNO (Response Assessment in Pediatric Neuro-Oncology) recommendation, the timing of the MRI is as follows [3]:

Pre-operative MRI of the Spine

- For all primary spinal tumours
- For brain tumours with known high risk for CSF dissemination like medulloblastoma,

ATRT, and leptomeningeal metastases at diagnosis, spine MRI is timed concurrently with brain MRI as per the recommended MRI protocol.

Immediate Post-op MRI 24–72 h

– To assess the extent of resection
– Serves as baseline for further treatment (pre-chemo or RT)
– To assess complications like hematoma, ischemia, CSF leak, to look for hardware position & integrity

Follow-up for Symptomatic Patients

– To assess tumour recurrence
– Hardware failure
– To assess delayed complications like compression fracture, post-RT myelitis, post-RT myositis.

Follow-up for Asymptomatic Patients

– MRI at 4–6 months to look for tumour recurrence or disease progression (Table 12.3).

Table 12.3 Reporting template

Number of lesions	<Single> <two> <multiple>
Location	<intramedullary> <intradural> <extradural> <bony> <soft tissue> <mixed>
Transverse extent	WBB zones: [1–12 clock position][a] WBB layers: <A: extraosseous soft tissue : clock position> < B: intraosseous superficial > <C: deep intraosseous> <D: extraosseous extradural> <E :extraosseous intradural>
Longitudinal extent	[--] to [--] vertebral level (counting done from C2 downwards)
Size	[--]x[--] x[--] cm
Parenchyma	<T1/T2 morphology> <solid/cystic/mixed> <calcification> <fat> <haemorrhage>
Enhancement	<none/mild/marked> <homogenous/ heterogenous/peripheral/ other: describe > <target sign +/–>
Margins	<smooth/ irregular/ill defined>
Cysts	<intratumoral: central/at periphery> <peritumoral> <intraspinal> <syrinx>
Intramedullary tumour	
Cysts	<intratumoral: central/ at periphery> <peritumoral> <intraspinal > <syrinx>
Haemorrhage	<present/ absent> <cap sign>
Tortuous flow void	<Present/absent>
Extramedullary tumour	
Relation with adjacent structures	<spinal cord> <nerve roots/conus/cauda equina> <neural foramina widening/ involvement> <spinal canal widening +/–> <bony invasion +/–> <vascular invasion +/–>
Spinal cord	<Cord compression> <Cord signal change> <cord/conus involvement>
Spinal canal	<canal widening> <nerve root> <cauda equina: thickened/involvement/ enhancement/displacement> <dural tail/ thickening>
Neural foramina	<widened> <involved> <extraforaminal involvement>
Other association	<intracranial lesions> <neurofibromatosis> <abdomino thoracic findings>
Vertebral scalloping	Yes/No
Presence of feeding vessels	Yes/No
Primary brain neoplasm	Present/absent
Other findings	
IMPRESSION	

[a]WBB (Weinstein, Boriani, Biagnini) Surgical Staging System. The transverse extension of the vertebral tumour is described with reference to 12 radiating zones (numbered 1–12 in clockwise order) and to five concentric layers: *A* paravertebral extraosseous compartment, *B* intraosseous superficial, *C* intraosseous deep, *D* extraosseous extradural, *E* extraosseous intradural. The longitudinal extent of the tumour is recorded according to the levels involved [4]

12.3 Intramedullary Tumours

General Considerations Intramedullary tumours account for 25% of paediatric spinal tumours, being more prevalent in children between 1 and 5 years of age without a gender prevalence. Astrocytomas are the most common, followed by gangliogliomas. Ependymomas are uncommon except in the setting of Neurofibromatosis II [5].

Intramedullary tumours pose a difficult diagnostic challenge as they can have varied clinical presentations and imaging appearances. Spinal tumours can present with vague symptoms, which can be misleading and lead to a delay in diagnosis. A biopsy is often necessary as imaging alone may not distinguish between low- and high-grade neoplasms, and tumours from demyelination [6].

Some features like location, bone remodelling and signal characteristics may help indicate tumour pathology. Accurate tumour extent may be difficult to determine as the T2 hyperintense signal in the cord could represent infiltration or oedema. DWI is useful in some situations to determine the lesion's presence and extent, assist in surgical grading, and guide resection [7, 8]. The main goal of surgical treatment is complete resection; however, partial resection is also accepted to avoid neurological injury. Polar cysts (juxta tumoral cysts) demonstrating peripheral enhancement need to be resected; however, those without enhancement can resolve spontaneously and may just be drained. Syrinx of the cord is often seen with cervical tumours and is caused by the obstruction to normal CSF flow. The presence of syrinx is favourable as it indicates displacement of parenchyma rather than infiltration [9].

12.3.1 Astrocytomas

In the paediatric age group, most intramedullary tumours are astrocytomas, with most being low-grade (pilocytic or fibrillary astrocytomas—WHO grade I and II tumours). Pilocytic astrocytomas are more often seen in children between 1 and 5 years of age, and fibrillary astrocytomas are seen in slightly older children, about 10 years of age [10].

On MRI, the lesions cause expansion of the cord, spanning multiple vertebral segments. They are typically located eccentrically in the cord and can have well-demarcated margins. Actual holocord tumours are rare, and most of the T2 hyperintense signal in the cord may be due to oedema rather than the tumour itself. The most common location is in the cervicomedullary junction and the cervicothoracic cord. Tumours can have varied appearances, including a cystic-necrotic appearance, a "cyst with a mural nodule", or a structurally solid lesion. Most of the lesions demonstrate some degree of contrast enhancement; however, the extent of enhancement does not correspond to tumour margins [5]. Tumour margins usually demonstrate enhancement in post-contrast studies, unlike with syrinx (Fig. 12.1).

High-grade gliomas (HGGs), defined by the WHO as grade III and IV, are uncommon. Infiltrative growth, non-demarcated margins, and dissemination through the cerebrospinal fluid (CSF) are more typical in high-grade tumours. pHGGs are more common in the cervical and thoracic spinal cord while involvement of the medulla is more rare. The neoplasm is usually inhomogeneous in signal on T1 and T2 sequences with inhomogeneous enhancement and may also have intralesional haemorrhage and cystic areas. The prognosis of pHGG is poor, with a mean survival of 12 months after diagnosis [10] (Fig. 12.2).

Diffusion tensor imaging (DTI) and diffusion tensor tractography (DTT) have been used in surgical planning in patients with spinal cord astrocytomas to minimise the morbidity associated with surgery with debatable efficacy. A suggested classification of astrocytomas of the cervical cord based on DTT was infiltrating type (type I) and displacement type (type II). Type I tumours were further subdivided into simple infiltrating (Type IA) and infiltrating with destruction (Type IB) [11].

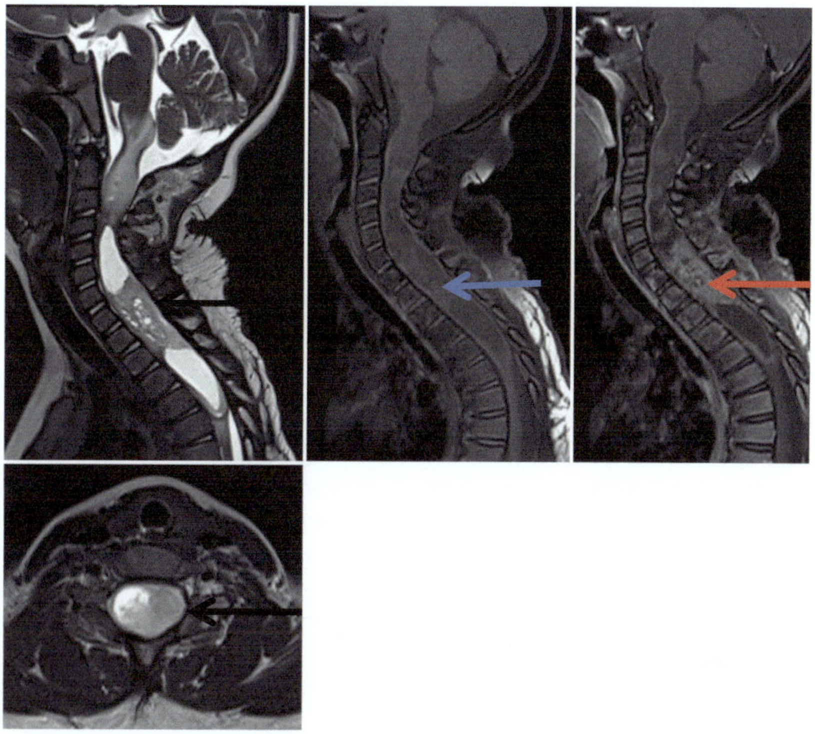

Fig. 12.1 Pilocytic astrocytoma. T2 sagittal and axial images of the cervicothoracic spine show an expansile intramedullary lesion with solid and cystic areas. The lesion is T1 hypointense (blue arrow) with heterogeneous post-contrast enhancement (red arrow)

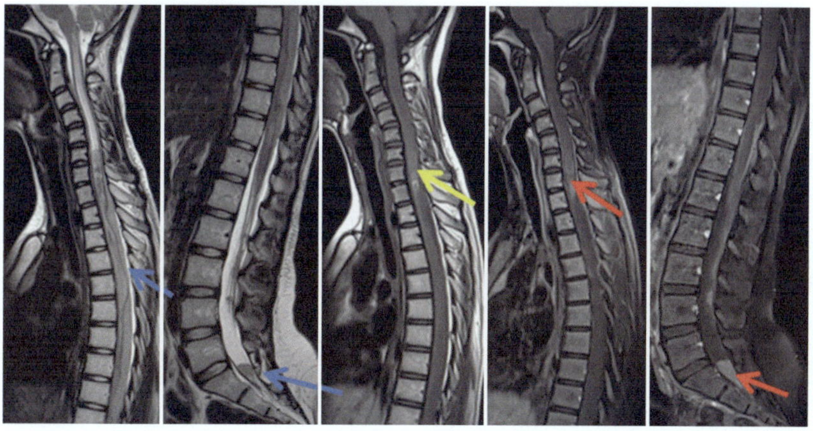

Fig. 12.2 High-grade glioma—H3K27M. T2 sagittal images show an ill-defined expansile T2 heterogeneously hyperintense lesion involving the entire spinal cord with evidence of drop metastases in the sacral canal at S1 level (blue arrows). The lesion is iso to mildly hypointense on T1W images with heterogeneous post-contrast enhancement (red arrows)

12.3.2 Ganglioglioma

Gangliogliomas are the second most common paediatric intramedullary tumours after pilocytic astrocytomas, being more common in children between 1 and 5 years of age [5]. Although low-grade, they have a significant propensity for local recurrence and high-grade transformation of the glial element. The commonest site of occurrence is the cervical and upper thoracic cord with extension into the medulla. Holocord involvement is more common than in other tumours. The tumours are primarily solid, with a propensity to have cystic areas. The presence of calcification is a feature that is suggestive of gangliogliomas and may help to distinguish it from pilocytic astrocytomas, the rest of the imaging features being quite indistinguishable from pilocytic astrocytomas [5]. It differs from ependymomas by being eccentric in location, the long segment cord involvement of more than four vertebral segments up to eight segments, and the lack of hemosiderin capping. Solid components are iso-hypointense on T1-weighted images and iso-hyperintense on T2-weighted images. A notable imaging feature is the absence of perilesional oedema, even when large and association with adjacent osseous erosion. Contrast enhancement rarely involves the whole tumour and can be patchy or focal [12].

12.3.3 Diffuse Leptomeningeal Glioneuronal Tumour (DL-GNT)

DL-GNT is a rare neuronal-glial tumour characterised by slow growth and leptomeningeal dissemination.

The most common imaging feature is diffuse abnormal nodular leptomeningeal growth without evidence of a primary intraparenchymal focus. Abnormal leptomeningeal enhancement is most commonly seen in the basal cisterns and posterior fossa and along the spinal cord. Small T2 hyperintense cystic nodules are sometimes seen along the leptomeninges. Intraparenchymal lesions are rare but are more commonly described in the spinal cord.

Differential diagnoses include infections like tuberculosis and neurocysticercosis, leptomeningeal dissemination of other neoplasms, lymphoproliferative diseases, and neurosarcoidosis (rare in paediatric age) [10].

Neurocysticercosis in the brain parenchyma is usually seen in varying stages with varied imaging appearances based on the stage—non-enhancing cyst, cyst with peripheral rim enhancement and perilesional oedema, nodular enhancing lesion, or a calcified granuloma. DL-GNT is a great mimicker of tuberculosis, as basal meningeal enhancement can be seen in both conditions. The presence of typical parenchymal lesions with central T2 hypointense signal in tuberculomas may help confirm the diagnosis of tuberculosis. Lack of constitutional symptoms and response to anti-tubercular drug therapy may be clues for an alternative diagnosis like DL-GNT.

12.3.4 Ependymomas

Ependymomas can occur during adolescence (13–14 years) and account for 30% of intramedullary spinal tumours in children. They are categorised into subependymoma (World Health Organization (WHO) grade 1), myxopapillary ependymoma (WHO grade 2), and classic or anaplastic ependymoma (WHO grade 2/3). The three distinct histopathological subtypes of spinal EP are subependymoma (SP-SE), myxopapillary ependymomas (SP-MPE), and classical EP (SP-EPN).

On MRI, ependymomas tend to occupy the central portion of the spinal cord and cause symmetric cord expansion with an average length of four vertebral body segments. Although unencapsulated, they are well-circumscribed lesions with tumoural and non-tumoural cysts, the latter being more common. Syringohydromyelia occurs in a variable proportion of cases. Calcification is

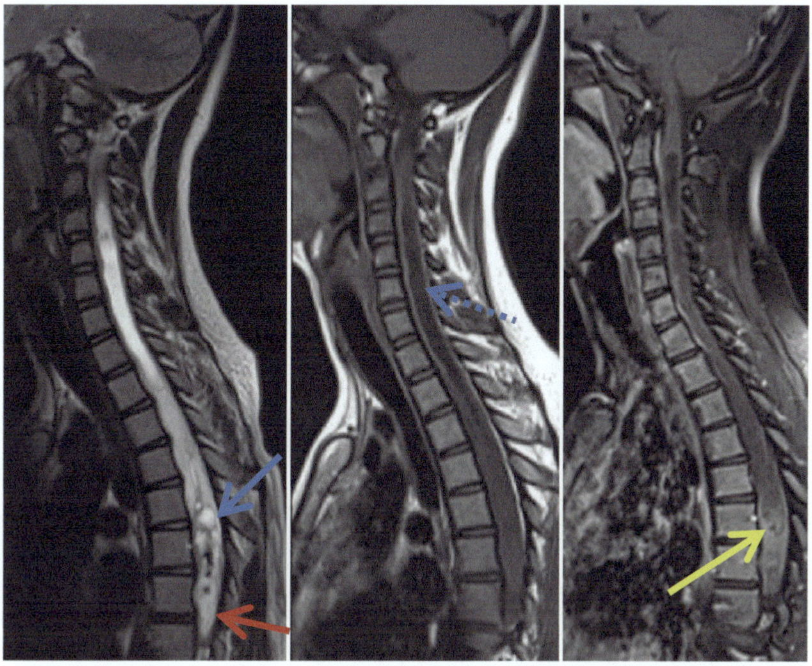

Fig. 12.3 Ependymoma. T2 sagittal images show a long segment expansile lesion in the thoracic cord with hemorrhagic areas (blue arrow) within and a hypointense "cap" inferiorly (red arrow). T1 sagittal image shows a long segment syrinx proximal to the lesion (dotted arrow) and heterogeneous enhancement on post-contrast images (yellow arrow)

uncommon in spinal ependymomas. The hemosiderin "cap sign", a cap of T2 hypointense hemosiderin above and/or below the tumour due to previous haemorrhage, is most often associated with spinal ependymomas. However, it can be seen in hemangioblastomas and paragangliomas as well [5] (Fig. 12.3).

Myxopapillary ependymomas (SP-MPE) occur most commonly at the filum terminale and/or along the conus medullaris. They are the most common tumours that occur in the cauda equina region. They can be large, spanning multiple vertebral levels, but small tumours are also seen. They are usually T2 hyperintense but can have areas of T2 hypointense signal within, possibly due to calcification or haemorrhage. A variable degree of enhancement is seen within the lesion (Fig. 12.4).

A distinctive type of spinal ependymoma with unique molecular characteristics and aggressive clinical behaviour is the SP-EPN-MYCN, characterised by anaplastic Grade III histology, *MYCN* amplification, an absence of *NF2* alterations, and a unique methylation classifier profile. They are found to be associated with dismal outcomes and malignant progression despite aggressive management [13].

Drop metastases are known to occur with ependymomas. Leptomeningeal spread in the cisternal and sulcal spaces can also be seen.

In association with neurofibromatosis 2, multiple spinal ependymomas can occur, and they usually have an indolent course, often being asymptomatic [14].

12.3.5 Hemangioblastomas

Hemangioblastomas are benign capillary-rich neoplasms, with the majority being intramedullary in location. They are rare in children and may occur sporadically or in association with Von Hippel-Lindau syndrome. They are usually intramedullary lesions occurring in the cervical or thoracic cord; however, they can also arise from the spinal roots and hence can be intradural extramedullary in location. Screening for muta-

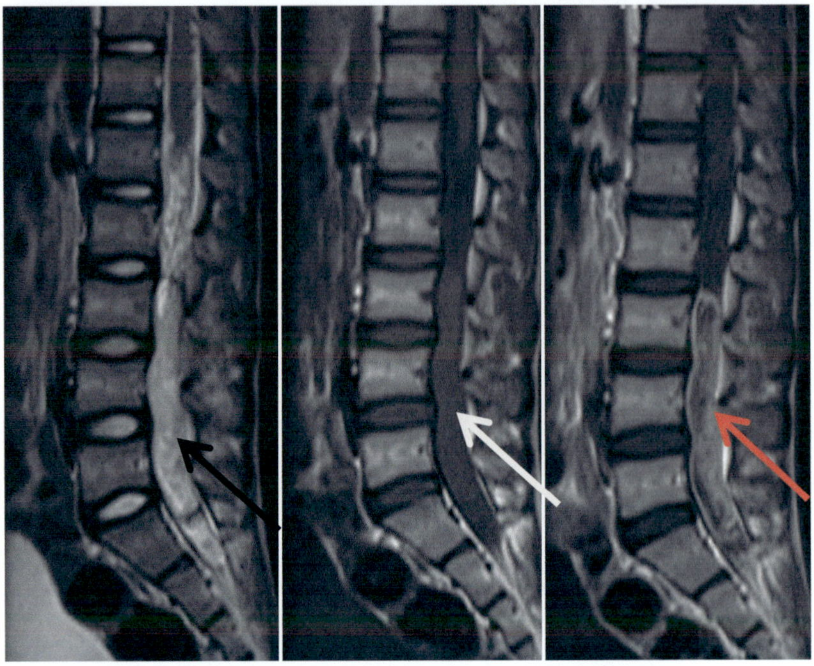

Fig. 12.4 Myxopapillary ependymoma. T2 sagittal image of the lumbosacral spine shows an intradural extramedullary lesion in the lumbosacral region of heterogeneous signal intensity, causing mild canal widening and posterior vertebral body scalloping. T1 sagittal images show an iso to mildly hyperintense lesion (white arrow) with heterogeneous post-contrast enhancement on the post-contrast images (red arrow)

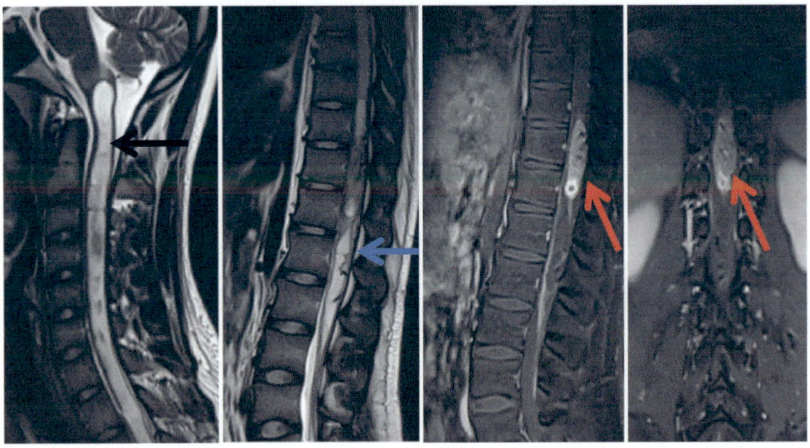

Fig. 12.5 Hemangioblastoma. T2 sagittal images show long segment syrinx in the cervicothoracic cord (black arrow) with a T2 heterogeneously hyperintense lesion in lower thoracic cord and conus with multiple tortuous flow void leading to it (blue arrow). T1 sagittal fat suppressed post-contrast images in the sagittal and coronal plane show intense enhancement of the lesion (red arrows)

tions in the VHL gene is recommended in children with hemangioblastomas.

On MRI, hemangioblastomas appear hypointense on T1 and hyperintense on T2 with intense enhancement. Flow voids, adjacent cysts and haemorrhage are also common findings. Long segment syrinx or long segment oedema without syrinx are commonly seen [15, 16] (Fig. 12.5).

12.4 Management and Post-op Imaging for Intramedullary Tumours

Intramedullary tumours are surgically challenging. Surgical techniques include gross total resection, subtotal resection or a biopsy, along with spinal canal surgery like laminectomy or laminoplasty.

Adjuvant treatments include radiotherapy (RT), chemotherapy like Temozolomide (TMZ), and anti-angiogenic therapy like Bevacizumab. These are reserved for high-grade tumours & partially resected tumours.

Immediate post-op MRI is done at 24–48 h (less than 72 h). Beyond 72 h, subacute haemorrhage and reactive post-op enhancement may be confused with residual tumour. Post-op changes like oedema with cord expansion and T2 hyperintensity may be challenging to differentiate from residual tumours. On post-contrast sequences, smooth and mild peripheral enhancement is due to post-op-related granulation tissue, whereas nodular enhancement is likely a residue. Enhancement pattern and location similar to the pre-op MRI strongly indicate a residue.

On surveillance MRI scans, the enhancement patterns due to post-treatment-related changes need to be differentiated from tumour recurrence or residue [17, 18].

12.5 Intradural Extramedullary Spinal Neoplasms

General Considerations About 10–15% of extramedullary paediatric spinal tumours are intradural [15]. Back pain, weakness and radicular pain are the most typical symptoms at presentation. The commonest cause of an intradural extramedullary lesion in the paediatric population is leptomeningeal metastasis from a primary brain tumour [19].

12.5.1 Nerve Sheath Tumours

These include schwannomas and neurofibromas, mostly in the setting of NF1 and NF2.

Spinal tumours in NF1 can be single/multiple/plexiform neurofibromas. They can also have few skin lesions. It is associated with mutations in the tumour suppressor gene NF1 located in chromosome 17.

Aggressive evolution of the neurofibroma can be suspected with the onset of new neurological symptoms/deficits, pain, changes in the growth and consistency, compression of the locoregional areas, and bleeding of the neurofibroma. Other spinal manifestations of NF1 include dysplasia (primary), lateral meningocoeles, dural ectasia and bony remodelling which are related to tumour growth (secondary). In addition to the supra and infratentorial FASI (foci of abnormal signal intensity), spinal UBOs (unidentified bright objects) can be seen.

Schwannomas occur rarely in children and are solitary. Multiple schwannomas can, however, be associated with NF2. Based on severity as well as clinical course, NF2 is classified into two types: the less aggressive late onset Feiling-Gardner phenotype with a single tumour in the central nervous system and the aggressive Wishart phenotype in young adults with multiple tumours in the central as well as the peripheral nervous system [20].

Schwannomas and neurofibromas may be challenging to differentiate on imaging. Both tumours can scallop the vertebrae, widen the neural foramina and erode bone [7]. On MRI, both neurofibromas and schwannomas appear hypointense on T1 and hyperintense on T2-weighted images. Schwannomas can have a heterogeneous hyperintense signal on T2-weighted imaging due to the presence of Antoni A and B cells. The "target sign" has been described with neurofibromas and may be seen as a central area of lower T2 signal on T2-weighted images. Post-contrast, various degrees of enhancement can be seen, but it is often intense. Haemorrhage, cystic change or fatty degeneration can be seen with schwannomas. Malignant transformation, although rare, occurs more often in neurofibromas and may be indicated by a rapid growth in size.

Giant invasive schwannomas are rare tumours, especially in the paediatric population, extending over two or more vertebral levels, eroding vertebral bodies, and extending into the extraspinal space, disrupting myofascial planes. Multi-stage operations may be required to resect the entire tumour [21].

12.5.2 Paragangliomas

Paragangliomas are WHO grade 1 neuroendocrine tumours that rarely occur in the spine, and if they do, they occur most commonly along the cauda equina nerve roots. On MRI, paragangliomas are well-defined lesions, appearing T2 hyperintense with intense post-contrast enhancement. As in head and neck paragangliomas, a "salt and pepper" appearance may be seen in these lesions. Due to their vascular nature, tortuous flow voids may be seen in and around the tumour. They can appear very similar to myxopapillary ependymomas with a hemosiderin rim, causing osseous remodelling.

Secretion of catecholamines is rare with spinal paragangliomas; however, preoperative screening is suggested to prevent a hypertensive crisis during surgery. As the tumours are very vascular, preoperative embolisation may be performed to reduce intraoperative bleeding [7].

12.5.3 Meningiomas

Meningiomas in the paediatric age group are rare except in the setting of neurofibromatosis 2. Isolated paediatric spinal meningiomas are typically histologically "clear cell meningiomas". They occur in the spinal canal and cerebellopontine angle and have a high propensity for recurrence and CSF dissemination.

On MR imaging, they are well-defined masses with moderate to intense homogeneous enhancement. A "dural tail" may not always be seen [22, 23].

12.5.4 Myxopapillary Ependymoma

Myxopapillary ependymomas are more common in the paediatric age group than in adults. They are thought to arise from the ependymal glia of the filum terminale, occurring as intradural extramedullary masses in the lumbar and sacral canal.

On MR imaging, the lesions are iso to hypointense on T1-weighted imaging and hyperintense on T2-weighted imaging with moderate to marked homogeneous or inhomogeneous enhancement. Large masses may widen the canal, scallop the vertebrae and sometimes extend through the neural foramina, mimicking schwannomas [15].

12.5.5 Atypical Teratoid Rhabdoid Tumours

Atypical teratoid rhabdoid tumours (ATRT) are highly malignant neoplasms that often affect the brain but can also involve the spine. Being aggressive tumours, although extra-axial, they can infiltrate the spinal cord. Hence, the origin of the tumour may be difficult to determine. They occur most often in the first 2 years of life and can be congenital.

Imaging appearances are similar to ATRTs involving the brain with intralesional haemorrhage, necrosis, cystic change and inhomogeneous post-contrast enhancement. Due to their high cellularity, solid components may be hypointense on T1- and T2-weighted images. The whole neuraxis must be imaged to identify possible secondary lesions or multi-centric involvement [5, 24, 25] (Fig. 12.6).

12.5.6 Primitive Neuroectodermal Tumours

Primitive neuroectodermal tumours (PNET) belong to a category of infantile aggressive neoplasms, including neuroblastoma or Ewing's sarcomas, which are cellular tumours, composed of small, round cells with hyperchromatic nuclei and scant cytoplasm. Intraspinal PNETs are rare and occur more often in older children and those that occur intracranially. Imaging appearances are non-specific and may appear isointense to the cord on T1 and T2-weighted images with homogeneous post-contrast enhancement [26].

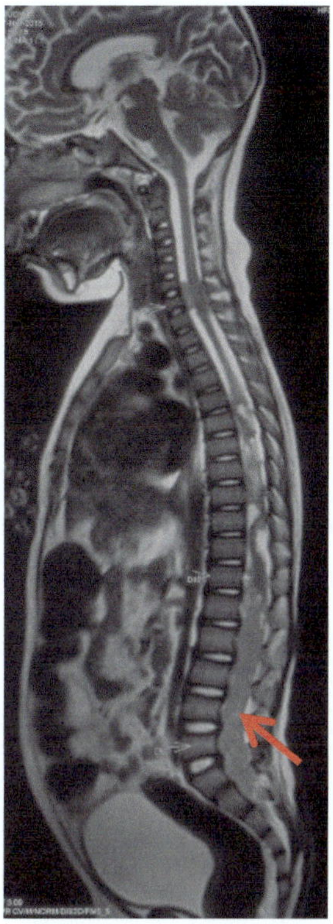

Fig. 12.6 ATRT with CSF seeding. T2 sagittal images show iso to mildly hyperintense lesions along the surface of the cord and within the spinal canal

12.5.7 Non-neoplastic IM/IDEM Lesions

12.5.7.1 Dermoids/Epidermoids

Dermoids are often associated with dermal sinuses and can occur in 10% of the paediatric population. Epidermoids are relatively uncommon in the paediatric age group. Dermoids are cystic lesions lined by squamous epithelium, containing dermal appendages like hair, sebaceous glands and sweat glands, whereas epidermoids, although lined by squamous epithelium, lack dermal appendages. Accumulation of keratin within these lesions can cause them to enlarge gradually. Complications like secondary infection or rupture leading to chemical meningitis can occur. (Epi)dermoids can have a signal similar to CSF and hence are better seen on FLAIR and proton density sequences rather than on routine T1- and T2-weighted sequences. Restricted diffusion may be seen in epidermoids. Lesions are non-enhancing; however, enhancement can be seen with super-added infections [5] (Figs. 12.7 and 12.8).

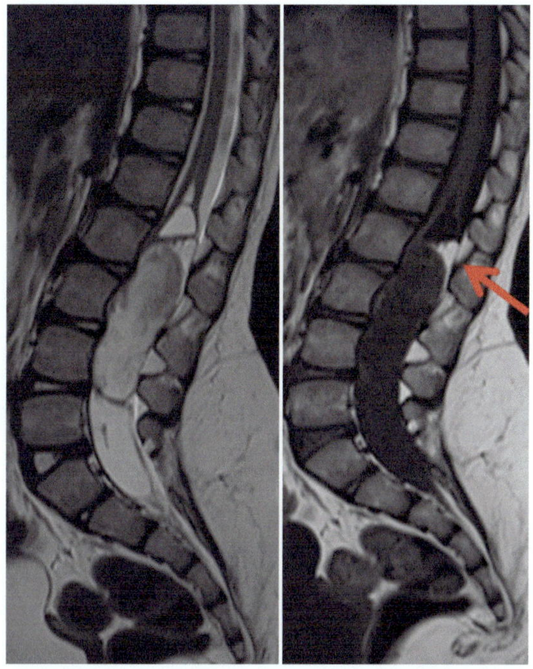

Fig. 12.7 Dermoid cyst. T2 sagittal and T1 sagittal images show a well-defined intradural extramedullary lesion with mixed signal intensities including fat (red arrow) in the lumbar canal

12.5.7.2 Neuroenteric Cysts

Neuroenteric cysts originate from embryonic remnants from the primitive streak during early embryonic development. They are lined by mucin-secreting cuboidal or columnar epithelium similar to the alimentary tract. Their signal intensity can be similar to CSF or vary based on their chemical composition. They are located most commonly in the cervico-thoracic spine, anterior to the cord.

12.5.7.3 Arachnoid Cysts

Arachnoid cysts are CSF loculations within a splitting of the arachnoid membrane that do not communicate with the subarachnoid space. They may be located in the subdural space or extradurally, dorsal to the cord. They may be congenital or arise due to adhesions secondary to infection

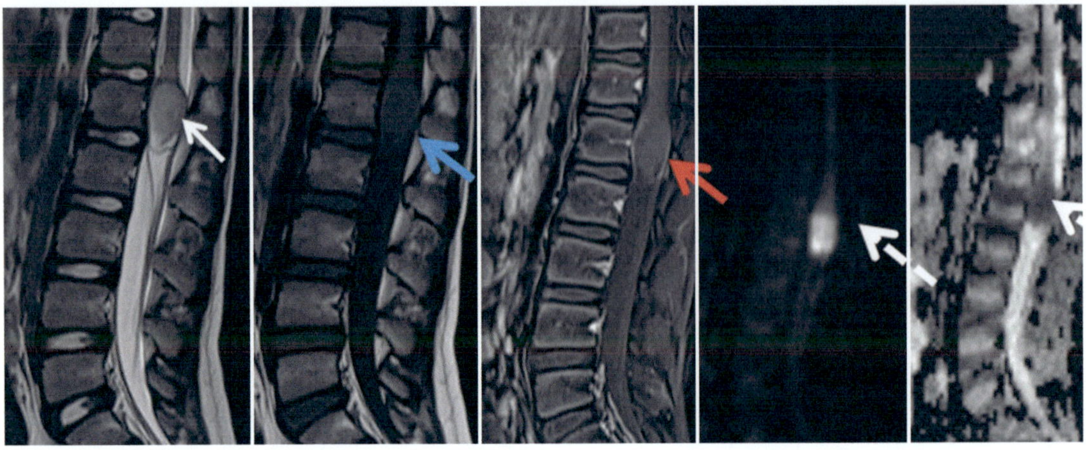

Fig. 12.8 Epidermoid. T2 sagittal image shows a well-defined T2 hyperintense lesion at the conus (white arrow). The lesion is hypointense on T1 W images (blue arrow) with a thin rim of peripheral enhancement and diffusion restriction

or previous trauma. On MR imaging, the signal intensity of these cysts is similar to CSF; however, their signal can vary if there is blood or proteinaceous fluid within the cysts. The cysts can enlarge, causing compression of the posterior aspect of the cord. Cine MR images help monitor surgical results and demonstrate their separation from the rest of the subarachnoid space.

12.6 Extradural Spinal Masses

General Considerations Extradural spinal masses account for about two-thirds of spinal masses in children. They are grouped into bone tumours, tumours of the epidural space and extraspinal tumours invading the spine. MRI and CT are required for imaging of extradural masses. MRI depicts the extradural soft tissue component, bone marrow infiltration, and cord signal changes secondary to compression. CT depicts the lesion's lytic or sclerotic nature and the extent of bone involvement.

12.6.1 Benign Bone Tumours and Tumour-like Conditions

12.6.1.1 Hemangioma

Hemangiomas are usually incidentally detected and may be solitary or multiple. Although most are dormant, some may behave aggressively, causing expansion of the involved bone, epidural extension and vertebral collapse, resulting in local pain and symptoms related to cord or nerve root compression. On radiographs and CT, hemangiomas can have a palisading appearance of vertical sclerotic densities in the vertebral body. End-stage dormant hemangiomas appear T1 and T2 hyperintense due to fatty and vascular components, with the rest of the vertebra remaining normal in morphology. Aggressive hemangiomas, on the other hand, appear hypointense on T1 and hyperintense on T2, expand the bone with extraosseous components, and are intensely enhancing [5].

12.6.1.2 Osteoid Osteoma

Approximately 10% of osteoid osteoma cases occur in the spine, with the posterior arch elements being the commonest location. The usual clinical presentation is nocturnal pain that responds to non-steroidal anti-inflammatory medication or painful scoliosis. A richly vascular nidus of osteoid bone containing a sclerotic centre surrounded by marked reactive osteosclerosis is seen on histopathology. Reactive inflammatory soft tissue masses involve the bone and the adjacent paravertebral regions [27].

Radionuclide scans are extremely sensitive in the detection of osteoid osteomas. On CT, a cen-

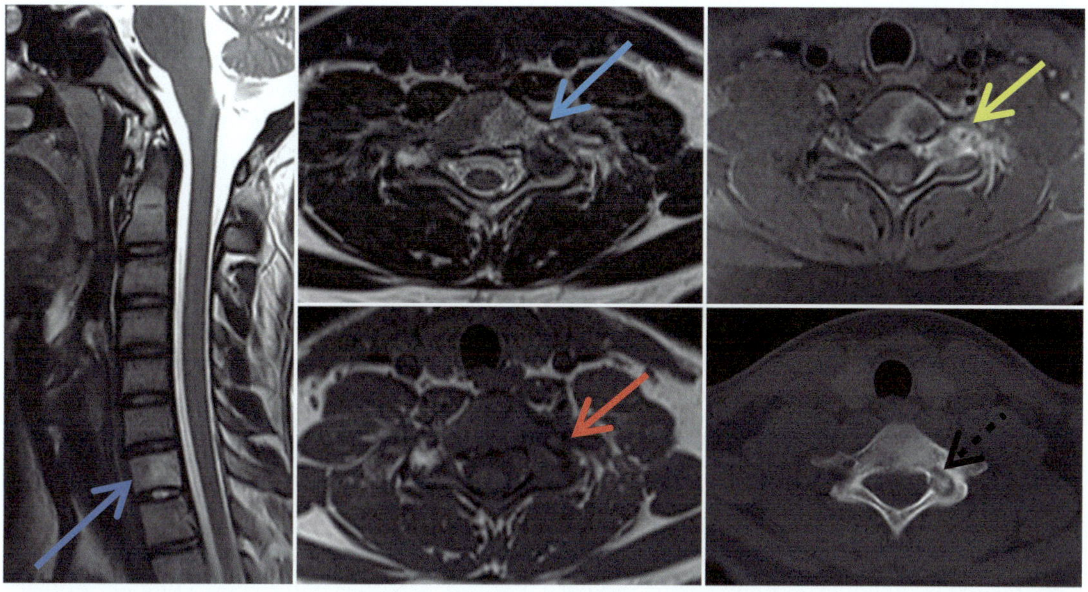

Fig. 12.9 Osteoid osteoma. T2 sagittal and axial images show edema in the posterior aspect of C7 vertebra (blue arrow) with T1 hypointense signal on T1W axial images (red arrow). Intense enhancement of the involved bone and the adjacent soft tissues on T1 FS post-contrast axial image (yellow arrow). CT axial sections of the cervical spine show a lucent nidus in the left C7 pedicle with a sclerotic focus in the centre and adjacent reactive sclerosis (dotted black arrow)

tral lucent nidus is seen with a surrounding sclerotic rim. A focus of central calcification in the nidus can give the appearance of a target. On MRI, the nidus appears T2 hyperintense with intense post-contrast enhancement. The rim appears hypointense due to the surrounding osteosclerotic bone. The associated soft tissue lesions are well-visualised on MRI. However, the accuracy of diagnosing an osteoid osteoma on MRI is not high (65%) and the lucent nidus may be better visualised on thin CT sections [28] (Fig. 12.9).

12.6.1.3 Osteoblastoma

Osteoblastomas differ from osteoid osteomas mainly in size, with the nidus measuring >2 cm in diameter. Although the two tumours are different histologically, osteoblastomas are more aggressive and tend to bleed profusely during surgery. They have a predilection for the neural arch but may extend into the vertebral body and paraspinal soft tissues. These patients present with non-specific pain, which does not respond to salicylates.

On CT, they are lytic expansile lesions with associated sclerotic components. Although they are histologically benign, they can appear aggressive, with bone destruction and haemorrhage and cause thecal sac and cord compression due to the soft tissue components. They enhance intensely on post-contrast images [29].

12.6.1.4 Aneurysmal Bone Cysts (ABCs)

Aneurysmal bone cysts are considered reactive lesions that result from trauma or co-exist with other benign or malignant bone lesions and are probably not neoplasms. ABCs have accounted for 42% of all benign bone tumours in children [5]. Most (~75%) are in the lower thoracic and lumbosacral spine. The site of origin is usually the neural arch. Still, they can extend to the body along one or both pedicles and cross intervertebral disc spaces to involve the adjacent vertebral levels [30]. The lesions are osteolytic with a multi-loculated structure containing unclotted blood in varying stages separated by thin calcified septae. They occur in older children or adolescents and present with local pain, which may be associated with radiculopathy or myelopathy [5].

On CT, they are lytic, expansile, often destructive lesions with multiple cystic spaces separated by thin calcified shells. On MRI, the signal intensity varies based on the stages of the blood degradation products within the spaces. Multiple blood-fluid levels within the lesion are the hallmark of ABCs. Other lesions that can have fluid-fluid levels are giant cell tumours (GCT) and telangiectatic osteosarcoma. Preoperative embolisation is performed to reduce intraoperative bleeding due to their hypervascularity.

12.6.1.5 Langerhans Cell Histiocytosis

Langerhans cell histiocytosis (LCH) is a rare disease involving multiple systems with varying clinical presentations. Historically, the condition was subdivided into three distinct entities—Letterer-Siwe disease, Hand-Schuller-Christian disease and eosinophilic granuloma. It is now divided into three groups based on the number of lesions and systems involved. The most common unifocal form occurs in about 70% of LCH cases. It is limited to a single or a few bones and may involve the lung. Patients are usually between the age group of 5 and 15 years [31].

In the spine, they affect the vertebral body, resulting in complete collapse. The end plates remain intact, and the discs are unaffected, showing compensatory swelling. As the growth plate is preserved, subsequent reconstitution of vertebral body height may occur, especially in younger children. Involvement of the posterior arch elements is rare. Pain, fever and weight loss are the usual clinical symptoms. Cervical spinal involvement is seen in almost three-fourths of cases.

On imaging, osteolytic vertebral body lesions have varying degrees of collapse and compensatory disc enlargement. The collapsed vertebra enhances intensely. Associated soft tissue components can involve the anterior epidural space and compress the thecal sac.

12.6.1.6 Sacrococcygeal Teratoma

Sacrococcygeal teratoma is the most commonly occurring congenital tumour seen mainly in neonates. They may be seen either in the setting of the Currarino triad, associated with anorectal malformations and caudal agenesis or in isolation. They are usually solid or partially cystic and may be large, sometimes larger than the neonate. Although most of them in the younger age group are benign, a tendency for malignant transformation is present as the child ages. Parenchymal tissue, fat and calcification are seen in the mature forms. The absence of fatty tissue, increased growth rate and metastases characterise immature forms [32].

12.6.2 Malignant Bone Tumours

12.6.2.1 Ewing's Sarcoma

Ewing's sarcoma is the most common primary bone tumour of the spine in children, the lumbosacral region being the most common location. Local pain, signs of compression, and radiculopathy are some clinical presentations, with other systemic symptoms like fever, weight loss, anaemia, and elevated erythrocyte sedimentation rates being common associations. On histopathology, they are hypercellular, composed of small rounded cells with prominent nuclei and scanty cytoplasm. Most lesions cause lytic destruction of the vertebra, which is associated with paravertebral soft tissue masses that extend into the epidural space. They can also spread across the intervertebral disc to the next vertebra, mimicking infection.

An osteolytic permeative lesion with sclerotic and calcific foci is seen on CT and radiographs. Large extraosseous soft tissue masses are seen on CT and MRI. This tends to envelop the involved vertebra, which is a useful diagnostic finding. On T1- and T2-weighted imaging, the lesion appears iso to hypointense and contrast enhancement may be minimal or absent. Extradural extension and thecal sac compression are best seen on MRI.

12.6.2.2 Osteosarcoma

Spinal involvement by osteosarcoma is rare in the paediatric age group. The body and sacral ala are predominantly involved in tumours of the sacrum, whereas non-sacral osteosarcomas arise mainly from the posterior elements with partial body involvement. The lesions are mixed sclerotic and lytic and are often accompanied by soft tissue masses.

12.6.2.3 Leukaemia and Lymphoma

Primary or secondary involvement of the vertebrae from leukaemia or lymphoma is known to occur. On MRI, diffuse marrow infiltration is seen as diffuse marrow signal alteration, appearing iso to hypointense on T1- and T2-weighted images. An epidural mass formation, thecal sac compression and vertebral collapse have been described with lymphoma.

12.6.3 Tumours of the Epidural Spaces

12.6.3.1 Lymphoma and Leukaemia

Chloromas are highly vascularised lesions composed of immature granulocytes, also called granulocytic sarcomas, and they are the most common extraosseous spinal masses in patients with acute myeloid leukaemia. On T1-weighted images, they are iso to hyperintense and iso to hypointense on T2-weighted images and show moderate to marked gadolinium enhancement. They respond well to chemotherapy, and hence, surgery is recommended only in cases of acute spinal cord compression.

Lymphoma can involve the epidural space in the setting of multi-system disease and is seen as epidural masses causing thecal sac and cord compression [5].

12.6.3.2 Germ Cell Tumours

Although rare, non-germinomatous germ cell tumours have been reported in the lumbosacral epidural space. In isolation, germ cell tumours can have non-specific findings, but the association of sacral agenesis with a large solid sacral mass is strongly suggestive. Tumour markers like B-human-chorionic gonadotropin, alpha-fetoprotein and placental alkaline phosphatase are helpful adjuncts in the diagnostic workup [5].

12.6.4 Extraspinal Tumours with Spinal Invasion

12.6.4.1 Neuroblastoma

Neuroblastomas originate from neural crest cells in the adrenal glands, the paravertebral sympathetic chain, the organ of Zuckerkandl and the carotid and aortic glomi. Neuroblastomas originating from the sympathetic chain can grow into the spinal canal through one or more neural foramina. They may compress the thecal sac and cord with extension cranially or caudally in the epidural space. Areas of necrosis, haemorrhage, and calcification within the lesion can result in heterogeneous signal intensities on MRI. Signal changes in the cord secondary to compressive myelopathy can be detected best on MRI [33].

12.7 Genomics of Spinal Tumours

The genetic and molecular alterations and mutations for spinal tumours are studied less than those for intracranial ones. A few critical recognised mutations involve KIAA1549-BRAF, BRAFV600E, PTPN11, H3F3A, TP53, FGFR1 and CDKN2A genes. Hemangioblastomas require evaluation for VHL mutation (Table 12.4).

Few Signs to Remember

Cap sign—Ependymoma
Dural tail sign—Meningioma
Feeding vessel sign—Hemangioblastoma
Target sign—Neurofibroma
Dumb-bell sign—Schwannoma
Corduroy cloth/polka-dot sign—Vertebral hemangioma

Brief algorithm to approach paediatric spine and cord lesions, based on MRI characteristics. (Design by Dr. Melwin Abishek).

Table 12.4 Few common spinal tumours and their associated genetic mutations

Tumours	Location	Genetics/mutations
LGG	Cervicothoracic level	KIAA1549-BRAF/BRAFV600E/NF1
HGG	No preferential location	H3K27M
DL-GNT	Leptomeningeal dissemination	KIAA1549-BRAF/NTRK1,2,3/ TRIM33:RAF1
Ependymomas	Cervical/lumbosacral	RELA/YAP-1/nMyc amp/NF2
Hemangioblastomas	Variable location	VHL mutation
Meningiomas	No preferential location	NF2/SMARCE1/SMARB1/SUFU
Mesenchymal chondrosarcomas	Thoracic spine	HEY1/NCOA2
Schwannomas	Nerve sheaths	NF2/LZTR1/SMARCB1
Plexiform neurofibroma	Nerve sheaths	NF1
ATRT	No preferential location	SMARCB1
Embryonal tumours with multilayered rosettes.	No preferential location	C19MC

Intradural Pediatric Spinal Tumors: An Overview from Imaging to Novel Molecular Findings. Marrazzo et al.

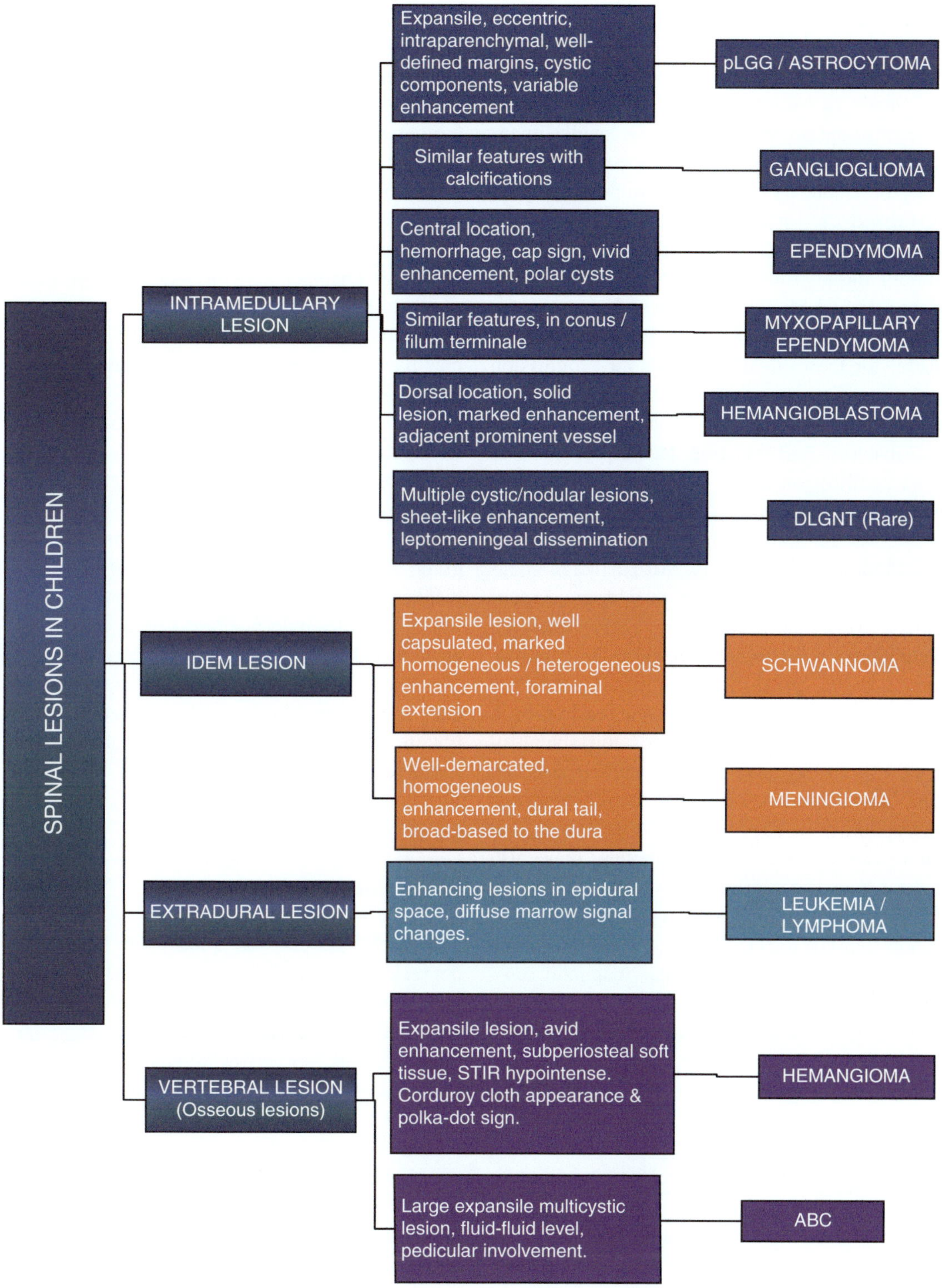
SPINAL LESIONS IN CHILDREN
INTRAMEDULLARY LESION
Expansile, eccentric, intraparenchymal, well-defined margins, cystic components, variable enhancement
pLGG / ASTROCYTOMA
Similar features with calcifications
GANGLIOGLIOMA
Central location, hemorrhage, cap sign, vivid enhancement, polar cysts
EPENDYMOMA
Similar features, in conus / filum terminale
MYXOPAPILLARY EPENDYMOMA
Dorsal location, solid lesion, marked enhancement, adjacent prominent vessel
HEMANGIOBLASTOMA
Multiple cystic/nodular lesions, sheet-like enhancement, leptomeningeal dissemination
DLGNT (Rare)
IDEM LESION
Expansile lesion, well capsulated, marked homogeneous / heterogeneous enhancement, foraminal extension
SCHWANNOMA
Well-demarcated, homogeneous enhancement, dural tail, broad-based to the dura
MENINGIOMA
EXTRADURAL LESION
Enhancing lesions in epidural space, diffuse marrow signal changes.
LEUKEMIA / LYMPHOMA
VERTEBRAL LESION (Osseous lesions)
Expansile lesion, avid enhancement, subperiosteal soft tissue, STIR hypointense. Corduroy cloth appearance & polka-dot sign.
HEMANGIOMA
Large expansile multicystic lesion, fluid-fluid level, pedicular involvement.
ABC

12.7.1 Recent Advances

Heterogeneity within primary spinal tumours may lead to a wrong estimation of the amount of tumour tissue on MR imaging. Molecular imaging with positron emission tomography of primary or secondary CNS spinal tumours may be performed to identify metabolically active tumour compartments, differentiate viable tumour tissue from necrosis, and predict treatment response by measurement of tumour perfusion or ischemia. 18F-FDG-PET imaging is useful for the evaluation of tumour progression and identification of the metabolically active components in spinal cord tumours [34].

Advanced MR imaging techniques such as DWI or diffusion tensor imaging (DTI) may be performed to assess the tumour's cellularity and its impact on longitudinal white matter tracts (tractography), respectively. MR perfusion imaging can provide information on tumoural vascularity. However, advanced MR imaging techniques encounter significant technical challenges in the spinal cord. The small voxel size (higher matrix) needs to be used for improved spatial resolution that decreases the signal-to-noise ratio. Image degradation can be caused by CSF flow/pulsation, breathing, swallowing, and susceptibility artefacts from the vertebral column. Local field inhomogeneities may also reduce image resolution by preventing efficient rephasing of proton spins, typically seen with echoplanar DWI/DTI. These technical issues also limit the acquisition of nuclear magnetic resonance (NMR) spectra with adequate signal-to-noise ratio for magnetic resonance spectroscopy of spinal cord lesions.

DTI metrics (e.g., ADC, fractional anisotropy [FA], radial diffusivity, axial diffusivity) are used to quantify water movement along the white matter fibre tracts. Low ADC values within intramedullary tumours suggest hypercellularity. Decreased FA values are seen in most intramedullary tumours compared with standard or reference regions, indicating infiltration by the tumour or destruction of standard fibre structure. Conversely, infiltrative growth of astrocytoma cells along fibres and encasement of the fibre tracts can result in increased FA values. The FA map helps detect the extent of a spinal cord tumour and distinguish it from the surrounding oedema.

Pre-operative DTI tractography can demonstrate the relationship between white matter fibres and spinal cord tumours, aiding surgical planning. Displacement of white matter fibres suggests benignity and increased possibility of complete resection. Because spinal ependymomas have only a slight likelihood of infiltrating the adjacent neural tissue and have a discrete capsule forming a cleavage plane between the tumour and the spinal cord, the fibres on tractography tend to be displaced. Spinal astrocytomas may demonstrate aggressive behaviour and infiltrate or encase the white matter tracts. The low-grade fibrillary or pilocytic astrocytomas tend to displace rather than infiltrate the cord. In addition to white matter fibre displacement and encasement by the tumour, fibres may also cross the tumour. An important clinical application of DTI tractography is for surgical guidance to obtain safer maximal resection of spinal cord tumours with the preservation of neurologic function [35].

12.8 Summary

Lesions of the cord & spine result in varying degrees of morbidity. Imaging and reporting them poses a great challenge to the radiologist. Knowledge about the common tumours in specific locations can narrow down our differentials and can help arrive at a specific diagnosis. Following strict protocols & optimising imaging parameters will result in good-quality MRI/CT scans. Multi-modality imaging should be performed whenever required. Adequate clinical input & discussion with the multi-disciplinary team is essential in reporting these cases. The role of the radiologist is very crucial in the management of these cases.

References

1. Shekdar KV, Schwartz ES. Imaging pediatric spine tumors. Appl Radiol. 2014;43:26–40.
2. Rogers SN, Udayasankar U, Pruthi S, Lai HA, Kadom N, Guerin J, et al. Imaging of pediatric spine and spinal cord tumors: a COG diagnostic imaging committee/SPR oncology committee/ASPNR white paper. Pediatr Blood Cancer. 2023;70(Suppl 4):e30150.
3. Kapadia T, Sahu A, Mahajan A, Ahuja A, Chatterjee A, Sahu A, et al. Imaging guidelines and recommendations for diagnosis, surveillance, and management of pediatric CNS and spinal tumors. Indian J Med Paediatr Oncol. 2023;44:039–46.
4. Boriani S. En bloc resection in the spine: a procedure of surgical oncology. J Spine Surg (Hong Kong). 2018;4:668–76.
5. Rossi A, Gandolfo C, Morana G, Tortori-Donati P. Tumors of the spine in children. Neuroimaging Clin N Am. 2007;17:17–35.
6. Palasis S, Hayes LL. Acquired pathology of the pediatric spine and spinal cord. Pediatr Radiol. 2015;45(Suppl 3):S420–32.
7. Smith AB, Soderlund KA, Rushing EJ, Smirniotopolous JG. Radiologic-pathologic correlation of pediatric and adolescent spinal neoplasms: Part 1, Intramedullary spinal neoplasms. AJR Am J Roentgenol. 2012;198:34–43.
8. Kothbauer KF. Neurosurgical management of intramedullary spinal cord tumors in children. Pediatr Neurosurg. 2007;43:222–35.
9. Samii M, Klekamp J. Surgical results of 100 intramedullary tumors in relation to accompanying syringomyelia. Neurosurgery. 1994;35:865–73. discussion 873.
10. Marrazzo A, Cacchione A, Rossi S, Carboni A, Gandolfo C, Carai A, et al. Intradural pediatric spinal tumors: an overview from imaging to novel molecular findings. Diagnostics (Basel). 2021;11 https://doi.org/10.3390/diagnostics11091710.
11. Ogunlade J, Wiginton JG 4th, Elia C, Odell T, Rao SC. Primary spinal astrocytomas: a literature review. Cureus. 2019;11:e5247.
12. Castillo M. Gangliogliomas: ubiquitous or not? AJNR Am J Neuroradiol. 1998;19:807–9.
13. Shatara M, Schieffer KM, Klawinski D, Thomas DL, Pierson CR, Sribnick EA, et al. Clinically aggressive pediatric spinal ependymoma with novel MYC amplification demonstrates molecular and histopathologic similarity to newly described MYCN-amplified spinal ependymomas. Acta Neuropathol Commun. 2021;9:192.
14. Plotkin SR, O'Donnell CC, Curry WT, Bove CM, MacCollin M, Nunes FP. Spinal ependymomas in neurofibromatosis type 2: a retrospective analysis of 55 patients: clinical article. J Neurosurg Spine. 2011;14:543–7.
15. Koeller KK, Rosenblum RS, Morrison AL. Neoplasms of the spinal cord and filum terminale: radiologic-pathologic correlation. Radiographics. 2000;20:1721–49.
16. Vougioukas VI, Gläsker S, Hubbe U, Berlis A, Omran H, Neumann HPH, et al. Surgical treatment of hemangioblastomas of the central nervous system in pediatric patients. Childs Nerv Syst. 2006;22:1149–53.
17. Sanghvi D. Post-treatment imaging of high-grade gliomas. Indian J Radiol Imaging. 2015;25:102–8.
18. Jecko V, Roblot P, Mongardi L, Ollivier M, Piccoli ND, Charleux T, et al. Intramedullary spinal cord lesions: a single-center experience. Neurospine. 2022;19:108–17.
19. Huisman TAGM. Pediatric tumors of the spine. Cancer Imaging. 2009;9 Spec No A:S45–8.
20. Das P, Singh GK, Prashantha GB, Barui S, Das DSR, Kushwaha S, et al. A rare case of aggressive phenotype (Wishart) of neurofibromatosis type 2. Indian J Dermatol Venereol Leprol. 2023;89:643.
21. Vadivelu S, Prasad P, Adesina AM, Kim E, Luerssen TG, Jea A. Giant invasive spinal schwannoma in children: a case report and review of the literature. J Med Case Rep. 2013;7:289.
22. Lee W, Chang KH, Choe G, Chi JG, Chung CK, Kim IH, et al. MR imaging features of clear-cell meningioma with diffuse leptomeningeal seeding. AJNR Am J Neuroradiol. 2000;21:130–2.
23. Yu KB, Lim MK, Kim HJ, Suh CH, Park HC, Kim EY, et al. Clear-cell meningioma: CT and MR imaging findings in two cases involving the spinal canal and cerebellopontine angle. Korean J Radiol. 2002;3:125–9.
24. Reddy AT. Atypical teratoid/rhabdoid tumors of the central nervous system. J Neuro-Oncol. 2005;75:309–13.
25. Rorke LB, Packer RJ, Biegel JA. Central nervous system atypical teratoid/rhabdoid tumors of infancy and childhood: definition of an entity. J Neurosurg. 1996;85:56–65.
26. Albrecht CF, Weiss E, Schulz-Schaeffer WJ, Albrecht T, Fauser S, Wickboldt J, et al. Primary intraspinal primitive neuroectodermal tumor: report of two cases and review of the literature. J Neuro-Oncol. 2003;61:113–20.
27. Woods ER, Martel W, Mandell SH, Crabbe JP. Reactive soft-tissue mass associated with osteoid osteoma: correlation of MR imaging features with pathologic findings. Radiology. 1993;186:221–5.
28. Davies M, Cassar-Pullicino VN, Davies AM, McCall IW, Tyrrell PNM. The diagnostic accuracy of MR imaging in osteoid osteoma. Skeletal Radiol. 2002;31:559–69.
29. Jackson RP, Reckling FW, Mants FA. Osteoid osteoma and osteoblastoma. Similar histologic lesions with different natural histories. Clin Orthop Relat Res. 1977;128:303–13.

30. Beltran J, Simon DC, Levy M, Herman L, Weis L, Mueller CF. Aneurysmal bone cysts: MR imaging at 1.5 T. Radiology. 1986;158:689–90.
31. Zaveri J, La Q, Yarmish G, Neuman J. More than just Langerhans cell histiocytosis: a radiologic review of histiocytic disorders. Radiographics. 2014;34:2008–24.
32. Diel J, Ortiz O, Losada RA, Price DB, Hayt MW, Katz DS. The sacrum: pathologic spectrum, multimodality imaging, and subspecialty approach. Radiographics. 2001;21:83–104.
33. Slovis TL, Meza MP, Cushing B, Elkowitz SS, Leonidas JC, Festa R, et al. Thoracic neuroblastoma: what is the best imaging modality for evaluating extent of disease? Pediatr Radiol. 1997;27:273–5.
34. Wilmshurst JM, Barrington SF, Pritchard D, Cox T, Bullock P, Maisey M, et al. Positron emission tomography in imaging spinal cord tumors. J Child Neurol. 2000;15:465–72.
35. Shah LM, Salzman KL. Conventional and advanced imaging of spinal cord tumors. Neuroimaging Clin N Am. 2023;33:389–406.

Orbital Tumors

13

Bhanupriya Singh, Ashish Verma,
and Ishan Kumar

13.1 Introduction

The evaluation of orbital masses in pediatric patients poses a unique set of challenges and opportunities for radiologists and clinicians alike. Unlike in adult populations, where the presence of tumors often aligns with more well-defined patterns of malignancy, pediatric orbital masses can represent a diverse array of conditions. These may include congenital anomalies, inflammatory processes, and a spectrum of both benign and malignant neoplasms.

The significance of precise imaging cannot be overstated, as it plays a pivotal role in the accurate diagnosis, informed treatment planning, and ongoing monitoring of these masses. Various imaging modalities—such as ultrasound, computed tomography (CT), and magnetic resonance imaging (MRI)—are employed to delineate the characteristics of these lesions. A thorough understanding of the distinctive imaging features associated with pediatric orbital masses is essential for guiding appropriate clinical management and ensuring the best possible outcomes for young patients navigating these complex conditions.

The foregoing text describes a combined "compartmentalized and patterned approach" to obtain an accurate early diagnosis of pediatric orbital masses and to classify them as non-neoplastic, benign, and malignant. The authors believe that such an approach may ensure the alleviation of delayed or erroneous diagnoses or treatments, hence reducing the burden of disability on the human race due to visual impairment.

13.2 Overview of Imaging Modalities

The structural complexities of the orbit and its content present an imaging challenge. Strides in radiologic modalities have allowed the clinician to obtain detailed and logistic information about orbital tumors [1].

- MRI: MRI offers exceptional soft-tissue resolution for structures within the orbit, including the eye, muscles, tendons, nerves, and blood vessels [2]. Both non-contrast and contrast-enhanced MRI are preferred techniques for assessing soft-tissue neoplastic conditions in and around the orbit. This imaging modality is particularly effective for characterizing masses, evaluating optic nerve pathology/

B. Singh
Department of Radiodiagnosis and Imaging, Sanjay Gandhi Post Graduate Institute of Medical Sciences, Lucknow, India

A. Verma · I. Kumar (✉)
Department of Radiodiagnosis and Imaging, Institute of Medical Sciences, Banaras Hindu University, Varanasi, Uttar Pradesh, India

I. Kumar et al. (eds.), *Practical Approach to Imaging in Pediatric Oncology*,
https://doi.org/10.1007/978-981-96-8158-7_13

involvement, and examining diseases affecting the globe and surrounding orbital tissues.

- The essential criteria for the diagnostic evaluation of retinoblastoma and lesions that may resemble it have been established through consensus among the members of the European Retinoblastoma Imaging Collaboration (ERIC). It recommends
  - 1.5/3T scanner
  - Orbits: Axial T2 (<2 mm slice thickness), heavily T2W (CISS/FIESTA/DRIVE).
  - Eyes and optic nerve:
    - Unilateral disease: T1 and T2 (axial/sagittal oblique), post contrast T1—no Fat saturation (axial and sagittal oblique).
    - Bilateral disease: T1 and T2 (axial), post contrast T1—no Fat saturation (axial and sagittal oblique).
  - Brain: axial T2 (slice thickness 4 mm or less), post-contrast T1.
- CT scans excel over MRI in assessing foreign bodies, detecting calcifications, and evaluating bony structures. Orbital CT serves as a complementary tool to MRI for patients with neoplasms involving the ocular region, orbit, and skull base. In cases where there is a clinical suspicion of an orbital mass, a contrast-enhanced orbital CT can provide valuable insights regarding adjacent bone involvement, such as erosion, sclerosis, or periosteal reactions, which may not be as easily identified on MRI.
- Ocular ultrasonography (US) can be used to visualize anterior and middle orbital lesions. A-scan ultrasonography allows for a one-dimensional description of echoes, while B-scan ultrasonography provides a two-dimensional image. C-scan ultrasonography affords coronal views, and D-scan ultrasonography creates three-dimensional orbital views. Doppler ultrasonography may be used to evaluate orbital vasculature and blood flow [3]. US is particularly useful for assessment of retinoblastoma, in detecting calcifications and retinal detachment.
- Fine needle aspiration biopsy (FNAB) is a technique used for diagnosing orbital lesions. This outpatient procedure allows for the retrieval of a cytological specimen through a well-controlled and minimally invasive technique. Disadvantages include poor cellular yield, cytopathologic and not a histologic diagnosis, difficulty in interpreting the specimen, and inadequate cellular yields requiring another biopsy procedure. Potential complications include retrobulbar hemorrhage, globe perforation, ptosis, extraocular motility dysfunction, and inadvertent entry intracranially. Patients with cystic lesions should not undergo FNAB. Common approach for obtaining tissue from an orbital lesion is open surgical biopsy, especially if FNAB is unable to obtain adequate tissue for pathologic assessment [4].

13.3 Approach to Diagnosis

The four steps of the compartmentalized and patterned approach to an orbital mass include:

(a) *Compartmentalization*: The human orbit may easily be divided into three compartments viz. the extra-conal space (outside the cone-shaped compartment formed by the extra-ocular muscles), the intra-conal extra-ocular space (within the above-cited muscle cone), and the intra-ocular space (originating from any of the layers of the eyeball). This approach aims to determine the epi-center (site of origin) of the pathology before attempting to characterize and define the spread or dissemination. The extraconal compartment consists of the lacrimal gland, fat, nerves, blood vessels, lymphatics, and bone. Intra-conal extra-ocular compartment contains the optic nerve, blood vessels and lymphatics, and fat. Intra-conal intra-ocular compartment is formed by the globe [5].

(b) *Focalization*: Intraconal lesions can be further focalized into the involvement of the optic nerve (optic nerve meningioma, glioma, etc.) or not (orbital varix, capillary hemangioma, lymphangioma, etc.).

(c) *Characterization*: MRI aids in the characterization of orbital lesions, with DWI/ADC sequence. Orbital lymphoma particularly shows low ADC and aids in differentiating malignant versus benign lesions. IVIM (intravoxel incoherent motion) takes acquisition at multiple B values and quantifies diffusion of mobile protons in intracellular, extracellular, and intravascular compartments. IVIM uses 3 major parameters: "True Diffusion Coefficient", "Pseudo-diffusion Coefficient", and "Perfusion Fraction". These parameters can differentiate with confidence: benign vs malignant and lymphoma vs inflammation. Imaging appearance of rhabdomyosarcomas and infantile hemangiomas are similar T2W and T1W + C images. ADC values of orbital rhabdomyosarcomas (mean ADC value 720 × 10^{-6} mm^2/s) were found to be significantly lower than infantile hemangiomas. Orbital lymphoma demonstrates ADC hypointensity with ADC values with similar range as rhabdomyosarcomas; however, it is a rare diagnosis in children. Selective usage of ADC in conjunction with the clinical information (including the age of the patient) and conventional MRI sequences is a much better approach, to differentiate benign from malignant lesions. ADC ratio of the lesion to the medulla and area under the curve are other potential parameters, to be documented.

(d) *Conceptualization*: Broadly dividing, orbital pathologies may be inflammatory (secondary to subperiosteal or para nasal sinus infections), congenital anomalies (entrapped ectoderm leading to dermoid and epidermoid cyst, Cephaloceles, Persistent Hyperplastic primary vitreous, Coloboma), vascular lesions (hemangioma, cavernoma), neoplasms (Rhabdomyosarcoma, Retinoblastoma, metastasis), trauma and foreign bodies, parasitic cysts [6].

Table 13.1 shows the common malignant and benign orbital lesions of the childhood.

Table 13.1 Common malignant and benign orbital lesions of the childhood

Extraconal compartment	Intraconal extraocular compartment	Intraconal intraocular compartment
Malignant lesions		
1. Myeloid sarcoma (chloroma)	1. Orbital rhabdomyosarcoma (RMS)	1. Retinoblastoma
2. Lymphoma	2. Optic nerve glioma	2. Ocular metastasis
3. Bony lesions	4. Myeloid sarcoma (Chloroma)	
	5. Orbital lymphoma & occular adnexal lymphoma	
Benign lesions		
1. Dermoid cyst	1. Optic nerve sheath & pathway glioma	1. Optic nerve glioma
2. Hemangioma	2. Optic nerve sheath meningioma	
3. Venolymphatic malformation	3. Venolymphatic malformation	
4. Neurofibroma	4. Optic nerve sheath schwannoma	
5. Orbital cavernous hemangioma.		
Tumor-like conditions		
1. Fibrous dysplasia	1.Cellulitis	1. Coat's disease
2. Cellulitis	2. Thyroid ophthalmopathy	2. Persistant hyperplastic primary vitreous
3. Non-specific orbital inflammatory disorder.		
4. Langerhans cell histiocytosis (LCH)		

13.4 Imaging Evaluation

Ultrasound of the eye provides dynamic evaluation, with the vascular status of lesions. It is essential to take a history of injury, diabetes mellitus or hypertension, and a history of active infection (Iridocyclitis) while doing an eye ultrasound. Because of the superficial location of the eye, linear high-frequency (7.5–13.0 MHz) transducers are used. While evaluation in B-mode, the gain settings are initially adjusted for superficial images (the anterior chamber), and then for the deeper area (the vitreous and posterior wall). During color Doppler evaluation, the parameters (pulse repetition frequency and filters) are adjusted for low velocities and a small Doppler gate. Pressure of the transducer should be reduced to avoid collapse of the anterior chamber, a precaution that is especially important in patients with traumatic eye injuries to avoid the risk for rupture [7].

CT scan is used to better evaluate calcification in the mass, with foraminal remodeling. But now, MRI susceptibility-weighted images provide nearly the same information. Although CT is still preferred modality in case of trauma, especially if a foreign body is suspected. CT is useful in bony pathologies (like fibrous dysplasia) and fat-containing lesions (dermoid) [8].

MRI evaluation of orbit can be done in 3 Tesla machines using 32 or 64-channel coils or 1.5 Tesla with the surface coils. MRI protocol should consist of axial SE T1W and TSE T2W sequences, coronal STIR sequences, and axial and coronal SE T1W sequences with fat saturation obtained after intravenous administration. Susceptibility and diffusion-weighted images are vital in characterization [9]. Optimal slice thickness should be 2–3 mm, with a volumetric 3D heavily T2W sequences (CISS, FIESTA, or DRIVE) and 3DFT T1W sequences with 0.6–1 mm thin slices (VIBE, THRIVE) after intravenous contrast material administration. The volumetric images allow multiplanar reconstructions in any given plane, thereby facilitating the evaluation of subtle findings. Orbit is a confined anatomical space, with a range of structures present within it that are often the site of origin of various pathologies, both in adults and children. While forming differentials, lesions with multicompartment involvement (veno-lymphatic malformation, plexiform neurofibroma, idiopathic orbital pseudotumor, IgG4 related disease, metastases). Brain should be included in scan, if retinoblastoma is suspected, to rule out trilateral disease, or possibility of metastasis [10]. Table 13.2 provides the structured reporting checklist in the evaluation of the orbital lesion.

Table 13.2 Reporting checklist for orbital masses (MRI-based with inputs from other modalities if available)

Compartment	*Extra-conal*: <extraorbital/bony> <Intra orbital> Intraconal: <intraocular> <extraocular>
Anatomical structure	*Extra-orbital*: < Sino-nasal bone/Orbito-sinonasal septum/Cranio-facial bone> *Extra-conal*: <Lachrymal apparatus> <Fat/fascia/Smallnerves/Small vessels> <Inferior ophthalmic vein> <Supra-orbital nerve> < Infraorbital nerve (CN5 V2)> <Trigeminal nerve – Optic division (CN5 V1)> <Trochlear nerve (CN 4)> *Intraconal*: <Extra-ocular muscles[a]> < Optic nerve-sheath complex (CN 2)> < Abducens nerve (CN 6)> <Oculomotor nerve (CN 3)> <Ophthalmic artery> <Superior ophthalmic vein> <Fat/ fascia/Small nerves/Small vessels> *Ocular*: <Globe> <Retrobulbar optic nerve> <Anterior segment> <Posterior segment>
Tumor size	[—x—x—]cm
Parenchyma	<T1/T2 signal> <Water suppression> <Fat suppression> <diffusion restriction> < post contrast enhancement> <calcification>
Extensions	<Paranasal sinus : Frontal/Ethmoid/Maxillary/Sphenoid> <Nasal Cavity> <Parapharyngeal space> <Pterygopalatine fossa> <oral cavity>
Intracranial	< anterior/middle cranial fossa: subarachnoid space/brain parenchyma> <sella turcica: pituitary/ infundibulum> <cavernous sinus> < cranial nerves
Vascular	<venous/arterial involvement> <part of artery/ vein encased> <thrombosis>
Other	<lymphadenopathy> <metastasis> <other findings>

[a]All seven extraocular muscles should be seen individually

13.5 Benign Tumors

Orbital Cavernous Hemangioma is one of the most common malformations in pediatric age group, with female gender predilection. One-third of them are present since birth, and most of them manifest by 6 months of age. Initially, they tend to grow till approx. 12 months of age, and rarely involutes. Common presentations include unilateral proptosis, diplopia, or painless diminished visual acuity. While hemangiomas are one of most common benign lesions, their close mimic orbital RMS is most common malignant lesion. ADC values of hemangioma are significantly higher than orbital RMS. It has phleboliths and shows remodeling of orbital bony walls. In contrast CT images, cavernous hemangioma enhances late on late venous images. It shows well-defined borders with honeycomb-like structures on USG. On MRI, presence of flow-voids, ADC hyperintensity, T1 iso and T2 hyperintensity is seen, with internal septation and progressive accumulation of contrast with homogeneous enhancement [11] (Fig. 13.1).

Orbital Dermoid is one of the most common benign tumors for pediatric age group, occurring in anterior extraconal orbit, upper temporal quadrant (lacrimal fossa), and occurring bilaterally. Proposed theories of origin include: either ectoderm gets trapped in bony sutures during embryogenic migration, or failure of surface ectoderm to separate from the neural tube [1]. It shows negative HU on CT, due to the presence of fat, and shows well-defined margins. Dermoid follows

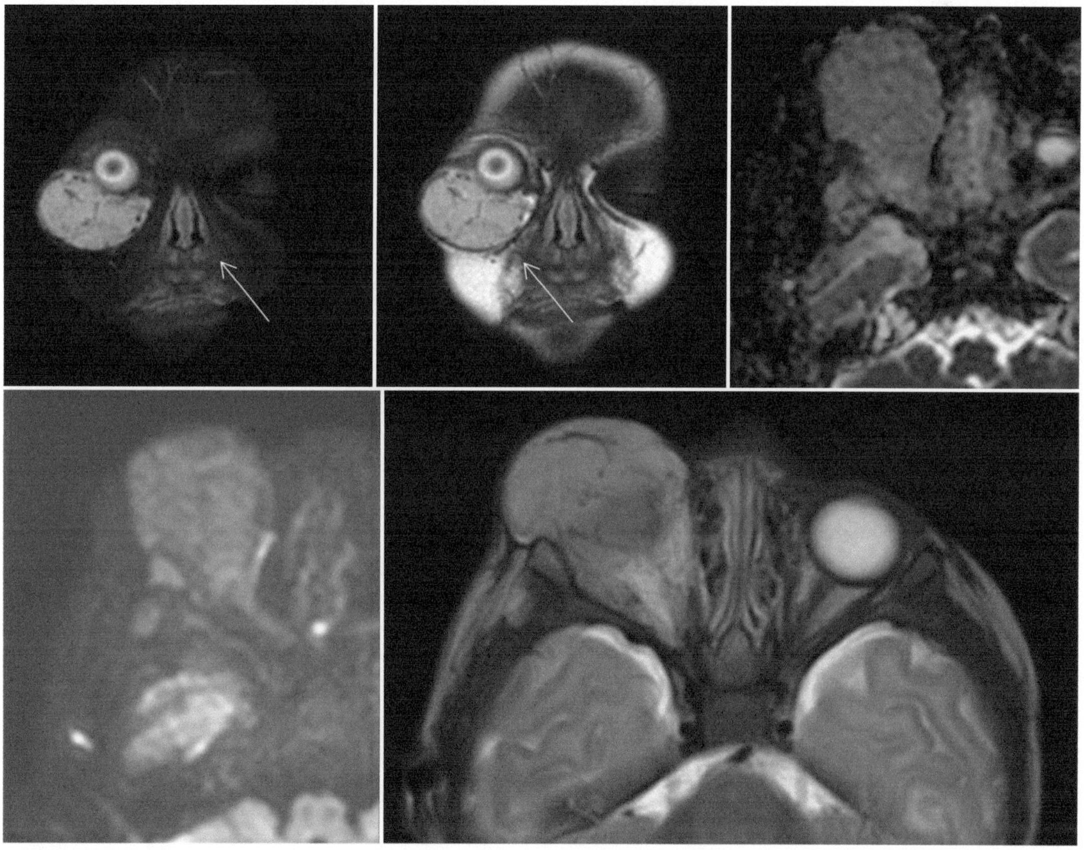

Fig. 13.1 A large T2 hyperintense, heterogeneously enhancing lobulated soft tissue at the infero-lateral aspect of intra-extraconal space of the right orbit (predominantly extraconal) involving the lower eyelid and showing peri-orbital extension (white arrow) as described above. Histopathology came out to be **Orbital Cavernous Hemangioma**

cystic features on USG & appears hyperintense on both T1 & T2 MR images, with thick well-defined capsule [11]. Bony remodeling and intracranial extension should be assessed. Differentials for such slow-growing lesions, causing increasing proptosis can be parasitic cysts (Neurocysticercosis, Hydatid). Epidermoid cysts present similarly but lack the dermal elements in the cyst wall.

Optic Nerve & Optic Pathway Glioma is common in the pediatric age group, and shows association with Neurofibromatosis 1 (Von Recklinghausen's disease), especially if present. Bilaterally. NF-1 association shows low-grade gliomas on histology. Poor prognosis is associated with intracranial extension [11]. Optic pathway gliomas can potentially involve any portion of the visual pathway, from the hypothalamus, optic disc, nerve, chiasm, and geniculate nucleus, to optic radiations. Imaging features of optic nerve glioma include fusiform enlargement of the optic nerve with widened optic canal, variable post-contrast enhancement, and rarely eccentric enlargement of nerve and cystic degeneration. MRI scores over CT, to evaluate intracranial extent of disease, as it shows nerve foramina better and avoids radiation. It appears T1 iso to hypointense, T2 hyperintense, and variable enhancement on postcontrast images.

Pathognomonic for neurofibromatosis 1 (Von Recklinghausen's disease) is the presence of plexiform neurofibroma, which originates from Schwann cells and fibroblasts, and is a hamartoma of neuroectodermal origin. When in orbit, it involves the upper eyelid, giving it a typical S shape, with exophthalmos and buphthalmos. Any peripheral nerve can be involved, but usually, sensory nerves in the orbit or eyelid are involved. Varying degrees of bony involvement can lead to the widening of superior orbital fissure, dysplasia of the greater sphenoid wing, expansion of middle cranial fossa, expansion of the anterior orbital rim, and expanded orbital foramina secondary to trigeminal nerve involvement [11] (Fig. 13.2).

Optic Nerve Sheath Meningioma is generally seen in adults. However, if present, they are slightly more aggressive in children, commonly presenting with insidious onset loss of visual acuity. Post-contrast tram track-like enhancement is seen on axial images, with a ring-like

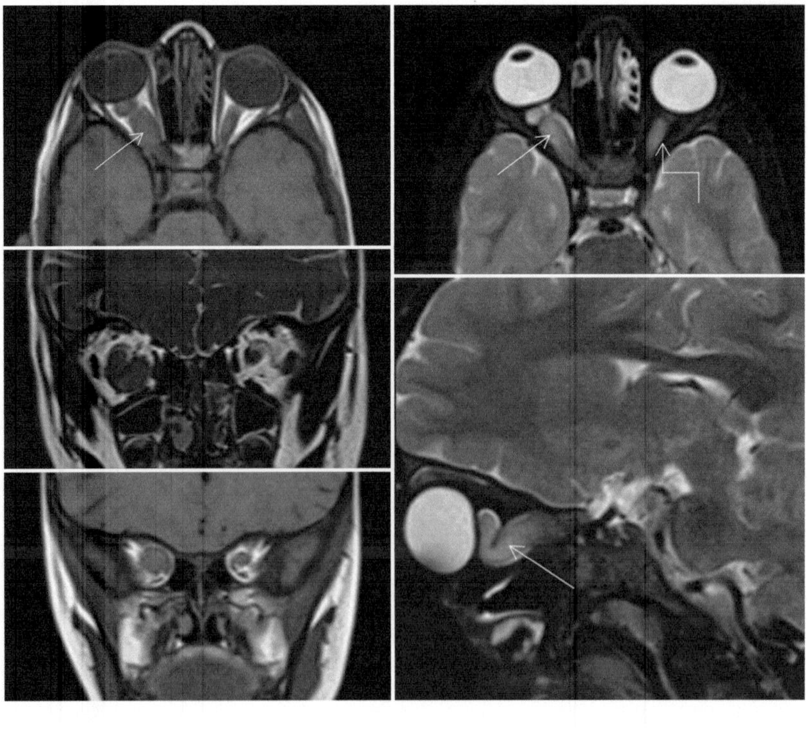

Fig. 13.2 A 6-year-old female presented with proptosis and difficulty of vision for 1.5 years. Diffusely enlarged T2W hyperintense entire right optic nerve (white arrow) & intraocular segment of left optic nerve (white elbow arrow connector) suggests **bilateral optic nerve glioma**. Proven case of **Neurofibromatosis Type I**

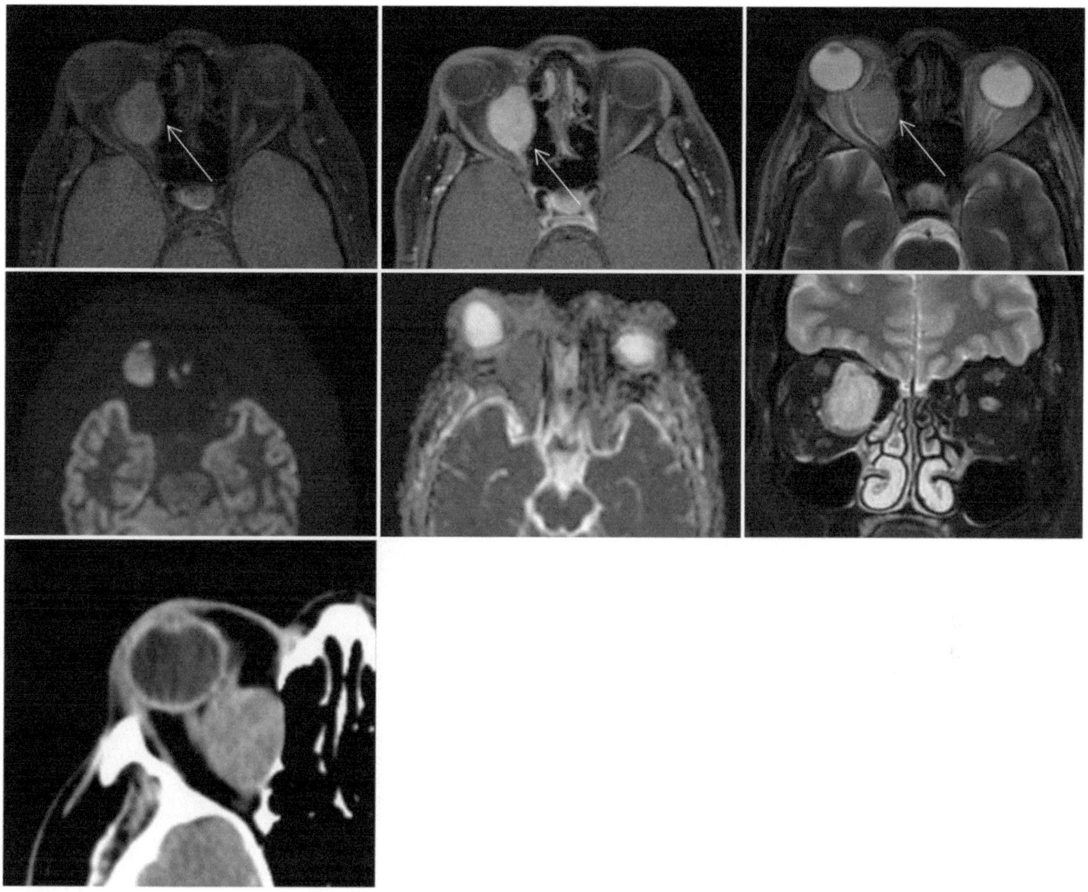

Fig. 13.3 A 7-year-old male presented with proptosis and difficulty of vision for 2 years. MRI shows a well-encapsulated, smoothly marginated homogeneously enhancing lesion in supero-medial extraconal compartment of right orbit (white arrow) projecting in intraconal space with resultant proptosis. CT also confirms the findings. Histopathology confirmed **Schwannoma (nerve sheath tumor)**

enhancement on coronal images [11, 12]. They appear T2 dark, and avid post-contrast enhancement.

Optic Nerve Schwannoma: Schwannoma is benign tumor of peripheral nervous system. Optic nerve Schwannoma is rare as optic nerve sheath lacks Schwann cells. The optic nerve gets stretched and may demonstrate solid-cystic intraconal mass [11, 12] (Fig. 13.3).

Orbital Lymphatic & Veno Lymphatic Malformation, earlier known as lymphangioma, can present with rapid onset proptosis, either due to lymphoid hyperplasia or intralesional hemorrhage. They're generally no to low flow malformations and can have intracranial components. Margins are poorly defined, with cyst-like areas showing rim enhancement. Proteinaceous fluid may show T1 hyperintensity. Blood products within lesion follow their intensity depending on age [13, 14]. Latest ISSVA classification should be followed for characterization and assessing vascularity. It's generally slow-growing. However, sudden increase can be due to internal bleeding or episode of cough. If this happens, it should be treated with steroids to save from potential complications of orbital compartment syndrome. Deep lesions are more commonly venous, while superficial lesions are more lymphatic (Fig. 13.4).

Fig. 13.4 **Orbital venous malformation:** An 8-year-old boy presented with C/o gradual loss of vision, proptosis in left eye since 2 years. A well-defined lobulated intensely enhancing altered signal intensity lesion along the medial & inferior aspect of left orbit (white arrow) with extension & displacement and associated proptosis of eyeball

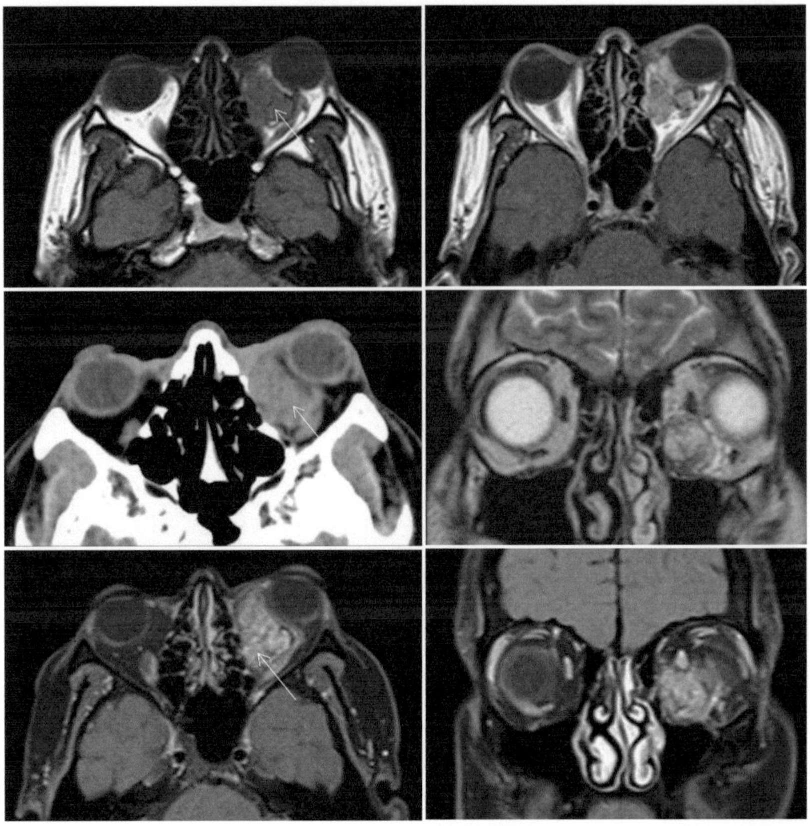

13.6 Malignant Tumors

Retinoblastoma comprises of approximately 4% of pediatric cancers and involves especially the very young age group, 0 to 5 years. It's most common intraocular malignancy and presents with leukocoria because these tumors are white. Calcification is the hallmark of the disease and most of the time is already detected on their ultrasound. Susceptibility-weighted MR images also demonstrate calcification equally well. Calcifications and necrotic mass arise from inner nuclear layer of retina [13]. Approximately 66% of them are non-heritable, including chromosomal anomaly (deletion of 13q) or sporadic post-zygomatic somatic mutation. The rest one-third of the cases are heritable mutations, with autosomal dominance transmission and 90% penetrance (showing loss of allele of RB1 tumor suppression gene: 13q14). The heritable form is more associated with bilateral disease. Trilateral retinoblastoma refers to the neuroectodermal tumor of the pineal gland with bilateral retinoblastoma. Quadrilateral retinoblastoma refers to fourth focus on suprasellar cistern in addition to trilateral retinoblastoma [14]. Hence other intracranial lesions should be looked for on MRI, demonstrating features similar to those of retinoblastoma (T2 hypointense with restricted diffusion). Any lesion in pineal gland region or suprasellar cistern showing wall thickening (>2 mm) and nodularity must raise suspicion. Neuroectoderm precursor of the pineal gland is prone to develop neoplasms in heritable retinoblastoma, and suprasellar lesions may occur, arising from ectopic pineal tissue or migrational rudiments of the retina [15].

The four morphological growth forms include endophytic, exophytic, mixed, and diffuse infiltrating. Unilateral retinoblastoma are more common, with involvement of posterolateral wall of globe. On ultrasound, they look as solid cystic mass with areas of tumor necrosis and fine focal calcification. It can be associated with vitreous hemorrhage or retinal detachment. Associated extraocular mass or thickened optic nerve can show intracranial extension, and whole brain should be screened on post-contrast images. Extensive retinoblastoma can metastasize into CNS and meninges. Post-contrast T1WI fat-saturated images can help separate normal orbital fat from abnormal enhancement. If subarachnoid spread of disease is suspected, a complete spinal survey to determine involvement of whole neuroaxis should be done [16].

In endophytic type of retinoblastoma growth, tumors are well visualized, with vessels coursing into the mass. Tumor extends from the deep retinal layer into the vitreous.

The morphological exophytic growth pattern extends from the retina outward into the subretinal space, with vessels coursing over the tumor. It can be associated with retinal detachment, which might underestimate the actual size of the tumor. The third pattern is the most common, which is a mixture of exophytic and endophytic growth [17]. A rare uncommon morphology seen in older children is diffuse anterior retinoblastoma, seen as plaque-like endophytic tumor, arising from peripheral retina and involving ocular structures anterior to the anterior vitreous margin such as the pars plicata, lens zonules, and iris.

The fourth pattern is a rare subtype, diffuse infiltrating retinoblastoma. This type accounts for 1–2% of retinoblastomas, and usually arises from the anterior retina in older children. Usually this form presents as a non-mass lesion and lacks calcium. Clinically, it may present as pseudohypopyon and floating vitreal tumor cells can be misdiagnosed with uveitis or endophthalmitis. Diffuse retinoblastomas start anteriorly and may enter the anterior chamber and fill the vitreous cavity but usually do not extend to the optic nerve. CT demonstrates smooth solid enhancing mass with calcification, dense vitreous, and extraocular/intracranial extension. MRI helps assess optic pathway better [16, 17]. Retinoblastoma appears mildly T1 hyperintense and T2 hypointense, with intralesional calcifications or hemorrhage appearing as signal void T2* images. Low T2* signal intensity can be peripheral & linear, suggesting intratumoral hemorrhage, or central and nodular signal voids generally representing calcification. Diffusion restriction and heterogenous post-contrast enhancement is also seen [15].

Larger lesions tend to involve prelaminar optic nerve (ON), seen on MRI when tumor interrupts the normal linear enhancement of the choroido-retinal complex at the disc. But postlaminar ON invasion is a high-risk feature for poor prognosis with increased risk of orbital recurrence after Enucleation. Imaging findings of postlaminar ON invasion include increased caliber of ON or abnormal triangular enhancement ($\geq$2 mm in diameter).

Choroid is a highly vascular and metabolically active layer, situated peripherally. Hence, its invasion makes hematogenous spread more likely. If choroid invasion is massive (more than 3 mm), significant increased risk of metastasis and mortality is seen. Similar another risk factor for hematogenous spread is abnormal anterior chamber enhancement (involvement of ciliary body, lens, iris, and/or cornea). Hemorrhage or hyphema is also a strong predictor of metastatic disseminations, as they're postulated to occur due to neoangiogenesis. Lungs, liver, and bone marrow are typical sites for systemic metastasis. Scleral invasion can be termed when tumor enhancement extends across the choroid, causing disruption of nonenhancing sclera, and/or extending into periocular tissues [15, 17]. Enucleation, followed by chemotherapy is indicated in such cases. Occurrence of glaucoma in the background of retinoblastoma is postulated due to displacement of the lens-iris diaphragm (angle closure), exudative retinal detachment, neoangiogenesis of iris, tumor seeding, and uveitis or pseudouveitis with tumor cells and/or inflammatory cells. Intraocular pressure of 34 mm Hg or more at the time of diagnosis has a significant poor prognosis [16, 17]. On MRI it's seen as increased globe size, contour deformity of the globe, and reduced anterior chamber depth [15]. A rare close mimic is retinoblastoma-associated orbital cellulitis, which also has poor prognosis, and patient will have aggressive symptoms. It is sterile inflammatory response to tumor undergoing autoinfarction. On MRI it's seen as nonenhancing necrotic

T2-hypointense tumor with periocular inflammatory changes. Lens subluxation can occur due to ciliary body necrosis. Occasionally, contrast enhancement may be seen in the postlaminar ON, secondary to inflammation, and not invasion. Post-contrast enhancement equal to or greater than choroid, covering the entire width of the lamina cribrosa, and postlaminar ON may suggest inflammation [15, 18].

Table 13.3 summarizes the imaging checklist (MRI) that should be assessed in suspected cases of retinoblastoma [17].

Treatment protocol for locally invasive retinoblastoma comprises neoadjuvant chemotherapy, followed by limited surgery and adjuvant chemotherapy. Smaller lesions can be treated with cryotherapy. In advanced retinoblastoma cases, with failed prior intravenous chemotherapy, Selective intra-arterial chemotherapy can provide eye-sparing treatment, with follow-up. No adverse cerebral ischemic events have been reported. However, in few cases, central and partial retinal artery occlusion and choroidal atrophy have been reported. Another potential risk due to heavy radiation exposure of this procedure is secondary malignancy. However, it's not yet been reported.

Chances of metastasis and post-treatment recurrence are predicted by massive choroidal invasion, postlaminar ON invasion, anterior segment involvement (seen as enhancing thickening), and scleral and extrascleral invasion. Abnormal enhancing thickening of choroid or any discontinuity is a marker of invasion [15] (Figs. 13.5, 13.6 and 13.7).

Rhabdomyosarcoma is one of the most common primary orbital malignancy, originating from undifferentiated pluripotent mesenchymal germ cells (and not extraocular muscles). An increased risk of rhabdomyosarcoma (RMS) is associated with the following rare inherited diseases: Li-Fraumeni Syndrome, Beckwith-Widemann Syndrome, Neurofibromatosis type 2, Noonan Syndrome, and Multiple Endocrine Neoplasia type 2a Syndrome. Clinically, the lesion may present with unilateral proptosis, lid discoloration, and edema. Embryonal (common

Table 13.3 Imaging checklist for the assessment in suspected cases of retinoblastoma

Tumor characteristic	Imaging features
Size and location	Risk factors for globe rupture and orbital seeding during enucleation Increased intraocular pressure: Globe enlargement, deformed shape, decreased anterior chamber depth (buphthalmos)
Growth pattern	Tumor location Relative to the eye's equator (anterior, posterior, combined) Proximity to the optic disc and macula (tumors near the optic disc that may invade the optic nerve)
Optic nerve and meningeal sheath	Optic nerve invasion Distal optic nerve enhancement ≥2 mm Disruption of normal enhancement at the optic disc Leptomeningeal metastases Postlaminar optic nerve/meningeal sheath invasion Recommended: Sagittal post-contrast whole spine imaging
Ocular wall and extraocular extension	Choroid invasion Discontinuities in choroidal enhancement Focal thickening of choroid Thickening of the entire uveal tract indicates uveitis secondary to tumor necrosis (not tumor invasion) Scleral invasion: Protrusion of enhancing tissue through the choroid into the sclera Extraocular extension: Protrusion beyond sclera
Anterior eye segment	Anterior segment invasion Tumor extension into the ciliary body or beyond Mere anterior segment enhancement: Indicates iris angiogenesis (not invasion) Use axial T2 image of both orbits to compare and identify decreased anterior chamber depth
Brain involvement	Evaluate midline structures (pineal gland and suprasellar area) Leptomeningeal spread Congenital brain malformations associated with 13q-deletion syndrome (posterior encephalocele, holoprosencephaly, corpus callosum agenesis, Dandy Walker variant)

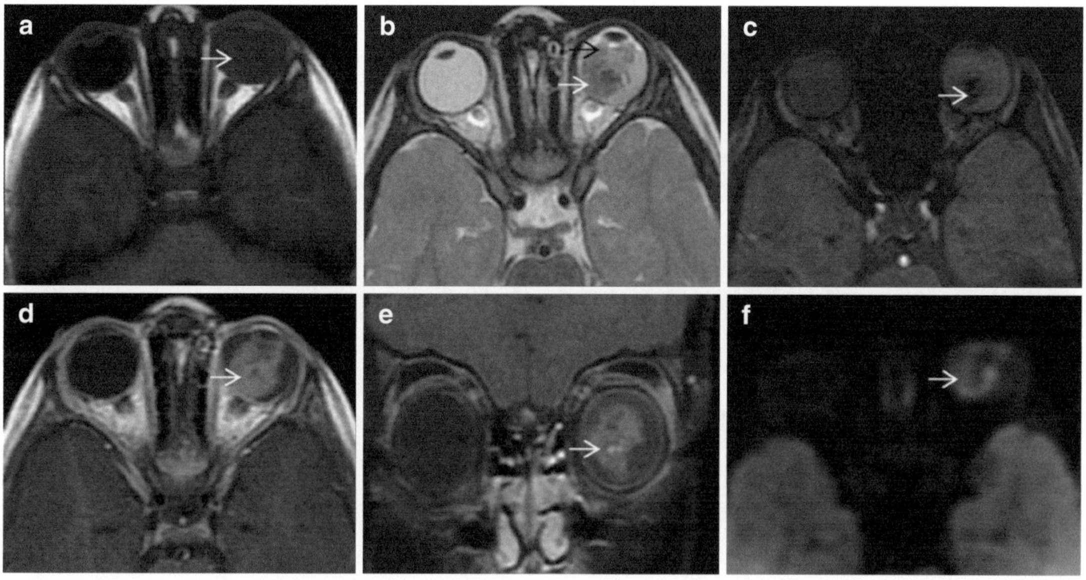

Fig. 13.5 MRI orbit. (**a**) Un-enhanced T1W image in axial plane demonstrates increased signals in the posterior chamber of left eye globe (white arrow) compared to normal hypointense signals in the right eye globe. (**b**) T2W image in axial plane shows fluid-fluid levels due to intravitreal hemorrhage (black arrow) in the posterior chamber of left eye globe with internal heterogenous lesion attached to the posterior part of the globe. (white arrow) (**c**) Susceptibility-weighted image in axial plane depicts blooming artifact in the lesion suggestive of calcification. (white arrow) (**d**, **e**) Contrast-enhanced T1W images in axial and coronal plane demonstrate heterogeneously enhancing lesion in the posterior chamber of the left eye globe, reaching up to the posterior surface of the lens. (white arrow) (**f**) Diffusion-weighted MRI image in the axial plane demonstrates diffusion restriction in the lesion which suggests hypercellularity of the lesion. (white arrow). Features are suggestive of **Retinoblastoma**

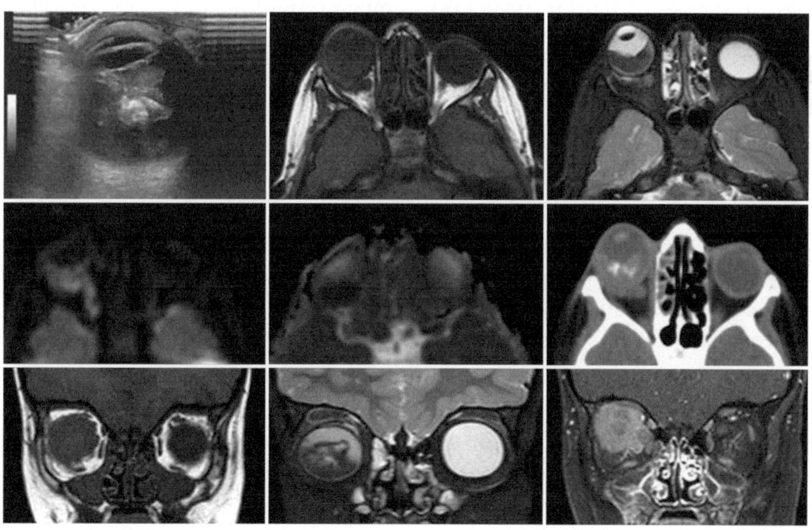

Fig. 13.6 **Retinoblastoma:** A 3-year-old girl presented with C/o gradual diminution of vision in right eye since 1 year. USG shows echogenic soft-tissue masses with variable shadowing due to calcifications and heterogeneity due to necrosis and hemorrhage. CT shows dense foci of calcification within the lesion. An inhomogeneously enhancing large lesion in posterior segment of right eyeball with calcification showing infiltration of sclera and along optic nerve in its intra-orbital, intracanalicular segment

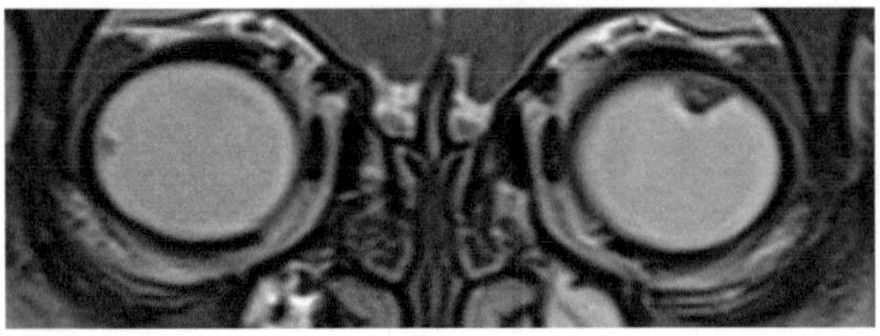

Fig. 13.7 In case of **bilateral Retinoblastoma**, a small intraretinal tumor (<3 mm), away from fovea and optic disc is seen on the right side. On left side, discrete tumor (>3 mm), confined to the retina is seen. Adjacent subretinal fluid is seen with no subretinal seeding

location being superior orbit) histopathologic type of RMS is most common, while alveolar (common location being inferior orbit) has poorest prognosis. Usually RMS occurs in extraconal (37–87%) location, followed by both intra- and extraconal location (13–47%), and more commonly along superonasal aspect [13].

It presents as well-defined heterogeneous extraocular mass with adjacent bony orbit erosion. Calcifications are seen only occurring with bony destruction. Orbital RMS appears isoattenuating to muscle on CT with moderate to marked post-contrast enhancement [14]. Necrosis, hemorrhage, and cavitation with ring enhancement are uncommon findings. MRI shows tumor is isointense to muscle on T1WI, hyperintense to muscle on T2WI, and demonstrates moderate to marked enhancement post-contrast. The lesion causes mass effect and distorts/displaces the globe and extraocular muscles, but rarely invades these structures. Incision biopsy confirms the diagnosis. PET-CT and WBMRI (whole body MRI) are the tools of choice for diagnosis, staging, and follow-up of the disease. Use of updated diffusion-weighted techniques improves the diagnostic accuracy of WBMRI [1]. RMS causes mass effect, by displacing globe, adjacent muscles, often forming indistinct border with adjacent muscles, and causing proptosis. Anteriorly RMS can extend into preseptal compartment. RMS can cause bone deformity, but frank bone destruction with bone involvement or posterior orbital canal extension is rare. If present, the diagnosis will change from orbital to parameningeal RMS. ADC values of orbital rhabdomyosarcomas (mean ADC value 720×10^{-6} mm^2/s) are significantly lower than a close mimic, infantile hemangiomas (Fig. 13.8).

Ocular Metastasis Neuroblastoma and Ewing's sarcoma are common malignancies in pediatric age group to cause ocular metastasis. Neuroblastoma is the most common extracranial solid malignancy of childhood and arises from neural crest cells. Orbital metastasis from neuroblastoma can present as early as infancy and generally has poor prognosis. A special paraneoplastic involvement of orbit in neuroblastoma is opsoclonus (saccadic intrusion). Choroidal and optic nerve metastasis is also a rarer subtype [16]. Morphologically metastases can be either well-circumscribed or ill-defined. CT scan shows increased attenuation compared to muscle, and can contain small calcifications.

CT can better show bony foramina, and demonstrate invasion of adjacent structures, including intracranial extension. On MR, neuroblastoma metastases appear low signal on T1WI, heterogeneous on T2WI due to hemorrhage or necrosis, and show heterogeneous post-contrast enhancement. If multiple metastatic lesions are suspected, radioiodinated metaiodobenzylguanidine (MIBG) scintigraphy can be used for diagnosis, staging, and monitoring therapy with high sensitivity and specificity. More recently, PET/CT has been shown to successfully stage the disease [1].

Orbital Lymphoma and Ocular Adnexal Lymphoma generally present in background of systemic disease. Commonly seen in older age groups, few cases have been documented in pediatric patients as well. It makes a heterogeneous group of tumors composing of non-Hodgkin's lymphomas (NHL) extranodal mucosa-associated lymphoid tissue (MALT) lymphomas [18]. Secondary ocular involvement occurs with advanced systemic NHL. Patients with Sjögren's syndrome have further high risk

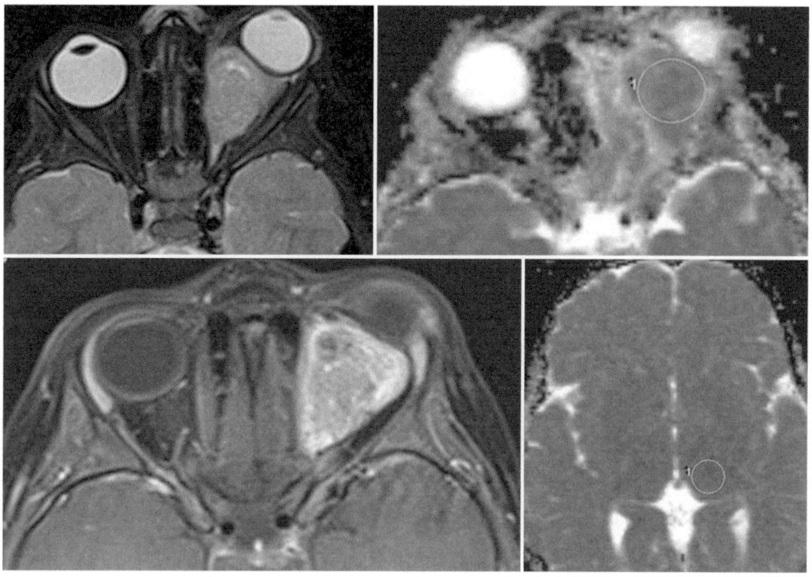

Fig. 13.8 A 3-year-old boy with rapidly progressive proptosis. On MRI mean ADC of 0.88 and ADC to thalamic ratio of 1.07. For distinguishing benign from malignant lesions, a lesion mean ADC cut-off value of 1.14 x 10–3 mm^2/s provided a sensitivity of 84% and specificity of 100%, while an ADC ratio of 1.4 provided a sensitivity of 81% and specificity of 89%. Histopathology came to be **Rhabdomyosarcoma**

in adult population. Typically, orbital lymphomas are known to have very low ADC values, usually between 0.44–0.92 x 10–3 mm^2/s (ADC values less than 1.0×10^{-3} mm^2/s). Lymphoid hyperplasia has overlapping imaging features with lymphoma; however, it is well-marginated as compared to more infiltrative pattern of lymphoma.

On the other hand, intraorbital pseudotumor or orbital inflammatory syndrome shows ADC range 1.02–2.28 × 10^{-3} mm^2/s (ADC values greater than 1.0×10^{-3} mm^2/s). Hence, high degree of accuracy using an ADC threshold of 1.0×10^{-3} mm^2/s and an ADC ratio of less than 1.2×10^{-3} mm^2/s [18]. Orbital pseudotumor is an uncommon, benign, non-infective, inflammatory pathology involving the orbital tissues, and diagnosis is usually clinched when a rapid response is seen to oral or systemic steroids. Histology shows polymorphous lymphoid infiltrate with varying degrees of fibrosis, and it is a diagnosis of exclusion after systemic and local causes have been thoroughly excluded [19, 20].

Chloroma/granulocytic sarcoma/myeloid sarcoma or extramedullary myeloid tumors can develop in children during the course of hematologic disorder or may precede it. These lesions are associated with leukemia. Leukemia is one of the common malignancies of childhood.

Few cases of acute myeloid leukemia develop extramedullary solid tumors of primitive granulocyte precursor cells. Orbit and orbital bones are commonly involved with multifocality. Temporal prediction with systemic disease is variable and should be evaluated with peripheral blood film and bone marrow biopsy [19] (Fig. 13.9).

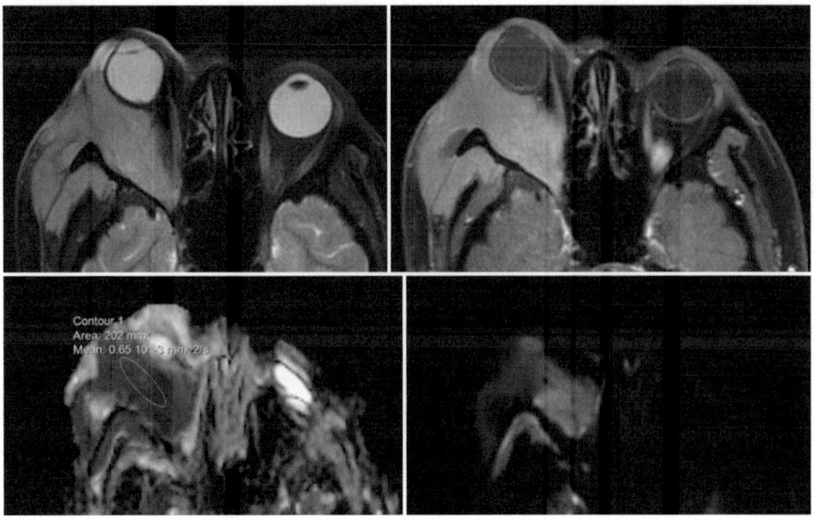

Fig. 13.9 Ocular adnexal lymphoma: Solid pliant homogeneously enhancing tumor that molds to the orbital contour. Tumor is minimally hypointense on T2-weighted images owing to its highly cellular nature. Lymphoma has quantifiable decreased signal on ADC maps

13.7 Tumor-Like Conditions

Fibrous Dysplasia is a developmental condition where bone is replaced by fibro-osseous tissue. Functional disability becomes of concern when the optic nerve gets compressed [19]. It replaces lamellar bone with abnormal metaplastic immature woven bone, forming irregular curvilinear trabeculae. CT and X-ray show bony expansion with ground glass matrix. Narrowing of bony foramina or canal is better demonstrated, optic nerve canal being one of the commonly affected areas. The narrowing can produce symptoms because of impingement of the optic nerve. The fibrous stroma and osteoid material appear hypointense on T1W images show mixed signal intensity on T2W images, with internal fluid-fluid level. Generally, marked enhancement is seen on CEMRI [18, 20].

Coat's Disease Retinal telangiectasia is a congenital nonhereditary primary vascular malformation of retina characterized by multiple abnormal telangiectatic retinal vessels that cause lipo-proteinaceous leakage into subretinal space. Clumpy particulate echoes are also appreciated on ultrasound. CT shows dense vitreous with linear V-shaped enhancement at anterior margin of subretinal exudate. T1/T2 hyperintense signal on MRI corresponds to these subretinal exudates. However, T2 heterogeneity may be seen because of hemorrhage and fibrosis [1, 14] (Fig. 13.10).

Persistent hyperplastic primary vitreous (PHPV) is a rare congenital non-hereditary disease, showing hyperplasia of fibrovascular system derived from the embryonic primary vitreous. Common cause of neonatal leukocoria, linear hypoechoic band is seen extending from the posterior surface of the lens to the posterior globe [3]. Vitreous also shows increased echogenicity. Cone-shaped enhancement is noted in the retrolental region, extending up to the optic nerve head. T1/T2 hyperintensity with triangular band near the base of optic disc and apex at the posterior surface of lens [14, 20]. Calcification is rare, and presence of calcification suggests the possibility of retinoblastoma. CT findings are absence of calcification, an increased density of the entire vitreous, tubular intravitreal density in Cloquet's canal or non-attached retina, fluid-fluid level in the subretinal space, a retrolental mass, and micro-ophthalmia (Fig. 13.11).

Orbital Cellulitis is generally spread of infection from adjacent paranasal sinuses, face, or teeth. It may also be a result of direct trauma. Abscess may appear T1/T2 hyperintense with DWI restriction and may require drainage. Orbital cellulitis appears hypointense on T1, hyperintense on T2, and shows post-contrast enhancement [1]. A clinical clue would be cellulitis that's not accompanied by erythema and warmth or periorbital ecchymosis with or without history of

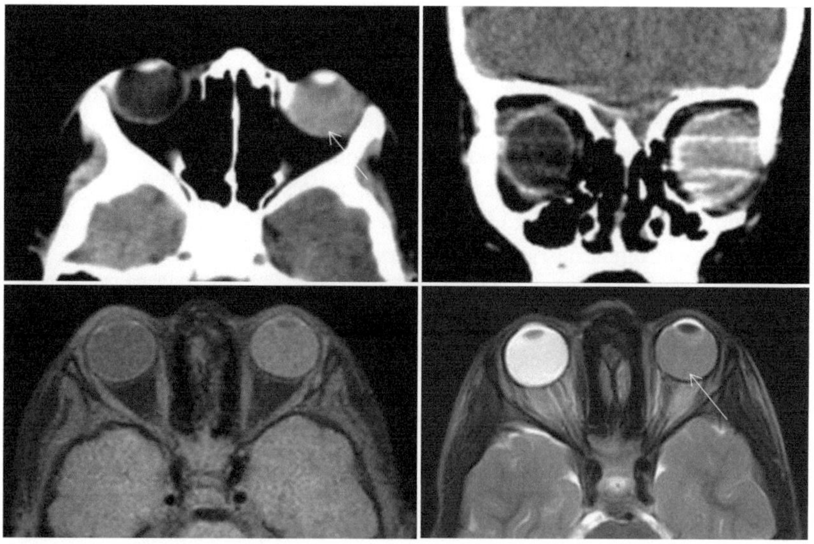

Fig. 13.10 **Coat's disease:** A 4-year-old boy presented with c/o leukocoria since one and half months. Retinal detachment with subretinal hemorrhagic/proteinaceous exudates (white arrow)

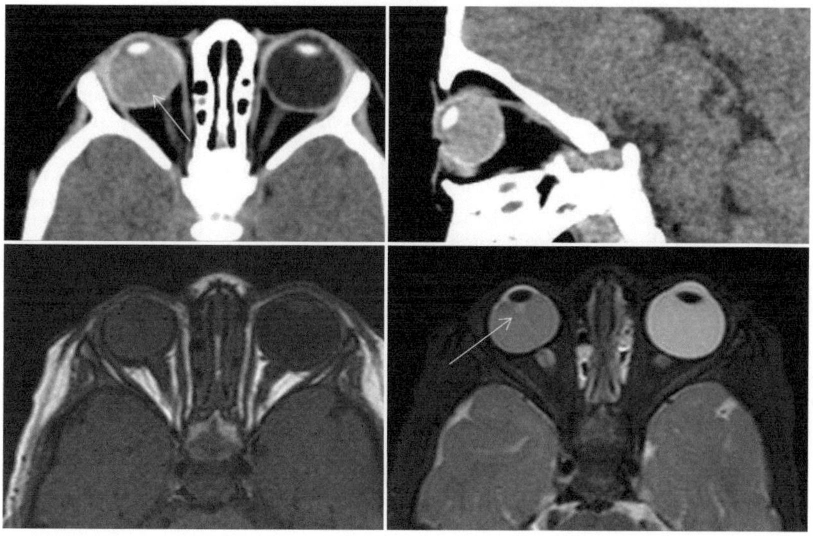

Fig. 13.11 **Persistent hyperplastic primary vitreous (PHPV):** A 3-year-old girl presented with C/o gradual loss of vision for 3 months. CT orbit reveals hyperdensity involving posterior chamber without evident calcification. Right-sided microphthalmos with linear retro-lental soft tissue extending from the head of the optic nerve to the posterior surface of the lens and associated homogeneous abnormal signal in the posterior segment (white arrow)

trauma. It can be ruled out if patient is afebrile and routine investigations are unremarkable [21].

Langerhans cell histiocytosis (LCH) includes a spectrum of disease ranging from benign unifocal bone disease to more aggressive multisystem disease. Eosinophilic granuloma, the most localized and benign form of LCH, usually presents in children less than 4 years of age as unifocal bone disease with possible orbital involvement. It's more commonly seen in males, with involvement of superior temporal orbit. Other associated clinical syndromes include: In infants, Letterer-Siwe disease, involving vital organs with often fatal outcome.

In young children, Hand-Schuller-Christian disease, associated with diabetes insipidus, osteolytic calvarial defects, exophthalmos. In older children or adults, eosinophilic granuloma, shows an indolent unifocal bone disease, with or without orbital involvement [1, 20].

Soft-tissue density eroding osseous structures can be well-defined or diffusely homogeneous, and shows moderate to marked enhancement. MRI shows extent of the disease better, including orbit, temporal fossa, forehead, face, and epidural space. T1 heterogeneous signal, T2 hyperintense or hypointense, and post-contrast enhancement on T1-weighted images. While evaluating intracranial extent, any abnormal thickening/enhancement pituitary gland and stalk should be looked for, or the absence of the posterior pituitary bright spot [20, 21].

References

1. Rao AA, Naheedy JH, Chen JY, Robbins SL, Ramkumar HL. A clinical update and radiologic review of pediatric orbital and ocular tumors. J Oncol. 2013;2013:975908.
2. Expert Panel on Pediatric Imaging, Maheshwari M, Ho ML, et al. ACR Appropriateness Criteria® orbital imaging and vision loss-child. J Am Coll Radiol. 2024;21(6S):S219–36.
3. Nayak BK, Desai S, Maheshwari S. Interpretation of magnetic resonance imaging of orbit: simplified for ophthalmologists (part I). J Clin Ophthalmol Res. 2013;1:29–35.
4. Brennan RC, Wilson MW, Kaste S, Helton KJ, McCarville MB. US and MRI of pediatric ocular masses with histopathological correlation. Pediatr Radiol. 2012;42(6):738–49.
5. Joseph AK, et al. Imaging findings of pediatric orbital masses and tumor mimics. Radiographics. 2022;42(3):880–97.
6. Castillo M, Mukherjee SK, Wagle NS. Imaging of the pediatric orbit. Neuroimaging Clin N Am. 2000;10:95–116.
7. Silva CT, Brockley CR, Crum A, Mandelstam SA. Pediatric ocular sonography. Semin Ultrasound CT MR. 2011;32(1):14–27.
8. Bord SP, Linden J. Trauma to the globe and orbit. Emerg Med Clin North Am. 2008;26(1):97–123, vi–vii.
9. Lee AG, Johnson MC, Policeni BA, Smoker WR. Imaging for neuro-ophthalmic and orbital disease: a review. Clin Experiment Ophthalmol. 2009;37(1):30–53.
10. Goh PS, Gi MT, Charlton A, Tan C, Gangadhara Sundar JK, Amrith S. Review of orbital imaging. Eur J Radiol. 2008;66:387–95.
11. Heran F, Berges O, Blustajn J, et al. Tumor pathology of the orbit. Diagn Interv Imaging. 2014;95:933–44.
12. Lope LA, Hutcheson KA, Khademian ZP. Magnetic resonance imaging in the analysis of pediatric orbital tumors: utility of diffusion-weighted imaging. J AAPOS. 2010;14:257–62.
13. Koch BL, Hamilton B, Hudgins P, Ric Harnsberger H. Diagnostic imaging: head and neck. 3rd ed. London: Elsevier; 2016.
14. Som PM, Curtin HD. Head and neck imaging. 5th ed. Missouri: Mosby; 2011.
15. Pai V, Muthusami P, Ertl-Wagner B, Shroff MM, Parra-Fariñas C, Sainani K, Kletke S, Brundler M-A, Mallipatna A. Diagnostic imaging for retinoblastoma cancer staging: guide for providing essential insights for ophthalmologists and oncologists. Radiographics. 2024;44:4.
16. de Graaf P, Pouwels PJW, Rodjan F, et al. Single-shot turbo spin-echo diffusion-weighted imaging for retinoblastoma: initial experience. Am J Neuroradiol. 2012;33(1):110–8.
17. de Graaf P, Göricke S, Rodjan F, et al. Guidelines for imaging retinoblastoma: imaging principles and MRI standardization. Pediatr Radiol. 2012;42(1):2–14.
18. Roe RH, Finger PT, Kurli M, Tena LB, Iacob CE. Whole body positron emission tomography/computed tomography imaging and staging of orbital lymphoma. Ophthalmology. 2006;113:1854–8.
19. Kumar J, Seith A, Bakhshi S, Kumar R, Kumar A, Sen S. Isolated granulocytic sarcoma of the orbit. Eur J Haematol. 2007;78:456.
20. Chung EM, Murphey MD, Specht CS, Cube R, Smirniotopoulos JG. From the archives of the AFIP. Pediatricorbit tumors and tumorlike lesions: osseous lesions of the orbit. Radiographics. 2008;28:1193–214.
21. Ginat DT, Meyers SP. Intracranial lesions with high signal intensity on T1-weighted MR images: differential diagnosis. Radiographics. 2012;32:499–516.

14 Head and Neck Tumors

Priya Singh and Surya Pratap Singh

14.1 Introduction

Imaging plays a crucial role in the diagnosis, staging, and management of pediatric head and neck tumors, which account for approximately 12% of all pediatric neoplasms. These tumors represent a diverse group of pathologies that can present significant diagnostic and therapeutic challenges [1]. Prompt and accurate diagnosis is essential, as many of these tumors are highly responsive to appropriate oncological treatment [2].

The evaluation of head and neck masses in children requires a comprehensive understanding of the complex anatomy and embryology of this region. The neck contains several critical structures within a relatively small volume, including the airway, major vessels, nerves, and cervical spine [3]. Familiarity with the fascia-defined compartments of the neck is essential for localizing lesions and assessing their extent [4, 5].

Imaging of pediatric head and neck tumors presents unique challenges compared to adult populations. Children have smaller anatomy, necessitating high-resolution techniques for accurate lesion characterization [6]. Radiation exposure is a key concern in pediatric imaging, given the increased radiosensitivity of developing tissues and the potential for long-term carcinogenic effects [7]. Sedation or general anesthesia is often required for cross-sectional imaging in young children, carrying additional risks and resource implications [8, 9].

A multimodality approach to imaging is often necessary, utilizing ultrasound, computed tomography (CT), magnetic resonance imaging (MRI), and nuclear medicine studies in a complementary fashion [10, 11]. The choice of imaging modality depends on the clinical presentation, suspected pathology, and patient factors such as age and ability to cooperate.

In this chapter, we aim to provide a practical, evidence-based approach to the imaging of pediatric head and neck tumors. We will review the key imaging features of common pathologies, discuss the advantages and limitations of various modalities, and present a structured algorithm for diagnostic interpretation.

14.2 Consensus Guidelines for Imaging

Several prominent radiological and oncological societies have published guidelines for the imaging of pediatric head and neck tumors. These guidelines aim to standardize imaging practices, optimize diagnostic accuracy, and minimize radiation exposure in children. Table 14.1 summarizes the existing recommendations for head and neck imaging in children.

P. Singh (✉) · S. P. Singh
Department of Radiodiagnosis, King George Medical University, Lucknow, India

I. Kumar et al. (eds.), *Practical Approach to Imaging in Pediatric Oncology*,
https://doi.org/10.1007/978-981-96-8158-7_14

Table 14.1 Existing recommendations for head and neck imaging in children

	Recommendations
American College of Radiology (ACR) appropriateness criteria [7, 12]	Ultrasound: initial imaging modality for superficial, palpable lesions Contrast-enhanced CT or MRI: for further characterization or suspicion of malignancy MRI: preferred for evaluating soft tissue extent, perineural spread, and intracranial extension CT: superior for assessing cortical bone involvement and detecting calcifications
Society for Pediatric Radiology (SPR) [13, 14]	Ultrasound: first-line modality CT or MRI: reserved for non-diagnostic ultrasound or concern for malignancy Child-specific protocols and optimized techniques to minimize radiation dose Sedation or general anesthesia for high-quality cross-sectional imaging in young children
Children's Oncology Group (COG)	*Lymphoma:* contrast-enhanced CT of the neck, chest, abdomen, and pelvis for initial staging; consider FDG-PET/CT in selected cases [15, 16] *Rhabdomyosarcoma*: MRI for local staging, contrast-enhanced CT of the chest, abdomen, and pelvis for metastatic disease; consider bone scintigraphy or FDG-PET/CT for distant staging [17, 18]
National Comprehensive Cancer Network (NCCN) [19, 20]	*Thyroid carcinoma:* ultrasound for primary tumor and regional lymph nodes Contrast-enhanced CT or MRI of the neck and chest for extrathyroidal extension or metastatic disease Radioactive iodine (RAI) imaging for residual disease and adjuvant therapy decisions

Ultrasound is the initial imaging modality of choice for superficial, palpable lesions in pediatric head and neck tumors. Contrast-enhanced CT or MRI is indicated for further characterization, suspicion of malignancy, or non-diagnostic ultrasound. MRI is preferred for evaluating soft tissue extent, perineural spread, and intracranial extension, while CT is superior for assessing cortical bone involvement and detecting calcifications. Child-specific protocols and optimized techniques should be used to minimize radiation dose. Sedation or general anesthesia may be necessary for high-quality cross-sectional imaging in young children. Specific imaging recommendations are provided by the COG and NCCN for lymphoma, rhabdomyosarcoma, and thyroid carcinoma, respectively. These guidelines provide a framework for the imaging of pediatric head and neck tumors, but imaging decisions must always be individualized based on the specific patient and clinical scenario.

14.3 Relevant Anatomy

A thorough understanding of the complex anatomy of the head and neck region is essential for accurate interpretation of imaging studies and localization of pathology. The neck is divided into various compartments and spaces by layers of fascia, with each space containing specific structures that can give rise to different pathologies. The fascial spaces and their contents provide a framework for understanding the pathways of disease spread and the differential diagnosis based on lesion location.

The important neck spaces, their boundaries, contents, and the common pathology arising from the space are summarized in Table 14.2 [21–29].

Other relevant anatomic structures in the head and neck include the lymph nodes, salivary glands, and thyroid gland. The lymph nodes of the neck are divided into seven levels based on their location relative to the hyoid bone and sternocleidomastoid muscle [30]. Each level has specific drainage pathways and is associated with different primary tumor sites. The salivary glands include the parotid, submandibular, and sublingual glands, as well as numerous minor salivary glands throughout the oral cavity and pharynx.

Table 14.2 Neck spaces, their boundaries, contents, and tumors arising from these spaces

Space	Boundaries	Contents	Common pathology
Parapharyngeal space.(PPS)	Medial: pharyngobasilar fascia Lateral: masticator space, parotid Anterior: pterygomandibular raphe Posterior: carotid fascia, retropharyngeal space	Fat Minor salivary glands Lymph nodes	1. Salivary gland tumors 2. Nodal metastases 3. Primarily affected by mass from adjacent space and structures causing deformity of PPS fat away from its origin
Pharyngeal mucosal space (PMS)	Suprahyoid space	Mucosa Waldeyer's ring Minor salivary glands, Constrictor, levator palatine muscles, Cartilaginous Eustachian tube	1. Malignant tumors (mucosal SCC or NPC and submucosal minor salivary tumors or lymphoma) 2. Infections 3. Congenital lesions (lingual thyroid, thyroglossal cyst)
Masticator (MS)	Skull base to mandibular angle, lateral to PPS	Muscles of mastication Posterior body and ramus of mandible CNV3	1. Odontogenic infections 2. Venous malformations 3. Sarcomas
Retropharyngeal space	Anterior: visceral fascia Posterior: alar fascia	Fat Lymph nodes	1. Nodal metastases 2. Lymphoma 3. Infection
Carotid space	Surrounded by all three layers of deep cervical fascia	Common carotid artery Internal jugular vein Vagus nerve	1. Paraganglioma 2. Nerve sheath tumors 3. Nodal metastases 4. Vascular pathology
Prevertebral space	Anterior: alar fascia Posterior: prevertebral fascia	Fat Prevertebral muscles	1. Chordoma 2. Lymphoma 3. Infection
Posterior triangle	Anterior: posterior border of sternocleidomastoid Posterior: anterior border of trapezius Inferior: clavicle	Fat Lymph nodes Spinal accessory nerve	1. Lymphoma 2. Nodal metastases 3. Venolymphatic malformations
Visceral space	Hyoid to mediastinum Enclosed by middle layer of deep cervical fascia	Thyroid Parathyroid Trachea Larynx Hypopharynx Cervical esophagus Recurrent laryngeal nerve	1. Neoplasm arising from the structures present in its content 2. Infection 3. Thyroglossal cyst 4. Ectopic thyroid tissue

14.4 Structured Radiological Reporting Template

Structured reporting template (Table 14.3) provides a standardized framework for radiological reporting, ensuring consistent and comprehensive communication of imaging findings. The use of checklists in these templates can help to minimize variability and reduce the risk of missing critical findings. We present a checklist-based reporting template for the interpretation of pediatric head and neck tumor imaging, with guidance on how to complete each section based on the imaging appearances.

Table 14.3 Suggested reporting template

Technique	<modality> <protocol> <contrast> <sedation>
Location	<oral cavity: Lip/tongue/check/ palate> <nasal cavity> <sinuses: frontal/ethmoid/maxillary/ sphenoid> <oto-mastoid> <pharynx> <larynx> <parapharyngeal> <retropharyngeal> <prevertebral> <thyroid/thyroglossal> <parotid space> <infratemporal fossa> <posterior triangle>
Size	[--x-x-x] cm <if unmeasurable: describe extent>
Depth	<subcutanous> <intermuscular> <intramuscular> <bone> <specific fascial space>
Laterality	<Right> <left> <midline> <crossing midline>
Shape	<round> <oval> <lobulated> <irregular>
Margins	<well circumscribed> <ill-defined> <infiltrative>
Parenchyma/ internal architecture	<solid> <cystic> <mixed> <homogeneous/heterogeneous> <calcification> <fat> <necrosis> <fluid-fluid levels> <hemorrhage> Describe <T1/T2/ADC/ other characteristics> <attenuation> <vascularity on color doppler/ flow voids/enhancing vessels>
Enhancement	<none> <mild/marked> <heterogenous/homogenous/peripheral> <cyst wall/septal>
Structures involved	<muscles> <bone> <cartilage> <nerves> <vessels>
Perineural spread	<enlarged nerves> <involved canals> <denervation edema/atrophy>
Vessels	<invasion/tumor thrombosis> <encasement> <bland thrombus>
Airway	<compression> <invasion> <effacement>
Intracranial extension	<skull base> <extraaxial> <intraaxial> <parasellar/cavernous sinus>
Lymph nodes	<size> <number> <location> <morphology> <necrosis> <calcification> <extracapsular extension>
Metastasis	Lung/bone/liver/other
Associated findings	<sinusitis> <mastoiditis> <other infections> <dental/periodontal disease> <congenital anomaly or anatomical variant>
Impression	<diagnosis/differential diagnosis> <staging> <recommendations for further imaging, biopsy, or clinical and pathological correlation>

To complete this checklist, the radiologist should systematically review the imaging study, assessing each of the above features. The lesion's location should be described in relation to specific anatomic landmarks and fascial spaces, as this can significantly impact the differential diagnosis.

By systematically applying this checklist to the interpretation of pediatric head and neck tumor imaging, radiologists can ensure a thorough and consistent approach to reporting, ultimately leading to improved patient care.

14.5 Imaging Algorithm for Interpretation and Approach to Diagnosis

Accurate diagnosis of pediatric head and neck tumors requires a systematic approach that integrates imaging findings with clinical information and histopathological data.

The common childhood head and neck malignancies with their imaging features are listed in Table 14.4 [1, 5, 11, 31–39].

We present a flow chart-based algorithm to guide the interpretation of imaging studies and facilitate the differentiation between benign and malignant lesions. (Fig. 14.5):

The first step in the algorithm is to determine the location of the lesion within the specific anatomic subsite and fascial space. This information can significantly narrow the differential diagnosis, as certain tumors have a predilection for specific locations [31].

Next, the imaging characteristics of the lesion should be assessed using the structured template described in the previous section. The internal architecture of the lesion is a key factor in determining its nature. Purely cystic lesions are more likely to be benign, such as branchial cleft cysts, thyroglossal duct cysts, or ranulas [5]. However, some cystic lesions may represent malignancies such as lymphoma or metastatic papillary thyroid

Table 14.4 Imaging features of common pediatric head and neck tumor

Type of mass	Imaging features on USG/CT	Imaging features on MRI
Benign neoplasms		
Infantile hemangioma	Ultrasound: Hypoechoic CT: well-defined, lobulated enhancing mass	Serpenginous flow voids having central feeding vessels and draining veins, T2 hyperintensity, shows intense enhancement May have high T1 signal in later stages due to fat replacement
Juvenile nasopharyngeal angiofibroma (Fig. 14.1)	Highly vascular mass, typically originating in the nasopharynx (sphenopalatine foramen), anterior displacement of posterior wall of maxillary sinus, pterygopalatine fossa involvement, intense enhancement, bony remodeling, destruction, and locally infiltrative. Typical affects adolescent male	Intense enhancement, hypervascular appearance
Schwannoma	Well-circumscribed, encapsulated mass; typically located along nerve pathways, may enhance	Well-defined, encapsulated, T1 isointense, T2 hyperintense, may enhance
Neurofibroma	Fusiform masses along nerve pathways CT: Well-defined, low-attenuation mass with mild enhancement	MRI: isointense to hypointense on T1-weighted images, hyperintense on T2-weighted images (target appearance), heterogeneous enhancement after contrast
Teratoma	Complex, heterogeneous masses with cystic and solid components. Contains fat (hypodense on CT) may have calcification	Variable degrees of cystic, fat, calcified, and solid enhancing components
Juvenile ossifying fibroma	Arise in craniofacial bones of children under the age of 15 years predominantly in maxilla and paranasal sinuses. Well-demarcated lesion with varying degrees of radiolucency and opacity depending on the stage On CT, usually an expansile mass, surrounded by thick or thin radiodense rimming	Low-to-intermediate signal intensity on T1-weighted images and hypointense signal intensity on T2-weighted MR images. There is moderate contrast enhancement on postgadolinium T1-weighted MRI scans
Paraganglioma (Fig. 14.2)	Highly vascular mass with typical location in neck at carotid bifurcation causing splaying of arteries. Other location are jugular foramen, along vagal nerve and middle ear Cause permeative erosion of bone	Salt-and-pepper appearance on T2 due to flow voids. High T2 signal, intermediate T1 signal, and intense enhancement
Dentigerous cysts	Well-circumscribed, unilocular radiolucent lesion associated with the crown of an unerupted tooth	MRI: cystic lesion, T2 hyperintense
Ameloblastoma	Multilocular radiolucent lesion with well-defined borders, may show expansion and thinning of cortical bone	T1 hypointense, T2 hyperintense, enhances post-contrast
Odontogenic keratocyst	Unilocular or multilocular radiolucent lesion, often shows cortical expansion, may recur	Variable signal intensity, T2 hyperintense, may show enhancement

(continued)

Table 14.4 (continued)

Type of mass	Imaging features on USG/CT	Imaging features on MRI
Melanotic neuroectodermal tumor of infancy (MNTI)	Rare, benign, and locally aggressive tumor of infants involving craniofacial bones maxilla. Well-demarcated radiolucent lesion with cortical bone expansion, tooth displacement, reactive sclerosis. Soft tissue lesions are slightly hyperdense	Inhomogeneously isointense to hyperintense on T1-weighted images and isointense or hypointense on T2-weighted images. Shows intense enhancement
Malignant neoplasms		
Rhabdomyosarcoma (Fig. 14.3)	Heterogeneous mass with areas of necrosis and hemorrhage; shows enhancement Two types: parameningeal (skull base, orbit, and nasopharynx) non-parameningeal (neck)	MRI: to assess intracranial extension involvement of vascular structures (internal carotid artery, jugular vein, and dural venous sinuses) cranial nerves or tumor along the skull base foramina
Nasopharyngeal carcinoma	Enhancing mass in the nasopharynx; may show invasion of adjacent structures CT: Useful for assessing bone involvement	MRI: Enhancing mass, useful for assessing neural and brain involvement
Neuroblastoma (Fig. 14.4)	Heterogeneous mass. May have calcification	MRI: T1 isointense to hypointense, T2 hyperintense, shows enhancement
Thyroid carcinoma (papillary thyroid carcinoma)	Solid, hypoechoic nodule, irregular borders, microcalcifications, cervical lymphadenopathy TI-RADS: not validated in pediatric age	T1: iso- to hypointense, T2: hyper- to isointense, heterogeneous enhancement, cervical lymphadenopathy
Ewing sarcoma/ peripheral primitive neuroectodermal tumor	Very aggressive mass, permeative destruction of bone, invasion into surrounding tissues	Variable signal intensity predominately moderate to mild hyperintensity on T2 and heterogeneous mild enhancement
Langerhans cell histiocytosis	Lytic bone lesions, with beveled edges often involving the skull	Variable signal intensity depending on lesion activity
Lymphoma	Homogeneous, enhancing non-necrotic masses present as diffuse and bulky lymphadenopathy	Isointense on T1 and hyperintense on T2-weighted images. Diffusion-weighted imaging (DWI) can help differentiate based on ADC values
Chloroma/myeloid sarcoma	Orbit, skull, and epidural spaces are common sites. Multiple lesions, iso-dense or hyper-dense to brain or muscle on NC CT, well-demarcated, and mildly and homogenously enhancing masses with adjacent bony invasion Can present as lymph nodal mass, or tonsillar enlargement	Hypo-intense or iso-intense on T1-weighted MR images, heterogeneously iso-intense or hyper-intense on T2-weighted MR images, and homogeneous enhancement

carcinoma, particularly if they demonstrate thick or irregular walls, septations, or solid components [32].

Solid lesions can be further characterized based on their attenuation or signal intensity, enhancement pattern, and presence of calcifications or fat. Lesions with macroscopic fat are most likely to represent benign entities such as lipomas or dermoid cysts [33]. The presence of calcifications can also favor benign lesions such as hemangiomas or teratomas, although some malignancies like thyroid carcinoma and metastatic sarcoma can also demonstrate calcifications [11].

The enhancement pattern of a solid lesion can provide valuable diagnostic clues. Homogeneous enhancement is more common in benign tumors such as pleomorphic adenomas or schwannomas, while heterogeneous or peripheral enhancement may indicate a malignancy such as rhabdomyosarcoma or squamous cell carcinoma [31]. The presence of necrosis or cystic degeneration is

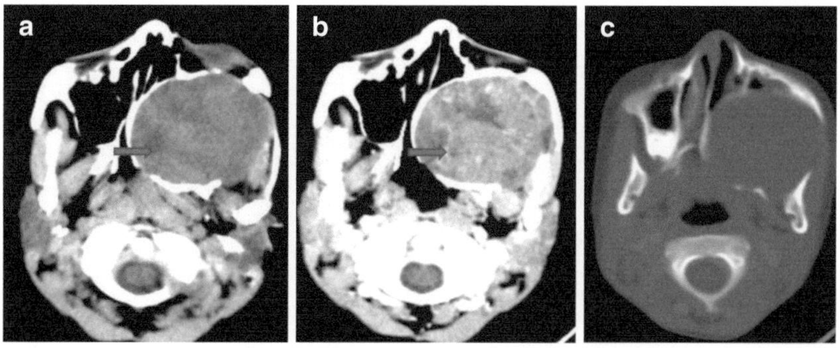

Fig. 14.1 Juvenile nasal angiofibroma. Axial non-contrast computed tomography (NCCT) (**a**); contrast-enhanced CT(CECT) (**b**); bone window (**c**) in a 14-year-old male boy shows a well-defined heterogeneously enhancing mass lesion (blue arrows) in left infratemporal fossa involving left pterygopataine fossa and sphenopalataine foramen with widening of left pterygomaxillary fissure and anterior scalloping of posterior wall of left maxillary sinus (white arrow). It causes erosion/rarefaction of left lesser, greater wing of sphenoid (white arrow) and left pterygoid plates

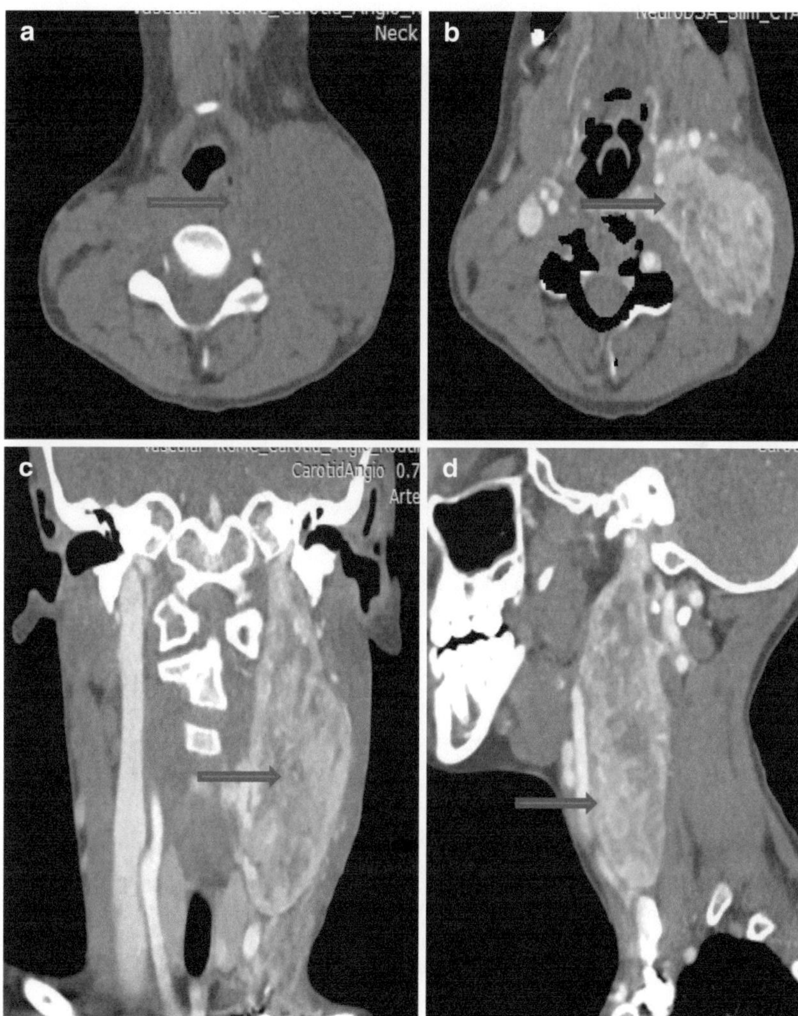

Fig. 14.2 Vagal paraganglioma. Non-contrast computed tomography (NCCT) axial (**a**); contrast-enhanced CT(CECT) axial (**b**); contrast-enhanced CT(CECT) coronal (**c**); contrast-enhanced CT(CECT) sagittal (**d**) in a 17-year-old male boy shows a well-defined intensely enhancing mass lesion (blue arrows) in left carotid space displacing left carotid vessels anteriorly and IJV posterior with its marked compression. It reaches upto the jugular foramen of skull base with its widening

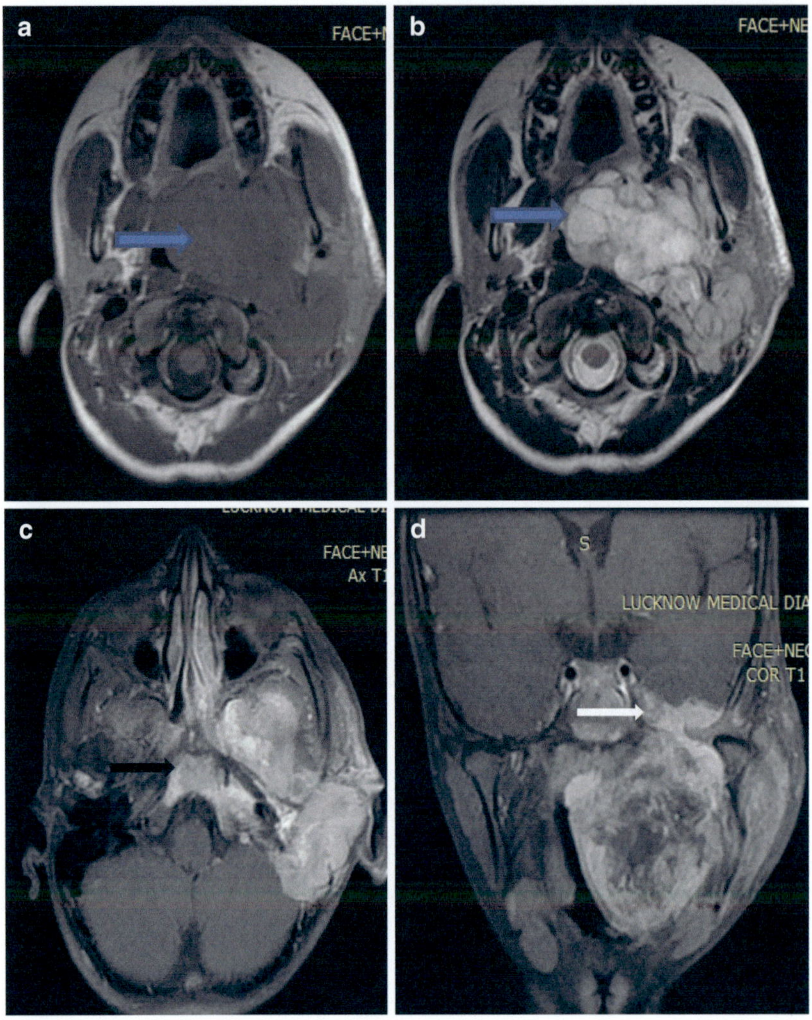

Fig. 14.3 Rhabdomyosracoma. Magnetic resonance imaging (MRI), T1-weighted axial image (**a**); T2-weighted axial image (**b**); post-contrast T1-weighted axial image (**c**); post-contrast T1-weighted coronal image (**d**) in a 6-year-old male boy shows a poorly defined heterogeneously enhancing mass lesion (blue arrows) with central necrosis in left parapharyngeal space involving left oropharynx, carotid space, masticator space, and left mastoid region. It involves the left greater wing of sphenoid (white arrow), left pterygoid plates, sphenoid bone (black arrow), and pertous bone. The mass shows perineural spread along foramen ovale into brain (white arrow) with parameningeal involvement in middle and posterior cranial fossa

another worrisome feature that suggests an aggressive or malignant process.

The vascularity of the lesion should also be considered. Hypervascular lesions with multiple flow voids on MRI or prominent vessels on contrast-enhanced CT are more likely to represent juvenile nasopharyngeal angiofibromas, hemangiomas, or hypervascular metastases such as those from thyroid carcinoma [34]. Lesions with a more moderate degree of enhancement may still be benign, but the possibility of a low-grade malignancy should be considered.

The extent of the lesion and its impact on adjacent structures is another critical factor in determining the likelihood of malignancy. Benign lesions tend to be well-circumscribed and do not typically invade or destroy adjacent tissues. Malignant tumors, on the other hand, often

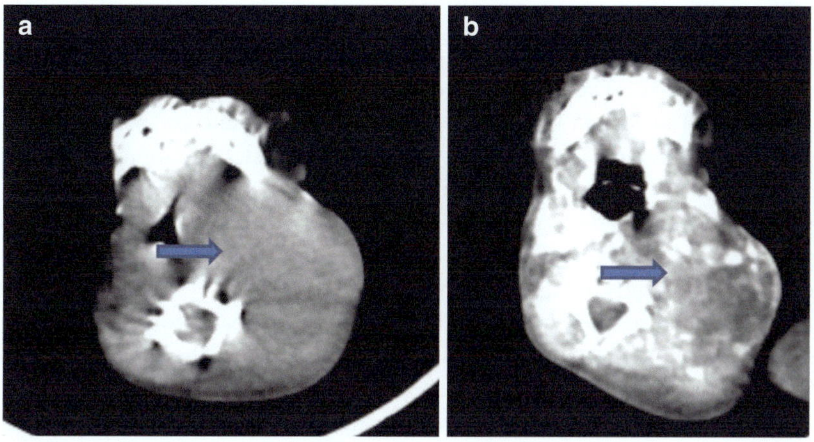

Fig. 14.4 Neuroblastoma. Axial non-contrast computed tomography (NCCT) (**a**); contrast-enhanced CT(CECT) (**b**) in a 2-year-old male child shows a poorly defined heterogeneously enhancing mass lesion (blue arrows) on the left side of neck involving left posterior triangle of neck, carotid, prevertebral, and parapharyngeal spaces with erosion of adjacent bones

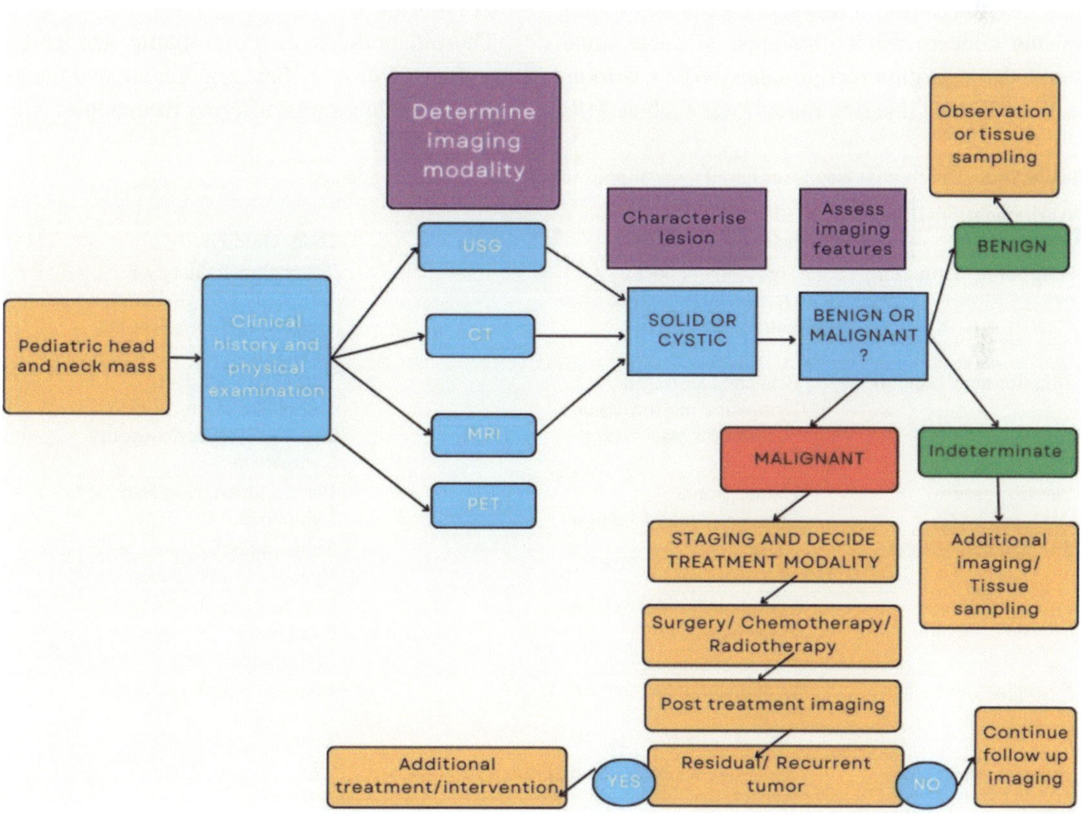

Fig. 14.5 Flowchart-based algorithm for the interpretation of pediatric head and neck tumor imaging and approach to diagnosis

demonstrate infiltrative margins, perineural spread, vascular encasement, airway invasion, or intracranial extension [35]. The presence of lymph node involvement or distant metastases is also a strong indicator of malignancy.

Based on the integration of these imaging features, the algorithm guides the radiologist towards a working diagnosis or differential diagnosis. If the lesion demonstrates clearly benign features such as a purely cystic nature, presence of fat or calcifications, and lack of aggressive characteristics, a confident diagnosis of a benign entity can be made. If the lesion shows definite signs of malignancy such as infiltrative margins, necrosis, or metastatic disease, a malignant diagnosis should be suggested, and the patient should be referred for immediate biopsy or resection.

However, in many cases, the imaging findings may be indeterminate or equivocal, with some features suggesting a benign process and others raising concern for malignancy. In these situations, the algorithm recommends further workup with additional imaging modalities, such as MRI for better soft tissue characterization or PET/CT for metabolic assessment. If the lesion remains indeterminate after additional imaging, tissue sampling should be performed to establish a definitive histopathological diagnosis [36].

It is important to emphasize that this algorithm serves as a general guide and should be used in conjunction with clinical judgment and multidisciplinary collaboration. Some lesions may not fit neatly into the benign or malignant categories, and the final diagnosis should be based on a combination of imaging, clinical, and pathological findings. By using this systematic approach, however, radiologists can improve the accuracy and consistency of their interpretations and guide appropriate management for children with head and neck tumors.

The differential diagnosis can be further narrowed based on the patient's age and lesion location (Table 14.5).

Thyroid nodules in the pediatric age group have more chances of being malignant and therefore their evaluation is different from adults. The

Table 14.5 Differential diagnoses based on anatomic subsite, fascial space, and age

Anatomic subsite/fascial space	Infant/neonate	Older children
Anterior neck (midline)	Thyroglossal duct cyst Dermoid/epidermoid cyst Ectopic thyroid	Thyroglossal duct cyst Dermoid/epidermoid cyst Thyroid lesions (adenoma, carcinoma)
Anterior neck (lateral)	Branchial cleft cyst Lymphatic malformation Neuroblastoma	Branchial cleft cyst Lymphatic malformation Reactive lymphadenopathy Lymphoma
Parotid space	Hemangioma Lymphatic malformation	Parotid gland neoplasm Lymphoma
Submandibular space	Ranula Hemangioma	Submandibular gland neoplasms Reactive lymphadenopathy
Posterior triangle	Lymphatic malformation Fibromatosis colli	Reactive lymphadenopathy Lymphoma Metastatic disease
Retropharyngeal space	Lymphatic malformation	Reactive lymphadenopathy Lymphoma Juvenile angiofibroma
Bony lesion	Melanotic neuroectodermal tumor of infancy (MNTI) Chloroma Neuroblastoma	Langerhans cell histiocytosis (LCH) Odontogenic keratocyst Ameloblastoma Dentigerous cysts Juvenile ossifying fibroma chloroma

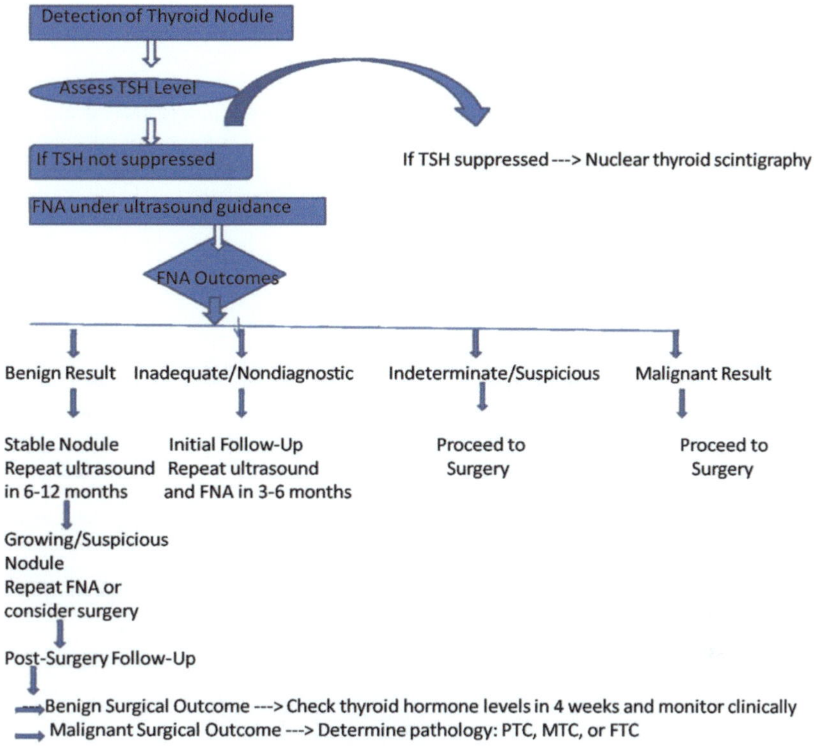

Fig. 14.6 Flowchart-based algorithm based on ATA guidelines for the pediatric solitary thyroid nodule evaluation

American Thyroid Association (ATA) has given guidelines on evaluation of solitary/suspicious thyroid nodule >=1 cm in pediatric age group which is summarized in Fig. 14.6.

14.6 Post-treatment Imaging

Imaging plays a crucial role in assessing treatment response, detecting complications, and identifying recurrence in children with head and neck tumors. The post-treatment imaging protocol and interpretation depend on the specific type of therapy administered, which may include surgery, chemotherapy, and/or radiation therapy. This has been summarized in the following (Table 14.6) as well as in the form of flowchart (Fig. 14.7). There are numerous complications that can arise following treatment of these tumors, which require specific imaging modality and imaging protocol for evaluation. The imaging of post-treatment complication has been summarized in Table 14.7. The structured reporting template is given in Table 14.8 for post-treatment imaging which reduces the variability and errors in reporting and helps in response assessment.

Table 14.6 Summarizes the post-treatment imaging and management in pediatric head and neck tumor

Treatment modality	Imaging goals	Imaging modalities	Key imaging features
Surgery [1, 31, 35, 37, 38]	Assess completeness of resection Identify residual tumor Detect complications (hematoma, infection, nerve injury)	Immediate post-op: CT or MRI Follow-up: modality based on tumor type and risk of recurrence	Residual tumor: Enhancing soft tissue in surgical bed (may be reactive in early post-op period) Complications: hematoma, abscess, nerve or vascular injury
Chemotherapy [39–42]	Assess treatment response (RECIST criteria) Detect residual or recurrent disease Identify treatment-related complications	CT MRI PET/CT	Response assessment: change in tumor size per RECIST Residual disease: persistent enhancing soft tissue (may represent necrosis/fibrosis rather than viable tumor) Complications: mucositis, neutropenic enterocolitis, venous thrombosis
Radiation therapy [43–46]	Assess treatment response Detect recurrent disease Identify radiation-induced complications	CT MRI PET/CT	Radiation changes: edema, fibrosis, necrosis of soft tissues; osteoradionecrosis and fatty marrow replacement in bones Recurrent tumor: growing enhancing mass, invasion of adjacent structures Complications: mucositis, xerostomia, trismus, radiation-induced vasculopathy

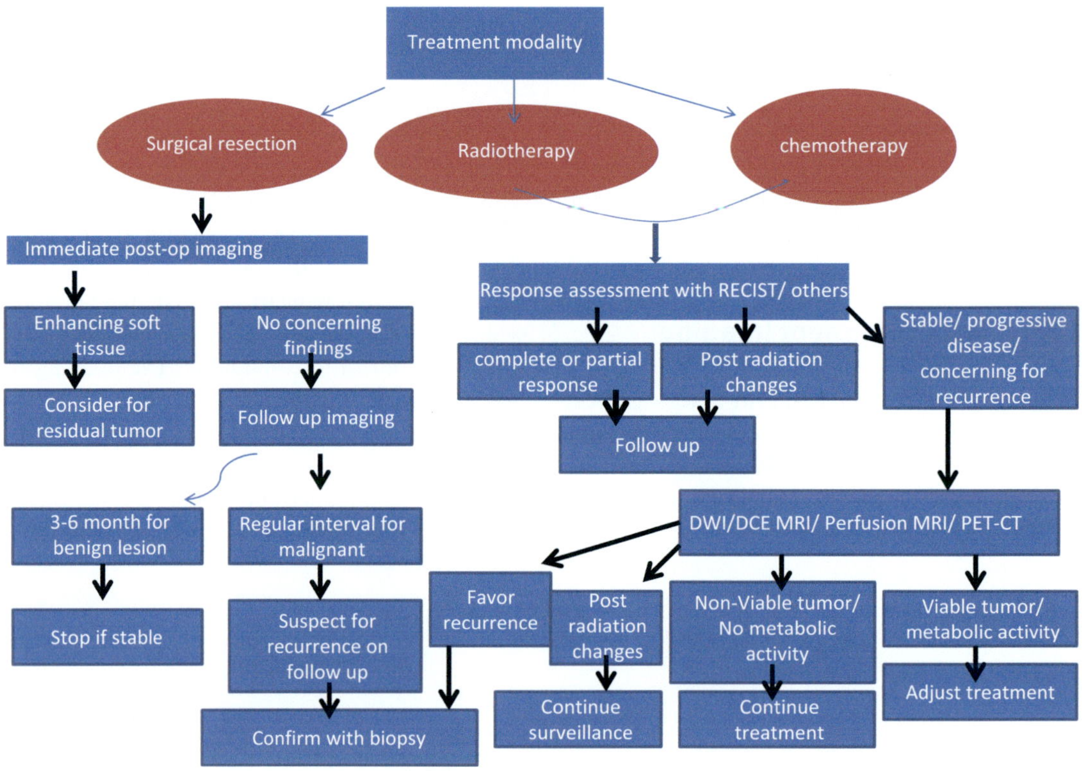

Fig. 14.7 Flowchart-based algorithm for posttreatment imaging protocol and interpretation

Table 14.7 Post-treatment complications and imaging protocols

Complication	Imaging findings	Preferred modality
Recurrent/residual disease	Enhancing soft tissue, restricted diffusion, hypermetabolic activity	MRI with DWI, PET/CT
Radiation-induced changes	Edema, fibrosis, necrosis, fatty marrow replacement	MRI
Surgical site infection	Fluid collections, rim-enhancing lesions, adjacent inflammatory changes	CT with contrast, MRI
Vascular injury	Pseudoaneurysm, arteriovenous fistula, venous thrombosis	CTA, MRA, Doppler ultrasound
Cranial neuropathy	Denervation changes in muscles, nerve thickening/ enhancement	MRI with high-resolution sequences

Table 14.8 Post-treatment imaging reporting template

Technique	<modality> <protocol> <contrast> <sedation>
Treatment history	<surgery> <chemotherapy> <radiation therapy>
Baseline imaging	<date> <modality> <key findings>
Tumor site	<location> <size>
Residual disease	<location> <size> <extent> <morphology> <enhancement pattern> <diffusion restriction (ADC value)> <metabolic activity (SUV on PET)>
Treatment changes	<edema> <necrosis> <fibrosis> <fat replacement> <atrophy> <hemorrhage> <calcification> <radiation-induced inflammation>
Complications	<infection> <fistula> <abscess> <nerve injury> <vascular injury> <bone necrosis> <secondary malignancy>
Lymph nodes	<size> <morphology> <enhancement patter> <necrosis> <extracapsular extension> <metabolic activity (SUV on PET)>
Metastases I	<location> <size> <enhancement pattern> <metabolic activity (SUV on PET)>
Impression	<treatment response (complete, partial, stable, progressive)> <presence and extent of residual/ recurrent disease> <complications> <recommendations for further management>

14.7 Tumor Recurrence

The early detection of tumor recurrence is critical for guiding further treatment and improving outcomes in children with head and neck malignancies. The imaging features of recurrent tumors vary depending on the specific histology and location but often include a growing enhancing soft tissue mass, invasion of adjacent structures, and new or enlarging lymphadenopathy [47].

To differentiate residual/recurrent tumor from post-treatment changes:

- Diffusion-weighted imaging (DWI): [45]
  - Residual/recurrent tumor shows restricted diffusion (low ADC)
  - Post-treatment changes show facilitated diffusion (high ADC)
- PET/CT:
  - Residual/recurrent tumor exhibits increased metabolic activity (high SUV)
  - Post-treatment changes are usually hypometabolic (low SUV) [48]
- However, false-positive findings can occur due to inflammation, infection, or treatment-related changes, and correlation with clinical findings and biopsy may be necessary to confirm the diagnosis.

Specific post-treatment imaging protocols for certain tumors:

- Lymphoma: PET/CT for response assessment and surveillance
- Rhabdomyosarcoma: MRI for primary site, CT chest/abdomen/pelvis for metastases; routine imaging every 3 months in year 1, every 4 months in years 2–3, annually for 2 more years [49]
- Thyroid carcinoma: Radioactive iodine (RAI) imaging to detect residual/recurrent disease and guide adjuvant therapy.

14.8 Tumor Mimics

Differentiating tumor mimics from true pediatric head and neck tumors is crucial for accurate diagnosis and appropriate management. Tumor mimics, such as congenital cysts, inflammatory, and infective lesions, can present with similar clinical and imaging features as malignant or benign tumors, leading to potential misdiagnosis [5, 32, 35]. Accurate identification of these mimics helps avoid unnecessary invasive procedures, reduces patient and family anxiety. Imaging techniques, such as ultrasound, CT, and MRI, play a key role in distinguishing these entities by highlighting their unique characteristics, which aids in formulating an accurate differential diagnosis. The common tumor mimics in the pediatric head and neck region are summarized in Table 14.9, with a focus on their imaging characteristics.

Table 14.9 The common tumor mimics in the pediatric head and neck region

Thyroglossal duct cyst	Congenital	Midline cystic lesion, typically near the hyoid bone. Anechoic or hypoechoic on USG with posterior enhancement; low attenuation on CT; high T2 signal on MRI with possible thin rim enhancement if infected
Branchial cleft cyst	Congenital	Lateral neck cyst near the sternocleidomastoid muscle. Anechoic or hypoechoic on USG; fluid-attenuation on CT; high T2 signal on MRI with rim enhancement if infected
Dermoid/epidermoid cyst	Congenital	Cystic lesion may contain internal debris or fat. Hypoechoic on USG; low density with possible fat and calcifications on CT; variable T1 signal on MRI, no enhancement
Lymphangioma (cystic hygroma)	Congenital	Multiloculated cystic mass, often with septations. Anechoic or hypoechoic on USG; low attenuation on CT; high T2 signal on MRI with internal septations and possible fluid-fluid levels
Ranula	Congenital	Cystic lesion in the floor of the mouth. Anechoic or hypoechoic on USG with posterior enhancement; fluid attenuation on CT; high T2 signal on MRI, no enhancement
Ectopic thyroid	Congenital	Homogeneous mass, usually in midline, resembling thyroid tissue. Hypoechoic on USG, similar to normal thyroid tissue; soft-tissue density on CT; iso- to hyperintense on MRI, with homogeneous enhancement
Inflammatory adenopathy	Inflammatory	Enlarged lymph nodes with preserved hilum. Hypoechoic on USG; homogeneous or heterogeneous enhancement on CT; low to intermediate T1 and high T2 signal on MRI
Suppurative lymphadenitis	Infective	Enlarged lymph nodes with central liquefaction. Hypoechoic with internal echoes on USG; low attenuation with rim enhancement on CT; high T2 signal with central necrosis on MRI
Tonsillar abscess (peritonsillar or retropharyngeal)	Infective	Hypoechoic or anechoic collection with internal debris and septations on USG; hypodense with rim enhancement on CT; high T2 signal with surrounding inflammatory changes on MRI
Fibromatosis colli	Congenital	Fusiform enlargement of the sternocleidomastoid muscle. Hypoechoic with striated appearance on USG; homogeneous enhancement on CT; iso- to hyperintense on MRI with mild enhancement

14.9 Recent Updates and Future Directions

Advances in imaging techniques and the application of artificial intelligence (AI) have significantly improved the diagnosis, treatment planning, and prognostication of pediatric head and neck tumors. These developments have the potential to revolutionize the management of these complex conditions.

1. Diffusion-weighted imaging (DWI):

   Quantitative apparent diffusion coefficient (ADC) values can help differentiate benign from malignant lesions and assess treatment response [50–52]. Malignant tumors typically demonstrate lower ADC values ($0.6–1.2 \times 10^{-3}$ mm^2/s) compared to benign lesions ($1.4–2.0 \times 10^{-3}$ mm^2/s). An increase in ADC values (>30%) after treatment suggests a favorable response, while a decrease or lack of change may indicate residual/recurrent disease.
2. Perfusion imaging and arterial spin labeling (ASL):

   Dynamic contrast-enhanced (DCE) MRI and ASL can provide quantitative measures of tumor vascularity and perfusion. Malignant tumors exhibit higher Ktrans (>0.2 min^{-1}) and kep (>0.5 min^{-1}) values compared to benign lesions [53]. ASL-derived tumor blood flow (TBF) values >100 mL/100 g/min are suggestive of malignancy [53]. Early changes in perfusion parameters (>20% decrease in Ktrans or TBF) after treatment may predict favorable outcomes.
3. Magnetic resonance spectroscopy (MRS):

   MRS can detect metabolic alterations in tumors, such as increased choline (Cho) and decreased N-acetylaspartate (NAA) levels [43]. Malignant tumors demonstrate higher Cho/Cr ratios (>2.0) and lower NAA/Cr ratios (<1.0) compared to benign lesions. A decrease in Cho/Cr ratio (>30%) after treatment suggests a favorable response.
4. Hybrid imaging:

   Another major development has been the increasing use of hybrid imaging modalities, such as PET/CT and PET/MRI, which combine the functional information of PET with the anatomic detail of CT or MRI [54].

   PET/CT has become the standard of care for staging and response assessment in pediatric lymphomas, while PET/MRI has shown promise in reducing radiation exposure and providing additional functional information in head and neck sarcomas [54].

   The development of novel PET tracers has also expanded the role of molecular imaging in pediatric head and neck tumors.

   In addition to the conventional FDG tracer, newer tracers such as 18F-fluorothymidine (FLT) and 18F-fluoromisonidazole (FMISO) have been used to evaluate tumor proliferation and hypoxia, respectively [55]. These tracers may help guide targeted therapies and predict treatment response.
5. Advances in ultrasound technology:

   High-frequency transducers, elastography, and contrast-enhanced ultrasound have improved the diagnostic accuracy of this modality in evaluating superficial head and neck lesions [56]. Ultrasound elastography has shown promise in differentiating benign from malignant thyroid nodules. Contrast-enhanced ultrasound has been used to evaluate tumor vascularity and response to treatment [57].
6. Radiomics and machine learning:

   Radiomics involves the extraction of quantitative features from medical images to create predictive models for diagnosis, prognosis, and treatment response [58]. Machine learning algorithms can analyze these radiomic features to develop automated classification systems for pediatric head and neck tumors. Preliminary studies have shown promising results, with accuracies ranging from 80% to 95% for differentiating benign from malignant lesions and predicting treatment outcomes.
7. Deep learning and convolutional neural networks (CNNs):

   CNNs are a type of deep learning architecture that can automatically learn hierarchical features from medical images [59]. These networks have been applied to various tasks in pediatric head and neck tumor imaging, such as tumor segmentation, detection, and classification. Recent studies have demonstrated the potential of CNNs to improve the accuracy and efficiency of tumor delineation for radiation therapy planning, with Dice similarity coefficients >0.8 [60].

8. Radiogenomics and multi-omics integration:

   Radiogenomics explores the relationship between imaging phenotypes and gene expression profiles in tumors [61]. The integration of radiomic, genomic, and other omics data (e.g., proteomics, metabolomics) may provide a more comprehensive understanding of tumor biology and behavior. This approach has the potential to identify novel imaging biomarkers and guide personalized treatment strategies for pediatric head and neck tumors.

   Finally, the increasing use of minimally invasive and image-guided interventions, such as biopsies, ablations, and drug delivery, may improve the safety and effectiveness of diagnostic and therapeutic procedures in children with head and neck tumors [62]. The development of new image guidance technologies, such as real-time MRI and 3D ultrasound, may further enhance the precision and accuracy of these procedures.

References

1. Sengupta S, Pal R. Clinicopathological correlates of pediatric head and neck cancer. J Cancer Res Ther. 2009;5(3):181–5.
2. Albright JT, Topham AK, Reilly JS. Pediatric head and neck malignancies: US incidence and trends over 2 decades. Arch Otolaryngol Head Neck Surg. 2002;128(6):655–9.
3. Mukherji SK, Chong V. Atlas of head and neck imaging. New York: Thieme; 2004.
4. Som PM, Curtin HD, Mancuso AA. An imaging-based classification for the cervical nodes designed as an adjunct to recent clinically based nodal classifications. Arch Otolaryngol Head Neck Surg. 1999;125(4):388–96.
5. Koeller KK, Alamo L, Adair CF, Smirniotopoulos JG. Congenital cystic masses of the neck: radiologic-pathologic correlation. Radiographics. 1999;19(1):121–46.
6. Vazquez E, Enriquez G, Castellote A, et al. US, CT, and MR imaging of neck lesions in children. Radiographics. 1995;15(1):105–22.
7. Siegel MJ. Neck masses. In: Siegel MJ, editor. Pediatric sonography. 5th ed. Philadelphia: Wolters Kluwer; 2018. p. 149–98.
8. Brenner DJ, Hall EJ. Computed tomography—an increasing source of radiation exposure. N Engl J Med. 2007;357(22):2277–84.
9. Machata AM, Willschke H, Kabon B, Kettner SC, Marhofer P. Propofol-based sedation regimen for infants and children undergoing ambulatory magnetic resonance imaging. Br J Anaesth. 2008;101(2):239–43.
10. Nour SG, Lewin JS. Pediatric head and neck malignancies. Neuroimaging Clin N Am. 2000;10(1):139–51, viii.
11. Brown RE, Harave S. Diagnostic imaging of benign and malignant neck masses in children-a pictorial review. Quant Imaging Med Surg. 2016;6(5):591–604.
12. Abdel Razek AAK, King A. MRI and CT of neck lesions in children. Eur Radiol. 2012;22(6):1089–100.
13. Goodwin A, Olson M, Tomich C, Carrico C, Elluru R. Pediatric neck masses: an evidence-based imaging approach. Pediatr Radiol. 2020;50(11):1575–87.
14. Strauss KJ, Kaste SC. The ALARA (as low as reasonably achievable) concept in pediatric interventional and fluoroscopic imaging: striving to keep radiation doses as low as possible during fluoroscopy of pediatric patients—a white paper executive summary. Pediatr Radiol. 2006;36(Suppl 2):110–2.
15. Flerlage JE, Kelly KM, Beishuizen A, et al. Staging evaluation and response criteria harmonization (SEARCH) for childhood, adolescent and young adult Hodgkin lymphoma (CAYAHL): methodology statement. Pediatr Blood Cancer. 2017;64(7):e26421.
16. Voss SD. Staging and following common pediatric malignancies: MRI versus CT versus functional imaging. Pediatr Radiol. 2018;48(9):1324–36.
17. Brindle M, Flerlage J, Krasin M, et al. Imaging of rhabdomyosarcoma: a multidisciplinary approach. Pediatr Radiol. 2021;51(9):1602–17.
18. Bhargava R, Shapeero LG. Imaging pediatric sarcomas. Radiol Clin North Am. 2016;54(6):1101–25.
19. Francis GL, Waguespack SG, Bauer AJ, et al. Management guidelines for children with thyroid nodules and differentiated thyroid cancer. Thyroid. 2015;25(7):716–59.
20. Parisi MT, Eslamy H, Mankoff D. Management of differentiated thyroid cancer in children: focus on the American Thyroid Association pediatric guidelines. Semin Nucl Med. 2016;46(2):147–64.
21. Gamss C, Gupta A, Chazen JL, Phillips CD. Imaging evaluation of the suprahyoid neck. Radiol Clin North Am. 2015;53(1):133–44.
22. Smoker WR, Harnsberger HR. Differential diagnosis of head and neck lesions based on their space of origin. 2. The infrahyoid portion of the neck. AJR Am J Roentgenol. 1991;157(1):155–9.

23. Guidera AK, Dawes PJ, Fong A, Stringer MD. Head and neck fascia and compartments: no space for spaces. Head Neck. 2014;36(7):1058–68.
24. Stambuk HE, Patel SG. Imaging of the parapharyngeal space. Otolaryngol Clin N Am. 2008;41(1):77–101, vi.
25. Debnam JM, Guha-Thakurta N. Retropharyngeal and prevertebral spaces: anatomic imaging and diagnosis. Otolaryngol Clin N Am. 2012;45(6):1293–310.
26. Vieira F, Allen SM, Stocks RM, Thompson JW. Deep neck infection. Otolaryngol Clin N Am. 2008;41(3):459–83, vii.
27. Meltzer DE, Shatzkes DR. Masticator space: imaging anatomy for diagnosis. Otolaryngol Clin N Am. 2012;45(6):1233–51.
28. Aygenc E, Kaymakci M, Karaca S, Ozdem C. Carotid body tumors and our surgical approaches. Kulak Burun Bogaz Ihtis Derg. 2003;11(2):47–52.
29. Policeni BA, Smoker WR, Reede DL. Anatomy and embryology of the thyroid and parathyroid glands. Semin Ultrasound CT MR. 2012;33(2):104–14.
30. Som PM, Curtin HD, Mancuso AA. Imaging-based nodal classification for evaluation of neck metastatic adenopathy. AJR Am J Roentgenol. 2000;174(3):837–44.
31. Robson CD. Imaging of head and neck neoplasms in children. Pediatr Radiol. 2010;40(4):499–509.
32. Restrepo R, Oneto J, Lopez K, Kukreja K. Head and neck lymph nodes in children: the spectrum from normal to abnormal. Pediatr Radiol. 2009;39(8):836–46.
33. Harnsberger HR. Diagnostic imaging: head and neck. 2nd ed. Salt Lake City: Amirsys; 2011.
34. Parikh ND, Chaudhry A, Gandhi D, et al. Imaging evaluation and management of pediatric head and neck tumors. Neuroimaging Clin N Am. 2000;10(1):153–67.
35. Vázquez E, Enríquez G, Castellote A, et al. US, CT, and MR imaging of neck lesions in children. Radiographics. 1995;15(1):105–22.
36. Cesmebasi A, Gabriel A, Niku D, Bukala K, Donnelly J, Fields PJ. Pediatric head and neck tumors: an intra-demographic analysis using the SEER* database. Med Sci Monit. 2014;20:2536–42.
37. Smoker WR. The postoperative neck. Radiol Clin North Am. 2000;38(4):667–88.
38. Abdel Razek AA, King A. MRI and CT of neck lesions in children. Eur Radiol. 2012;22(6):1089–100.
39. Sandlund JT, Downing JR, Crist WM. Non-Hodgkin's lymphoma in childhood. N Engl J Med. 1996;334(19):1238–48.
40. Eisenhauer EA, Therasse P, Bogaerts J, et al. New response evaluation criteria in solid tumours: revised RECIST guideline (version 1.1). Eur J Cancer. 2009;45(2):228–47.
41. Marcus KJ, Tishler RB. Head and neck carcinomas across the age spectrum: epidemiology, therapy, and late effects. Semin Radiat Oncol. 2010;20(1):52–7.
42. Kaste SC. Imaging pediatric head and neck cancer. Cancer Treat Res. 2008;143:135–61.
43. Alfouzan AF. Radiation therapy in head and neck cancer. Saudi Med J. 2021;42(3):247–54. https://doi.org/10.15537/smj.2021.42.3.20210660.
44. Glastonbury CM, Parker EE, Hoang JK. The post-radiation neck: evaluating response to treatment and recognizing complications. AJR Am J Roentgenol. 2010;195(2):W164–71.
45. King AD, Thoeny HC. Functional MRI for the prediction of treatment response in head and neck squamous cell carcinoma: potential and limitations. Cancer Imaging. 2016;16(1):23.
46. Gensheimer MF, Liao JJ, Garden AS, et al. Submandibular gland-sparing radiation therapy for locally advanced oropharyngeal squamous cell carcinoma: patterns of failure and xerostomia outcomes. Radiat Oncol. 2014;9:255.
47. Vaid S, Chandorkar A, Atre A, Shah D, Vaid N. Differentiating recurrent tumours from post-treatment changes in head and neck cancers: does functional imaging help? Clin Radiol. 2017;72(2):96–111.
48. Marcus C, Ciarallo A, Tahari AK, et al. Head and neck PET/CT: therapy response interpretation criteria (Hopkins criteria)-interreader reliability, accuracy, and survival outcomes. J Nucl Med. 2014;55(9):1411–6.
49. Freling NJ, et al. Imaging findings in craniofacial childhood rhabdomyosarcoma. Pediatr Radiol. 2010;40(11):1723–38. https://doi.org/10.1007/s00247-010-1787-3.
50. Rao A, Sharma C, Parampalli R. Role of diffusion-weighted MRI in differentiating benign from malignant bone tumors. BJR|Open. 2019;1(1):20180048. https://doi.org/10.1259/bjro.20180048.
51. Abdel Razek AA, Gaballa G, Elhawarey G, Megahed AS, Hafez M, Nada N. Characterization of pediatric head and neck masses with diffusion-weighted MR imaging. Eur Radiol. 2009;19(1):201–8.
52. Driessen JP, Caldas-Magalhaes J, Janssen LM, et al. Diffusion-weighted MR imaging in laryngeal and hypopharyngeal carcinoma: association between apparent diffusion coefficient and histologic findings. Radiology. 2014;272(2):456–63.
53. Lee SK, et al. Multiparametric quantitative analysis of tumor perfusion and diffusion with 3T MRI: differentiation between benign and malignant soft tissue tumors. Br J Radiol. 2020;93(1115):20191035. https://doi.org/10.1259/bjr.20191035.
54. Purz S, Sabri O, Viehweger A, et al. Potential pediatric applications of PET/MR. J Nucl Med. 2014;55(Supplement 2):32S–9S.
55. Arens AIJ, Troost EGC, Schinagl D, et al. FDG-PET/CT in radiation treatment planning of head and neck squamous cell carcinoma. Q J Nucl Med Mol Imaging. 2017;61(2):257–68.
56. Bhatia KS, Yuen EH, Cho CC, et al. A pilot study evaluating real-time shear wave ultrasound elastography of miscellaneous non-nodal neck masses in a routine head and neck ultrasound clinic. Ultrasound Med Biol. 2012;38(6):933–42.

57. Rifai K, Cornberg J, Mederacke I, et al. Clinical feasibility of liver elastography by acoustic radiation force impulse imaging (ARFI). Dig Liver Dis. 2011;43(6):491–7.
58. Huang YQ, Liang CH, He L, et al. Development and validation of a radiomics nomogram for preoperative prediction of lymph node metastasis in colorectal cancer. J Clin Oncol. 2016;34(18):2157–64.
59. Kann BH, Aneja S, Loganadane GV, et al. Pretreatment identification of head and neck cancer nodal metastasis and extranodal extension using deep learning neural networks. Sci Rep. 2018;8(1):14036.
60. Wei Z, et al. Towards interactive deep-learning for tumour segmentation in head and neck cancer radiotherapy. Phys Imaging Radiat Oncol. 2023;25:100408. https://doi.org/10.1016/j.phro.2022.12.005.
61. Pinker K, et al. Background, current role, and potential applications of radiogenomics. J Magn Reson Imaging. 2017;47(3):604–20. https://doi.org/10.1002/jmri.25870.
62. Yuen HY, et al. A short review of basic head and neck interventional procedures in a General Radiology Department. Cancer Imaging. 2013;13(4):502–11. https://doi.org/10.1102/1470-7330.2013.0043.

Part III

Thoracic and Musculoskeletal Systems

15 Mediastinal Masses in Children

Deeksha Bhalla and Manisha Jana

15.1 Introduction

The mediastinum is a complex anatomical region with a wide range of differential diagnoses for masses arising in this region, including congenital, neoplastic, and inflammatory lesions. The classification for these has been based on anatomic compartment, according to the International Thymic Malignancy Interest Group (ITMIG) classification [1], which is to be applied to cross-sectional imaging studies. In this chapter, we will restrict ourselves to the discussion of neoplastic lesions in children and their imaging appearance.

15.2 Consensus Guidelines

Mediastinal masses in children are usually detected incidentally on radiographs performed for symptoms such as chest pain or shortness of breath. The ITMIG considers CT as the gold standard for the definition of mediastinal compartments. For this reason, and due to the challenges of sedation in children with mediastinal masses, CT forms the mainstay of imaging. Contrast-enhanced imaging is the norm.

The indications of MRI are limited. These include distinguishing cystic lesions such as thymic cysts from solid masses, or for determining the presence of solid component/septa within cysts. Further, it may be used for differentiation of thymic hyperplasia using in and opposed-phase imaging. In patients allergic to IV contrast or with renal dysfunction, non-contrast MR may be used as a substitute for CT. For paravertebral masses, MRI is recommended to allow for simultaneous spinal canal evaluation. The suggested MRI protocol is summarized in Table 15.1 [2].

D. Bhalla (✉)
Department of Radiodiagnosis, Postgraduate Institute of Child Health, Noida, Uttar Pradesh, India

M. Jana
Department of Radiodiagnosis and Interventional Radiology, All India Institute of Medical Sciences, New Delhi, India

I. Kumar et al. (eds.), *Practical Approach to Imaging in Pediatric Oncology*,
https://doi.org/10.1007/978-981-96-8158-7_15

Table 15.1 Recommended MRI protocol for evaluation of mediastinal masses. All sequences are recommended in breath hold, which is preferred over respiratory gating

MRI protocol
1. Axial ultrafast spin echo T2w
2. Coronal/sagittal STIR
3. Axial SSFP (balanced gradient echo)
4. Axial in and out of phase T1 gradient echo
5. Axial DWI
6. 3D ultrafast gradient echo pre gadolinium
7. 3D ultrafast gradient echo dynamic post gadolinium at 20 s, 1, 3, and 5 min of injection

15.3 Structured Radiological Reporting

The ITMIG classification is a standardized classification scheme for cross-sectional imaging, which divides the mediastinum into three compartments, prevascular, visceral, and paravertebral (Fig. 15.1). The prevascular compartment lies between the sternum anteriorly and the anterior border of the pericardium. This contains the thymus and lymph nodes. The visceral compartment lies between the anterior border of the pericardium and a line that passes one centimeter posterior to the anterior border of the thoracic vertebral bodies. This compartment contains the heart, great vessels, trachea, and esophagus. The paravertebral compartment begins where the visceral compartment ends and contains the thoracic spine and paravertebral soft tissue [3].

On radiographs, it is possible to estimate the compartment of the lesion based on the silhouette sign, which refers to obliteration of margins between structures that are in contact with each other. Prevascular lesions show obliteration of the retrosternal fat triangle on lateral radiographs. Visceral compartment lesions cause airway displacement and narrowing, obliteration of cardiac borders, or the aortic knuckle. Paravertebral lesions on the other hand show increase in the posterior rib space, and may be accompanied by scalloping of vertebral column or scoliosis (Fig. 15.2).

On cross-sectional imaging such as CT or MRI, it is essential to follow a systematic approach to reporting of mediastinal masses, including compartment of origin, extension, and internal characteristics. A sample format and its application in a 12-year-old boy with a mediastinal mass is shown in Table 15.2.

The reporting must begin with designating location of the mass according to the ITMIG classification (Fig. 15.3). The location of the mass is determined based on organ of origin and displacement of structures. Prevascular space masses will displace structures such as ascending aorta, aortic arch, or trachea posteriorly. Visceral space masses usually arise from lymph nodes or the hollow viscera, and cause obliteration of retrosternal fat due to mass effect. Paravertebral masses are in close relation to the vertebral column. When a mass traverses more than one compartment, it is termed 'multicompartmental'. Further description includes the size, in all three dimensions. In lymphomas particularly, a size cut-off of 7 cm (maximum transverse or coronal dimension) is often used for labeling disease as 'bulky', which is an independent poor prognostic factor. Tumor margins or contour are described as smooth, when margins are well defined with no edge irregularity, when undulations are seen in the margin, it is referred to as lobulated and when the margins cannot be well defined or are uneven, they are referred to as irregular. Lobulated and irregular margins are more often seen in malignant lesions.

Intratumoral characteristics including composition (solid versus cystic) and density are to be noted, as well as intratumoral fat or calcification (Fig. 15.4). Cystic lesions show uniform low attenuation (<20 HU) in cases of fluid content, though higher attenuation may be seen with proteinaceous content. On MR, there is uniform intense T2 hyperintensity and T1 hypointensity. The differential diagnosis varies based on each of these characteristics, for instance, cystic lesions are usually benign, may be thymic cysts or foregut duplication cysts. Intratumoral fat and calcification are characteristic of teratomas. Diffusion restriction is labeled when ADC value is $<1000 \times 10^{-6}$ mm²/s. This is seen in malignant lesions, however it must be noted that normal lymph nodes also show diffusion restriction. Next, enhancement characteristics are noted, when enhancement resembles vascular structures, it is called avid, else categorized as mild. Avid enhancement is seen in

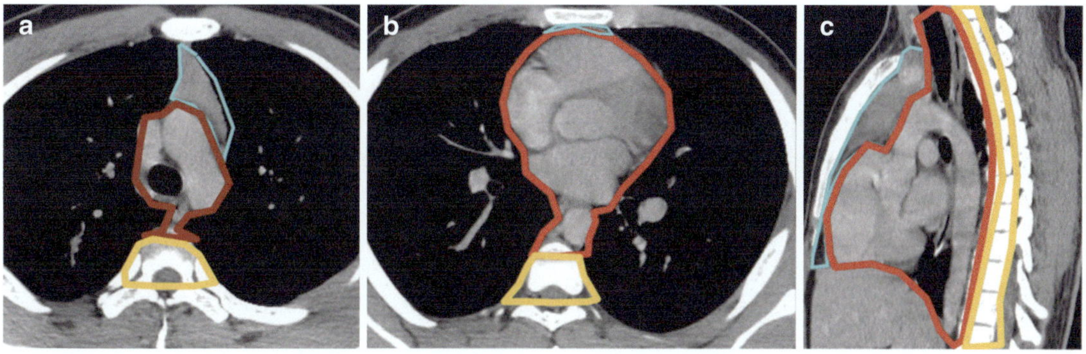

Fig. 15.1 Classification of mediastinal compartments into prevascular (blue), visceral (red), and paravertebral (yellow) as per the ITMIG system. (**a** and **b**). Axial sections depict the division in the upper and lower thorax, respectively. (**c**). Sagittal section depicting the division in craniocaudal orientation.

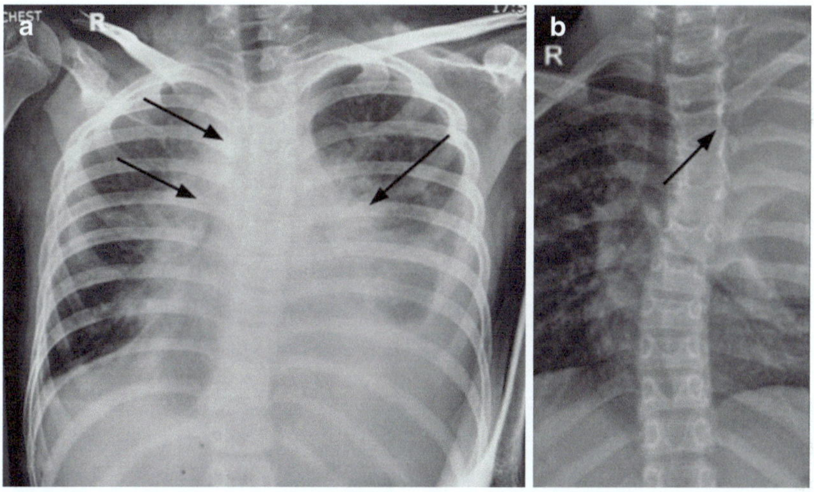

Fig. 15.2 Radiographic localization of mediastinal masses. (**a**). There is mediastinal soft tissue seen on both sides, which is silhouetting the right as well as left heart border (arrow), and the paratracheal stripe suggesting a visceral space origin. (**b**). A large mass is seen on the left side causing vertebral scalloping, scoliosis, and increase in posterior rib space suggesting a paravertebral space origin

vascular tumors or Castleman disease. Uniform enhancement throughout the lesion is called homogeneous, else it is labeled heterogenous. When only a rim of tissue along the margin shows enhancement, it is labeled peripheral. Peripheral enhancement is seen in infections, necrotic tumors. Fat infiltration, if present, will be seen as stranding in the fat abutting the lesion.

Following this, a detailed description of involvement of surrounding structures is essential, since the mediastinum contains many critical structures and hence meticulous surgical planning is of paramount importance (Fig. 15.5). Contiguous tumor extension into the lung parenchyma is recorded. Non-contiguous lesions such as lung nodules are considered metastatic and are recorded in the section on 'metastases'. Any other lung changes such as those secondary to infection or aspiration are mentioned as such.

Description of vascular involvement is usually based on angle of contact. Angle of contact <180 degrees is referred to as abutment while >180 degrees is called encasement. Attenuation means decrease in the luminal caliber. In some tumors,

Table 15.2 Structured reporting format for mediastinal masses

Parameters	Assessment
Location	<prevascular> <visceral> <paravertebral> <multicompartmental>
Size	—
Contour	<smooth> <lobulated> <irregular>
Parenchyma	<solid/cystic/mixed> <homogeneous/heterogeneous> <calcification> <intratumoral fat> <T1/T2 signal> <diffusion restriction: ADC>
Enhancement	<mild/avid> <homogeneous/heterogeneous/peripheral)
Infiltration of surrounding fat	<present> <absent>
Involvement of surrounding structures	
Lungs	<yes> <no> < other abnormalities in adjacent lung parenchyma>
Trachea	<normal> <abutment> <displacement> <attenuation>
Esophagus	<normal> <compressed> <infiltrated>
Aorta/pulmonary artery	<normal> <abutment> <encasement> <attenuation>
Superior vena cava	<normal> <encased/narrowed/infiltrated > <collaterals: SVC syndrome>
Pulmonary veins	<normal> <encased/attenuated/obliterated>
Pleura	<normal> <effusion> <involved>
Pericardium	<normal> <effusion> <involved> <cardiac chambers>
Expected site of phrenic nerve	<free> <involved> <elevated hemidiaphragm>
Direct bony invasion	<sternum> <ribs> <chest wall> <vertebra> <intraspinal extension>
Lymph nodes	<axillary> <mediastinal> <intrapulmonary> <other>
Metastasis	<none> <lung> <bone> <other>
Impression	<diagnosis/differential> <further suggestion>

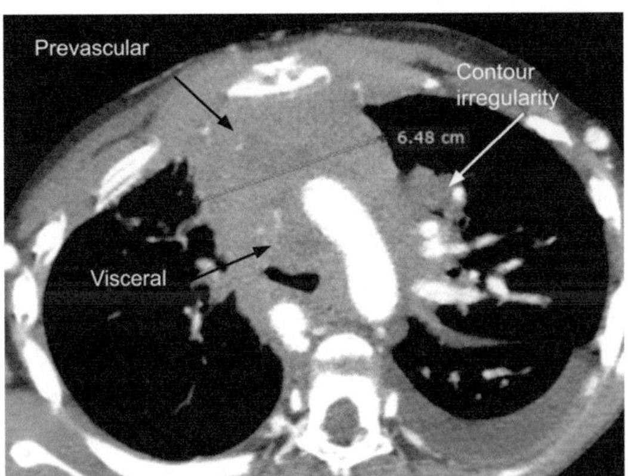

Fig. 15.3 12-year-old boy with mediastinal T cell lymphoma. Location, size, and contour characteristics are labeled

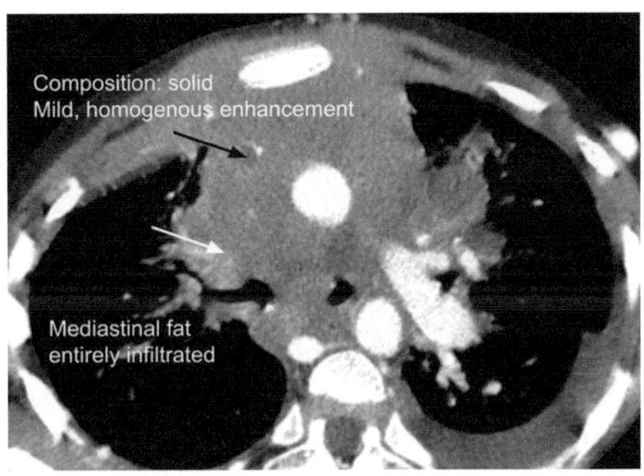

Fig. 15.4 Same patient as Fig. 15.2. Parenchymal characteristics and fat invasion depicted

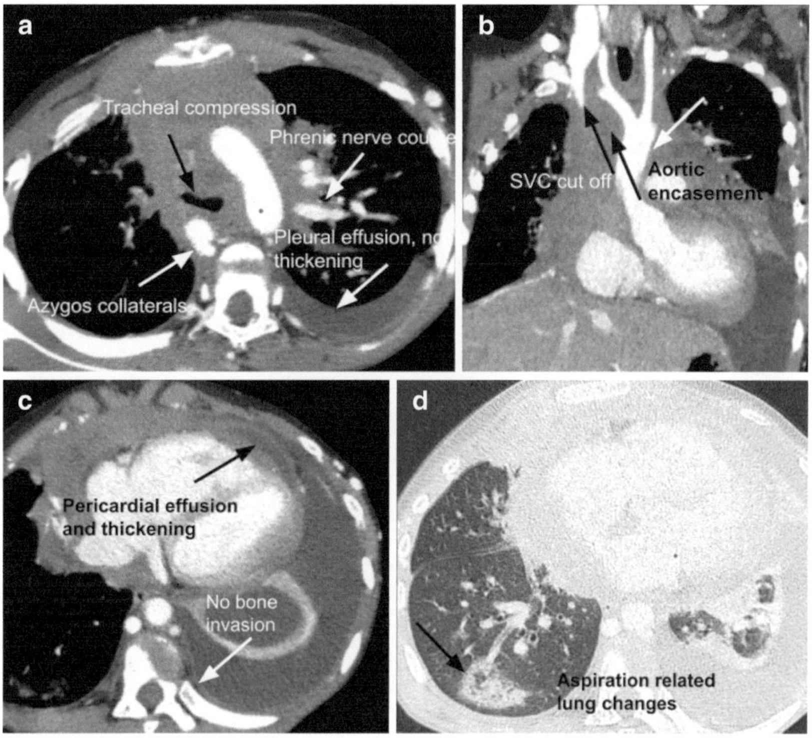

Fig. 15.5 Same patient as Fig. 15.2. Depiction of assessment of surrounding structures in mediastinal masses. (**a**). Azygous collaterals are seen due to SVC compression, soft tissue is seen in the course of the phrenic nerve as well as causing tracheal compression. Pleural involvement is also present. (**b**). Coronal image depicting vascular involvement. (**c**). Axial image depicting pericardial invasion. Bones are spared. (**d**). Lung window shows aspiration related changes

direct venous infiltration may be seen as contiguous extension of tumor into the venous lumen with expansion of the lumen. In cases of venous infiltration or complete luminal obliteration, venous collaterals may be seen.

Pleural or pericardial chambers are to be assessed for the presence of effusion and involvement. Thickening of the lining, particularly if it shows a nodular or irregular contour, is considered a sign of involvement. Effusion without thickening would need to be proven malignant by cytology. An important additional site of assessment is along the expected course of the phrenic nerve. The phrenic nerve at the thoracic inlet is posterior to subclavian vein, and descends laterally, lying anterior to the hilum on each side. On the right side, it is in contact with the lateral margin of SVC, right atrium, and ventricle while on the left side it is in contact with lateral margin of subclavian artery, left atrium, and left ventricle. Inclusion of phrenic nerve in the resection may cause postoperative pulmonary compromise.

Similar to lung involvement, in cases of contiguous tumor extension causing bone erosion, it is labeled direct bony erosion. Intraspinal extension, and percentage diameter of spinal canal involved must be recorded. Non-contiguous lesions are considered metastatic. For nodal involvement, a cut-off of 10 mm short axis diameter is applied on both CT and MRI. All nodal sites including intrapulmonary and axillary must be assessed. In metastatic assessment, lung nodules which are round and random in distribution are considered metastatic and recorded. Bone lesions may be lytic, occasionally sclerotic metastases are seen in children with neuroblastoma and lymphoma. Distant lymph nodal involvement is also considered metastatic.

Finally, an assessment of the diagnosis (including benign or malignant nature), or a set of close differential diagnoses as well as further sampling/imaging recommendations if required must be given as a conclusion to the report. The filled sample format is depicted in Table 15.3.

Table 15.3 Sample report for patient in Figs. 15.3, 15.4, and 15.5

Parameters	Assessment
Location	✓ <prevascular> <visceral> <paravertebral> <multicompartmental>
Size	6.5 cm
Contour	✓ <smooth> <lobulated> <irregular>
Parenchyma	<solid/cystic/mixed> : solid <homogenous/heterogenous> : heterogenous <calcification> : absent <intratumoral fat> : absent <T1/T2 signal> : NA <diffusion restriction: ADC> : NA
Enhancement	<mild/avid> : mild <homogenous/heterogenous/peripheral) : heterogenous
Infiltration of surrounding fat	<present> ✓ <absent>
Involvement of surrounding structures	
Lungs	✓ <yes> <no> <other abnormalities in adjacent lung parenchyma>
Trachea	✓ <normal> <abutment> <displacement> <attenuation>
Esophagus	✓ <normal> <compressed> <infiltrated>
Aorta/pulmonary artery	✓ <normal> <abutment> <encasement> <attenuation>
Superior vena cava	✓ ✓ <normal> <encased/narrowed/infiltrated > <collaterals: SVC syndrome>
Pulmonary veins	✓ <normal> <encased/attenuated/obliterated>
Pleura	✓ <normal> <effusion> <thickening>
Pericardium	✓ <normal> <effusion> <thickening> <cardiac chambers>
Expected site of phrenic nerve	✓ <free> <involved> <elevated hemidiaphragm>
Direct bony invasion	**None** <sternum> <ribs> <chest wall> <vertebra> <intraspinal extension>
Lymph nodes	**None** <axillary> <mediastinal> <intrapulmonary>
Metastasis	✓ <none> <lung> <bone> <other>
Impression	Multicompartmental solid mediastinal mass, likely malignant hematolymphoid neoplasm CT CT-guided biopsy from the mass is advised

15.4 Approach to Diagnosis

15.4.1 Prevascular Compartment

15.4.1.1 Thymic Lesions

Normal thymus may be mistaken for a mediastinal mass on radiographs, particularly in young children. Several signs have been described to help in this differentiation. The thymus is soft in consistency and shows wavy contour due to indentation by the ribs. This is referred to as 'wave sign'. Further, the thymus shows a sharp inferior margin and convex right margin, resembling the sail of a ship, known as the 'sail sign' (Fig. 15.6). A normal thymus does not cause mass effect on airway or vasculature. On CT, the normal thymus has quadrilateral shape and convex borders till 5 years of age, following which it gradually flattens. There is gradual involution of the gland, by puberty it shows concave borders and is triangular in shape. Similar to radiographs, there is no vascular or airway compromise secondary to a normal thymus. True thymic neoplasms such as thymomas and thymic carcinoma are rare in children.

Thymic hyperplasia (TH), which usually occurs secondary to stress such as infection or chemotherapy, is a common cause of thymic enlargement (Fig. 15.7). It can be differentiated from thymic neoplasms by the characteristic 'starry sky' appearance on ultrasonography (US). This refers to the hypoechogenicity of the gland with interspersed hyperechoic foci. Further, in-and-opposed phase MRI can be used to differentiate thymic hyperplasia from neoplasms, there is marked signal loss on opposed phase due to the fat component in the normal thymus [4]. The chemical shift ratio (CSR) is calculated as follows:

$$\text{CSR} = \left(\text{Thymus SIopp} / \text{paraspinal muscle SIopp}\right) / \left(\text{Thymus SIin} / \text{paraspinal muscle SIin}\right)$$

A cut-off of CSR <0.9 is taken as an indicator of benign thymic tissue [5].

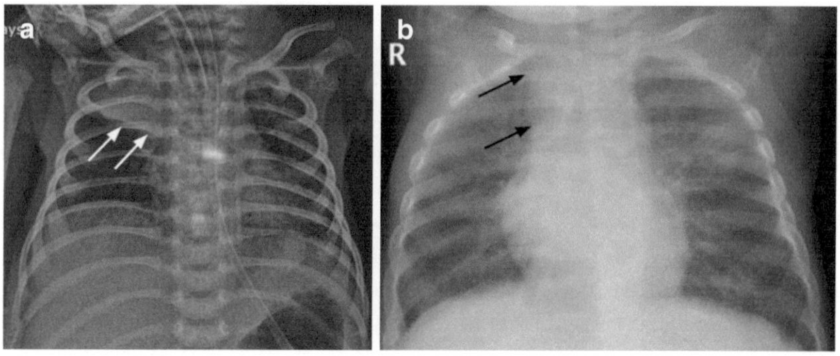

Fig. 15.6 Normal thymus on radiographs. (**a**). The thymic sail sign is seen when thymus projects to the right side of midline with a convex lateral margin and sharp inferior margin (arrow). (**b**). The wave sign is formed when there are undulations due to indentation by the ribs (arrow)

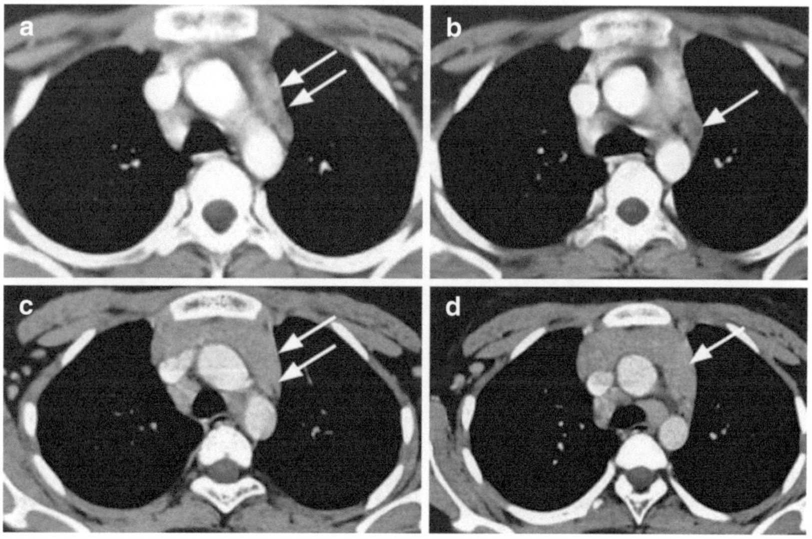

Fig. 15.7 Rebound thymic hyperplasia in a 15-year-old girl post recovery from sepsis. (**a** and **b**). Initial scan shows minimal thymic tissue in anterior mediastinum which is heterogeneous in attenuation due to interspersed fat (arrow). (**c** and **d**). Scan done at 12 weeks shows diffuse increase in the thymic tissue with homogeneous attenuation suggesting thymic hyperplasia

There is association of thymic hyperplasia as well as thymomas with immune disorders such as myasthenia gravis, with TH seen in up to 65% and thymoma seen in 15% of patients with myasthenia at disease onset [6]. Further, other systemic disorders such as lymphoma and Langerhans cell histiocytosis also show thymic involvement. In children with primary immune deficiency disorders, particularly DiGeorge syndrome, thymic hypoplasia or aplasia may be seen.

Certain thymic lesions may also be incidentally detected during imaging for other causes. These include thymic cysts, which may be primary or secondary. Primary cysts are congenital in origin, while secondary cysts are seen post radiotherapy and surgery, or inflammation such as in autoimmune disorders. A unilocular mass with homogenous fluid attenuation and no enhancement is seen on CT. Another incidentally detected benign thymic lesion is a thymolipoma. They are seen in older children or young adults. They are often large at diagnosis. There is predominant fat density seen within the mass on CT, with intervening fibrous septae. On MRI, there is T1/T2 hyperintensity due to the fat component with intervening low signal intensity fibrous septae.

15.4.1.2 Germ Cell Neoplasms

Germ cell tumors (GCTs) are the third most common pediatric mediastinal tumour [7] (Fig. 15.8). These are classified into seminomatous and non-seminomatous GCTs. In patients with mediastinal non-seminomatous GCTs, it is essential to perform imaging of the testis at the time of presentation, since imaging differentiation of primary mediastinal GCT and metastatic GCT is not possible.

The imaging and laboratory features of major subtypes are summarized in Table 15.4.

15.4.1.3 Hematolymphoid Neoplasms

Lymphoma is the most common malignant mediastinal mass in children. There are two forms, Hodgkin lymphoma (HL) and non-Hodgkin lymphoma (NHL). Non-Hodgkin lymphoma is more common in younger children. The NHL subtypes most common in the chest are large B cell lymphoma, anaplastic large cell lymphoma, and Burkitt lymphoma (Fig. 15.9). T cell acute lymphoblastic leukemia (T ALL) may also present with a mediastinal mass.

Prior to performing CT of the chest in children with lymphoma, it is essential to evaluate for airway compression on chest radiographs, since sedation for CT may not be safe in these children. HL presents as a lobulated, homogeneous mediastinal mass while NHL presents as thymic enlargement. Further, cervical lymphadenopathy as well as involvement of abdominal solid organs such as liver or spleen is more common in NHL. High-grade tumors such as T-ALL often show central necrosis. Vascular encasement is often seen without attenuation of the vascular caliber, due to the soft nature of these tumors.

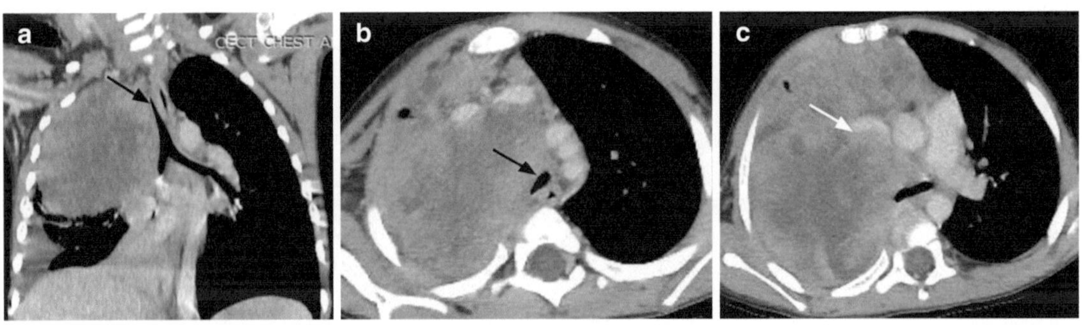

Fig. 15.8 Mixed germ cell tumor in an 8-year-old boy. (**a**–**c**). Contrast CT shows a large invasive mass with central hypodense areas. There is posterior displacement and flattening of the airway suggesting anterior mediastinal origin (black arrow). Infiltration into the lumen of SVC is also noted (white arrow)

Table 15.4 Clinical and imaging features of mediastinal GCTs

Pathological subtype	Age/gender	Laboratory markers	Imaging features-CT	Imaging features-MRI
Seminoma	Adolescent or older Male	Raised LDH, normal AFP	Homogeneous mass on both sides of mediastinum	Homogeneous T2 hyper/T1 hypointense
Mature teratoma	Older children/ young adults	–	Calcification in ~25% cases. Combination of fat, fluid components, and calcification is characteristic. Tooth or fat-fluid level is diagnostic	Cystic component hyperintense on T1/T2w images due to sebaceous material, dark line seen on chemical shift imaging (CSI) at fat-fluid interface, enhancing mural projections (Rokitansky protuberances)
Immature teratoma	Infants/young children	Raised AFP is ~50%	Fat/calcification present, evolved structures (teeth/bone) usually not seen. Larger solid areas than mature teratomas	Smaller fat foci show suppression on fat-sat images, mural calcification, enhancement in solid components
Yolk sac tumor	Adolescent or older Male>female	Raised AFP	Infiltrative masses, hemorrhage, and necrosis. Frequent metastases at presentation.	Heterogeneous enhancement, restricted diffusion
Embryonal carcinoma	Adolescent or older Male>female	Raised AFP	Ill-defined, infiltrative masses. Metastases often at presentation.	Heterogeneous enhancement, restricted diffusion
Choriocarcinoma	Adolescent or older Male>female	Raised beta-HCG (may present with gynecomastia)	Infiltrative masses, hemorrhage, and necrosis. Frequent metastases often at presentation.	Heterogeneous enhancement, restricted diffusion

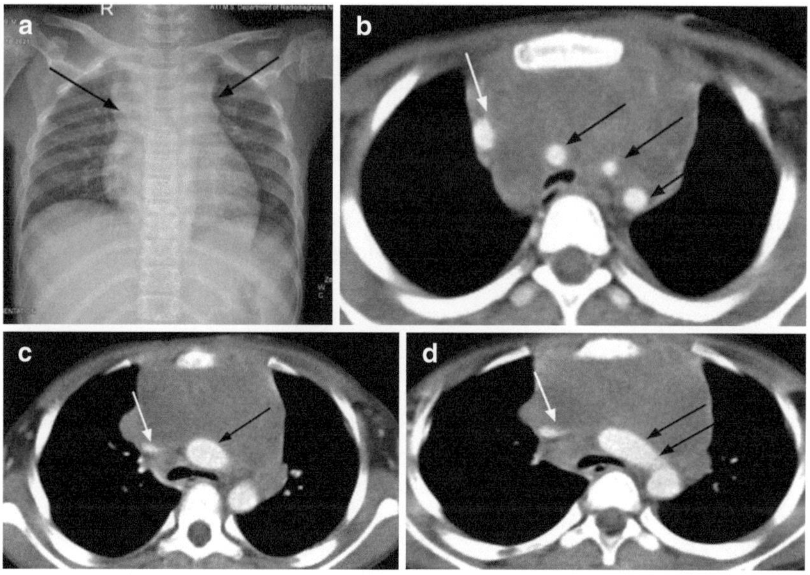

Fig. 15.9 Mediastinal B cell lymphoma in a 13-year-old boy. (**a**). Chest radiograph shows mediastinal widening with silhouetting of the right paratracheal stripe, and the aorta suggesting visceral space involvement. (**b**–**d**). Heterogeneous mass is seen in prevascular and visceral space with encasement of the aortic arch vessels (black arrow) as well as the SVC (white arrow) causing tracheal narrowing

Table 15.5 Clinical and imaging features of mediastinal vascular neoplasms

	Infantile hemangioma	Kaposiform hemangioendothelioma
Thrombocytopenia (Kasabach-Meritt phenomenon)	Absent	Present
MRI	Intensely T2 hyperintense	T2 hyperintensity with speckled T2 hypointense foci
Enhancement	Avid, homogenous Large feeding artery often seen	Avid, heterogeneous Large feeding artery often seen
Margins	Sharp	Ill-defined, invasion of adjacent structures may be present
Pleural/pericardial effusion	Absent	Present (Chylous)

15.4.1.4 Vascular Neoplasms

Vascular neoplasms are also rarely seen in the mediastinum. These may be benign (hemangioma) or aggressive (Kaposiform hemangioendothelioma).

Based on their natural history, they usually present in the first few months of life, with 90% being diagnosed by 1 year of age [8].

Their clinical and imaging features are summarized in Table 15.5.

Table 15.6 Differentiating features of unicentric and multicentric CD

	Unicentric CD	Multicentric CD
Age at presentation	Older (5–18 year)	Younger (2–15 year)
Association with HHV 8	Absent	Strong
Mediastinal involvement	Less common	More common
Treatment	Surgical resection	Chemotherapy

15.4.2 Visceral Compartment

The visceral compartment lesions may be classified into

(a) Cystic: Foregut duplication cysts (bronchogenic cyst, esophageal duplication cyst, neurenteric cyst), pericardial cysts.
(b) Solid: Lymphadenopathy (tuberculosis, sarcoidosis, Castlemann disease).
(c) Vascular: Aortic aneurysm.
(d) Hernias: Para-esophageal hernia, Morgagni hernia.

15.4.2.1 Castleman Disease

Castleman disease (CD) is a rare lymphoproliferative disorder which may involve the mediastinum in 11–16% cases [7]. There are two forms of the disease, unicentric and multicentric. The differences in these two forms are summarized in Table 15.6. There are two pathological forms as well, the hyaline vascular type which is seen in ~90% cases and the plasma cell type. The hyaline vascular type has hyalinized germinal centers with abundant capillaries between the follicles. Plasma cell variant has hyperplastic germinal centers with plasma cells between follicles [9].

In the mediastinum, it presents as a lobulated soft tissue mass, which is hyperattenuating on unenhanced CT. On contrast-enhanced CT, avid enhancement is seen. On MR, these masses are hyperintense on T2w and iso-hyperintense on T1w images with enhancement due to their vascular nature. Calcification may also be seen within the masses.

15.4.3 Paravertebral Compartment

15.4.3.1 Neurogenic Tumors

These include tumors that arise from the sympathetic ganglia or paraganglia. Tumors arising from the sympathetic ganglia or neural crest are neuroblastomas (NB), ganglioneuroblastomas (GNB), and ganglioneuromas (GN).

The neural crest tumors form a spectrum, NB is a malignant lesion, GNB is intermediate, while

GN is a benign lesion. NB is seen in children <5 years of age. The prognosis of thoracic NB is better than NB at other sites. Presentation may be non-specific, however certain syndromes such as opsoclonus-myoclonus or Horner's syndrome (in case of superior mediastinal lesions) are often associated. Spinal cord compression is a deadly complication. On radiographs, a posterior mediastinal mass with rib erosion and calcification is seen. The radiological staging of NB is performed according to the International Neuroblastoma Risk Group Staging System (INRGSS), which defines image-defined risk factors (IDRFs) for each body region [10]. The IDRFs in the thorax are:

- Aortic and/or major branch vessel encasement.
- Tracheal compression.
- Invasion of spinal canal (>1/3rd diameter) or spinal cord compression.
- Lower costovertebral junction (T9-T12) invasion.
- Brachial plexus root encasement.

MRI is mandatory for staging of thoracic NBs to look for spinal canal extension (Fig. 15.10). I123 metaiodobenzylguanidine (MIBG) is essential for metastatic workup. 90% of NB and 66% of GNB are MIBG avid [11].

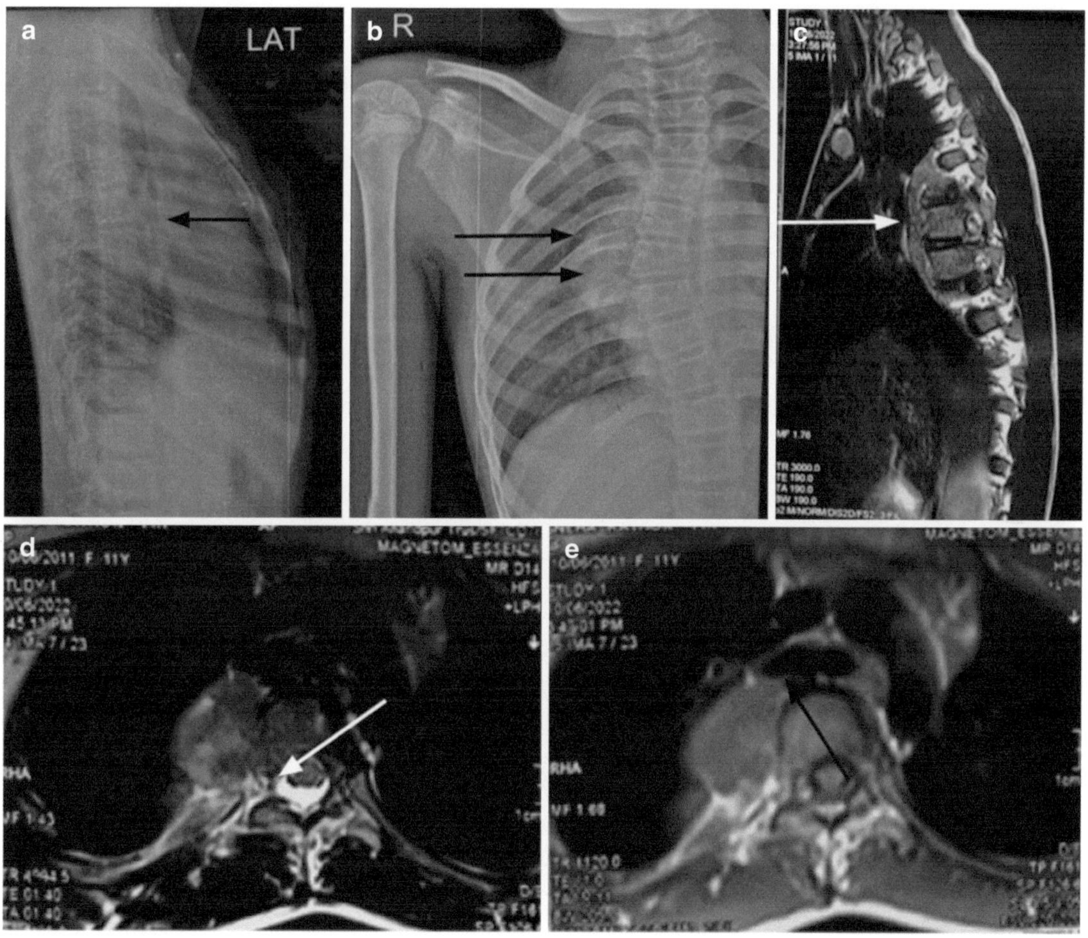

Fig. 15.10 Thoracic neuroblastoma in an 11-year-old girl. Lateral (**a**) and frontal (**b**) radiographs show a posterior mediastinal lesion with widening of posterior rib space (arrow). (**c**). On the sagittal MRI, the longitudinal extent of tumor is greater than transverse extent, suggesting neural crest origin. (**d**). T2w axial MRI shows the foraminal extension of the lesion, with no intraspinal extension. (**e**). There is also a fat plane with the tracheal bifurcation (arrow) on the T1w images and no aortic contact. This lesion is IDRF negative

GNBs are seen in older children, between 5 and 10 years old, while GN are seen in children >10 years old. It is usually not possible to differentiate GNB or GN from NB on imaging, though aggressive features are seen in NB and GNB and not seen in GN. Further, spontaneous regression of NB may be seen in children <2 years old.

15.4.3.2 Nerve Sheath Tumors

These include neurofibromas, schwannomas, and malignant peripheral nerve sheath tumors (MPNST). These are uncommon in the pediatric population, sporadic occurrence is seen in patients >20 years age. In the setting of neurofibromatosis 1 (NF-1), multiple thoracic neurofibromas may be seen. Similarly, in the setting of NF-2, thoracic schwannomas may be seen. On imaging, these are seen along spinal nerve roots or intercostal nerves. The long axis of these tumors is, therefore, oriented in a transverse direction. On CT, a 'split fat' sign may be seen. This refers to the displacement of fat around the normal neurovascular bundle, around the lesion. On MRI, the lesions are hyperintense on T2w images and typically show homogenous enhancement. The 'target' appearance, with central T2 hypointensity due to collagen and peripheral T2 hyperintensity is characteristic of neurofibromas.

MPNST is usually seen secondary to malignant transformation of nerve sheath tumors in the setting of NF-1. Rapid growth, heterogeneity, and invasion of surrounding structures suggest the development of malignancy in a previously benign lesion.

Summary of imaging approach is provided in Fig. 15.11.

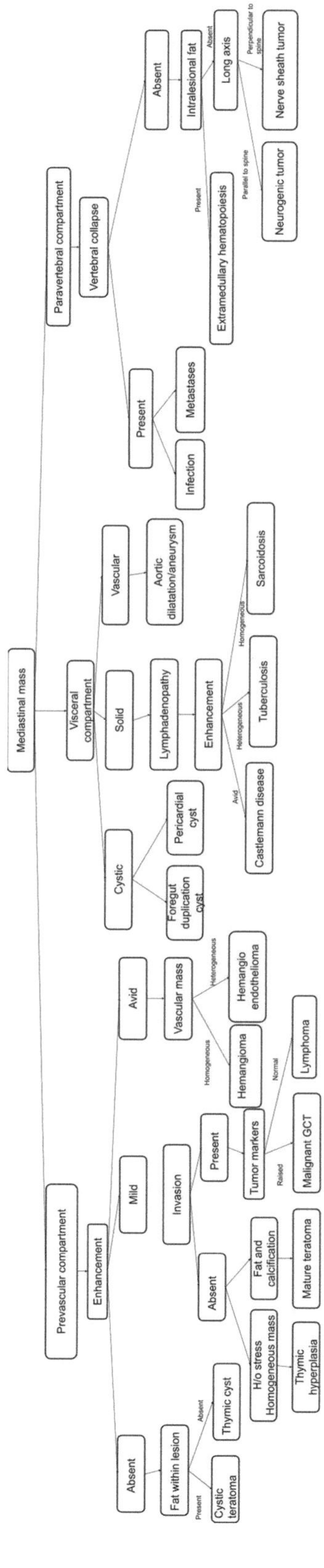

Fig. 15.11 Summary of imaging approach to mediastinal masses in children

15.5 Post-treatment Imaging

The role of post-treatment imaging is vital in children with malignant mediastinal masses, particularly those who undergo chemotherapy either as definitive therapy or as adjuvant to surgery.

In mediastinal lymphomas, particularly HL, it is not uncommon to encounter residual masses which may represent fibrotic tissue. The differentiation of these sterile masses from residual active lesions may be done using MRI. Homogenous T2 hypointensity is seen in fibrotic masses. Sharp decrease in gadolinium enhancement also represents remission in these patients [12]. However, due to nearly uniform avidity of HL on PET-CT, it remains the modality of choice for assessment of interim and post-therapy response in these patients.

Similarly, FDG-PET CT has shown 94.2% sensitivity and 85.8% accuracy for determining post-therapy response in malignant germ cell tumors, in a study by Sharma and colleagues [13].

As previously mentioned, 90% of NBs show avidity on I^{123} MIBG, and thus it remains the imaging modality of choice for post-treatment response evaluation in these patients as well. For patients who are not MIBG avid in the initial scan, FDG PET is used for pre- and post-therapy evaluation along with MRI for preoperative assessment.

15.6 Advances

Newer MRI sequences such as 'cine MRI' have emerged for preoperative evaluation of mediastinal tumors, particularly to image adherence or invasion of critical structures such as the pericardium or diaphragm. This is essentially a balanced SSFP (steady-state free precession sequence) which may be used for real-time imaging of various structures in motion. For evaluation of the heart, ECG-gated acquisition is essential. For structures such as the diaphragm, where respiratory motion is to be evaluated, cardiac gating is not required [14].

MR lymphangiography is a technique for indirect evaluation of the thoracic duct anatomy and pathology by injection of gadolinium contrast into inguinal lymph nodes. This has shown great promise in the evaluation of children with cervico-thoracic masses who present consequently chylous pleural effusion or ascites. This helps to display the lymphatic duct in its entirety, including pathology such as obstruction or invasion.

Further, an MRI sequence called REACT (relaxation enhanced angiography without contrast and triggering) has been developed for non-gadolinium-enhanced MR angiography. This sequence uses a T2 and STIR prep pulse to suppress signal from tissues, followed by a DIXON readout which additionally suppresses fat signal, while preserving signal from arteries and veins [15]. This may be employed for the detection of vascular invasion and thrombosis.

15.7 Conclusion

The key to differential diagnosis of mediastinal masses in children lies in compartment-based localization. Following this, a combination of factors including age, tumor marker levels as well as imaging features such as internal architecture, enhancement, intralesional fat, and calcification as well as other organ changes are analyzed to reach a probable diagnosis. Radiologists must be familiar with this approach and seek to follow structured reporting formats that allow accurate description of lesions on cross-sectional imaging.

References

1. Carter BW, Tomiyama N, Bhora FY, et al. A modern definition of mediastinal compartments. J Thorac Oncol. 2014;9(9 Suppl 2):S97–101. https://doi.org/10.1097/JTO.0000000000000292.
2. Ackman JB. MR imaging of mediastinal masses. Magn Reson Imaging Clin N Am. 2015;23(2):141–64. https://doi.org/10.1016/j.mric.2015.01.002.
3. Carter BW, Benveniste MF, Madan R, et al. ITMIG classification of mediastinal compartments and multidisciplinary approach to mediastinal masses.

Radiographics. 2017;37(2):413–36. https://doi.org/10.1148/rg.2017160095.
4. Takahashi K, Al-Janabi NJ. Computed tomography and magnetic resonance imaging of mediastinal tumors. J Magn Reson Imaging JMRI. 2010;32(6):1325–39. https://doi.org/10.1002/jmri.22377.
5. Jb A, Cc W. MRI of the thymus. AJR Am J Roentgenol. 2011;197(1):W15. https://doi.org/10.2214/AJR.10.4703.
6. Priola AM, Priola SM. Imaging of thymus in myasthenia gravis: from thymic hyperplasia to thymic tumor. Clin Radiol. 2014;69(5):e230–45. https://doi.org/10.1016/j.crad.2014.01.005.
7. Biko DM, Lichtenberger JP, Rapp JB, Khwaja A, Huppmann AR, Chung EM. Mediastinal masses in children: radiologic-pathologic correlation. Radiographics. 2021;41(4):1186–207. https://doi.org/10.1148/rg.2021200180.
8. Ji Y, Yang K, Peng S, et al. Kaposiform haemangioendothelioma: clinical features, complications and risk factors for Kasabach-Merritt phenomenon. Br J Dermatol. 2018;179(2):457–63. https://doi.org/10.1111/bjd.16601.
9. Sopfe J, Endres A, Campbell K, et al. Castleman disease in pediatrics: insights on presentation, treatment, and outcomes from a two-site retrospective cohort study. Pediatr Blood Cancer. 2019;66(5):e27613. https://doi.org/10.1002/pbc.27613.
10. Monclair T, Brodeur GM, Ambros PF, et al. The international Neuroblastoma risk group (INRG) staging system: an INRG task force report. J Clin Oncol. 2009;27(2):298–303. https://doi.org/10.1200/JCO.2008.16.6876.
11. Sreedher G, Tadros SS, Janitz E. Pediatric mediastinal masses. Pediatr Radiol. 2022;52(10):1935–47. https://doi.org/10.1007/s00247-022-05409-4.
12. Rahmouni A, Divine M, Lepage E, et al. Mediastinal lymphoma: quantitative changes in gadolinium enhancement at MR imaging after treatment. Radiology. 2001;219(3):621–8. https://doi.org/10.1148/radiology.219.3.r01jn06621.
13. Sharma P, Jain TK, Parida GK, et al. Diagnostic accuracy of integrated (18)F-FDG PET/CT for restaging patients with malignant germ cell tumours. Br J Radiol. 2014;87(1040):20140263. https://doi.org/10.1259/bjr.20140263.
14. Raptis CA, McWilliams SR, Ratkowski KL, Broncano J, Green DB, Bhalla S. Mediastinal and pleural MR imaging: practical approach for daily practice. Radiographics. 2018;38(1):37–55. https://doi.org/10.1148/rg.2018170091.
15. Thacker PG. Magnetic resonance imaging of the pediatric mediastinum: updates, tips and tricks. Pediatr Radiol. 2022;52(2):323–33. https://doi.org/10.1007/s00247-021-05041-8.

Cardiac and Vascular Tumors

16

Surya Pratap Singh and Sanjeev Kumar

16.1 Introduction

Cardiac tumors are rare in the pediatric population, with a prevalence ranging from 0.0017 to 0.28% in autopsy studies [1]. Despite their rarity, cardiac tumors can have significant clinical implications and may lead to life-threatening complications if not diagnosed and managed promptly. The most common primary cardiac tumors in children are benign, with rhabdomyoma and fibroma accounting for the majority of cases [2]. Malignant cardiac tumors, such as sarcomas and lymphomas, are exceedingly rare in children [3].

The clinical presentation of cardiac tumors in children varies depending on the size, location, and type of tumor. Some children may be asymptomatic, and the tumor may be detected incidentally during routine imaging or physical examination. Others may present with symptoms such as dyspnea, chest pain, palpitations, or syncope [4]. In some cases, cardiac tumors may lead to life-threatening complications, such as arrhythmias, valve obstruction, or cardiac failure [5].

The diagnosis of cardiac tumors in children relies heavily on imaging modalities, as the clinical presentation is often nonspecific. Echocardiography is typically the first-line imaging modality for the detection and initial characterization of cardiac tumors [6]. However, advanced imaging techniques such as magnetic resonance imaging (MRI) and computed tomography (CT) play a crucial role in further delineating the extent of the tumor, evaluating its impact on cardiac function, and guiding treatment decisions [7].

Accurate diagnosis and timely management of cardiac tumors in children require a multidisciplinary approach involving pediatric cardiologists, radiologists, oncologists, and cardiac surgeons. The choice of treatment depends on various factors, including the type of tumor, its location, size, and associated symptoms. While some benign tumors may regress spontaneously and require only close monitoring, others may necessitate surgical resection to alleviate symptoms or prevent complications [8].

This chapter aims to provide a comprehensive overview of the imaging approach to cardiac tumors in children, with a focus on the role of advanced imaging techniques in diagnosis, risk stratification, and management. The chapter will discuss the epidemiology and clinical features of pediatric cardiac tumors, provide consensus guidelines for imaging, describe relevant cardiac anatomy, and present a structured reporting template for radiological interpretation. An imaging algorithm for the differential diagnosis of cardiac

S. P. Singh (✉)
Department of Radiodiagnosis, King George Medical University, Lucknow, India

S. Kumar
Department of Cardiovascular Radiology & Endovascular Interventions, AIIMS, Delhi, India

I. Kumar et al. (eds.), *Practical Approach to Imaging in Pediatric Oncology*,
https://doi.org/10.1007/978-981-96-8158-7_16

tumors will be proposed, and the role of imaging in posttreatment follow-up and surveillance will be highlighted. The chapter will also discuss recent updates and future directions in the field, including the application of novel imaging techniques, risk stratification models, and targeted therapies.

16.2 Consensus Guideline(s) for Imaging

Several prominent radiological and oncological societies have provided consensus guidelines and recommendations regarding the indications, preferred modalities, and techniques for imaging cardiac and vascular tumors in children. The American College of Radiology (ACR) Appropriateness Criteria and the Society for Pediatric Radiology (SPR) Guidelines offer valuable guidance in this regard.

Echocardiography is universally recommended as the initial imaging modality of choice for suspected cardiac tumors in pediatric patients [9, 10]. Its wide availability, lack of ionizing radiation, and ability to assess cardiac structure and function in real time make it an ideal first-line tool. MRI is the preferred modality for further characterization of cardiac tumors and assessment of extracardiac extension [10]. MRI provides superior soft-tissue contrast and multiplanar capabilities, allowing for detailed evaluation of tumor morphology, tissue characteristics, and relationship to adjacent structures.

CT may be utilized when MRI is contraindicated or unavailable [10]. Although CT provides excellent spatial resolution, its use should be judicious in children due to the risks associated with ionizing radiation exposure. Catheter angiography is typically reserved for preoperative planning or interventional procedures and is not routinely used for diagnostic purposes [9].

For the initial diagnosis and staging of suspected malignant cardiac tumors, a multimodality approach is often necessary. In addition to echocardiography and MRI, CT of the chest, abdomen, and pelvis may be indicated to assess for metastatic disease [11]. Positron Emission Tomography (PET) may provide additional functional information in select cases [12].

Regarding follow-up imaging after treatment, the same modality used for initial diagnosis is generally recommended, typically every 3–6 months for the first year and then annually thereafter [9]. More frequent surveillance may be necessary based on the specific tumor type, stage, and response to treatment.

Echocardiography and MRI form the backbone of imaging for pediatric cardiac tumors, with CT and PET serving as adjunctive tools in specific scenarios. Adhering to these guidelines can help optimize diagnostic accuracy, minimize radiation exposure, and guide appropriate management in this vulnerable patient population (Table 16.1).

Table 16.1 Imaging modalities for cardiac and vascular tumors in children

Modality	Advantages	Disadvantages
Echocardiography	First-line imaging tool Widely available No ionizing radiation Assesses cardiac structure and function	Limited field of view Operator-dependent Limited tissue characterization
Cardiac MRI	Superior soft-tissue contrast Multiplanar imaging No ionizing radiation Provides functional assessment	Requires sedation in young children Less available than echocardiography Contraindicated with certain implants
CT	Rapid acquisition Useful for assessing calcification and coronary arteries May be used when MRI is contraindicated	Ionizing radiation exposure Limited soft-tissue contrast compared to MRI
PET/CT	Evaluates tumor metabolism Useful for detecting metastatic disease	Ionizing radiation exposure Limited experience in pediatric cardiac tumors

16.3 Relevant Anatomy

A comprehensive understanding of the normal cardiac and vascular anatomy is crucial for accurately characterizing and assessing the extent of cardiac and vascular tumors in children. The heart is a complex organ composed of four chambers (right and left atria and right and left ventricles), four valves (tricuspid, pulmonary, mitral, and aortic), and great vessels (aorta, pulmonary arteries, pulmonary veins, superior and inferior vena cavae), all of which can be affected by neoplastic processes [1].

Cardiac tumors can arise from any of these structures and may involve multiple chambers, valves, or great vessels. Rhabdomyomas, the most common pediatric cardiac tumor, are often multiple and can be found in any cardiac chamber, with a predilection for the ventricles, particularly the septum and free walls. Fibromas typically arise from the ventricular septum or free wall [4], while myxomas are usually attached to the atrial septum near the fossa ovalis [13]. Pericardial teratomas are often attached to the ascending aorta and pulmonary artery (Table 16.2).

Table 16.2 Implications of cardiac tumors according to the location

Anatomic structure	Potential tumor implications
Right atrium	Tricuspid valve obstruction Superior/inferior vena cava obstruction
Right ventricle	Outflow tract obstruction Tricuspid valve dysfunction
Left atrium	Mitral valve obstruction Pulmonary vein obstruction
Left ventricle	Outflow tract obstruction Mitral valve dysfunction
Tricuspid valve	Regurgitation Stenosis
Pulmonary valve	Outflow tract obstruction
Mitral valve	Regurgitation Stenosis
Aortic valve	Outflow tract obstruction
Aorta	Compression Wall invasion
Pulmonary arteries	Compression Invasion Obstruction
Superior/inferior vena cava	Compression Invasion Obstruction
Pericardium	Invasion Compression Effusion Tamponade

Vascular tumors can affect any component of the vascular system, including capillaries, veins, arteries, and lymphatics. Hemangiomas, the most common vascular tumor in children, can occur anywhere but are frequently found in the skin and subcutaneous tissues of the head and neck region [14]. Kaposiform hemangioendotheliomas and tufted angiomas often arise in the skin and subcutaneous tissues of the trunk and extremities. Vascular malformations, though not true neoplasms, can mimic vascular tumors and may involve any combination of capillaries, veins, arteries, and lymphatics [15] (Tables 16.3 and 16.4).

Table 16.3 Common vascular tumors in children

Tumor type	Characteristic features	Associated conditions
Infantile hemangioma	Most common vascular tumor in infancy Rapid growth phase followed by gradual involution Typically occurs in the skin and subcutaneous tissues Rarely requires imaging unless complicated	PHACE syndrome (posterior fossa malformations, hemangiomas, arterial anomalies, cardiac defects, eye abnormalities)
Kaposiform hemangioendothelioma (KHE)	Locally aggressive vascular tumor Typically occurs in the skin and subcutaneous tissues Associated with Kasabach-Merritt phenomenon (consumptive coagulopathy) MRI is the modality of choice for evaluation	Kasabach-Merritt phenomenon
Tufted angioma	Benign vascular tumor, often considered a milder form of KHE Typically occurs in the skin and subcutaneous tissues May be associated with Kasabach-Merritt phenomenon MRI is useful for evaluation	Kasabach-Merritt phenomenon
Pyogenic granuloma	Benign vascular tumor Typically occurs in the skin and mucous membranes Rapid growth followed by stabilization Imaging is rarely required	None

Table 16.4 Imaging findings of common vascular tumors in children

Tumor type	Ultrasound	MRI
Infantile hemangioma	Well-defined hypoechoic or heterogeneous mass Internal vascularity on color Doppler Hyperechoic areas may represent fibrosis or involution	T1: Isointense to muscle T2: Hyperintense to muscle Avid enhancement on post-contrast images Flow voids may be present
Kaposiform hemangioendothelioma (KHE)	Ill-defined heterogeneous mass Possible decreased vascularity compared to infantile hemangioma	T1: Isointense to muscle T2: Hyperintense to muscle Heterogeneous enhancement on post-contrast images Infiltrative growth pattern Possible associated lymphedema and soft-tissue edema
Tufted angioma	Ill-defined hypoechoic or heterogeneous mass Internal vascularity on color Doppler	T1: Isointense to muscle T2: Hyperintense to muscle Homogeneous enhancement on post-contrast images Less aggressive appearance compared to KHE
Pyogenic granuloma	Well-defined hypoechoic mass Internal vascularity on color Doppler	Rarely imaged with MRI T1: Isointense to muscle T2: Hyperintense to muscle Homogeneous enhancement on post-contrast images

16.4 Structured Radiological Reporting and Interpretation

A structured reporting template is essential for consistent, comprehensive, and accurate interpretation of imaging studies in children with cardiac tumors. The following template outlines the key elements to be included in the radiological report, along with their diagnostic, prognostic, and therapeutic significance (Table 16.5).

Certain imaging features can provide valuable insights into the tumor type and guide differential diagnosis. For example:

- Rhabdomyomas are typically well-circumscribed, homogeneous, and hyperechoic on echocardiography and demonstrate isointense T1 and hyperintense T2 signal on MRI [3].
- Fibromas are often large, solitary, and heterogeneous, with areas of calcification and cystic degeneration. They demonstrate intermediate T1 and low T2 signal on MRI [8].
- Myxomas are usually pedunculated, mobile, and heterogeneous, with areas of hemorrhage and necrosis. They show intermediate T1 and high T2 signal on MRI [16].
- Malignant tumors, such as sarcomas, often demonstrate invasive growth, ill-defined margins, and heterogeneous enhancement on MRI [17] (Table 16.6).

The assessment of cardiac function and hemodynamic impact is crucial in the evaluation of cardiac tumors. Echocardiography plays a central role in assessing ventricular size and function, valvular competence, and the presence of outflow

Table 16.5 Structured radiological reporting and interpretation

Element	Description	Significance
Protocol	Modality, technique, sequences	Ensures appropriate imaging protocol for accurate diagnosis
Location	Chambers, valves, great vessels, pericardium	Guides surgical approach and predicts potential complications
Local involvement	Myocardial wall thickness, lumen, pericardium, outflow tract, papillary muscles	Assesses extent of tumor invasion and guides surgical planning
Size	Dimensions in cm	Monitors tumor growth and response to treatment
Shape	Round, oval, elongated	Suggests tumor type and guides differential diagnosis
Margins	Irregular/smooth, lobulated, well-/ill-defined	Indicates tumor invasiveness and guides surgical planning
Parenchyma	Echogenicity, signal intensity, fat suppression, cystic changes, calcification, hemorrhage	Characterizes tumor tissue and guides differential diagnosis
Enhancement	Mild, marked, homogeneous/heterogeneous, peripheral/septal	Reflects tumor vascularity and guides differential diagnosis
Vascularity	Color Doppler, feeding vessels, draining veins	Assesses tumor blood supply and guides surgical planning
Impact on cardiac function	Chamber compression, outlet obstruction, valvular dysfunction, ventricular size and function, wall motion abnormality	Predicts hemodynamic consequences and guides management
Associated findings	Pleural effusion, pericardial effusion, lungs, mediastinum, ascites	Indicates tumor extension and guides management
Metastatic disease	Intrathoracic, extrathoracic	Guides staging and treatment planning
Complications	Thrombosis, rupture, infarction, others	Guides management and predicts prognosis
Impression	Differential diagnosis, further recommendations	Summarizes key findings and guides further management

Table 16.6 Common benign cardiac tumors in children

Tumor type	Characteristic features	Associated conditions
Rhabdomyoma	Most common pediatric cardiac tumor Often multiple Typically located in ventricles Spontaneous regression is common	Tuberous sclerosis complex
Fibroma	Second most common pediatric cardiac tumor Usually solitary Typically located in the ventricular septum or free wall Surgical resection is often required	Gorlin syndrome
Myxoma	Rare in children Usually solitary Typically located in the atria, attached to the interatrial septum Surgical resection is recommended	Carney complex
Teratoma	Rare in children Usually located in the pericardial cavity Composed of multiple germ cell layers Surgical resection is recommended	None

tract obstruction. Cine MRI sequences can provide additional information on tumor mobility and its impact on cardiac function throughout the cardiac cycle. The reporting template should include quantitative measures of ventricular size and function, such as ejection fraction and wall motion abnormalities, to guide management and monitor response to treatment.

16.5 Imaging Algorithm for Interpretation and Approach to Diagnosis

An imaging-based algorithm for the interpretation and approach to the diagnosis of cardiac and vascular tumors in children is essential for guiding clinical decision-making. The algorithm is based on the imaging features described in the structured reporting template (Table 16.7).

1. Determine the location of the tumor (intracardiac or extracardiac).
   (a) If intracardiac, assess the number of lesions (single or multiple).
      (i) If single:
         - Well-defined margins in the ventricular septum or free wall suggest fibroma or rhabdomyoma.
         - Well-defined margins in the atrial septum suggest myxoma.

Table 16.7 Imaging findings suggestive of malignancy in cardiac tumors

Imaging modality	Findings suggestive of malignancy
Echocardiography	Invasive growth pattern Ill-defined borders Heterogeneous echogenicity Associated pericardial effusion
Cardiac MRI	Heterogeneous signal intensity Heterogeneous enhancement Extracardiac extension Associated lymphadenopathy or metastases
CT	Irregular borders Invasion of adjacent structures Lymphadenopathy or metastases
PET/CT	Increased FDG uptake Extracardiac uptake suggestive of metastases

      (ii) If multiple:
         - Small, intramural lesions suggest rhabdomyoma.
         - Large, infiltrative lesions raise suspicion for metastatic disease or malignant primary tumor.
   (b) If extracardiac, determine if the tumor is pericardial or intramyocardial.
      (i) If pericardial:
         - Multilocular, with cystic and solid components, suggests teratoma.
         - Homogeneous and cystic appearance suggests pericardial cyst.

(ii) If intramyocardial, assess vascularity.
- High vascularity suggests hemangioma or malignant vascular tumor.
- Low vascularity suggests fibroma or rhabdomyoma.

2. Evaluate tumor tissue characteristics and enhancement patterns.
   (a) Benign tumors (e.g., rhabdomyoma and fibroma) tend to have homogeneous signal intensity and enhancement.
   (b) Malignant tumors often demonstrate heterogeneous signal intensity and enhancement, with areas of necrosis or hemorrhage.
3. Assess the effect of the tumor on cardiac function and hemodynamics.
   (a) Benign tumors may cause obstruction or valvular dysfunction, but cardiac function is often preserved.
   (b) Malignant tumors are more likely to cause significant hemodynamic compromise and impaired cardiac function.
4. Look for associated findings and complications.
   (a) Pericardial effusion, metastatic disease, or tumor-related complications (e.g., thrombosis and infarction) raise suspicion for malignancy.
   (b) Absence of these features supports a benign etiology.
5. If the imaging features are indeterminate or suggestive of malignancy, consider additional work-up:
   (a) Further imaging with CT or PET to assess for metastatic disease.
   (b) Tissue biopsy for definitive histopathological diagnosis [18].
   (c) Genetic testing for associated syndromes (e.g., tuberous sclerosis complex and Carney complex) (Table 16.8).

Table 16.8 Imaging algorithm for interpretation and approach to diagnosis

Imaging features	Criteria	Findings	Implications
Location	Intracardiac	Single lesion	Well-defined margins in ventricular septum/free wall: Fibroma or rhabdomyoma
			Well-defined margins in atrial septum: Myxoma
		Multiple lesions	Small, intramural: Rhabdomyoma
			Large, infiltrative: Metastatic disease or malignant primary tumor
	Extracardiac	Pericardial	Multilocular with cystic and solid components: Teratoma
			Homogeneous and cystic: Pericardial cyst
		Intramyocardial	High vascularity: Hemangioma or malignant vascular tumor
			Low vascularity: Fibroma or rhabdomyoma
Tissue characteristics	Signal intensity	Homogeneous	Suggestive of benign tumors
		Heterogeneous	Suggestive of malignant tumors
	Enhancement pattern	Homogeneous	Suggestive of benign tumors
		Heterogeneous	Suggestive of malignant tumors
Cardiac function	Preserved	Minimal impact	More likely benign
	Impaired	Significant hemodynamic compromise	More likely malignant

(continued)

Table 16.8 (continued)

Imaging features	Criteria	Findings	Implications
Associated findings	Present	Pericardial effusion, metastases, complications	Raise suspicion for malignancy
	Absent	No additional findings	Support benign etiology
Additional work-up	Indeterminate or suspicious features	CT or PET	Assess for metastatic disease
		Tissue biopsy	Definitive histopathological diagnosis
		Genetic testing	Evaluate for associated syndromes

16.6 Treatment Options for Pediatric Cardiac Tumors

Management of pediatric cardiac tumors requires a multidisciplinary approach, with treatment choices depending on tumor type, location, size, and associated symptoms.

Surgical Resection is the primary treatment for most pediatric cardiac tumors, especially benign ones. While complete resection is preferred, partial resection may be necessary in some cases. The surgical approach depends on tumor location and extent, with median sternotomy being most common. Intraoperative echocardiography guides resection and assesses postoperative function [4].

Chemotherapy is used primarily for malignant tumors such as sarcomas and lymphomas. It can serve as adjuvant, neoadjuvant, primary, or palliative treatment, with agents chosen based on tumor type and extracardiac malignancy protocols. Careful cardiac function monitoring is essential due to potential cardiotoxicity [2].

Radiotherapy is rarely used as primary treatment due to potential long-term effects on the developing heart. However, it may be considered as adjuvant or palliative therapy in specific cases. Advanced techniques, like intensity-modulated radiation therapy or proton beam therapy, are preferred to minimize healthy tissue exposure. Regular follow-up is necessary to monitor for late adverse effects [19].

Treatment decisions are individualized based on tumor characteristics and patient factors, with close monitoring and follow-up essential for all treatment modalities.

16.7 Posttreatment Imaging

Posttreatment imaging is crucial for assessing the response to therapy, identifying complications, and detecting tumor recurrence in children with cardiac and vascular tumors. The imaging protocol and findings vary depending on the type of treatment employed, including surgery, chemotherapy, and radiation therapy.

16.8 Surgical Treatment

1. Follow-up protocol.
   - Echocardiography: Perform within 1–2 weeks post-surgery, then every 3–6 months for the first year, and annually thereafter [13].
   - Cardiac MRI: Perform at 3–6 months post-surgery and then annually, or as clinically indicated [13].
2. Normal post-surgical imaging appearances.
   - Absence of residual tumor.
   - Intact surgical repairs or reconstructions.
   - Preserved cardiac function.
3. Abnormal post-surgical imaging appearances and complications.
   - Residual or recurrent tumor.
   - Valvular dysfunction or stenosis.

- Ventricular dysfunction or aneurysm.
- Pericardial effusion or tamponade.
- Thrombosis or infarction.

4. Tumor recurrence.
   - New or enlarging mass at the surgical site or distant locations.
   - Associated hemodynamic compromise or symptoms.

16.9 Chemotherapy

1. Follow-up protocol.
   - Echocardiography: Perform at baseline, every 3 months during treatment, and then every 6–12 months after completion of therapy [20].
   - Cardiac MRI: Perform at baseline, end of treatment, and then annually, or as clinically indicated [20].
2. Normal post-chemotherapy imaging appearances.
   - Reduction in tumor size or complete resolution.
   - Stable or improved cardiac function [20].
3. Abnormal post-chemotherapy imaging appearances and complications.
   - Persistent or progressive tumor.
   - Cardiotoxicity (e.g., left ventricular dysfunction and heart failure).
   - Valvular dysfunction.
   - Pericardial effusion.
4. Tumor recurrence.
   - Increase in tumor size or new lesions after initial response to chemotherapy.
   - Associated hemodynamic compromise or symptoms.

16.10 Radiation Therapy

1. Follow-up protocol.
   - Echocardiography: Perform at baseline, every 6 months for the first 2 years after treatment, and then annually [21].
   - Cardiac MRI: Perform at baseline, 6–12 months after treatment, and then every 1–2 years, or as clinically indicated [21].
2. Normal postradiation imaging appearances.
   - Reduction in tumor size or complete resolution.
   - Stable cardiac function [21].
3. Abnormal postradiation imaging appearances and complications.
   - Persistent or progressive tumor.
   - Radiation-induced cardiac dysfunction (e.g., myocardial fibrosis, valvular stenosis, and pericardial thickening) [22].
   - Coronary artery stenosis or occlusion.
   - Secondary malignancies.
4. Tumor recurrence.
   - Increase in tumor size or new lesions after initial response to radiation therapy.
   - Associated hemodynamic compromise or symptoms.

16.11 Identifying Tumor Recurrence

- Compare current imaging studies with prior exams to assess for interval change [14, 15].
- Look for new or enlarging masses, either at the primary site or at distant locations [15, 16].
- Evaluate for associated complications, such as ventricular dysfunction, valvular abnormalities, or pericardial effusion [4, 8, 17].
- Correlate imaging findings with clinical symptoms and markers (e.g., elevated tumor markers, arrhythmias, and heart failure) [13, 14, 23].

Posttreatment imaging is essential for monitoring the response to therapy, identifying complications, and detecting tumor recurrence in children with cardiac and vascular tumors. The choice of imaging modality and follow-up protocol depends on the type of treatment employed and the patient's clinical status. By recognizing the normal and abnormal posttreatment imaging appearances, radiologists and clinicians can effectively guide management decisions and optimize patient outcomes.

16.12 Recent Updates and Future Directions

In recent years, significant advancements have been made in the diagnosis, characterization, and management of pediatric cardiac tumors.

16.13 MRI Techniques and Their Potential Applications

The development of MRI techniques, such as T1 and T2 mapping, diffusion-weighted imaging (DWI), and perfusion imaging, has opened new avenues for the characterization of pediatric cardiac tumors. T1 and T2 mapping techniques provide quantitative measurements of tissue relaxation times, which can help differentiate between benign and malignant tumors. For example, Suna et al. demonstrated that malignant cardiac tumors exhibit significantly lower T1 and T2 values compared to benign tumors [23]. DWI and perfusion imaging techniques offer insights into tumor cellularity and vascularity, respectively, which can further aid in the differential diagnosis and assessment of treatment response [24].

16.14 3D Printing Technology for Surgical Planning and Patient Education

The integration of 3D printing technology into the management of pediatric cardiac tumors has shown promising results. By creating patient-specific 3D models of the heart and tumor, surgeons can better visualize the spatial relationships between the tumor and surrounding structures, facilitating preoperative planning and intraoperative guidance. Bhatla et al. highlighted the successful use of a 3D-printed model in the surgical planning for a complex cardiac fibroma in a 3-month-old infant [25]. Additionally, 3D-printed models can be used as educational tools to help patients and their families better understand the nature of the tumor and the proposed treatment plan [25].

16.15 Risk Stratification and Prognostication Using Imaging Features and Genetic/Molecular Markers

The identification of imaging features and genetic/molecular markers associated with tumor behavior and prognosis is an active area of research in pediatric cardiac tumors. Recent studies have explored the potential of imaging features, such as tumor size, location, and enhancement pattern, in predicting patient outcomes. For example, Beroukhim et al. found that tumors larger than 5 cm and those involving the ventricular septum were associated with a higher risk of adverse events [3]. Additionally, the integration of genetic and molecular profiling with imaging data has shown promise in refining risk stratification and guiding personalized treatment approaches [26].

16.16 Integration of Artificial Intelligence and Machine Learning in Tumor Diagnosis and Management

The application of artificial intelligence (AI) and machine learning techniques in the field of pediatric cardiac tumors holds great promise for improving diagnostic accuracy, predicting patient outcomes, and optimizing treatment strategies. Recent studies have demonstrated the potential of AI algorithms in the automated segmentation and classification of cardiac tumors on imaging studies [27, 28]. For example, a study by Xue et al. developed a deep learning model that achieved high accuracy in the automatic detection and segmentation of cardiac tumors on MRI images [29]. Furthermore, machine learning algorithms have been used to identify imaging features and biomarkers associated with tumor prognosis and treatment response.

16.17 Conclusion

Pediatric cardiac tumors, although rare, present significant diagnostic and therapeutic challenges. A comprehensive understanding of their epidemiology, clinical presentation, and imaging characteristics is crucial for accurate diagnosis, risk stratification, and management. This chapter has provided an overview of the practical approach to imaging pediatric cardiac tumors, emphasizing the key role of advanced imaging modalities in guiding clinical decision-making.

Echocardiography remains the first-line imaging modality for initial evaluation, while cardiac MRI has emerged as the gold standard for further characterization. The use of a structured reporting template and an imaging algorithm based on tumor location, morphology, and tissue characteristics aids in the differential diagnosis of benign and malignant tumors.

Management of pediatric cardiac tumors requires a multidisciplinary approach, with surgical resection being the primary treatment for most benign tumors causing hemodynamic compromise or refractory arrhythmias. Advances in imaging technology, such as novel MRI techniques and 3D printing, have improved preoperative planning, intraoperative guidance, and patient education.

Recent updates focus on integrating imaging data with genetic and molecular profiling to refine risk stratification and guide personalized treatment. Future research should focus on validating novel imaging biomarkers, optimizing imaging protocols, and developing standardized guidelines for follow-up and surveillance. International registries and collaborative research networks will be crucial for advancing our understanding of these rare tumors and improving patient outcomes (Figs. 16.1, 16.2 and 16.3).

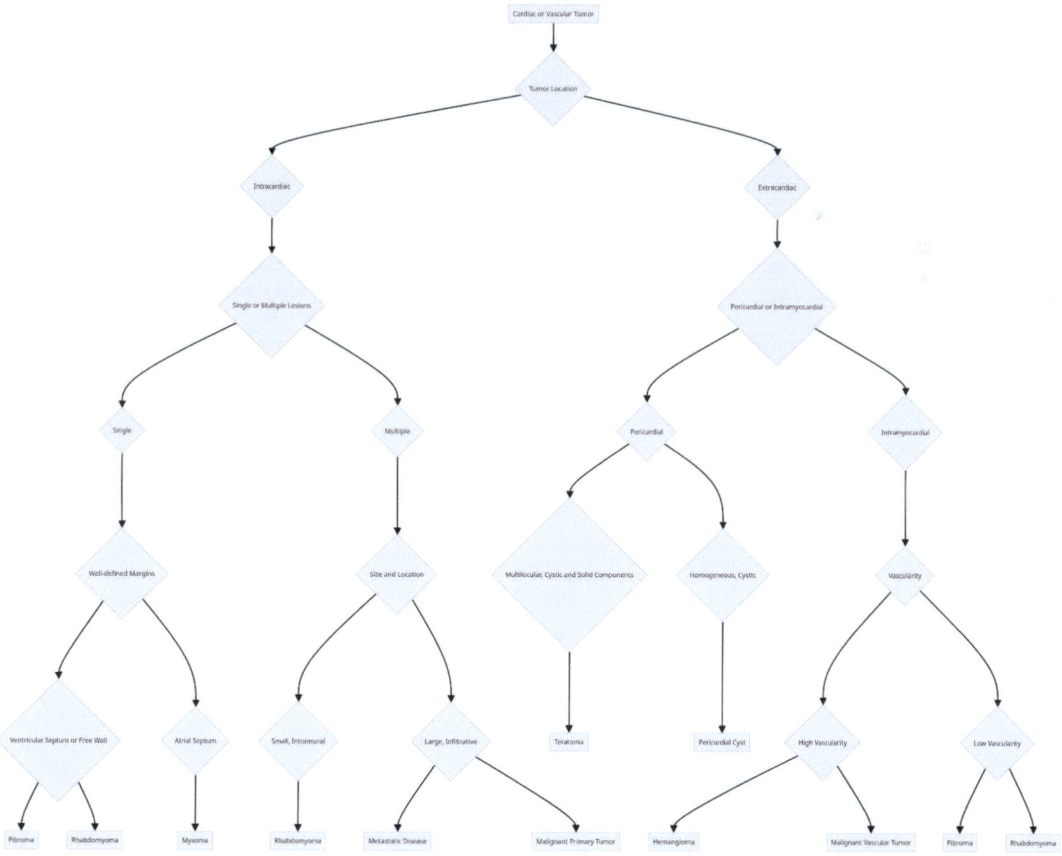

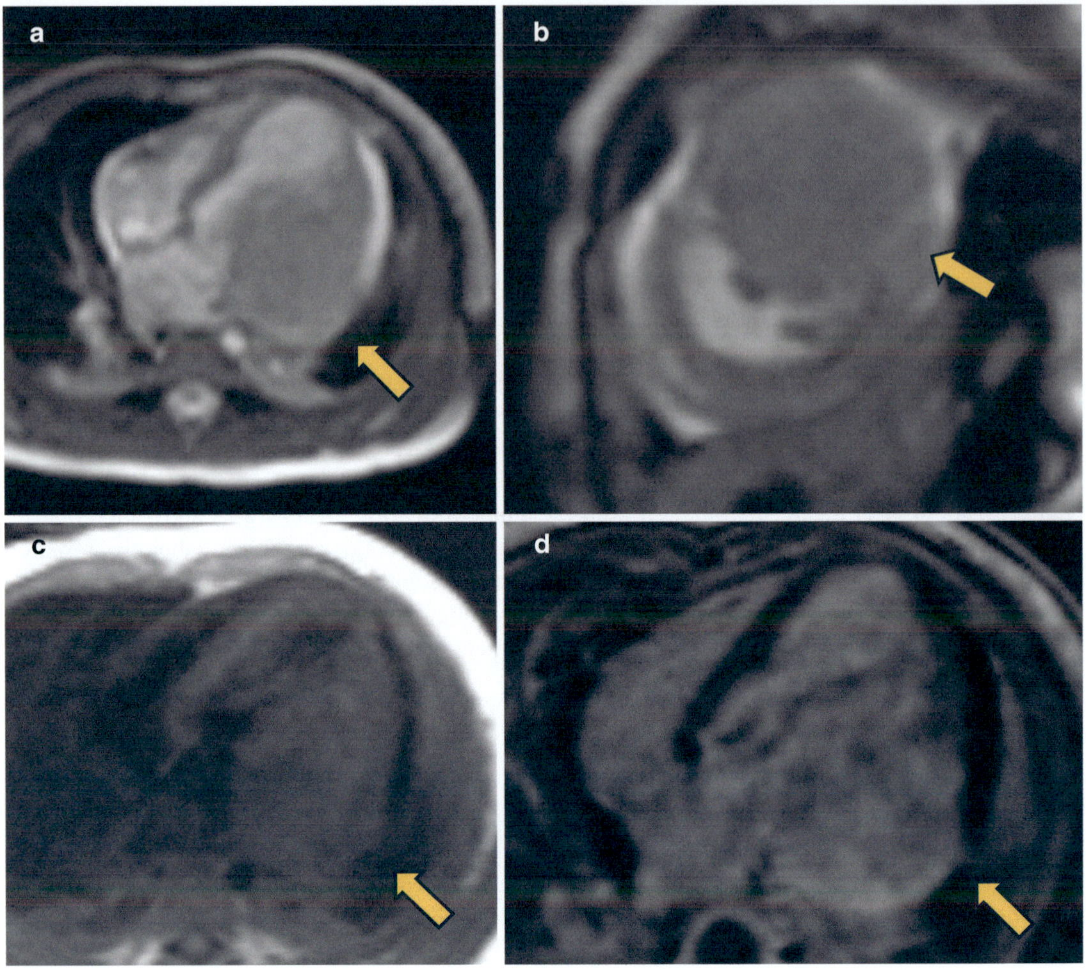

Fig. 16.1 Cardiac MRI of a 3-year-old male child showing large well-defined myocardial mass (yellow arrow) causing LV lumen compromise (**a**) True fast imaging with steady-state precession (TrueFISP) 4-chamber (**b**) TrueFISP SA show T2-isointense mass lesion which is hypointense on (**c**) T1 4ch. PSIR post-contrast shows heterogeneous post-contrast enhancement of the lesion. Imaging characteristics are in favor of benign lesion: cardiac fibroma

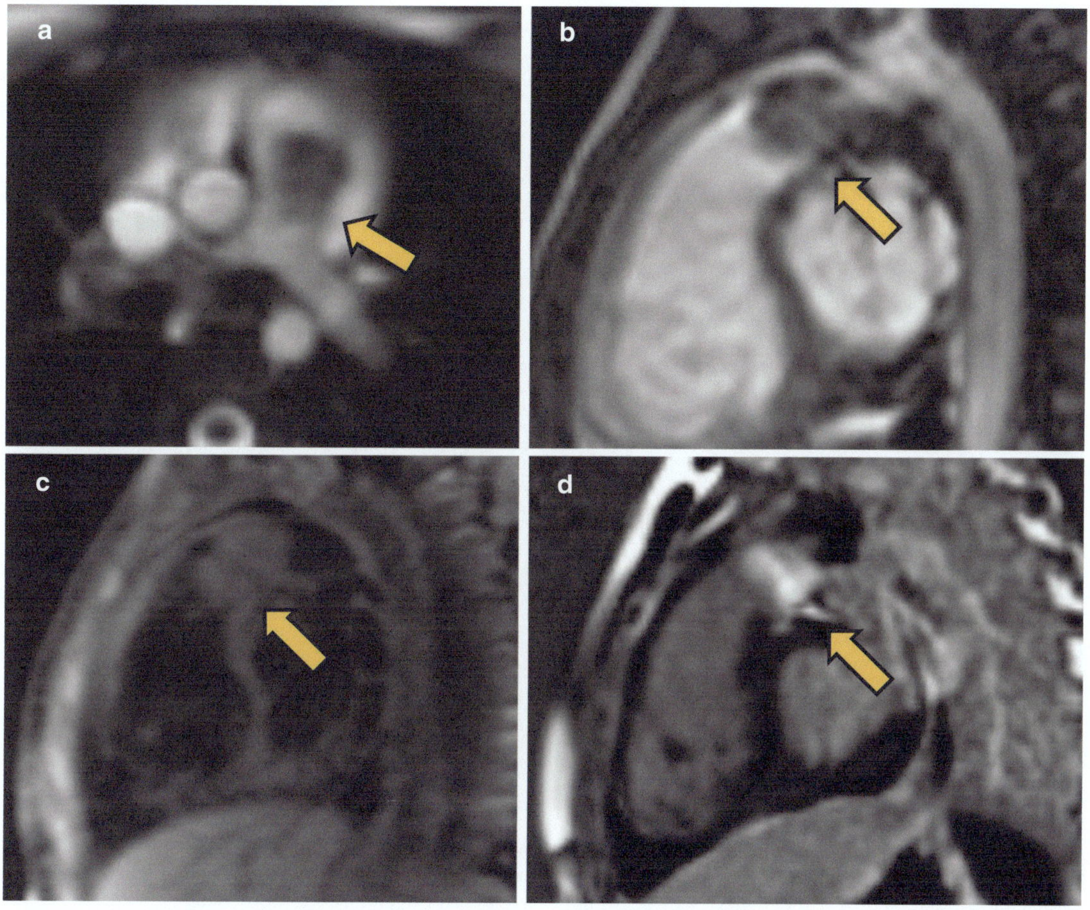

Fig. 16.2 Cardiac MRI of a 4-year-old male child showing 17 × 11 mm mass lesion (yellow arrow) in the region of RVOT, adjacent to the pulmonary annulus. Mass is hyperintense on T2WI [(**a**) TrueFISP axial section and (**b**) TrueFISP RVOT view]. Mass is hypointense on T1WI (c). Post-contrast enhancement in the midpart of the lesion. Imaging characteristics are in favor of benign lesion: pulmonary wall myxoma

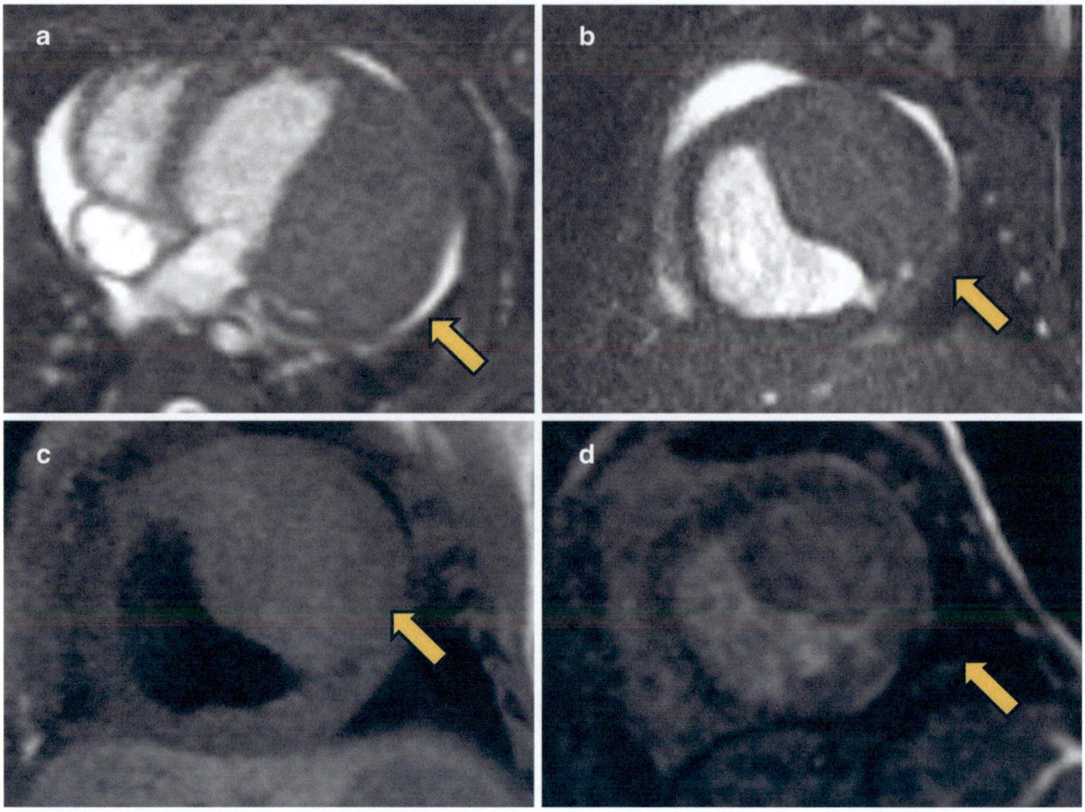

Fig. 16.3 Cardiac MRI of a 5-year-old male child who is the known case of tuberous sclerosis showing intramyocardial mass lesion (yellow arrow) in the LV myocardium. Mass is isointense on T2WI [(**a**) 4ch and (**b**) SA] images. Mass is also isointense on T1WI (**c**). No significant contrast enhancement in the lesion. Imaging characteristics are in favor of cardiac rhabdomyoma

References

1. Uzun O, Wilson DG, Vujanic GM, Parsons JM, De Giovanni JV. Cardiac tumours in children. Orphanet J Rare Dis. 2007;2:11.
2. Shi L, Wu L, Fang H, Han B, Yang J, Ma X, et al. Identification and clinical course of 166 pediatric cardiac tumors. Eur J Pediatr. 2017;176(2):253–60.
3. Beroukhim RS, Prakash A, Buechel ER, Cava JR, Dorfman AL, Festa P, et al. Characterization of cardiac tumors in children by cardiovascular magnetic resonance imaging: a multicenter experience. J Am Coll Cardiol. 2011;58(10):1044–54.
4. Ying L, Lin R, Gao Z, Qi J, Zhang Z, Gu W. Primary cardiac tumors in children: a center's experience. J Cardiothorac Surg. 2016;11(1):52.
5. Miyake CY, Del Nido PJ, Alexander ME, Cecchin F, Berul CI, Triedman JK, et al. Cardiac tumors and associated arrhythmias in pediatric patients, with observations on surgical therapy for ventricular tachycardia. J Am Coll Cardiol. 2011;58(18):1903–9.
6. Sánchez Andrés A, Insa Albert B, Carrasco Moreno JI, Cano Sánchez A, Moya Bonora A, Sáez Palacios JM. Cardiac tumors in children: a review of 15 years' experience. Rev Esp Cardiol. 2008;61(10):1113–6.
7. Ghadimi Mahani M, Lu JC, Rigsby CK, Krishnamurthy R, Dorfman AL, Agarwal PP. MRI of pediatric cardiac masses. AJR Am J Roentgenol. 2014;202(5):971–81.
8. Padalino MA, Vida VL, Boccuzzo G, Tonello M, Sarris GE, Berggren H, et al. Surgery for primary cardiac tumors in children: early and late results in a multicenter European congenital heart surgeons association study. Circulation. 2012;126(1):22–30.
9. Winkler MA, et al. ACR appropriateness criteria® known or suspected congenital heart disease in the adult. J Am Coll Radiol. 2017;14(11S):S166–76.
10. Dorfman AL, et al. Use of cardiovascular magnetic resonance imaging in children. Pediatrics. 2019;143(3):e20182602.

11. Beroukhim RS, et al. Characterization of cardiac tumors in children by cardiovascular magnetic resonance imaging: a multicenter experience. J Am Coll Cardiol. 2011;58(10):1044–54.
12. Poterucha JT, et al. Imaging of pediatric cardiac masses. Pediatr Radiol. 2019;49(12):1516–30.
13. Shi L, Wu L, Fang H, et al. Identification and clinical course of 166 pediatric cardiac tumors. Eur J Pediatr. 2017;176(2):253–60.
14. Darrow DH, Greene AK, Mancini AJ, Nopper AJ. Diagnosis and Management of Infantile Hemangioma. Pediatrics. 2015;136(4):e1060–104.
15. Wassef M, Blei F, Adams D, et al. Vascular anomalies classification: recommendations from the International Society for the Study of vascular anomalies. Pediatrics. 2015;136(1):e203–14.
16. Grebenc ML, Rosado-de-Christenson ML, Green CE, Burke AP, Galvin JR. Cardiac myxoma: imaging features in 83 patients. Radiographics. 2002;22(3):673–89.
17. Truong PT, Jones SO, Martens B, Alexander C, Paquette M, Joe H, et al. Treatment and outcomes in adult patients with primary cardiac sarcoma: the British Columbia Cancer Agency experience. Ann Surg Oncol. 2009;16(12):3358–65.
18. Biswas S, Almond CS, Blume ED. Transcatheter intracardiac biopsies in the evaluation of cardiac masses. Catheter Cardiovasc Interv. 2011;78(1):143–50.
19. Veeragandham RS, Goldin MD. Surgical management of radiation-induced heart disease. Ann Thorac Surg. 1998;65(4):1014–9.
20. Armenian SH, Hudson MM, Mulder RL, et al. Recommendations for cardiomyopathy surveillance for survivors of childhood cancer: a report from the international late effects of childhood cancer guideline harmonization group. Lancet Oncol. 2015;16(3):e123–36.
21. Mulrooney DA, Yeazel MW, Kawashima T, et al. Cardiac outcomes in a cohort of adult survivors of childhood and adolescent cancer: retrospective analysis of the childhood cancer survivor study cohort. BMJ. 2009;339:b4606.
22. Schellong G, Riepenhausen M, Bruch C, et al. Late valvular and other cardiac diseases after different doses of mediastinal radiotherapy for Hodgkin disease in children and adolescents: report from the longitudinal GPOH follow-up project of the German-Austrian DAL-HD studies. Pediatr Blood Cancer. 2010;55(6):1145–52.
23. Suna G, Özsaraç M, Yener Ö, Börekci S, Akyürek N, Karabulut N. Diagnostic value of magnetic resonance imaging in the differentiation of benign and malignant cardiac tumors. Turk Kardiyol Dern Ars. 2019;47(6):475–82.
24. Esposito A, De Cobelli F, Ironi G, Marra P, Canu T, Mellone R, et al. CMR in the assessment of cardiac masses: primary malignant tumors. JACC Cardiovasc Imaging. 2014;7(10):1057–61.
25. Bhatla P, Tretter JT, Ludomirsky A, Argilla M, Latson LA, Chakravarti S, et al. Utility and scope of rapid prototyping in patients with complex muscular ventricular septal defects or double-outlet right ventricle: does it alter management decisions? Pediatr Cardiol. 2017;38(1):103–14.
26. Morin DP, Mauer AC, Atallah J, Dubin AM, Erickson CC, Rosenthal DN, et al. Treatment of ventricular arrhythmias in patients with congenital heart disease: a multicenter study. J Am Heart Assoc. 2019;8(14):e012731.
27. Dey D, Slomka PJ, Leeson P, Comaniciu D, Shrestha S, Sengupta PP, et al. Artificial intelligence in cardiovascular imaging: JACC state-of-the-art review. J Am Coll Cardiol. 2019;73(11):1317–35.
28. Martin-Isla C, Campello VM, Izquierdo C, Raisi-Estabragh Z, Baebler K, Petersen SE, et al. Image-based cardiac diagnosis with machine learning: a review. Front Cardiovasc Med. 2020;7:1.
29. Xue W, Islam A, Bhaduri M, Li S. Direct multitype cardiac indices estimation via joint representation and regression learning. IEEE Trans Med Imaging. 2017;36(10):2057–67.

Pulmonary, Pleural, and Chest Wall Masses

17

Poonam Sherwani and Namrata Bagchi

17.1 Introduction

Primary lung tumors are extremely uncommon in the pediatric population and have a limited diagnostic spectrum. In children, metastatic disease resulting from extracranial solid neoplasms is far more common than primary pulmonary malignancy, and it is primarily linked to hepatoblastoma, sarcomas, and Wilms tumors. Hancock et al. published the biggest study series, which included 383 cases in total, 76% of which were malignant. Since the tumors in neonates and infants are quite different from the children, age is an important crucial factor in the diagnosis of tumors. In neonates and infants, the most common tumors are pleuropulmonary blastoma, infantile fibrosarcoma, and fetal lung interstitial tumor while in children, the most common tumors are inflammatory myofibroblastic tumors (IMTs), carcinoid salivary gland tumors, recurrent respiratory papillomatosis (RRP), and other rare entities. In a published study review spanning 90 years of experience at a single institution, Yu et al. identified 14 distinct pathologic types of pediatric primary lung tumors, with pleuropulmonary blastoma (PPB) accounting for 15% of cases, inflammatory myofibroblastic tumor (IMT) for 17.5% of cases, and carcinoid tumor (20%) for 50% of cases. The location and size of the lesion determine the clinical presentation of primary malignant lung tumors in children, and the nonspecificity of the lesion may cause a delay in diagnosis. Pneumonia (23%), fever (18%), respiratory distress (12%), cough (35%), and hemoptysis (11%) are all present in the patients. Six percent of children with malignant pulmonary lesions do not exhibit any symptoms.

Meanwhile, chest wall masses in children broadly include bone or soft-tissue tumors, latter being divided into vascular tumors, peripheral nerve sheath tumors, fibroblastic-myofibroblastic tumors, with benign and malignant counterparts; examples such as osteochondroma, fibrous dysplasia, osteoid osteoma, Langerhans cell histiocytosis, Ewings sarcoma and family of tumors, osteosarcoma, soft tissue tumors such as infantile hemangioma, neurogenic tumors, and Malignant peripheral nerve sheath tumor (MPNST), rhabdomyosarcoma, and metastasis. Although there is a lot of overlap in the imaging features of various tumors, some tumors have characteristic imaging features, various genetic markers are specific to tumors, and few tumors have specific pathological findings.

In this chapter, we will review how to approach the common pediatric lung, pleural, and chest wall masses in children depending on the epidemiology with their specific imaging features and reporting format to narrow down the diagnosis.

P. Sherwani (✉) · N. Bagchi
AIIMS, Rishikesh, Uttarakhand, India

I. Kumar et al. (eds.), *Practical Approach to Imaging in Pediatric Oncology*,
https://doi.org/10.1007/978-981-96-8158-7_17

17.2 General Guidelines for Imaging

A chest radiograph is often the preliminary investigation for patients with nonspecific respiratory complaints and recurrent symptoms. It is recommended that chest radiographs be obtained in frontal and lateral views to help in identifying lesion localization to the airway, lung parenchyma, mediastinum, or as a multicompartmental pathological process. Few lesions may be difficult to identify on a radiograph because atelectasis or pneumonia may mask the tumor. Moreover, tiny endobronchial neoplasms and small pulmonary metastases are frequently occult on radiographs.

Owing to its rapidity, high spatial resolution, and excellent representation of lung parenchyma, a chest CT scan is the gold standard for the diagnosis as well as the local-regional staging of pediatric pulmonary cancers. Therefore, as part of the initial assessment of primary pediatric lung cancer, chest CT should be done following the recommended protocol by Thacker et al. as elaborated in the table below [1].

Series name	Coverage	Reconstructed slice thickness	Reformat plane/types/ reconstruction kernel	Comment(s)
Chest axial for lungs	Top of lungs through bottom of the lungs	1–3 mm	Axial plane Lung kernel	Mixed pulmonary arteriographic and venous phase (iodinated contrast should be administered in the evaluation of primary tumors unless contraindicated) Contrast unnecessary, if only assessing for lung metastases
Chest axial Soft tissue	Top through bottom of the lungs	3–5 mm	Axial plane Soft-tissue kernel	
Chest Coronal reformat	Anterior skin through posterior skin	2–4 mm	Coronal plane Soft-tissue kernel	
Chest MIPs	Top of lungs through bottom of the lungs	5–15 mm	Axial or coronal plane Lung kernel	Best series for depicting small pulmonary nodules

Guidelines have been developed by the pediatric cancer group for PPB; however, for the evaluation of non-PPB pediatric chest malignancies, magnetic resonance imaging (MR) is preferred over CT if the mediastinal mass is detected on radiographs, especially if the mass is located in the posterior compartment to look for the invasion of the spinal cord and neural foramina. Magnetic resonance imaging (MR) outperforms computed tomography (CT) in this regard with superior soft tissue contrast resolution. However, MR is not helpful for pulmonary parenchymal involvement because tiny pulmonary nodules, particularly calcified nodules, as in the case of metastatic osteosarcoma, may go undetected.

Extrathoracic Imaging for Staging When there is a high likelihood of metastatic disease following a pediatric lung malignancy, a comprehensive diagnostic imaging search should be conducted to identify the most likely affected locations. The EXPeRT group recommends that if a patient has type II or III PPB, they should have radionuclide bone scans, brain MR, and abdominal CT scans [2].

Additionally, 18F-FDG PET/MRI shows a high degree of sensitivity for bone marrow invasion. In certain situations, 18F-FDG PET/CT or PET/MRI can be considered as an alternative to radioactive bone scintigraphy.

10–15% of pediatric bronchial carcinoids develop metastatic disease; the liver, adrenal glands, brain, and bones are the most frequently affected organs. It is advised using the somatostatin receptor radiotracers, when available, for PET/CT or PET/MR for the staging of carcinoids.

17.3 Suggested Structured Reporting Template

The first step is to look at the age of the child. Suggested structured reporting template for thoracic pediatric masses (Table 17.1).

17.3.1 Lung Tumors in Neonates and Infants

Primary lung tumors are very few in neonates and infants and must be differentiated from congenital lung lesions. As a rule, a lung lesion detected in the neonate is a mass if antenatal ultrasound in the second or third trimester is normal; nevertheless, lung cysts are echogenic and resemble lung tissue and can be missed on antenatal ultrasound. Figure 17.1 shows the radiological approach to diagnosis in pleural and pulmonary tumors.

17.3.2 Pleuropulmonary Blastoma (PPB)

Pleuropulmonary blastoma (PPB) is an aggressive dysodontogenic neoplasm and is common pediatric lung neoplasm and is seen in 0.25–0.5% of children under 6 years. Dehner classified PPB into three subtypes.

- Type1: Purely cystic
- Type II: Cystic and solid
- Type III: Solid

It is also added as one of the PPBs that was introduced in 2006 and resembles Type I PPB histologically without malignant cells and is believed to have regressed from Type I.

PPB can either arise from the lung or pleura and have both epithelial and mesenchymal components in which epithelial component is not

Table 17.1 Suggested structured reporting template for thoracic pediatric masses

Origin	<chest wall> <pleural> <pulmonary> <diaphragm> <mixed>
Size	[---x—x--] cm
Pleural and pulmonary masses	
Number of lesions	<single> <multiple> <innumerable>
Location	<central> <peripheral>
Parenchyma	<cystic> <solid> <mixed> <fat> <calcification> <hemorrhage>
Enhancement	<none> <mild> <marked>
Pattern of enhancement	<homogenous> <heterogenous> <peripheral> <cyst wall/septa enhancement>
Local invasion	<mediastinal: fat/vessels/pericardiac/cardiac> <trachea/bronchi: craniocaudal extent> <chest wall: ribs/intercostal muscles/subcutaneous/ others> <diaphragm>
Lymph nodes	<mediastinal> <hilar> <pulmonary> <others>
Associated changes	<collapse> <consolidation> <pleural effusion> <pleural thickening/nodularity> <pneumothorax> <others>
Chest wall lesion	
Origin and extent of involvement	<bone: ribs/vertebra> <intercostal/ pectoral/other muscles> <subcutaneous tissue> <diaphragm> <subcutaneous fat> <intermuscular> <extrapleural>
Number	<single> <multiple>
Parenchyma	<Cystic> <matrix: osseous/cartilaginous/fibrous/soft tissue> <fat> <fluid-fluid levels> <MR signal: T1/T2/ADC/Other>
Enhancement	<none/mild/marked> <homogenous/heterogenous>
Bone involvement	<expansion> <endosteal scalloping> <reactive sclerosis> <geographical/permeative destruction> <periosteal reaction> <pathological fracture>
Spread	<Extrathoracic> <neural foraminal> <intraspinal extension>
Metastasis	<present> <absent>

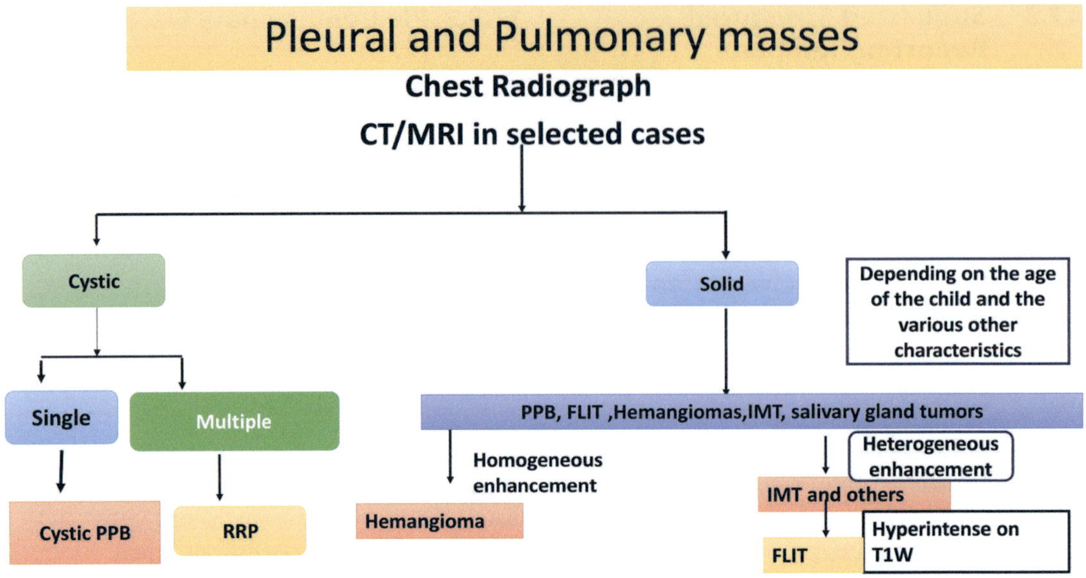

Fig. 17.1 Radiological approach to pleural and pulmonary masses

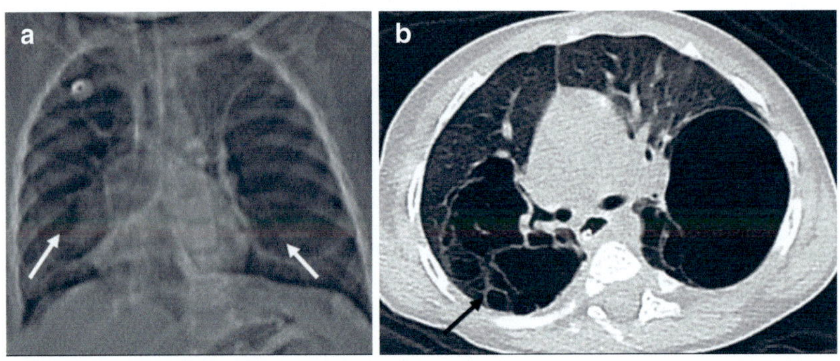

Fig. 17.2 (**a**) Frontal chest radiograph of a neonate shows the large globular lucent areas in both middle and lower lung zones with absent bronchovascular markings (white arrows). No significant mediastinal shift. (**b**) Axial non-contrast CT thorax in lung window shows well-defined oval-shaped cystic lesions in basal segments of lower lobes with multiple locules on right side (black arrow).—Cystic Type I PPB

malignant while the mesenchymal component is malignant.

17.3.2.1 Type 1 Pleuropulmonary Blastoma (PPB)

Type 1 PPB is seen in younger children as compared to type II and III, seen in infants <3 years in 97% of cases, and is seen more commonly in males and manifests with pneumothorax in 30% of cases (Fig. 17.2). Prognosis is good with 5-year survival of 91% however few may progress to type II and III [3]. Type I PPB appears as a large (>5 cm) well-demarcated cyst with thin septa without any nodule. Type 1r is the variant of Type I which shows either regression or failure of progression of the disease.

17.3.2.2 Type II Pleuropulmonary Blastoma

Type 2 PPB is the intermediate tumor between I and III with solid and cystic components, present later than Type I at around 35 months. Symptoms consist of breathlessness and chest pain and present with pneumothorax and pleural effusion and

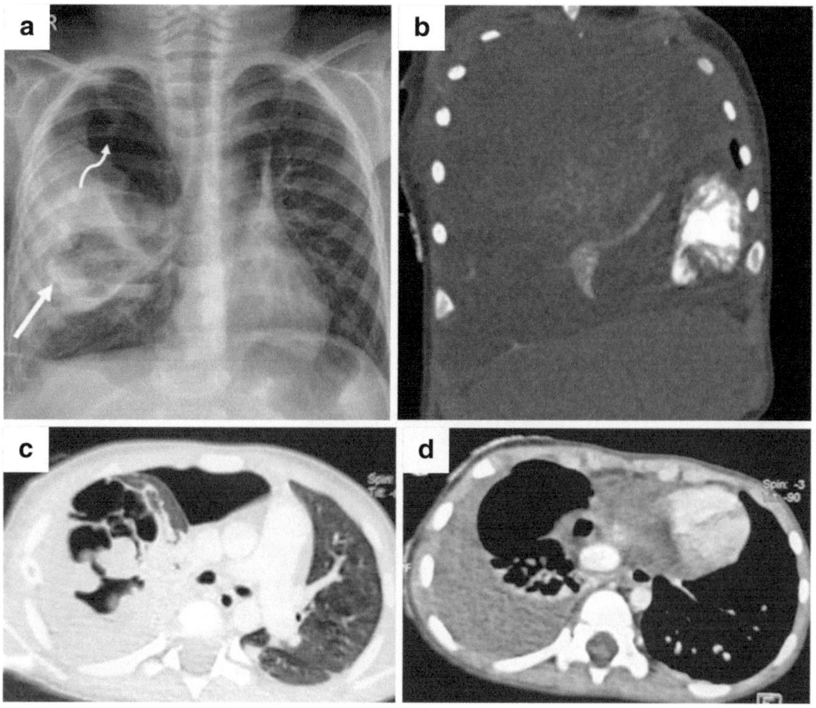

Fig. 17.3 (**a**) Frontal chest radiograph of a 4-year-old male child with recurrent chest infections shows large well-defined heterogenous radioopacity (white arrow) in the right hemithorax with broad-based towards the lateral chest wall causing contralateral cardiomediastinal shift. Crescentic pneumothorax along the right apical lung zone is seen (curved white arrow). (**b**) Coronal reformatted contrast CT thorax in mediastinal window shows a large heterogenously enhancing mass with hypodense areas, mediastinal shift. (**c**, **d**) Axial reformatted CT thorax images in lung and mediastinal window show the heterogenous mass with mixed solid-cystic internal morphology, right hydropneumothorax, and evident mass effect of the lesion-Type II PPB

have a propensity to show mediastinal invasion and metastases to bone and brain are seen in 10% of cases. [4] (Fig. 17.3).

17.3.2.3 Type III Pleuropulmonary Blastoma

Occurrence of Type III PPB is seen at around the age of 40 months and is entirely solid with a propensity for mediastinal invasion and metastasis in 10% cases and has a worse prognosis than Type II with a 5-year survival of 53%. [3] Chest wall invasion is very rarely seen with PPB [5] (Fig. 17.4).

Clinically cystic ones remain asymptomatic or present with either rupture as pneumothorax or superimposed infection and present with non-specific symptoms as fever or respiratory distress delaying the diagnosis.

PPB are associated with DICER1 gene which is associated with chromosome 14q.32.13 which is associated with numerous benign and malignant neoplasm like cystic nephroma, pineoblastoma, pituitary blastoma, differentiated thyroid cancer, ovarian sex-cord stromal tumor, embryonal rhabdomyosarcoma, and others.

Radiograph: Depending on the type of PPB, chest radiograph shows large cystic lesion with solid components to complete opacification of hemithorax. Associated imaging findings like pleural effusion and pneumothorax can also be seen (Figs. 17.3a, and 17.4a).

CT: Cystic lesions unilateral or bilateral with or without solid component or large solid heterogeneously enhancing mass lesions involving

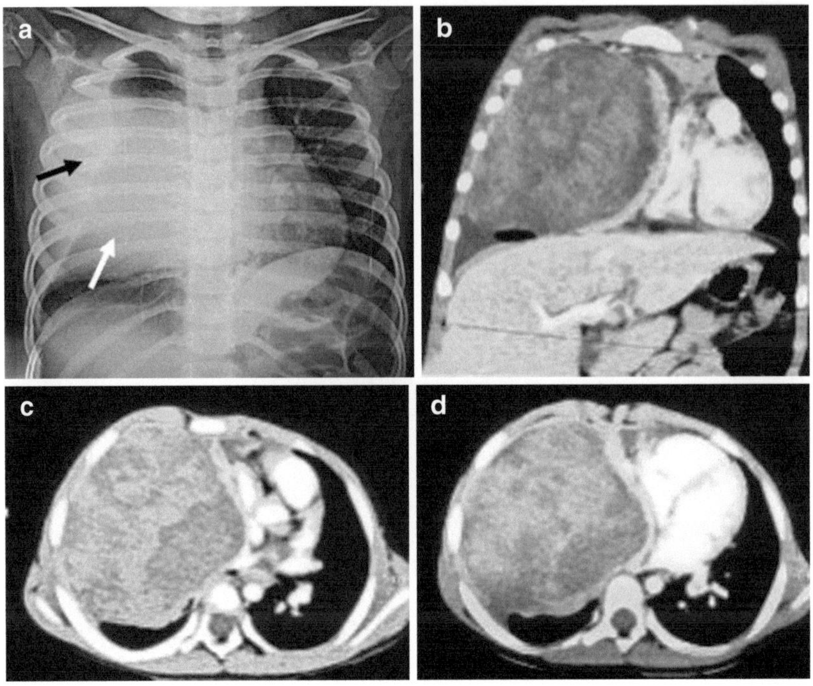

Fig. 17.4 (**a**) Frontal chest radiograph of a 5-year-old male child with recurrent chest infections shows large well-defined homogenous radioopacity in the right hemithorax with broad-based toward the lateral chest wall causing contralateral cardiomediastinal shift (white arrow). Effacement of the extrapleural lucent fat along the lateral chest wall with a crescentic opacity underlying right second to -sixth ribs and their intercostal spaces (black arrow). (**b**) Coronal reformatted images show evident mass effect of the lesion and compression of mediastinal structures. (**c**, **d**) Axial contrast CT thorax in mediastinal window shows a large heterogenously enhancing mass with central hypodense areas, mediastinal invasion. -Type III PPB

the entire hemithorax with mediastinal invasion are the predominant findings. Type 1 PPB is difficult to differentiate from CPAM radiologically; however, bilateral cystic lesions and normal antenatal ultrasound favor PPB. Involvement of the chest wall is uncommon and its invasion suggests other malignancy (Figs. 17.2b, 17.3b–d, and 17.4b–d).

MRI: MRI is not routinely indicated and appears heterogeneously hypointense on T1W and hyperintense on T2W and appears hyperintense due to hemorrhage on T1W with or without mediastinal invasion.

CT-PET: Shows increased uptake in Type III PPB.

Imaging staging: Currently, PPB is the only primary pediatric pulmonary malignancy for whom a pediatric cancer cooperative group has recommended imaging staging. These were developed using the Consensus Conference Standard Operating Procedure technique by the European Cooperative Study Group for Pediatric Rare Tumors (EXPeRT).

Chest CT is required for all PPB types. CT of the abdomen is recommended for Type II and III. Chest CT with contrast enhancement is required for the evaluation of the original tumor and any locoregional extension. Evaluation of the lymph nodes, mediastinum, cardiac and pericardial involvement, and potential tumor extension to the liver and diaphragm are all dependent on this. Thoracic MRI may be useful in defining regional tumor extension in Types II and III PPB. When evaluating a patient with Type II or III PPB for distant metastases, radionuclide bone scan and brain MRI should be performed. To determine intra-cardiac involvement and vascular invasion, an echocardiogram is also necessary. At present, no tumor markers are available. Additional examinations may be necessary for synchronous DICER1-related diseases.

Treatment strategies: Broadly include surgery, different multi-agent chemotherapy regimen including Vincristine, Actinomycin-D, Ifosfamide, and/or Cyclophosphamide. Radiotherapy is recommended only in the case of residual viable tumor after chemotherapy and second look surgery in PPB type II-III.

Post-treatment Assessment: Clinical and radiological evaluations should be performed on patients both throughout and after their course of treatment. Typically, CT scans with contrast enhancement are used. Assessment should be carried out to determine the patient's reaction to the initial chemotherapy after two to three cycles and before surgery to determine the potential residuals and make the decision for radiation therapy. In the event of metastatic disease in the initial phase, all known metastatic locations should be included in the imaging evaluation.

Surveillance: All PPB cases should be referred for genetic consultation with screening for *DICER1* mutation. Diligent follow-up and active surveillance of children and adolescents having the germline DICER1 pathogenic variation is required as recommended by Schultz et al. Proposed imaging surveillance procedures for patients with predisposed DICER1 pathogenic gene variations involve employing CT and CXR to test for the development of PPB. Specifically, abdominal ultrasonography is advised to rule out ovarian tumors and cystic nephromas.

Differential Diagnosis: The differential for cystic PPB is CPAM or bronchogenic cyst or pneumatocele while thoracic neuroblastoma is the differential for solid PPB; however, chest wall involvement and neural foramina extension will be seen in neuroblastoma.

17.4 Fetal Lung Interstitial Tumor (FLIT)

FLIT is a rare tumor seen in infants less than 3 years and very few cases have been reported so far [6]. Histologically resembles primitive lung tissue.

Imaging: Antenatal ultrasound shows echogenic mass with posterior acoustic shadowing. The mass appears hypodense and resembles PPB on CT, but no cystic variants are seen and no mediastinal invasion. Due to hemorrhage, the lesion is hyperintense on T1W.

Lobectomy and wedge resection is done and the prognosis is good.

17.4.1 Infantile Hemangioma

Infantile hemangiomas are commonly seen in the skin and liver and very rarely involve the lungs. According to the International Society of Vascular Anomalies, hemangiomas are either congenital or infantile. Infantile ones are present after birth and are endothelial glucose transport uptake inhibitor (GLUT) positive.

Imaging: Homogeneously enhancing mass which shows avid enhancement. Cystic masses and multiple enhancing masses can be seen. Associated pulmonary hypertension can also be seen.

17.4.2 Inflammatory Pseudotumor (IMT)

IMT is also known as inflammatory myofibrohistiocytic proliferation, plasma cell histiocytoma complex, and plasma cell granuloma. IMT is a rare mesenchymal benign tumor consisting of myofibroblast spindle cells with infiltration of plasmocytes and lymphocytes, although benign however shows aggressive features with adjacent organ invasion. IMT can be seen from head to toe; however, it is more common in the lungs in children. It is the most common lung lesion seen in younger children. Symptoms are non-specific and include cough, chest, and hemoptysis with

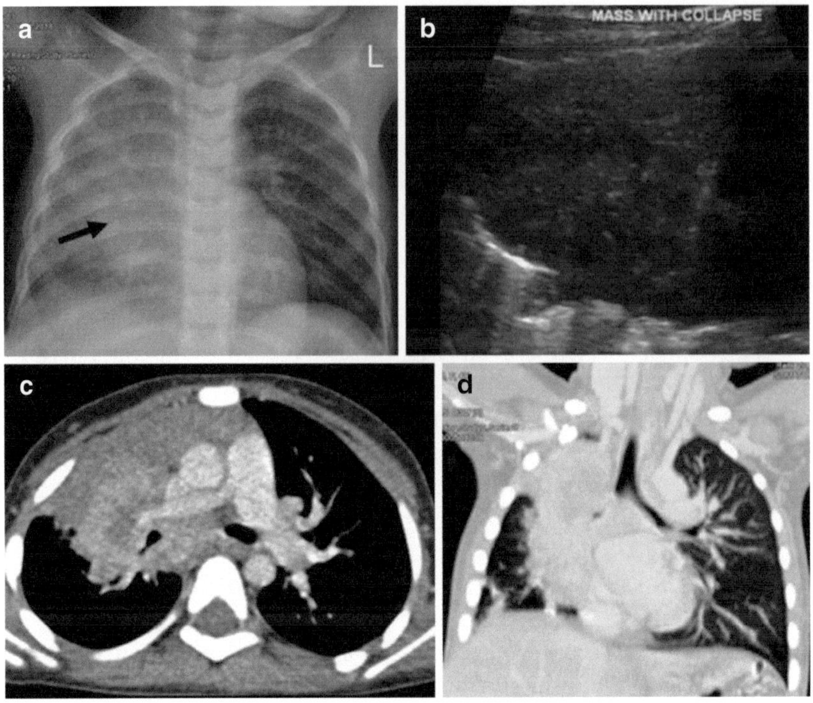

Fig. 17.5 (**a**) Frontal chest radiograph of a 3-year-old male with recurrent pneumonia and fever shows focal ill-defined soft tissue radioopacity (black arrow) in the right middle and lower lung zone with broad based towards the mediastinum, spiculated lateral and superior margins along with a veil-like homogenous radioopacity in right hemithorax. (**b**) Ultrasound thorax shows a solid heterogenous mass with adjacent collapsed lung. (**c**) Axial reformatted contrast CT thorax in mediastinal window shows an ill-defined hypoenhancing mass with collapse of apical and anterior segments of right upper lobe and encasement of SVC and right main pulmonary artery. Normal thymus is seen anteriorly. (**d**) Coronal reformatted lung window images shows the narrowing of the right main stem bronchus. Biopsy of the mass revealed inflammatory myofibroblastic tumor

anaplastic lymphoma kinase (ALK) which is a receptor protein tyrosine kinase is elevated in 50%, however not in cases of lung IMT [7].

Imaging Nonspecific and can range from intrapulmonary mass to endobronchial lesion or multicentric disease and can invade into the mediastinum and chest wall. Calcification is more prevalently seen in the pediatric age group than in the adult population, and cavitation and lymphadenopathy are very uncommon. [8] (Fig. 17.5a–d).

17.4.3 Neuroendocrine Tumors of the Lung

Neuroendocrine malignancies arise from the epithelial cells of neuroendocrine origin. Various subtypes of NEC according to the WHO Classification of lung tumors 2015 are typical carcinoid, atypical carcinoid, small cell lung cancer, and large cell lung cancer. Among the various subtypes, typical carcinoids are more common in children and the rest of the subtypes are very uncommon [9].

Imaging The most common finding is para hilar mass with distal atelectasis or collapse. On radiographs, calcifications are rarely visible and cavitation is extremely uncommon. On CT, the mass is located in the central airway lumen with either small or extensive extra bronchial components and lung extension with distal atelectasis or bronchiectasis with mucous impaction. The mass shows avid enhancement with evidence of calcification in 30% of cases. [10] Mediastinal lymph nodes are seldom seen in typical carcinoids.

Although MRI is rarely performed for carcinoids, however appears very much hyperintense on T2W. Unlike other tumors, FDG PET shows variable findings. Ga DOTATATE is performed to look for the identification of the site and predict the response from octreotide hormonal therapy.

17.4.4 Salivary Gland Tumors

The majority of salivary gland malignancies are derived from seromucinous submucous glands of the airways, which include mucoepidermoid and adenoid cystic tumors. Both tumors do not exhibit avid enhancement, but they do cause shortening of the airways and distal collapse akin to carcinoid tumors. Adenoid cystic carcinoma is less common in children; it affects the trachea and central bronchus with extension into the lung and is relatively larger with craniocaudal extension. Mucoepidermoid carcinoma is more common in children and involves the trachea and central or lobar bronchus with distal collapse and bronchiectasis [11, 12].

17.4.5 Recurrent Respiratory Papillomatosis (RRP)

RRP is caused by Human Papillomavirus 6 and 11 and there is growth of benign squamous papilloma in the aerodigestive tract and clinically present as hoarseness of voice. These papillomas tend to recur despite surgical resection. Spread to the lower respiratory tract is rare around 5% and pulmonary involvement is about 3.3% and is through the aerial route either due to tracheostomy or surgical resection. Therefore, the lower lobe, posterior, and peripheral lung are more commonly involved.

Imaging Multiple sessile or polypoid lesions can be seen involving the upper airway which can be detected on CT or virtual bronchoscopy. CT is better than radiograph in delineating the extent and severity of lesions and shows multiple small well-defined nodules in the previously mentioned region which can cavitate or transform into cysts later. Multiple small cysts can coalesce to form larger cysts or air fluid levels can be seen if the cysts become infected. Malignant transformation can be seen if there is development of large and heterogeneous with mediastinal invasion accompanied by pleural effusion, and mediastinal and cervical lymphadenopathy [13]. RRP guidelines state that imaging is not necessary for a diagnosis in the early stages but should be performed if malignant change is suspected.

Nut Midline Carcinoma Uncommon tumor that affects the head, neck, and thorax and is observed in all age groups. This particular kind of aggressive squamous cell carcinoma exhibits a large heterogenous mass with a substantial mediastinal invasion and pleural effusion. Final diagnosis is biopsy.

17.5 Chest Wall Masses

Based on the WHO classification in 2002, primary chest wall tumors can be broadly classified as bone or soft-tissue tumors, with the latter being further subclassified into adipocytic tumors, vascular tumors, peripheral nerve sheath tumors, cutaneous lesions, fibroblastic-myofibroblastic tumors, and so-called fibrohistiocytic tumors with malignant and benign subparts. A systematic approach based on few criteria such as (a) patient age and demographics, (b) clinical features, (c) lesion location in the chest wall, and (d) characteristic imaging findings such as matrix mineralization pattern, fat attenuation on CT and signal intensities on MRI imaging often help narrow down the differentials for a particular puzzling diagnosis. Figure 17.6 provides an approach to diagnosis in chest wall masses.

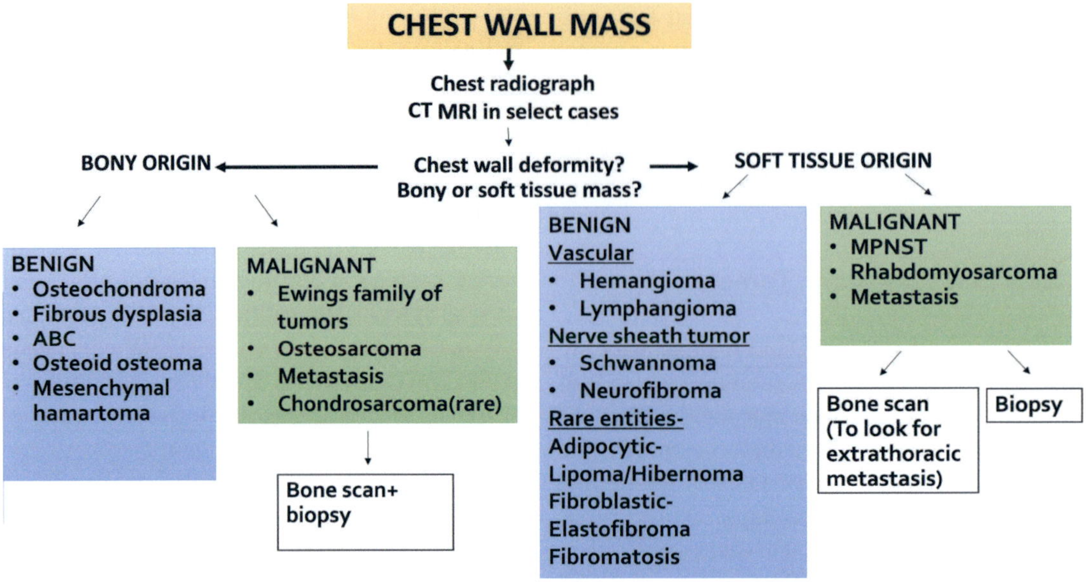

Fig. 17.6 Approach to chest wall masses

17.6 Benign Bone Tumors

17.6.1 Osteochondroma

Solitary osteochondroma is the most common benign bone tumor of the chest wall occurring in patients younger than 20 years, often presenting as a nontender, painless indolent mass. Usually originating from the surface of the underlying bone, these tumors grow until the bone reaches maturity, often beginning to develop before puberty. They most commonly appear near the costochondral junction of the ribs. Males are more likely to develop solitary lesions.

Imaging An osteochondroma appears on radiographs as an osseous protuberance that is continuous with the originating bone's surface. The lesion's attachment to the bone determines whether it is sessile or pedunculated. Osteochondroma is particularly common near the costochondral junction in the ribs [14].

CT is better for demonstrating the typical continuity of the medullary cavity of the osteochondroma and the affected bone. Cartilage cap (if calcified) can be well detected on CT.

MRI provides the most accurate assessment of the cartilaginous cap due to its distinctive T2-hyperintensity. The thickness of the cartilage cap is a crucial marker of the transition from osteochondroma to sarcoma. It is important to consider malignant transformation if an adult's cartilage cap is thicker than 2 cm, and a child's thicker than 3 cm (Fig. 17.7c, d).

Complications In these patients, enlargement, pain, and edema are markers of the progression to chondrosarcomatous disease. Compared to a rate of less than 1% in a single exostosis, malignant transition to chondrosarcoma happens more commonly (5–25%) in multiple hereditary exostoses [4]. The rate of chondrosarcomatous transformation is thought to be much lower in the pediatric population, but juvenile patients with several inherited exostoses need to be closely monitored by a skeletal survey on a regular basis.

Costal osteochondromas are characterized by an inward growth pattern, resulting in decreased range of motion, discomfort, and an irregular appearance.

An osteochondroma may compress nearby neurovascular structures, can also result in peri-

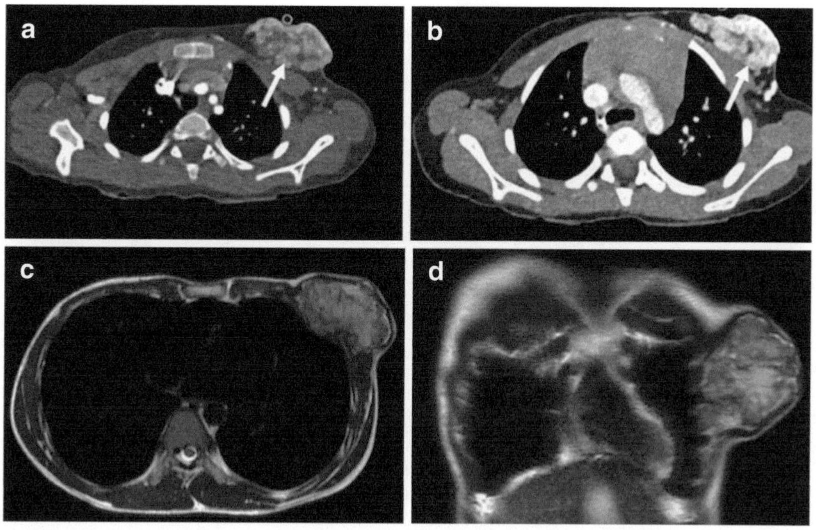

Fig. 17.7 Axial reformatted contrast CT thorax in arterial and venous phases (**a**) avidly enhancing left anterior chest wall lesion (white arrows in **a**, **b**) with peripheral nodular pattern of arterial hyperenhancement in subcutaneous plane (**b**) in venous phase, the lesion shows central pooling with homogenous enhancement- Infantile hemangioma. (**c**, **d**) T2W axial and coronal T1W FS non-contrast MRI of the thorax of a different patient shows an exophytic bony growth arising from the left seventh rib showing hyperintense cartilage cap—rib osteochondroma

cardial effusion, hemothorax, pneumothorax, pseudoaneurysm development, and overlying bursitis.

17.6.2 Fibrous Dysplasia

Fibrous dysplasia is a benign bone lesion in which the normal cancellous bone is replaced by immature fibro-osseous tissue that undergoes calcification. It is typically asymptomatic and incidentally detected.

Depending on the quantity of lesions, fibrous dysplasia has historically been divided into monostotic and polyostotic categories. While polyostotic disease is linked to other disorders, monostotic fibrous dysplasia is typically discovered by accident.

Mazabraud syndrome is characterized by an intramuscular myxoma that develops in a patient with polyostotic fibrous dysplasia, a rare nonhereditary condition. The clinical triad of fibrous dysplasia, café-au-lait pigmentation, and endocrine abnormalities (early onset puberty) characterize McCune-Albright syndrome. Fibrous dysplasia within the chest wall typically results from the lateral or posterior arc of the ribs [15].

Imaging Typically seen as a single, large, multilocular lesion on plain radiography, usually on the posteromedial part of the rib. It may at times present as fusiform expansion affecting the entire rib along with the ground glass matrix. The matrix can occasionally be lucent or sclerotic. Rarely, a cystic lesion with fluid-fluid levels is also seen. On CT, the fibrous dysplasia matrix may show peripheral trabeculation or appear to be solely osteolytic. Amorphous mineralization in fibrous dysplasia is indicative of woven bone growth and gives the characteristic ground-glass look seen on radiography. Moreover, cartilage nodules that exhibit normal cartilaginous mineralization may be present in fibrous dysplasia [15]. Fibrous dysplasia on MRI usually exhibits heterogeneous enhancement and isointense to skeletal muscle on T1-weighted images and heterogeneously hyperintense on T2-weighted sequences. The sclerotic rim that is frequently visible on radiographs corresponds with a hypointense rim seen on both T1- and T2-weighted sequences (Fig. 17.8).

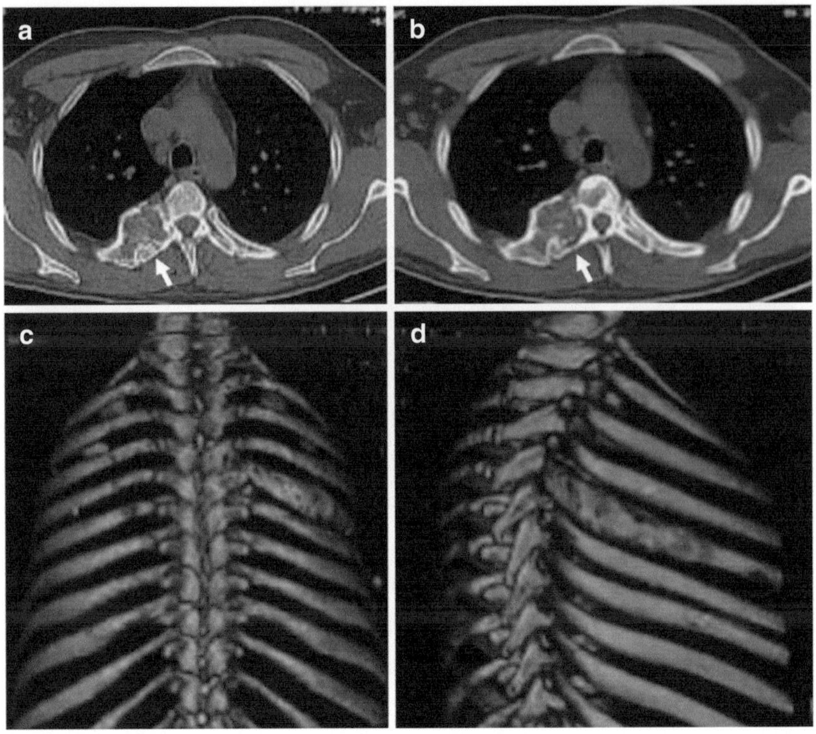

Fig. 17.8 Axial non-contrast CT thorax in bone window and volume rendered images of an adolescent patient. (**a**, **b**) Shows the medullary expansion of posterior segment of right fifth rib with an internal ground glass matrix (white arrow) involving the costovertebral and costotransverse joints. (**c**, **d**) Confirm the same findings on volume rendered images—cystic FD

Complications McCune-Albright syndrome is more common in women and is seen in 2–3% and is linked to a modest rate of malignant transformation (0.4–4.0%) [15] (Fig. 17.9).

17.6.3 Aneurysmal Bone Cyst

Aneurysmal bone cysts are uncommon benign lumps that can spread into nearby soft tissues and expand quickly, destroying bone.

An eccentric, expansile lytic lesion with septa that is clearly defined by a thin shell of periosteum is commonly seen on plain radiography. Intraosseous and extraosseous components are well-delineated by CT and MR scans. A lobulated or septated mass with a narrow, distinct rim of low T2 signal is typically visible on MR imaging [14]. ABCs frequently show fluid levels, which point to hemorrhage. However, other osseous tumors such as telangiectatic osteosarcoma, giant cell tumor, simple bone cyst, and chondroblastoma may also exhibit fluid levels.

17.6.4 Osteoid Osteoma

Osteoid osteomas typically are benign tumors of long bones, [14] however can originate from the ribs, sternum, or vertebral column, albeit they are less prevalent in the thorax. It occurs frequently between the ages of 7 and 25, more commonly in male population.

Imaging A well-defined lytic lesion often small (<2 cm) with a radiolucent center (nidus) encircled by reactive sclerosis on radiography. CT is done in cases of non-visualization of the lesion on radiograph and for delineating the nidus. The nidus's center frequently has mineralization. A recent report on radiologic findings to enhance the accuracy of diagnosis describes the "CT vessel sign," where a feeding vessel is observed approaching or entering the nidus (vascular nidus). The only benefit of using MRI is that it can occasionally show the nidus and surrounding sclerosis and surrounding edema. Even though the nidus greatly enhances when gadolinium is used, a typical double-density sign is shown in

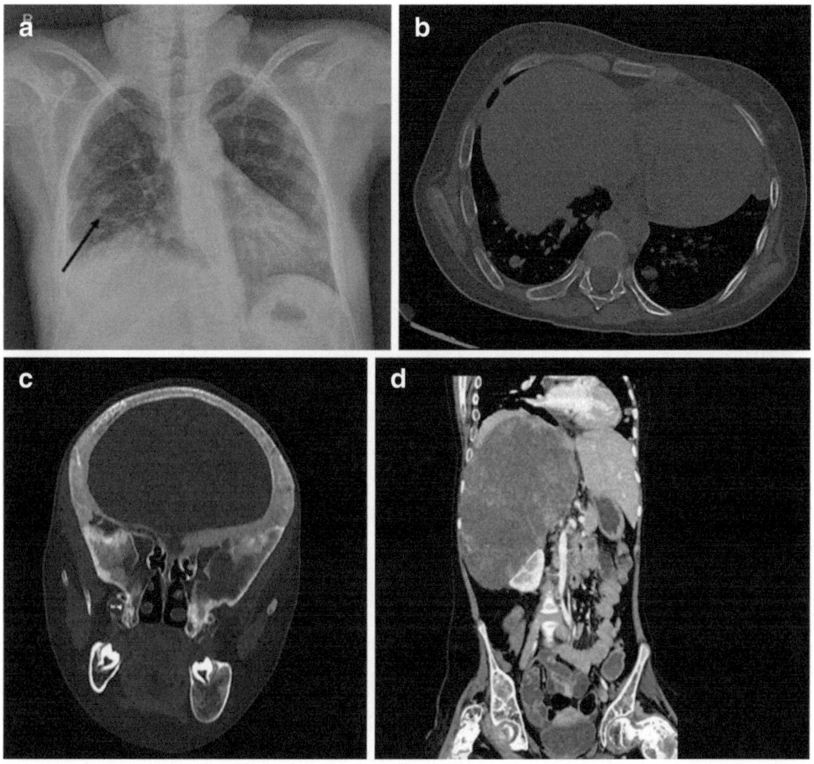

Fig. 17.9 (**a**) Frontal chest radiograph shows the expansion of multiple ribs on the right side with an internal ground glass matrix (black arrow). (**b**) Axial non-contrast CT thorax in bone window confirms the findings. Note is also made of bilateral multiple lung nodules. (**c**) Coronal reformatted non-contrast CT of face in bone window show the medullary expansion and diploic widening of the calvarial bones namely frontal, biparietal bones, maxilla and left hemimandible. (**d**) Coronal reformatted images of contrast CT abdomen of the same patient show a large heterogenous lesion in the right adrenal and multiple variable-sized intraosseous fibrous dysplasia in both iliac bones and proximal femur along with pathological fracture of neck of right femur—polystotic fibrous dysplasia in a patient with McCune Albright Syndrome

the 99mTc methylene diphosphonate (MDP) bone scan, where a greater area of enhanced uptake is superimposed over an intense tracer uptake in the nidus.

17.6.5 Mesenchymal Hamartoma

An uncommon tumor that develops antenatally is called mesenchymal hamartoma of the chest wall. This tumor is frequently found as a hard, immovable mass during birth or shortly thereafter. With time, it could grow, stabilize, or retreat during infancy [10]. As mesenchymal hamartomas are not classified as real neoplasms, there is no chance of metastasis or local invasion. Multifocality and bilaterality have been reported.

Imaging Mesenchymal hamartoma of the chest wall appears as an expansile chest mass involving one or more ribs on radiography and CT. There have been reports of subsequent aneurysmal bone cyst development and speckled popcorn-like calcifications. Patients with subsequent aneurysmal bone cysts have been shown to have hemorrhagic fluid-fluid levels within the lesion, which is a useful distinguishing characteristic.

The internal contents of mesenchymal hamartomas determine their MRI signal characteristics. The components of an aneurysmal bone cyst exhibit variable degrees of internal bleeding and are hyperintense on fluid-sensitive sequences. A low T1 signal is indicative of areas that have been calcified. Fetal MRI can occasionally be used to diagnose mesenchymal hamartoma prenatally based on these imaging features.

17.6.6 Enchondroma

A benign bony cartilaginous lesion which appears as a well-defined central medullary lesion with a lobulated shape and endosteal scalloping/erosion is shown on the plain radiograph.

Typical configurations of calcifications include "popcorn" and annular type. An enchondroma in the rib might result in significant osseous growth [14].

17.6.7 Langerhans Cell Histiocytosis

Depending on the systems and number of lesions, LCH can be divided into three types: Unifocal, multifocal unisystem, and multifocal multisystem [16] The radiologic appearance depends on the site of involvement and the phase of disease.

Imaging depends on the stage of the disease. Early bone lesions have a lytic appearance with either well-defined borders or poorly demarcated margins associated with ambiguous reactive sclerosis. Aggressive lesions may cause bone destruction and can mimic osteomyelitis or malignant neoplasms, such as Ewing sarcoma and lymphoma. Chronic lesions may resolve completely or have a sclerotic appearance. Remodeling of bone could cause expansion of the affected bone.

17.7 Malignant Bone Tumors

17.7.1 Ewing Sarcoma Family of Tumors

The classical Ewing sarcoma, atypical Ewing sarcoma, peripheral primitive neuroectodermal tumor, and Askin tumor are among the high-grade tiny round cell tumors that make up the Ewing sarcoma family of cancers. Tumors in the Ewing sarcoma family are more frequent in the second decade of life. There is a palpable mass seen in children with these tumors which may cause edema, elevated local temperatures, and rapid growth of the mass and hence could resemble an infection.

Imaging On radiography, a permeative lytic bone lesion, extra pleural in a location with the aggressive periosteal reaction which is typically a multi-lamellated or onion-ring pattern is observed. As seen in such tumors elsewhere in the body, surrounding soft tissue is frequently disproportionately larger than the osseous component [11], this is due to the cortical permeation phenomenon. In 5–8% of patients, extraosseous Ewing sarcoma family tumors are present [11]. CT is useful in determining the complete degree of the tumor's cortical involvement as well as internal calcifications that are not visible on radiography (Fig. 17.10).

MRI On T1-weighted scans, the tumor is isointense to slightly hyperintense to muscle, and hyperintense on T2-weighted sequences, post-contrast enhancement is heterogenous and non-uniform. Extra skeletal Ewing sarcoma appears as large soft tissue with multiple consecutive rib involvement on CT, however no marrow involvement is seen (Fig. 17.11).

17.7.2 Osteosarcoma

Osteosarcoma is a peculiar high-grade tumor of mesenchymal origin that is commonly found in long bones, however can arise within the soft tissue, or pleura as well. Ribs, manubrium, sternum, and clavicle are shown to have 1–2% of these tumors. Adolescence and young adulthood is the most common age group second only being the elderly >60 years with other predisposing conditions as well.

Imaging Chest wall osteosarcoma usually appears on radiography as a large lytic destructive bone lesion with concomitant osteoid type of matrix mineralization in the soft tissue mass and frank ossification. The sunburst pattern that is commonly linked to osteosarcomas of the

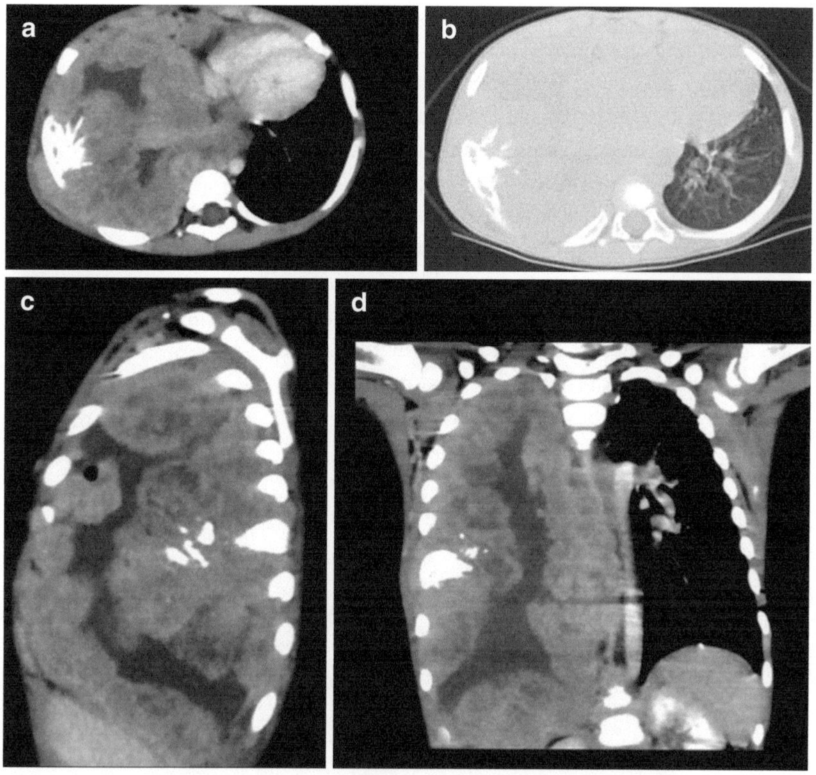

Fig. 17.10 Axial contrast enhanced CT thorax in soft tissue and lung window (**a**, **b**) shows large heterogenously enhancing mass with central non-enhancing necrotic core with circumferential growth within the right hemithorax and medially collapsed right lung. Associated aggressive periosteal reaction seen in right seventh rib with sun-burst pattern and extension beyond the right lateral chest wall. Mass effect is seen in the form of cardio-mediastinal shift to left side. (**c**, **d**) Sagittal and coronal reformatted mediastinal window confirms the findings—Ewings sarcoma

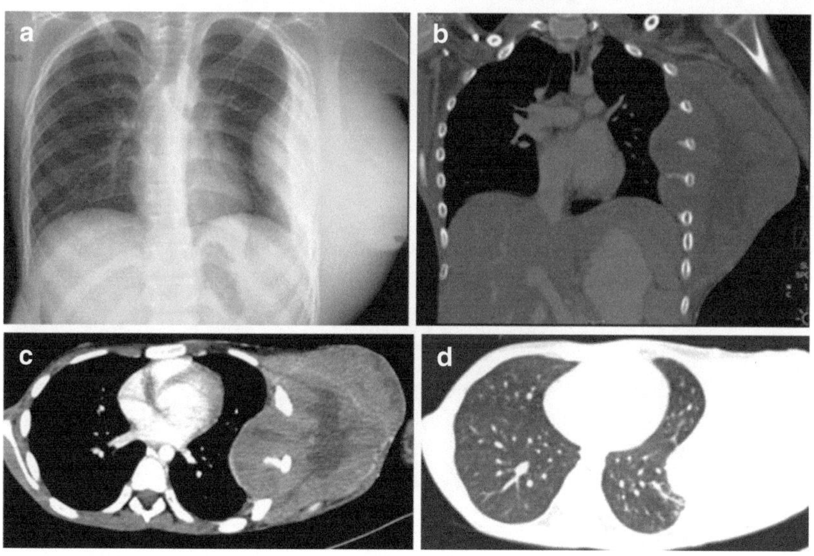

Fig. 17.11 Frontal chest radiograph of 13 year-old male with (**a**) large soft tissue opacity along the left lateral chest wall with intrathoracic extension from left third to seventh intercostal spaces. (**b**) Coronal reformatted contrast enhanced CT chest in bone windows show associated periosteal reaction seen in left fourth and fifth rib. (**c**, **d**) Axial contrast enhanced CT thorax in soft tissue and lung window shows large heterogenously enhancing mass with central non-enhancing necrotic area seen overhanging in left lateral chest wall with intrathoracic extension. Associated periosteal reaction seen in left fourth and fifth rib with solid interrupted pattern. Mass shows well-defined medial margins. No evident lung parenchymal infiltration—extraskeletal Ewings sarcoma

extremities is often absent in the chest wall rather an interrupted spiculated, buttress, or Codman triangle appearance with single or multiple laminae is seen. This imaging appearance often confuses radiologists with those seen in other benign conditions with an aggressive pattern of bony destruction such as osteomyelitis.

CT is useful as a problem-solving tool in localizing the origin of the mass and often better determining areas of cortical bone involvement and areas of matrix mineralization that are ambiguous on radiography. The lesion is hyperintense to muscle on sequences on both T1 and T2WI. On all MRI sequences, low signal intensity foci are indicative of internal calcification and show enhancement on post-contrast scans.

17.7.3 Metastasis

Although uncommon in the pediatric age group, metastasis is a significant cause of chest wall malignancies. Primary malignancy such as a posterior mediastinal primary neuroblastoma can directly invade the chest wall, or it may present as destructive metastatic lytic lesions in the ribs or thoracic spine. Other tumors include rhabdomyosarcoma, and hematologic malignancies, such as lymphoma or leukemia. Chest wall metastatic disease is frequently ambiguous, but it usually manifests as lytic lesions with periostitis and an underlying cortical disruption (Figs. 17.11 and 17.12).

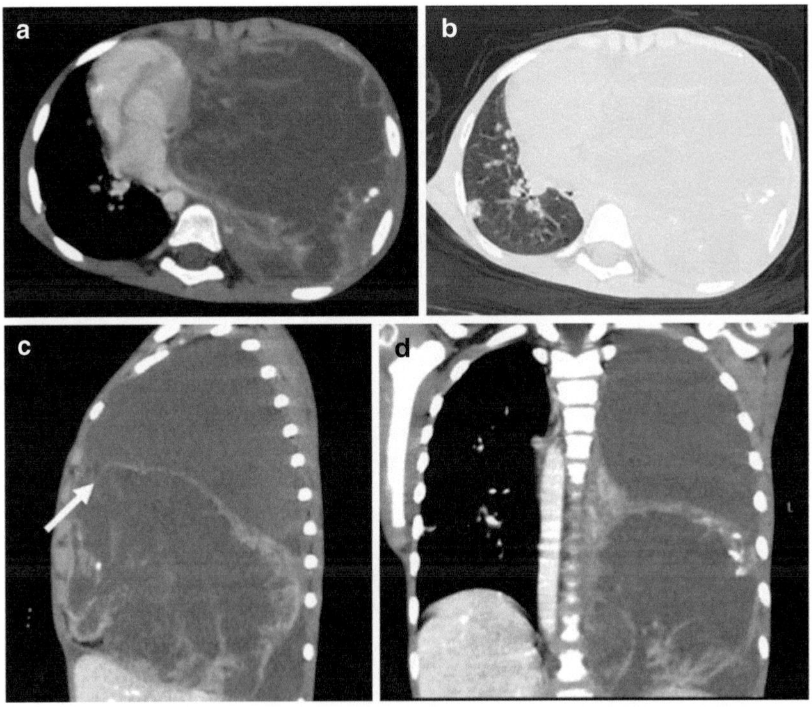

Fig. 17.12 Axial contrast enhanced CT thorax of an adolescent patient with right femoral osteosarcoma in soft tissue (**a**) and lung window (**b**). Large heterogenously enhancing mass with central non-enhancing areas in the left hemithorax showing mass effect in the form of contralateral mediastinal shift and collapse of left lung. Peripheral coarse calcifications seen within mass. (**b**) Another small well-defined solid soft tissue metastatic deposit seen in the subpleural region of the lateral basal segment of right lower lobe with internal calcifications. (**c**, **d**) Sagittal and coronal reformatted contrast CT thorax in mediastinal window confirms the findings (white arrow in **c**) in the anterosuperior aspect of the mass with communication of the hypodense contents into the left hydrothorax.—Metastasis from osteosarcoma

17.8 Benign Soft Tissue Tumors

17.8.1 Vascular Origin

17.8.1.1 Infantile Hemangioma

Infantile hemangiomas are one of the most common vascular tumors of infancy, affecting 2–3% of the general population with female predisposition. These are common in the face and neck region with only 25% of cases seen to originate from the chest. The lesion is typically heterogeneously hyperechoic compared to the adjacent muscle on ultrasound. They often show phasic pleomorphism with varied appearances. In the proliferative phase, they characteristically show a hypervascular mass with multiple small vessels of low-resistance arterial waveforms and one or more draining veins. In the involuting phase, most of the hypervascular soft tissue is now replaced with fatty tissue giving it a diffusely echogenic and more heterogenous appearance.

A well-demarcated mass that is isodense to the surrounding soft tissue and with significant postcontrast enhancement is the hallmark of an infantile hemangioma on CT. On MRI, the lesion may or may not show well-defined boundaries, however multiple flow voids consistent with high-flow vessels are well appreciated. It is T2 hyperintense and has an intermediate signal intensity on T1-weighted imaging with avid enhancement on T1 postcontrast fat saturation images. Due to intrinsic areas of necrosis and fatty replacement, the mass on T1-weighted imaging becomes increasingly heterogeneous and hyperintense as the child gets older and the infantile hemangioma starts to involute [17] (Fig. 17.12a, b).

Different vascular neoplasms known as kaposiform hemangioendotheliomas might resemble infantile hemangiomas. In addition to having the potential to be malignant, these tumors are more aggressive than infantile hemangiomas and, in over 50% of instances, are linked to the Kasabach-Merritt phenomenon, in which the patient experiences significant thrombocytopenia-induced coagulopathy. It is possible to distinguish between nonmalignant infantile hemangiomas and kaposiform hemangioendotheliomas by looking for minor signs of local invasion and poorly defined boundaries.

17.8.1.2 Lymphangioma

Lymphangioma is a congenital tumor that typically affects the neck and lymphatic systems. It is made up of dilated lymphatic channels. It is seen in the axilla, mediastinum, and cervicothoracic junction in children [18]. The lesion displays low signal intensities on T1-weighted images on MRI comparable to or lower than those of muscle, while on T2-weighted images, they often exhibit high signal intensities greater than those of fat. After gadolinium injection, there is thin peripheral and septal enhancement.

17.8.1.3 Peripheral Nerve Sheath Tumor

Schwannoma

Radiograph may reveal secondary changes such as erosion or scalloping of the bone. The CT scan shows a uniform, well-defined mass with attenuation comparable to or slightly less than that of muscle. Attenuation of lesion on postcontrast scan is comparable to or marginally greater than the muscle. The lesion is notably bright on T2WI and is isointense or slightly hyperintense than muscle on T1W. The nerve that leads into the tumor could be visible ("entry nerve root sign"). Postcontrast enhancement is variable with smaller tumors showing homogeneous enhancement, in larger tumors, heterogeneous enhancement. "Fascicular sign" is described on imaging as multiple small ring-like low T2W signal intensity structures with peripheral hyperintensity representing the fascicular bundles within the nerves. It is more commonly observed than in neurofibroma.

Neurofibroma

Widening of the neural foramina is seen on Radiograph. Neurofibromas have multiple types such as localized, plexiform ("bag of worms" appearance), and diffuse forms. They appear as well-defined hypodense lesions with variable heterogeneous contrast enhancement on CT scans. On MRI, it shows a target-like appearance

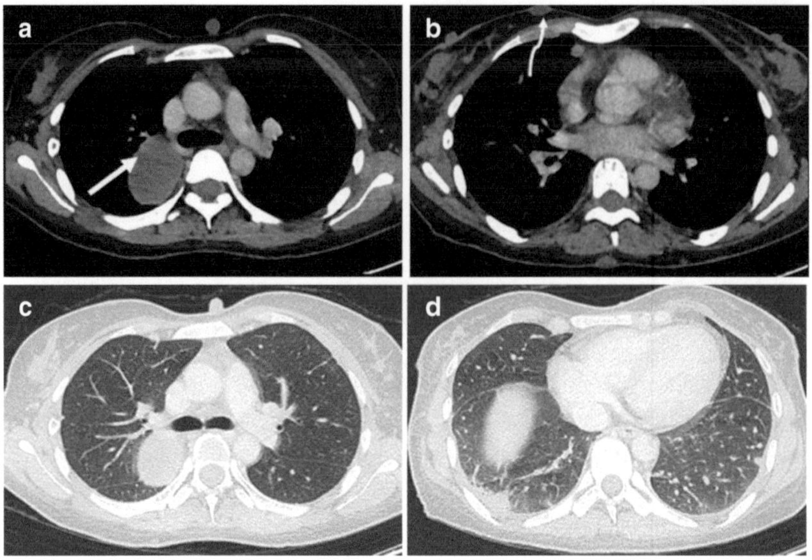

Fig. 17.13 Axial contrast CT thorax in mediastinal window (**a**) well-defined oval-shaped homogenous lesion in the right paravertebral and vascular compartment, homogenously isodense to skeletal muscle with no significant postcontrast enhancement (white arrows in **a**). No obvious intraspinal/intraforaminal extension. (**b**) Innumerable variable sized, homogenously isodense round to oval lesions diffusely scattered in skin and subcutaneous tissue of visualized anterior, posterior and lateral chest walls and bilateral breasts (curved white arrow)—Neurofibromas. (**c**, **d**) Axial contrast CT thorax in lung window shows multifocal subsegmental areas of atelectasis and fibrotic bands seen in anterior and lingular segments of left upper lobe and dependent basal segments of bilateral lower lobes with few fibrotic small solid random nodules—Neurofibromatosis-1

(rim of hyperintensity on T2WI with central lower signal intensity) (Fig. 17.13). A reverse target sign is seen on postcontrast images with marked enhancement of the core in comparison to the penumbra. This sign is more commonly seen than in Schwannoma.

17.9 Malignant Soft Tissue Tumors

17.9.1 Malignant Peripheral Nerve Sheath Tumors

These tumors can arise within plexiform neurofibromas in patients with neurofibromatosis type 1 (NF1), or they can arise sporadically. A significant male predominance is present. The "split fat sign," which depicts a rim of fat encircling the neurovascular bundle, and the "target sign," are two distinguishing features that aid in defining the neurological origin of the tumor. When these indicators are absent, it signals malignant transformation. Edema within the surrounding structures on T2-weighted imaging further implies that an MPNST is malignant. Other MRI characteristics that support MPNST above benign equivalents include rapid interval expansion, ill-defined margins, and big size (>5 cm) [19]. Large heterogeneous mass on CT with bony destruction and erosion suggest malignant transformation. On MRI, a large, aggressive tumor runs along the course of a peripheral nerve. Hyperintense and heterogeneous appearance on T2WI, iso to hypointense on T1WI, and with heterogeneous enhancement on postcontrast scan suggests malignant transformation. Seldom are target and fascicular signs observed [20].

17.9.2 Rhabdomyosarcoma

Rhabdomyosarcoma has three histologic subtypes: pleomorphic, alveolar, and embryonal. Chest wall involvement is often connected with the alveolar subtype, which is linked to the worse clinical outcome. Pertinent to the pediatric population, the embryonal subtype also potentially affects the mediastinum and lower chest wall.

The presence of metastatic disease at the time of diagnosis is the single most significant prognostic factor for patients with chest wall rhabdomyosarcoma, regardless of subtype.

The ultrasound image displays a distinct, heterogeneous mass that is primarily hypoechoic and appears hypervascular on Doppler. CT is done to look for the anatomic extent of the lesion, adjacent bone and soft tissue invasion, and pulmonary metastases. Mass displays isointense to hyperintense signal on T2w, and intermediate signal on T1-weighted sequences and shows intense contrast enhancement. FDG PET is the most effective imaging modality for staging rhabdomyosarcoma, outperforming CT or MRI for pure anatomic imaging [17].

17.9.3 Metastasis

In children, metastatic lesions make up a minor but significant portion of chest wall lesions. Direct neuroblastoma can emerge as deadly metastatic lytic lesions in the ribs or thoracic spine, or they may originate from a posterior mediastinal tumor that largely invades the chest wall. [21] Hematologic malignancies like lymphoma or leukemia, as well as rhabdomyosarcoma that originates outside the chest wall, are other tumors that have the potential to spread to the chest wall. Metastasis affecting the chest wall commonly manifests as lytic lesions with overlying cortical disruption and periosteal reaction on imaging, although the majority have non-specific features.

References

1. Thacker PG, Iyer RS, Pace E, States LJ, Guillerman RP. Imaging of pediatric pulmonary tumors: a COG diagnostic imaging committee/SPR oncology committee white paper. Pediatr Blood Cancer. 2023;70(S4):e29964.
2. Bisogno G, Sarnacki S, Stachowicz-Stencel T, Minard Colin V, Ferrari A, Godzinski J, et al. Pleuropulmonary blastoma in children and adolescents: the EXPeRT/PARTNER diagnostic and therapeutic recommendations. Pediatr Blood Cancer. 2021;68(S4):e29045.
3. Messinger YH, Stewart DR, Priest JR, Williams GM, Harris AK, Schultz KAP, et al. Pleuropulmonary blastoma: a report on 350 central pathology-confirmed pleuropulmonary blastoma cases by the international pleuropulmonary blastoma registry. Cancer. 2015;121(2):276–85.
4. Leung SS, Donuru A, Kandula V, Parekh MR, Saul D. Multimodality imaging of pleuropulmonary blastoma: pearls, pitfalls, and differential diagnosis. Semin Ultrasound CT MRI. 2022;43(1):61–72.
5. Biyyam DR, Chapman T, Ferguson MR, Deutsch G, Dighe MK. PEDIATRIC IMAGING congenital lung abnor-malities: embryologic features, prenatal diagnosis, and postnatal radiologic-pathologic correlation 1. Available from: http://radiographics.rsna.org/lookup/suppl/doi:10.1148/rg.306105508/-/DC1
6. Dishop MK, Mckay EM, Kreiger PA, Priest JR, Williams GM, Langston C, et al. Fetal lung interstitial tumor (FLIT) a proposed newly recognized lung tumor of infancy to be differentiated from cystic pleuropulmonary blastoma and other developmental pulmonary lesions [internet]. 2010. Available from: www.ajsp.com
7. Coffin CM, Hornick JL, Fletcher CDM. Inflammatory myofibroblastic tumor comparison of clinicopathologic, histologic, and immunohistochemical features including ALK expression in atypical and aggressive cases. Am J Surg Pathol. 2007;31:509.
8. Lee EY, Vargas SO, Park HJ, Plut D, Das KM, Winant AJ. Thoracic Multidetector computed tomography evaluation of inflammatory myofibroblastic tumor of the lung in pediatric patients in the era of modern diagnosis. J Thorac Imaging. 2021;36(5):310–7.
9. Travis WD, Brambilla E, Nicholson AG, Yatabe Y, Austin JHM, Beasley MB, et al. The 2015 World Health Organization classification of lung tumors: impact of genetic, clinical and radiologic advances since the 2004 classification. J Thorac Oncol. 10, 2015:1243–60.
10. Lichtenberger JP, Biko DM, Carter BW, Pavio MA, Huppmann AR, Chung EM. Primary lung tumors in children: radiologic-pathologic correlation. Radiographics. 2018;38(7):2151–72.
11. El Nayal A, Moran CA, Fox PS, Mawlawi O, Swisher SG, Marom EM. Primary salivary gland-type lung cancer: imaging and clinical predictors of outcome. Am J Roentgenol. 2013;201(1):W57.
12. Wang YQ, Mo YX, Li S, Luo RZ, Mao SY, Shen JX. Low-grade and high-grade mucoepidermoid carcinoma of the lung: Ct findings and clinical features of 17 cases. Am J Roentgenol. 2015;205(6):1160–6.
13. Knepper BR, Eklund MJ, Braithwaite KA. Malignant degeneration of pulmonary juvenile-onset recurrent respiratory papillomatosis. Pediatr Radiol. 2015;45:1077–81.
14. Tateishi U, Gladish GW, Kusumoto M, Hasegawa T, Yokoyama R, Tsuchiya R, et al. Chest wall tumors: radiologic findings and pathologic correlation – part 1. Benign tumors. Radiographics. 2003;23:1477–90.
15. Kushchayeva YS, Kushchayev SV, Glushko TY, Tella SH, Teytelboym OM, Collins MT, et al. Fibrous dysplasia for radiologists: beyond ground glass bone matrix. Insights Imaging. 2018;9:1035–56.

16. Zaveri J, La Q, Yarmish G, Neuman J. More than just langerhans cell histiocytosis: a radiologic review of histiocytic disorders. Radiographics. 2014;34(7):2008–24.
17. Baez JC, Lee EY, Restrepo R, Eisenberg RL. Chest wall lesions in children. Am J Roentgenol. 2013;200(5):W402.
18. Lee TJ, Collins J. MR imaging evaluation of disorders of the chest wall. Magn Reson Imaging Clin N Am. 2008;16:355–79.
19. Kransdorf MJ, Murphey MD. Neurogenic tumors. In: Kransdorf MJ, Murphey MD, editors. Imaging of soft tissue tumors. 2nd ed. Philadelphia, Pa: Lippincott Williams & Wilkins; 2006. p. 328–80. 2nd ed. Philafdelhia: Wolters Kluwer Health Adis (ESP; 2006. 328–330p.).
20. Tateishi U, Gladish GW, Kusumoto M, Hasegawa T, Yokoyama R, Tsuchiya R, et al. Chest wall tumors: radiologic findings and pathologic correlation – part 2. Malignant tumors. Radiographics. 2003;23:1491–508.
21. Chung WJ, Park YB, Jeon CH, Jung JW, Ko KP, Choi SJ, et al. Baseline characteristics of the Korean registry of pulmonary arterial hypertension. J Korean Med Sci. 2015;30(10):1429–38.

18 Hematological Malignancies

Priyanka Naranje and Manisha Jana

18.1 Introduction

Hematological malignancies in children encompass a broad spectrum of cancers that affect the blood, bone marrow, and lymphatic system. These can be broadly categorized into leukemias, lymphomas, and other less common malignancies such as myeloproliferative and myelodysplastic syndromes. Leukemia and lymphoma account for half of all childhood malignancies. Radiology plays a crucial role in the diagnosis, staging, response assessment, and follow-up of hematological malignancies in children. Radiographs, ultrasound (US), CT (computed tomography), MRI (magnetic resonance imaging), and PET-CT (positron emission tomography-computed tomography) have specific roles depending on the type of malignancy and the clinical question being addressed which will be discussed subsequently. In addition, interventional radiology plays an important role in image-guided procedures such as biopsies, drainages, line placement, and management of vascular complications. In leukemia, sometimes findings on imaging may be the first indication of the diagnosis; however, mainly imaging is utilized in the detection of treatment complications. In cases of lymphoma, CT and PET-CT predominantly play role in staging and treatment response evaluation.

18.2 Classification of Hematological Malignancies

The 5th Edition of the World Health Organization Classification of Hematolymphoid Tumors (the online version available since August 2022) provides a comprehensive and updated classification system for hematolymphoid neoplasms. This edition represents a significant revision from the previous edition (4th edition, published in 2008) and includes new entities, updates to existing classifications, and changes in terminology and diagnostic criteria. Table 18.1 shows the WHO classification terminologies of the common malignancies occurring in childhood.

P. Naranje (✉) · M. Jana
Department of Radiodiagnosis and Interventional Radiology, All India Institute of Medical Sciences, New Delhi, India

I. Kumar et al. (eds.), *Practical Approach to Imaging in Pediatric Oncology*,
https://doi.org/10.1007/978-981-96-8158-7_18

Table 18.1 WHO classification terminologies of the common malignancies occurring in childhood

Myeloid	B-cell lymphoid proliferations and lymphomas	T-cell and NK-cell lymphoid proliferations and neoplasms
Myeloid precursor lesions Acute myeloid leukemia (AML) Myeloid sarcoma	Precursor B-cell neoplasms (*B-lymphoblastic leukemia/ lymphoma*)	Precursor T-cell neoplasms (T-*lymphoblastic leukemia/ lymphoma)*
Mature myeloid cell Myeloproliferative neoplasms Myelodysplastic neoplasms	Mature B-cell neoplasms *Large B-cell lymphomas* Diffuse large B-cell lymphoma ALK-positive large B-cell lymphoma Primary mediastinal large B-cell lymphoma High-grade B-cell lymphoma *Burkitt lymphoma*	Mature T-cell and NK-cell leukemias *T-prolymphocytic leukemia* *Hepatosplenic T-cell lymphoma* *Anaplastic large cell lymphoma* *EBV-positive T-cell and NK-cell lymphoid proliferations and lymphomas of childhood*
Secondary myeloid neoplasms (post-cytotoxic therapy/associated with germline predisposition/with down syndrome)	Hodgkin lymphoma	

18.3 Lymphoma

Hodgkin's lymphoma (HL) and non-Hodgkin's lymphoma (NHL) account for 10–15% of all childhood malignancies. HL has a bimodal age distribution, peaking in the 20 s and after the age of 50 years, mostly occurring in adolescents and young adults. HL is associated with Epstein-Barr virus and immunosuppression. NHL is more common than HL in children younger than 10 years and often presents with symptomatic masses in the chest or abdomen. In children, NHL constitutes predominantly mature B-cell lymphoid proliferations/lymphoma such as Burkitt lymphoma and diffuse large B-cell lymphoma [DLBCL], anaplastic large cell lymphoma, and lymphoblastic lymphoma [1]. Indications of imaging include initial diagnosis, staging, response assessment, and follow-up to monitor for recurrence or progression of disease.

Among the available imaging modalities for anatomical and metabolic assessment, several oncological societies, including Children's Oncology Group (COG), the European Network for Pediatric Hodgkin Lymphoma (EuroNet-PHL), and the Indian Council of Medical Research (ICMR), recommend F^{18}-FDG PETCT or F^{18}-FDG PETMR for both staging evaluation and response assessment in HL [2, 3]. Currently, the accessibility of F^{18}-FDG PET/MRI is limited; however, where available it may be used as an alternative imaging modality to PET/CT.

PET-CT may also allow to forgo a bone marrow aspirate/biopsy in patients with HL as routine assessment. In NHL, if PET-CT is negative for bone marrow uptake then a bone marrow biopsy is indicated.

Most NHL show FDG avidity, however false positivity and false negativity of the FDGPET is higher in NHL. Other imaging modalities play an important adjunct role in diagnostic algorithm. Chest radiographs performed as PA and erect lateral views are used as initial screening investigation for presenting symptoms such as dyspnea or chest pain; may reveal the mediastinal mass, airway compromise, or lung lesions. Chest radiographs are valuable in the assessment of bulky mediastinal disease. Ultrasound helps to detect the nodes and guide the biopsy procedure in case the node is not accessible for excision biopsy. CT and MRI form the modalities of choice for anatomical imaging. A contrast-enhanced CT of neck, chest,

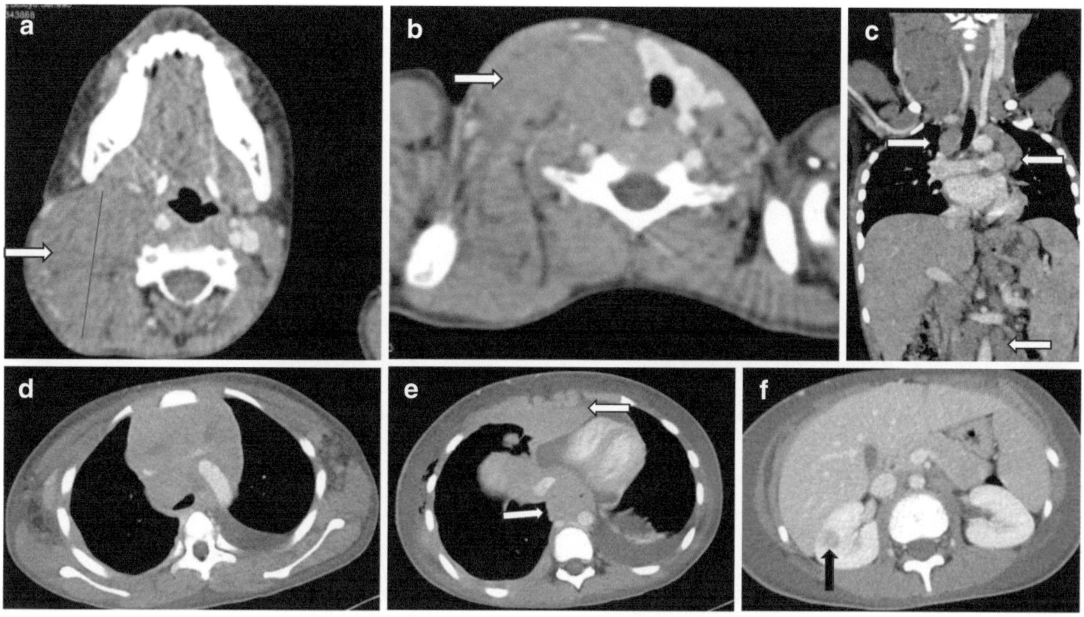

Fig. 18.1 Bulky, homogenous lymphadenopathy seen in right lower cervical stations (**a**, **b**) and right paratracheal and prevascular regions of the mediastinum, retroperitoneum (arrows) with hepatosplenomegaly (**c**) in a child with Hodgkin's lymphoma. (**d**, **e**, **f**). 8-year-old male with non-Hodgkin's lymphoma (NHL) showing conglomerating, sheet-like contiguous soft tissue (white arrows) in prevascular and visceral mediastinal compartments, left pleural effusion and right renal focal hypodense lesion (black arrow)

and abdomen is recommended for initial staging and also delineates lung involvement, splenic focal lesions, and GI involvement (positive oral contrast may be given), following the ALARA/Image Gently guidelines (Fig. 18.1). MRI may be valuable in the assessment of brain, bone marrow involvement, thymic, and splenic lesions.

Short Tau Inversion Recovery (STIR)-whole body (WB)-MRI and WB-DWI (images resembling PET image) have also been evaluated in the staging of pediatric lymphoma, with very good agreement between WB-MRI and FDG PET/CT examination [4] The high cellularity in lymphomas leads to diffusion restriction and low ADC values. A change in ADC value has been used for response assessment. WB-DWI has been reported to be superior to PET-CT in lymphoma subtypes with variable FDG avidity. WB-MRI can be used for assessment of nodal and extranodal disease and hence used for staging at baseline, treatment response, and detection of relapse [5] (Fig. 18.2).

Though MRI has a promising role in the evaluation of pediatric lymphoma owing to the advantages of being radiation free modality and providing high-quality anatomical information, the prolonged examination times, need for prolonged sedation, low detectability for small lung lesions, and underestimation of disease response and cost make it less favorable modality. Repeated CTs and FDG-PET CTs are associated with high radiation doses and predisposes children to secondary radiation-induced malignancies.

Post-treatment Follow-Up

In cases of Hodgkin's lymphoma, Children's Oncology Group protocol suggests to perform targeted CT (as per original disease sites) at the end of therapy. FDG PET/CT imaging is performed only in children showing residual FDG avidity during interim response evaluation. Further imaging surveillance is done at 6 months and 1 year. Beyond a year, clinical follow-up

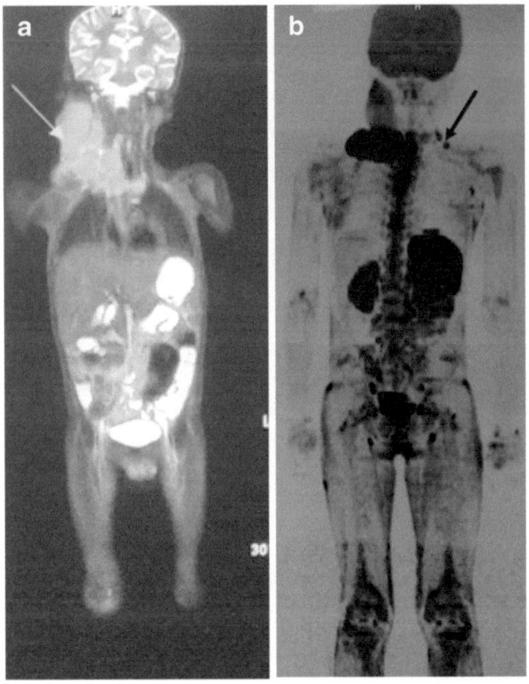

Fig. 18.2 WB-MRI, STIR coronal (**a**) and inverted DWI (**b**) in a patient with lymphoma show multiple, conglomerated lobulated, enlarged lymph node masses (white arrow) in the right lower cervical region showing intense diffusion restriction T2 hyperintensity. Few diffusion restricting lymph nodes also seen in left lower cervical region (Black arrow). Rest of the body regions did not show nodal involvement

with routine labs and chest radiograph is recommended. No further CT or PET/CT imaging is advised for routine follow-up [6, 7].

There are no clear guidelines on surveillance imaging in non-Hodgkin lymphoma in children. The aggressive NHL subtypes, such as primary mediastinal B-cell lymphoma and anaplastic large cell lymphoma, have higher rates of recurrence and require close follow-up. Whereas NHL types such as T lymphoblastic lymphoma, mature B-cell histology lymphoma subtypes, including Burkitt lymphoma, diffuse large B-cell lymphoma show excellent survival rates between 80% and 97% and as such the follow-up imaging plays little role in off-therapy management. In general, follow-up by CT or MRI depends on initial sites of involvement at 6-month intervals for 2 years, with subsequent clinical follow-up. It is further being suggested that the clinical indications should prompt the follow-up scans [6].

18.3.1 Imaging Approach and Structured Reporting Format for Suspected/Histologically Proven Lymphoma

For appropriate patient care, the accurate reporting of imaging data is of utmost importance and must be conveyed to the referring pediatric oncologist in the most comprehensive manner. The radiology report affects the decision-making and further management of the patient and hence a concise structured format for reporting the findings eases both radiologist and physician of the imaging interpretations.

One of the suggested formats for lymphoma is shown in Table 18.2. (Adapted from [8]).

Imaging approach to diagnosis is summarized in flowchart 1.

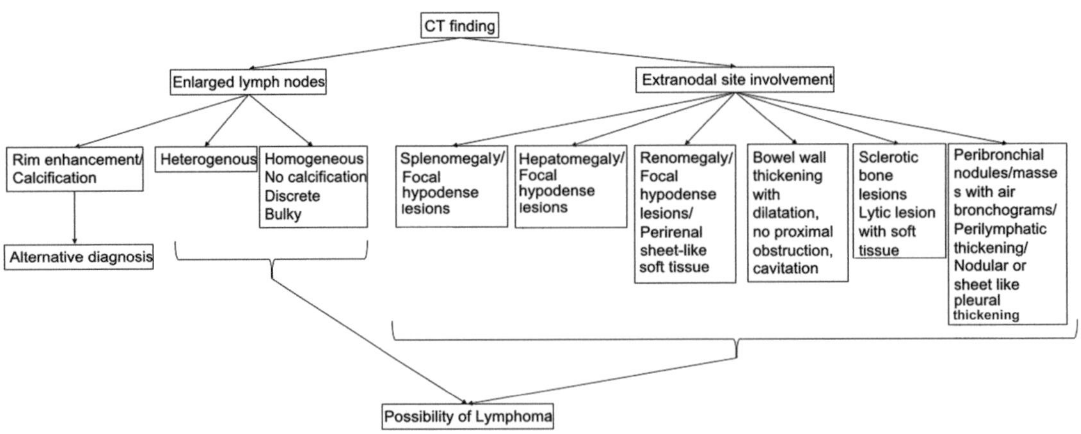

Table 18.2 Suggested structured reporting format for lymphoma

Patient clinical information	
Age	
Gender	
Presenting symptoms	
Family history of cancers	
Allergies	
Biopsy Bone marrow biopsy/ Other site	YES/NO If yes—results (date)
TLC	
RFT	
Clinical indication	Primary staging
CT Report	
Sites	Lymph node disease Bulky disease Spleen Extranodal disease
Lymph node disease description	
Number	
Site (select up to 2 target lesions)	Stage I-III (limited disease)/stage III-IV(advanced disease) If limited disease – Subdiaphragmatic sites Supradiaphragmatic sites If advanced disease- Site
Size	Largest dimension on axial plane (mm) Dimension perpendicular to largest diameter (mm)
CT appearance	Enhancement pattern Necrosis Conglomeration Calcification Relation with adjacent vessels and other structures
Bulky disease description	
Site	Chest Abdomen Other
Largest dimension	AP X CC X ML
CT appearance	Enhancement pattern Necrosis Complications Airway compression/displacement/infiltration Vascular compression/displacement/infiltration Bowel compression/displacement/infiltration
Spleen description	
Largest dimension (measured on MPR)	___in cm Normal Splenomegaly
CT appearance	Homogenous Heterogenous Presence of focal lesions (number)

(continued)

Table 18.2 (continued)

If focal lesion, select 2 target lesions	For each measure Largest dimension on axial plane (mm) Dimension perpendicular to largest diameter (mm)
Extranodal disease description	
Site Select up to 2 target lesions	Liver GI tract Kidney Lung Muscles/skin Orbit CNS Bone Other
Liver	Hepatomegaly (Y/N) Focal lesions (number); select 2 target lesions—two dimensions for each lesion* CT appearance
Kidney	Bilateral or unilateral involvement Focal lesions (number); select 2 target lesions—two dimensions for each lesion* Hilar/perirenal involvement
Lung	Lobe/segment involved CT pattern Single nodule/mass (two dimensions*) Multiple nodules/masses (dimensions for up to 2 target lesions) Consolidation Interstitial thickening
GI tract	Bowel segment involved Focal lesion CT appearance Ulcerated lesions Stenosing lesions Aneurysmal dilatation of segment involved Any obstruction
CNS	Site Focal lesions (number); select 2 target lesions—two dimensions for each lesion* Leptomeningeal enhancement
Muscles/skin	Site Focal lesions (number); select 2 target lesions—two dimensions for each lesion* CT appearance (text)
Orbit	Site Focal lesions (number); select 2 target lesions—two dimensions for each lesion* CT appearance (text)
Bone	Site Focal lesions (number); select 2 target lesions with soft tissue component—two dimensions for each lesion* CT appearance (text)
Other extranodal sites	Site Focal lesions (number); select 2 target lesions—two dimensions for each lesion* CT appearance (text)

(continued)

Table 18.2 (continued)

Non-measurable lesions	Pleural (effusion/thickening/nodules) Pericardium (effusion/thickening/nodules) Peritoneal (effusion/thickening/nodules)
Selected target lesions (Number)	For each: Nodal/Extranodal Site Size and CT appearance
Total lesion burden	Sum product diameter (mm) Volume of target lesions (mm^3)
Any other finding	Thrombosis Pneumonia Other
Suggest likely site for excision or image-guided biopsy if not done prior	Site
Conclusion (Lugano revision of Ann Arbor criteria)	Stage I-III (limited disease)/stage III-IV(advanced disease) Any other

18.4 Leukemia

Leukemia is the most common childhood malignancy. Leukemia usually presents in the acute form and children often show signs of bone marrow suppression, such as pallor, petechiae, bruising, and fever. Approximately 11–50% of children would present with extremity or spine-related complaints, including joint or bone pain, and limping. Leukemia is classified into acute lymphoblastic leukemia (ALL) and acute myeloid leukemia (AML). ALL peaks between 2 and 3 years of age, whereas AML peaks during the first 2 years of life and then gradually increases again during adolescence. The World Health Organization (WHO) subclassifies ALL as B-lymphoblastic or T-lymphoblastic, with pre–B-cell ALL being the most common form. The less common T-cell-derived ALL can be considered the disseminated form of T-cell lymphoblastic lymphoma with regard to imaging appearance as well as treatment.

Routine imaging evaluation is not indicated for diagnostic purposes in leukemias; however, occasionally when patient present with extramedullary manifestations such as soft tissue masses in orbital regions, extremities, CNS, or testicular enlargement, site-specific imaging are indicated. Such presentations are more frequent in relapse cases rather than at baseline. Chest X-ray for mediastinal mass, USG, CT, and MRI are utilized depending on the presenting symptoms [9].

Imaging rather plays a vital role in the detection of post-treatment complications and surveillance of post-transplant patients. CT of chest and abdomen is recommended in pre-transplant evaluation. Post-transplant imaging in the form of CT sinuses/neck/chest abdomen is often directed in the evaluation of infective complications, GVHD, and bronchiolitis obliterans.

18.4.1 Imaging of Leukemia

Radiological patterns of involvement in leukemia may be categorized into marrow involvement and extramedullary involvement (Table 18.3).

18.4.2 Musculoskeletal Involvement in Leukemia

Lucent metaphyseal bands or "leukemic lines" are seen in 10–55% of cases [10]. The bands represent the disrupted endosteal mineralization resulting in thin trabeculae adjacent to the zone of provisional calcification, and are most promi-

Table 18.3 Radiological patterns of involvement in leukemia

Marrow involvement	Extramedullary involvement
Periosteal reaction	Head and neck Sinus masses Parotid enlargement Hypertrophy of Waldeyer ring
Leukemic infiltration of marrow Vertebral body signals on MRI T1 hypointense or isointense to intervertebral disks and skeletal muscle T2-weighted fat-suppressed or STIR hyperintense Post-contrast enhancement of the abnormal marrow	Central nervous system Parenchymal mass Pachymeningeal/leptomeningeal enhancement Spinal epidural masses
Lucent metaphyseal bands or "leukemic lines"	Abdomen Soft tissue masses in retroperitoneum, mesentery, peritoneum, UB Nephromegaly Hepatosplenomegaly Ascites Bowel wall thickening.
Permeative vertebral lesions on CT/radiographs	Chest Pleural/pericardial deposits Perilymphatic thickening due to leukemic infiltration Mediastinal sheet-like soft tissue
	Testicles/ovaries Diffuse infiltration causing enlargement and hypoechoic on USG Focal hypoechoic lesions Enhancing deposits in ovaries
	Breast, skin, and soft tissues Masses, nodules, plaques
	Orbital involvement Masses Hemorrhage More frequently in granulocytic sarcoma

nent at sites of rapid growth, such as the knees and wrists. Acute lymphoblastic leukemia is more frequently associated with these lines. Most often these lines are seen in distal femur, proximal tibia (around knee), proximal humerus, distal radius, and ulna. After treatment, the lucent zones may become dense [11].

Periosteal reactions of laminated and aggressive forms may also be seen due to marrow infiltration in leukemia. The infiltrating cells traverse through the Haversian canals till the periosteum and elevate it off the bone cortex. Such involvement is more evident in lower limb long bones, especially tibia, fibula. Underlying marrow sometimes may show permeative osteolysis, osteopenia, or pathological fractures (Fig. 18.3).

Normal red marrow and yellow marrow in the long bones appear as hyperintense to skeletal muscle on T1-weighted image(T1WI) [yellow marrow > red marrow] and hyperintense to intervertebral discs in spine. The diseased marrow appears hypointense or isointense on T1WI, and may be difficult to distinguish from normal marrow in younger children. The diseased marrow also appears heterogeneously hyperintense on T2WI and shows post-contrast enhancement, causing the intervertebral discs to appear as darker against the enhancing abnormal marrow of vertebrae.

18.4.3 Extramedullary Involvements

Extramedullary involvement in leukemia is an uncommon manifestation occurring in up to 10–15% of the patients, either at the onset of the

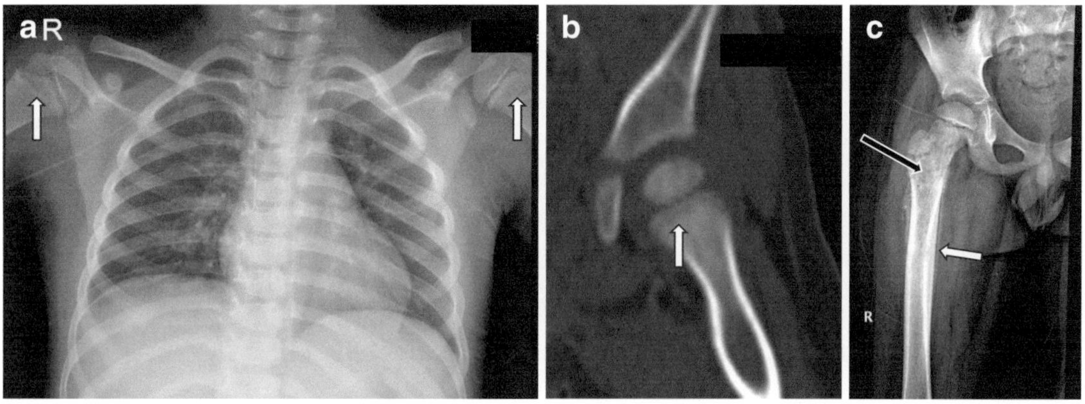

Fig. 18.3 A 7 year/M, presented to emergency with bone pains, abdominal distension, bleeding manifestations and detected to have cytopenias and subsequently diagnosed as acute lymphoblastic leukemia (ALL). Chest radiograph (**a**) and CT bone window (**b**) showed metaphyseal lucent bands in bilateral humeri and proximal femur. (**c**). Periosteal reaction and permeative osteolysis is noted in metaphysis and proximal diaphyseal regions of the right femur as a feature of leukemic involvement in a different child with ALL

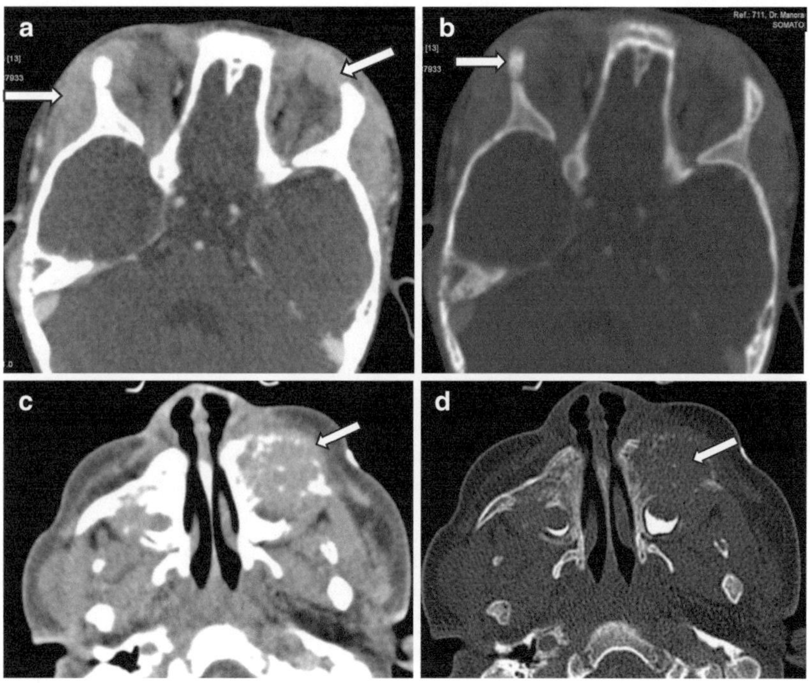

Fig. 18.4 Two different children with acute myeloid leukemia presenting with extramedullary involvement of orbits/PNS. (**a** and **b**). Homogenous enhancing soft tissues seen involving bilateral periorbital regions and extraocular spaces (arrows). No definite bone erosions seen in this case. (**c** and **d**). Enhancing soft tissues seen in bilateral maxillary sinuses with associated bone erosions (arrows)

disease or more likely during the relapse. These patients present with atypical clinical features causing delay in the diagnosis and further management. Several sites of extra medullary involvement are reported such as orbits, testicles, CNS, retroperitoneum, gastrointestinal tract, pleura, skin, and soft tissues, and the major imaging appearances are summarized in Table 18.3. Periorbital soft tissues and involvement of sinuses can present as homogeneously intensely enhancing soft tissue masses presenting with proptosis and external soft tissue swellings. Associated bone erosions and extension into the extradural intracranial regions may also be seen (Fig. 18.4). Testicular involvement may be seen in the form of enlargement of the testis or presence of multiple focal lesions or irregular diffuse hypoechoic testicular parenchyma on ultrasound. Testicular biopsies are indicated to prove the involvement by leukemia [12]. *Leukostasis* presents in the form of multifocal areas of ground glass opacities in both the lungs in a background of hyperleukocytosis (WBC count >1,00,000 cells per microliter). Leukemic infiltration in the lungs presents as perilymphatic thickening or irregular interlobular septal thickening with the presence of perilymphatic nodules.

18.5 Treatment-Related Complications

The predominant management of the hematological malignancies consists of chemotherapy and bone marrow transplantation. The resultant immune suppression predisposes the patient to multiple infective complications involving various organs. Overall, the treatment-related complications may be of infectious or non-infectious forms. Imaging plays an important role in the identification of these complications and early management to improve the overall treatment outcomes. Contrast-enhanced CT chest and abdomen are frequently ordered in case of a febrile neutropenia to identify the source of infection. CT of paranasal sinuses is indicated in case of any facial swelling or clinical suspicion of sinusitis. MRI of the perianal region is indicated in case of perianal tenderness or swelling or pus discharge.

Common organs affected are lungs, GI tract, and paranasal sinuses. Pulmonary complications include infectious acute pulmonary complications and several forms of non-infectious lung involvement [13]. Pulmonary infection is the most common and dreadful complication in patients with hematologic malignancy. The management of these infections is complicated and mostly the diagnosis needs to be made on imaging and supported by other blood investigations. Obtaining a diagnostic sample in the form of lavage or biopsy is mostly not feasible in view of cytopenias as a part of treatment complication. Hence, radiology plays a vital role in predicting the likely organism as well as assessment of the extent of involvement. Fungal pneumonia, bacterial pneumonia, Pneumocystis jiroveci pneumonia, CMV pneumonia, and other viral pneumonias are the predominant forms of respiratory infections encountered. The imaging patterns of these infections are summarized in Table 18.4.

18.5.1 Non-infectious Lung Involvement

Alveolar hemorrhage, pulmonary edema, drug-induced pulmonary complication [all-trans retinoic acid (ATRA) syndrome], bronchiolitis obliterans, and organizing pneumonia are some of the common non-infectious pulmonary complications in patients with hematological malignancies [14]. The imaging patterns in these conditions often overlap in acute presentations, and some of the subtle imaging features help in differentiating amongst these conditions. Combination of CT appearances may suggest the most possible diagnosis based on the background of appropriate clinical scenario [15].

Table 18.4 Pulmonary infectious complications (Fig. 18.5)

Pulmonary infection	Imaging features
Angioinvasive fungal	Nodules or segmental consolidations with surrounding ground glass opacities "halo sign". Reversed halo sign Cavitation in the nodules or consolidation is seen with improvement in neutropenia
Airway invasive fungal	Peribronchovascular consolidation Centrilobular nodules
Bacterial	Lobar or segmental consolidation Multiple subpleural cavitary nodules (septic emboli)
Pneumocystis Jiroveci pneumonia	Peri-hilar diffuse ground glass opacities
Viral	Ground glass opacities Micro nodules Consolidations Interstitial thickening

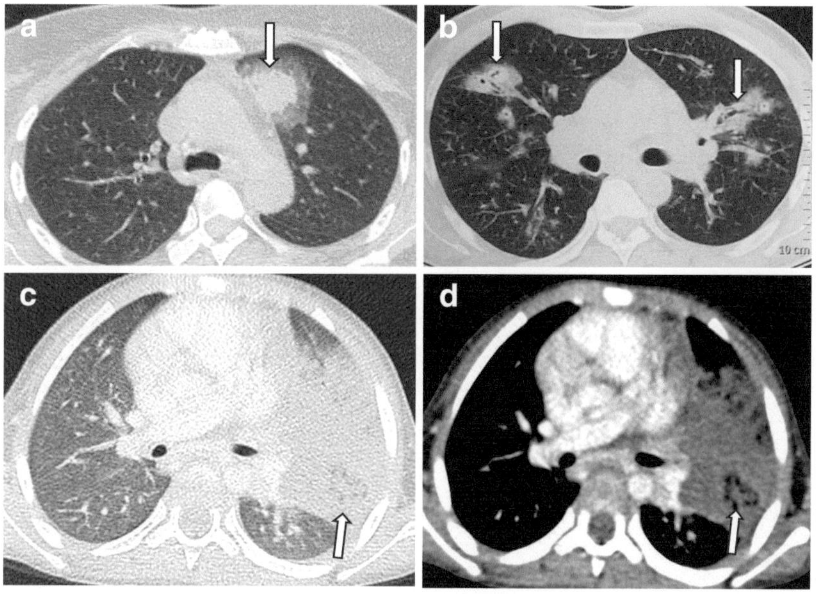

Fig. 18.5 Pulmonary infectious complications. (**a**). Nodules with surrounding ground glass opacities producing a "halo sign "(arrow)—in an adolescent of febrile neutropenia suggestive of angioinvasive fungal infection. (**b**). Peribronchial nodules and peribronchial thickening with surrounding ground glass opacities(arrows) suggestive of airway invasive fungal infection. (**c** and **d**). Lobar consolidation in left upper lobe with areas of central necrosis/ hypodensities (arrows) in a child of ALL with mucormycosis

Where the infections mostly present on imaging in a pattern of nodules or focal consolidations, the non-infectious complications present with diffuse pulmonary involvement in the form of ground glass opacities predominantly. *Pulmonary edema* classically presents with perihilar or peribronchovascular ground glass opacities with subpleural interlobular smooth septal thickening and associated plural or pericardial effusions. The pulmonary edema in such patients occurs due to the high volume fluid or blood products transfusion, due to renal impairment, or chemotherapy-induced cardiac dysfunction. *Diffuse alveolar hemorrhage* is usually associated with thrombocytopenia, underlying pulmonary infection, and peri-hematopoietic stem cell transplantation (HSCT). Characteristically, the radiographs show rapidly progressing diffuse ground glass opacities and patching consolidations. On CT the ground glass opacities are seen as involving diffusely both the lungs with the presence of reticulation and subpleural sparing. Patients of APML, when treated with all trans retinoic acid (ATRA), may show pulmonary complication (*Differentiation syndrome*) characterized by fever respiratory distress and pulmonary opacities which occurs after the onset of therapy from day 2 to day 21 with elevated WBC count. The CT shows the presence of multifocal or diffuse ground glass opacities and pleural effusion with bronchial wall thickening. These findings show resolution with steroids (Fig. 18.6).

Post-HSCT graft versus host disease can occur as an acute form (within 3 months of transplant) or late form (after 3 months). Early forms involvement is more commonly seen involving the gastrointestinal tract and the lung involvement is very rare. In the late engraftment phase, bronchiolitis obliterans and organizing pneumonia are the common forms of involvement. These are seen in allogenic form of bone marrow transplantation. CT shows the presence of bronchial wall thickening with mosaic attenuation and air trapping in case of bronchiolitis obliterans. Sometimes bronchiectasis may also develop in the later stages. Whereas organizing pneumonia on HRCT shows the presence of bilateral peribronchovascular or subpleural con-

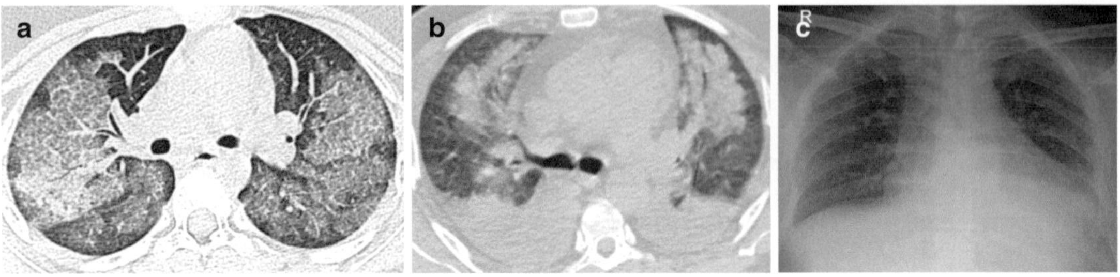

Fig. 18.6 Non-infectious pulmonary complications. (**a**) Difffuse alveolar hemmorhge in a thrombocytopenic child with ALL characterised by crazy paving appreance and subpeural sparing. (**b**) Differentiation syndrome in young adult with APML treated with ATRA; presented with acute shortness of breath and peribronchvascular consolidations in bilateral lungs with effusions (& negative infective workup). These resolved after steroids (**c**) Follow-up chest radiograph

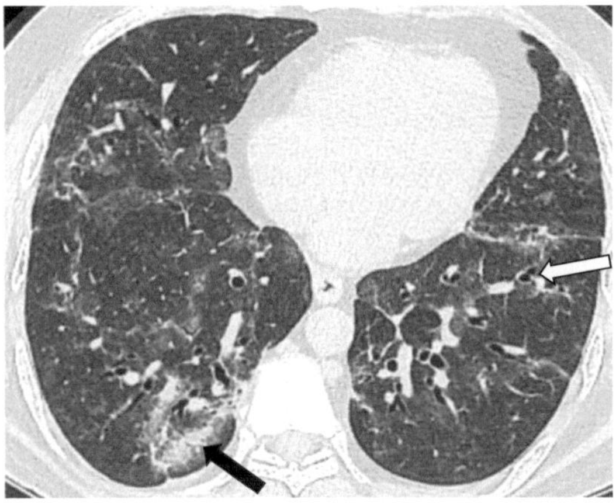

Fig. 18.7 HRCT in a patient 2 years after allogenic HSCT shows presence of bilateral peribronchovascular consolidations and ground glass opacities in lower lung zones with central clearing suggestive or areas of organizing pneumonia (black arrow). Associated bronchial wall thickening mild bronchiectasis is also seen (white arrow)

solidations in lower lung zones with central clearing giving an atoll sign. Small nodules and ground glass opacities may also be seen sometimes (Fig. 18.7).

18.5.2 Gastrointestinal Involvement

Gastrointestinal involvement may be of infectious or non-infectious etiology. Therapy-induced toxic mucositis, viral/fungal enteritis, and pseudomembranous colitis are the common forms of bowel involvement. Necrosis and ulceration of the intestinal wall, graft versus host disease, bowel hemorrhage or bowel wall hematomas, Typhlitis pneumatosis intestinalis and perforation are some of the non-infectious complications [16]. Neutropenic colitis is a life-threatening necrotizing enteropathy associated with therapy-induced neutropenia. The caecum and the ascending colon are most commonly affected sites with possible involvement of the terminal ileum. Ultrasound or CT is helpful in identifying the wall thickening (>6 mm) (Fig. 18.8). Early identification is essential as the progressive involvement may lead to perforation. Proctitis and perianal abscesses are another common sites of infection. MRI helps to delineate the extent of involvement of the perianal region and the presence of fistulas or sinuses [17].

In conclusion, radiology serves as a cornerstone in the comprehensive care of pediatric patients with hematological malignancies. From the initial clinical suspicion to diagnosis, staging, treatment monitoring, and long-term surveillance, imaging provides vital, non-invasive insights that guide clinical decision-making and improve outcomes. Each imaging modality—whether ultrasound, radiography, CT, MRI, nuclear medicine, or PET-CT—has unique advantages tailored to specific clinical scenarios. Advances in imaging technology, including low-dose protocols, whole-body MRI, and functional imaging, continue to enhance diagnostic precision while maintaining safety.Furthermore, radiology is not limited to diagnosis and follow-up alone. Interventional radiology has an increasingly important role in the management of com-

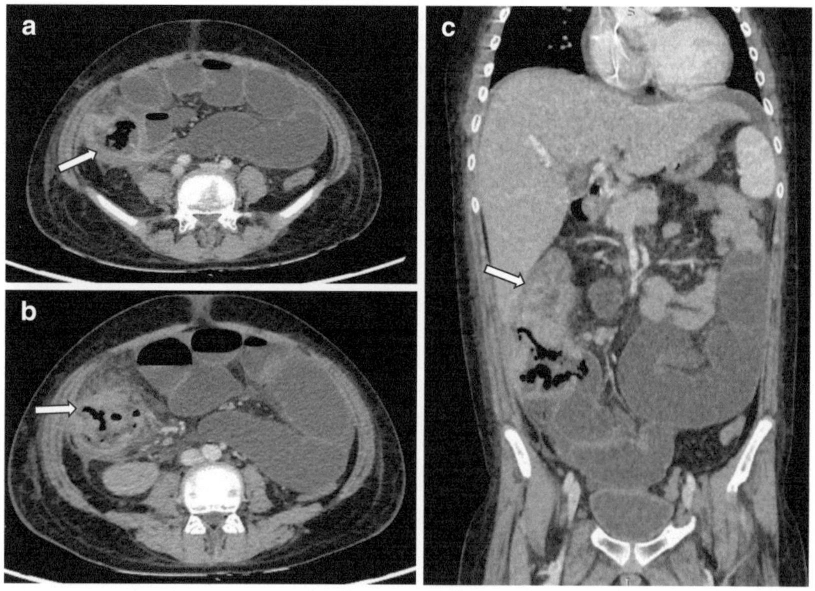

Fig. 18.8 (a–c) Neutropenic colitis involving the caecum and the ascending colon showing irregular enhancing wall thickening with pericolonic fat stranding (arrows) in a child on therapy for B-ALL and febrile neutropenia. Proximal small bowel dilatation (secondary to ileus or obstruction) is also noted

plications, facilitating biopsies, central venous access, and therapeutic procedures with minimal invasiveness. Incorporating radiological findings into a multidisciplinary framework—alongside clinical, pathological, and molecular data—ensures a holistic approach to care. In summary, imaging is integral to every phase of managing hematological malignancies in children. As technology evolves and our understanding of these diseases deepens, radiology will continue to play a dynamic and indispensable role in improving pediatric oncology care.

References

1. McCarten KM, Nadel HR, Shulkin BL, Cho SY. Imaging for diagnosis, staging and response assessment of Hodgkin lymphoma and non-Hodgkin lymphoma. Pediatr Radiol. 2019;49(11):1545–64.
2. Mhlanga J, Alazraki A, Cho SY, Lai H, Nadel H, Pandit-Taskar N, et al. Imaging recommendations in pediatric lymphoma: a COG diagnostic imaging committee/SPR oncology committee white paper. Pediatr Blood Cancer. 2023;70(Suppl 4):e29968.
3. main.icmr.nic.in. PEDIATRIC_LYMPHOMAS_AND_SOLID_TUMORS_0 [
4. Marie E, Navallas M, Katz DS, Farajirad E, Punnett A, Davda S, et al. Non-Hodgkin lymphoma imaging spectrum in children, adolescents, and young adults. Radiographics. 2022;42(4):1214–38.
5. Di Giuliano F, Picchi E, Pucci N, Minosse S, Ferrazzoli V, Pizzicannella G, et al. Comparison between diffusion-weighted magnetic resonance and positron-emission tomography in the evaluation of treated lymphomas with mediastinal involvement. Egypt J Radiol Nucl Med. 2022;53(1):149.
6. Voss SD, Cairo MS. Surveillance imaging in pediatric lymphoma. Pediatr Radiol. 2019;49(11):1565–73.
7. Flerlage JE, Hiniker SM, Armenian S, Benya EC, Bobbey AJ, Chang V, et al. Pediatric Hodgkin lymphoma, version 3.2021. J Natl Compr Cancer Netw. 2021;19(6):733–54.
8. Granata V, Pradella S, Cozzi D, Fusco R, Faggioni L, Coppola F, et al. Computed tomography structured reporting in the staging of lymphoma: a Delphi consensus proposal. J Clin Med. 2021;10(17)
9. Agrwal S, Sahi PK. National comprehensive cancer network guidelines for pediatric acute lymphoblastic leukemia. Indian Pediatr. 2020;57(6):561–4.
10. Tannenbaum MF, Noda S, Cohen S, Rissmiller JG, Golja AM, Schwartz DM. Imaging musculoskeletal manifestations of pediatric hematologic malignancies. AJR Am J Roentgenol. 2020;214(2):455–64.
11. Sinigaglia R, Gigante C, Bisinella G, Varotto S, Zanesco L, Turra S. Musculoskeletal manifestations in pediatric acute leukemia. J Pediatr Orthop. 2008;28(1):20–8.
12. Mejia M, Royero Arias M, Santiago Pacheco V, Pimiento FJ. Extramedullary imaging manifestations of leukemia/lymphoblastic lymphoma in pediatrics: a case series. Cureus. 2024;16(2):e54714.
13. Choi MH, Jung JI, Chung WD, Kim YJ, Lee SE, Han DH, et al. Acute pulmonary complications in patients with hematologic malignancies. Radiographics. 2014;34(6):1755–68.

14. Harris B, Geyer AI. Diagnostic evaluation of pulmonary abnormalities in patients with hematologic malignancies and hematopoietic cell transplantation. Clin Chest Med. 2017;38(2):317–31.
15. Singh R, Naranje P, Bhalla AS, Manchanda S, Mahapatra M. Evaluation of non-infectious pulmonary complications in hematological malignancies on MDCT: decoding imaging markers. Indian J Hematol Blood Transfus. 2021;37(4):669–74.
16. Kurucay M, Kloth C, Bethge W, Faul C, Horger M. Gastrointestinal complications in hematological patients. Rofo. 2016;188(7):619–24.
17. Ashkar C, Britto M, Carne P, Cheung W, Mirbagheri N. Perianal sepsis in neutropaenic patients with haematological malignancies: the role of magnetic resonance imaging and surgery. ANZ J Surg. 2020;90(9):1642–6.

Bone Tumors

19

Vaishali Upadhyaya and B. T. Pushpa

19.1 Introduction

In children, benign tumors are more common than malignant lesions. Initially radiographs are obtained for assessment of suspected osseous tumors, but subsequently cross-sectional imaging can be done for further characterization of these lesions and evaluation of their extent [1, 2]. Imaging is important at each step in the management of children with bone tumors. It helps to identify the tumor, provide information to prepare a list of differentials for the lesion, stage the tumor, and helps guide biopsy procedures. It can assess response to radiotherapy and chemotherapy, follow-up lesions, and identify recurrent disease after completion of treatment [3].

19.2 Consensus Guidelines for Imaging

The American College of Radiology (ACR) Appropriateness Criteria, updated in 2020, guide the imaging of osseous lesions across six variants.

V. Upadhyaya (✉) · B. T. Pushpa
Department of Radiology, Apollomedics Superspeciality Hospitals, Lucknow, India

Department of Radiology, Ganga Hospital, Coimbatore, India

- Initial imaging typically involves radiographs to assess tumor location, size, shape, margins, matrix type, and periosteal reactions [4].
- For radiographically occult lytic lesions such as those with mineralization loss under 30–50%, MRI is recommended as next modality. Contrast-enhanced MRI should be done for biopsies and treatment response evaluation.
- CT with or without contrast may be employed for complex bony anatomy or if MRI is contraindicated, with non-contrast CT preferred for suspected osteoid osteoma.
- Benign lesions seen on X-ray and associated with pain or swelling should also undergo contrast-enhanced MRI.
- Lesions appearing indeterminate or aggressive on radiographs should also be evaluated by contrast-enhanced MRI because of its ability to identify extent of marrow involvement, relationship of the tumor to adjacent soft tissues, adjacent joint involvement, and neurovascular bundle involvement.
- For incidentally found lesions on MRI or CT that are not clearly benign, radiographs should be done [5].
- For post-treatment follow-up, both radiographs and contrast-enhanced MRI are recommended as per guidelines provided by the COG Diagnostic Imaging Committee/SPR Oncology Committee to monitor outcomes, complications, and recurrence, with MRI

I. Kumar et al. (eds.), *Practical Approach to Imaging in Pediatric Oncology*,
https://doi.org/10.1007/978-981-96-8158-7_19

providing superior soft tissue detail. If metallic hardware is present, MRI with metal artifact reduction sequences (MARS) or FDG-PET/CT may be useful.

- For pulmonary follow-up, non-contrast chest CT is recommended to identify metastases and assess nodules.
- For whole-body imaging, FDG-PET/CT or PET/MRI is preferred.

19.3 Structured Radiology Reporting and Interpretation

It is considered appropriate to label osseous tumors as aggressive/non-aggressive on imaging and not malignant/benign. Mostly, malignant lesions will look aggressive and benign lesions will not look aggressive on radiographs but there are exceptions such as an eosinophilic granuloma which is benign but can appear aggressive. Also, radiographs acquired for assessment of bone tumors should include two projections of the lesion obtained perpendicular to each other [3].

The following features can be used to describe bone tumors which will help to characterize the lesion and arrive at a differential diagnosis. It cannot be overemphasized however that the radiologist must be aware of the clinical presentation of the patient which can provide important clues to reaching the right diagnosis!

1. Location:
   (a) Tumors can involve flat bones/long bones and axial skeleton/appendicular skeleton. Some tumors occur in characteristic locations such as osteosarcomas which commonly involve the metaphysis of long bones. Enchondromas are commonly seen in the small bones of the hand.
   (b) The location can be described in both longitudinal (epiphysis/metaphysis/diaphysis) and transverse axis (cortical/medullary—central or eccentric/surface) [6]. A chondroblastoma has a characteristic epiphyseal location.
2. Number of lesions: Bone tumors are mostly solitary lesions. Some conditions in which there may be multiple osseous lesions include metastases, leukemia, and eosinophilic granuloma [7].
3. Size of the lesion: Although there are many differences between an osteoid osteoma and osteoblastoma, lesion size is also a helpful criterion. Osteoid osteomas are usually smaller than 1.5 cm while osteoblastomas are larger lesions, measuring more than 1.5 cm [8].
4. Margins and zone of transition: As per the modified Lodwick-Madewell grading system, lesions can be classified into three grades [9].
   - Grade IA and IB lesions: well-defined geographic lytic lesions with sclerotic rim and without sclerotic rim respectively.
   - Grade II lesions: geographic lytic lesions with circumferential or partial ill-defined margins.
   - Grade IIIA lesions: changing margins with the lesions showing transition from well-defined sclerotic margins to ill-defined margins at a point in time or change in margins when serial radiographs are compared.
   - Grade IIIB lesions: non-geographic lesions which show moth-eaten and permeative patterns of bone destruction.
   - Grade IIIC lesions: radiographically occult lesions where radiographs are normal/near normal and the lesion can be seen by other modalities such as MRI or PET/CT. Increasing grade of the lesion increases the risk of malignancy.

   Grade I lesions are benign, Grade II lesions carry a moderate risk of malignancy, and Grade III lesions are likely to be malignant.
5. Zone of transition: In tumors with well-defined margins, the junction between the lesion and normal bone is sharp and this is called a narrow zone of transition. This suggests that the tumor is a slowly growing lesion and non-aggressive. However, when

tumors are growing rapidly and aggressive, they are not sharply marginated and such lesions have a wide zone of transition. Both radiographs and CT can be used to determine the zone of transition [3].

6. Matrix: Different tumors produce different patterns of matrix mineralization and although this does not indicate whether the lesion is benign/malignant, it helps to identify the histology of the lesion [10].

   Osteoid matrix has a fluffy and cloudlike or ivory and dense appearance. Cartilaginous matrix produces a pattern of arcs and rings or can look stippled. Fibrous lesions can show mildly increased density or ground-glass appearance or homogeneous/heterogeneous pattern of dense mature mineralization [11]. MRI can additionally determine whether the lesion is solid or cystic and identify fat or fluid-fluid levels suggestive of hemorrhage or necrosis within the lesion [12]. Fluid-fluid levels have a prevalence of 2.7% in bone tumors. They are most seen in aneurysmal bone cyst but can also be seen in other lesions such as fibrous dysplasia, osteoblastoma, simple bone cyst, and chondroblastoma [13].
7. Cortical involvement: Cortical changes in response to tumors include scalloping, thickening, or thinning and destruction. Endosteal scalloping can be seen with lesions such as enchondroma and chondrosarcoma, while outer cortical scalloping can be seen with lesions such as periosteal osteosarcoma. Cortical thickening is seen with lesions such as osteoid osteoma while lesions such as clear cell chondrosarcoma can cause cortical thinning. Malignant mass lesions cause destruction of the cortex [7].
8. Periosteal reaction: Any insult to the cortex results in the periosteum producing new bone. This periosteal reaction differs according to the biological activity of the tumor [12]. A thin or thick type of solid periosteal reaction is usually associated with slowly growing benign lesions such as osteoid osteoma. There can be single layered or multilayered laminated periosteal reaction. The single-layered type is commonly seen with benign conditions such as infection or healing fractures while the multilayered type is commonly associated with malignant conditions such as Ewing's sarcoma or osteosarcoma. Spiculated type of periosteal reaction can have a hair-on-end or sunburst appearance. These are commonly seen with malignant conditions such as Ewing's sarcoma, osteosarcoma, hematologic malignancies, or metastases. The Codman's triangle is a type of interrupted periosteal reaction which is commonly seen with malignant conditions such as osteosarcoma [7].
9. Pathological fracture: Pathological fractures are seen in about 18% of pediatric bone tumors and tumor-like lesions. Most of these lesions are benign, commonest being simple bone cyst and non-ossifying fibroma and humerus is the commonest site of involvement. About 10% of cases are seen in malignant tumors [14].
10. Peritumoral edema: Marrow edema is seen with both benign and malignant tumors such as osteoid osteoma, osteoblastoma, chondroblastoma, Ewing's sarcoma, and osteosarcoma. Causative factors for the development of edema include destruction of trabeculae, increased intramedullary pressure, and increased prostaglandin level. Edema can also be seen after a pathological fracture has occurred. On MRI, edema associated with tumors appears ill-defined with homogeneous intermediate signal intensity in T1W images and appears hyperintense in T2W fat saturated/STIR images. Dynamic contrast-enhanced imaging helps to distinguish the tumor from the surrounding edema [15].
11. Extra-osseous component, neurovascular bundle involvement, and adjacent joint involvement: Malignant lesions can destroy the cortex with extra-osseous soft tissue component, infiltrate adjacent structures including the neurovascular bundle, and extend into adjacent joints. Assessment of adjacent joints should always be included in the scan for proper staging of the lesion. MRI is the best modality for local staging of malignant lesions and facilitates planning of

appropriate surgical procedures [16]. In case MRI cannot be done for some reason, CT is the next preferred option. Advantage of CT in children is that it enables rapid imaging and sedation can be avoided even if the child is not cooperative.

12. Skip lesions: Skip metastases in osteosarcoma suggest a poor prognosis [17]. The affected bone must be imaged in MRI along its entire length in longitudinal axis to enable identification of skip lesions [3].

Figure 19.1 depicts Imaging algorithm in a suspected bone tumor.

Table 19.1 provides a sample suggested reporting checklist [18].

Imaging features of common benign tumors and tumor-like lesions as well as malignant and quasi-malignant tumors are given in Tables 19.2 and 19.3.

19.4 Marrow Signal in Children

Bone marrow is classified into two types: red marrow, which is active in hematopoiesis, and yellow marrow, which is not. Red marrow comprises about 40% water, 40% fat, and 20% protein, while yellow marrow consists of approximately 15% water, 80% fat, and 5% protein. The transition from red to yellow marrow begins after birth and is typically complete by age 25, starting in the appendicular skeleton and progressing to the axial skeleton. Changes first occur in the hands and feet, then in long bones (distal to proximal), flat bones, and vertebral bodies. In tubular bones, changes move from the diaphysis to the metaphysis.

Marrow reconversion, the reversal of this process, primarily affects the spine and flat bones before tubular bones, moving from proximal to distal. This can occur in conditions like anemia,

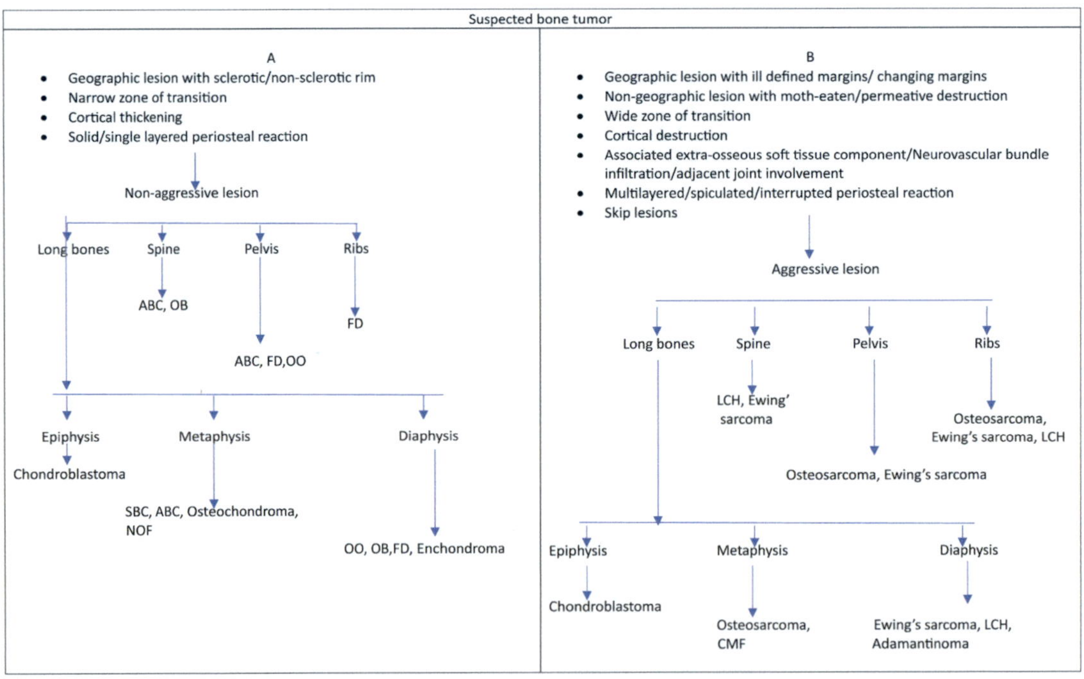

Fig. 19.1 Imaging algorithm in a case of suspected bone tumor [2, 3]. This helps to differentiate non-aggressive lesions from aggressive lesions. *ABC* aneurysmal bone cyst, *SBC* simple bone cyst, *OO* osteoid osteoma, *OB* osteoblastoma, *FD* fibrous dysplasia, *NOF* non-ossifying fibroma, *LCH* langerhans cell histiocytosis, *CMF* chondromyxoid fibroma

Table 19.1 Reporting check list (based on radiographs, MRI, and CT)

Size	---x---x—cm
Bone involved	Specify <bone> <part of bone> <side>
Location in bone	<Epiphysis> <metaphysis> <diaphysis> <epi-metaphyseal> <meta-diaphyseal>
Depth	<cortical> <medullary> <periosteal>
Orientation	<central> <eccentric>
Number of lesions	<single> <multifocal> <skip lesions>
Margin	Type < IA/IB> <II> <IIIA/IIIB/IIIC>
Zone of transition	<Narrow> <wide>
Parenchyma	<cystic> <solid> <mixed>
Matrix	<osteoid> <chondroid> <fat> <calcification> <fluid-fluid levels>
ADC value	ADC cut-off value $\geq 1.10 \times 10^{-3}$ mm^2 (benign),$< 1.10 \times 10^{-3}$ mm^2/s (malignant)
DCE	Type of signal intensity time curve <I/II/III/IV/V>
Pathological fracture	<Present> <absent>
Peritumoral edema	<absent> <marrow edema> <muscular/soft tissue edema>
Cortex	<thickening> <scalloping> <destruction>
Periosteal reaction	<none> <present: solid/Laminated (single layered/multilayered)/Spiculated/ Interrupted>
Extra-osseous spread	<absent> <extraosseous extension without muscle invasion> <muscular involvement>
Neurovascular bundle involvement	<present> <absent>
Other bony findings	<red marrow> <other anatomical findings>

Table 19.2 Benign tumors and tumor-like lesions

Lesion	Common locations	Imaging findings	Advanced imaging role	Pitfalls and precautions
Osteoid osteoma (Fig. 19.2)	Diaphysis of long bones (femur, tibia), small bones, vertebral posterior elements	CT: hypodense nidus with calcification and surrounding sclerosis MRI: hypointense on T1, variable on T2; surrounding edema is hyperintense	CT is preferred for detection and treatment planning. MRI shows surrounding edema	Has to be differentiated from intraosseous abscess and stress fracture
Osteoblastoma	Diaphysis of long bones, vertebral posterior elements	Round or oval lytic lesion (>1.5–2 cm), with calcification, sclerosis, and possible cortical destruction	MRI shows variable signal intensity; edema is hyperintense on fluid-sensitive sequences	Aggressive lesions can mimic other conditions
Ossifying fibroma/ osteofibrous dysplasia	Mid tibial diaphysis, may involve fibula	Intracortical lytic lesions with sclerosis, possible cortex expansion, and bowing	MRI shows intermediate T1 signal, intermediate to hyperintense T2 signal	May be associated with pathological fractures
Chondroblastoma	Epiphysis/ apophysis of long bones (femur, humerus, tibia), small bones (talus, calcaneus)	Eccentric lytic lesion with sclerotic margin; foci of calcification in 30–50% of cases	MRI shows hypointense on T1, variable on T2, and post-contrast lobular enhancement	Secondary aneurysmal bone cysts may develop

(continued)

Table 19.2 (continued)

Lesion	Common locations	Imaging findings	Advanced imaging role	Pitfalls and precautions
Chondromyxoid fibroma	Long bones of the lower limb (tibia, femur)	Eccentric metaphyseal lytic lesions, potential cortical expansion, and endosteal sclerosis	MRI shows intermediate T1 signal, heterogeneously hyperintense T2 signal, and peripheral nodular enhancement	Calcification and periostitis are usually absent
Osteochondroma (Fig. 19.3)	Long bones (femur, humerus, tibia)	Osseous outgrowth with cortical and medullary continuity; cartilage cap with potential for malignant transformation	MRI: cartilage cap is intermediate on T1, hyperintense on T2	Cap thickness >3 cm in children, >2 cm in adults, may indicate malignancy
Hereditary multiple exostoses	Femur, tibia, fibula, humerus	Bilateral or unilateral exostoses with deformities and higher risk of malignant transformation	Imaging assesses for complications similar to solitary osteochondroma	Higher frequency of malignant transformation (2–5%)
Simple bone cyst (Fig. 19.4)	Metaphysis of long bones (humerus, femur, tibia); calcaneus in small bones	Central radiolucent lesion with mild expansion, cortical thinning, and thin sclerotic margin	MRI: hypointense on T1, hyperintense on T2, with peripheral and internal septal enhancement	Pathologic fracture may show "fallen fragment sign"
Aneurysmal bone cyst (ABC)	Long bones (tibia, femur, humerus), spine	Expansile lytic lesion with internal trabeculation and fluid-fluid levels on MRI	Solid variant may show aggressive features; secondary ABCs associated with other lesions	Distinguish from aggressive bone lesions
Fibrous dysplasia	Rib, femur, tibia, jaw bone, skull, humerus	Eccentric or central diaphyseal lesions with ground-glass appearance; bone expansion and cortical thinning	MRI: intermediate to hypointense on T1, heterogeneous on T2, with variable enhancement	Involvement of craniofacial bones shows expansile radiolucency. McCune-Albright syndrome may be present
Nonossifying fibroma	Long bones (tibia, femur)	Well-defined lytic lesions with sclerotic rim; larger lesions may be expansile and multiloculated	MRI: hypointense on T1, hypo to hyperintense on T2, marginal enhancement	Nonossifying fibromas may be associated with Jaffe-Campanacci syndrome

physiological stress, high-altitude living, myelofibrosis, and metastases. Marrow infiltration may also happen due to infections, inflammation, or treatments like chemotherapy.

On T1-weighted MRI images, yellow marrow appears hyperintense due to its fat content, while red marrow shows variable intensity. Differentiating between the two on T2-weighted images is difficult. Fat-saturated images can better highlight yellow marrow. Marrow diseases typically show hyperintense signals on fluid-sensitive sequences, and since both red marrow and diseases enhance with contrast, contrast imaging is less effective. Chemical-shift imaging is useful, as non-neoplastic lesions often exhibit significant signal loss on out-of-phase images [19].

Table 19.3 Malignant and quasi-malignant tumors

Tumor	Common locations	Imaging findings	Advanced imaging role	Pitfalls and precautions
Osteosarcoma	Long bones (femur, tibia, humerus)	Ill-defined, metaphyseal lesion; lytic, sclerotic, or mixed with cortical destruction. MRI: Hypointense lytic areas on T1, hyperintense on T2; mineralized areas hypointense on both. Heterogeneous enhancement	Large field of view T1W images can reveal skip metastases	Telangiectatic osteosarcoma shows fluid-fluid levels. Misdiagnosis with other conditions possible
Ewing's sarcoma (Fig. 19.5)	Lower skeleton (femur, tibia, ilium, ribs, sacrum)	Metadiaphyseal or diaphyseal lesion with permeative destruction, cortical destruction, and periosteal reaction (laminated, onion-skin). MRI: Heterogeneous intensity on T1 and T2, variable contrast enhancement	MRI distinguishes from osteomyelitis by detecting soft tissue mass and cortical saucerization	Confusion with osteomyelitis; look for serpiginous tracts and penumbra sign in osteomyelitis
Leukemia and lymphoma	Bones around knee, pelvis, spine	Osteopenia, medullary widening, cortical thinning, bilateral metaphyseal bands MRI: hypointense marrow on T1, hyperintense on T2/STIR, with post-contrast enhancement	MRI aids in evaluating marrow involvement and differentiating from other conditions	Epiphyseal osteonecrosis and pathologic fractures may complicate diagnosis
Langerhans cell histiocytosis	Skull, mandible, spine, ribs, pelvis, long bones (femur, humerus)	Well-defined lytic areas in tubular bones; beveled margins in the skull; button sequestrum possible. MRI: Aggressive lesions with surrounding edema and intense post-contrast enhancement	MRI reveals extent of marrow edema and cortical erosion	Lesions can mimic other bone pathologies; look for characteristic features

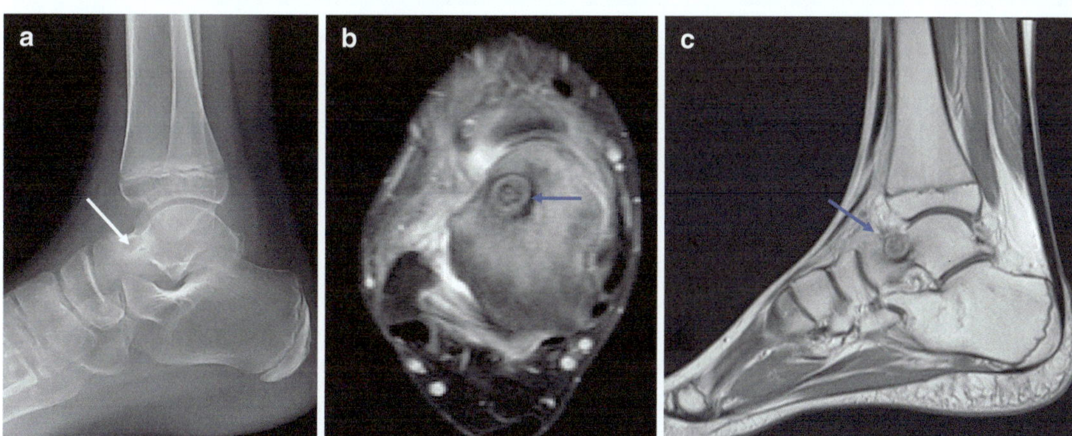

Fig. 19.2 Lateral radiograph of the right ankle joint (**a**) showing a lucent lesion with marginal sclerosis in the neck of talus (white arrow). Axial PD fat saturated MR image (**b**) and sagittal T1W MR image (**c**) showing an osteoid osteoma in the talar neck (blue arrows) with surrounding marrow edema and joint effusion

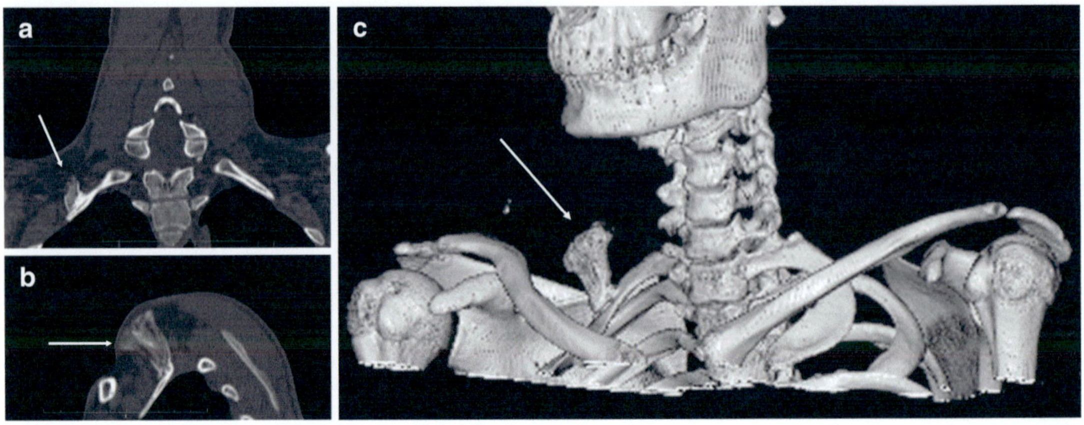

Fig. 19.3 Coronal (**a**) and sagittal (**b**) reformatted CT images showing an osteochondroma arising from the right first rib (white arrows), which is well depicted in the 3D reconstructed image (**c**)

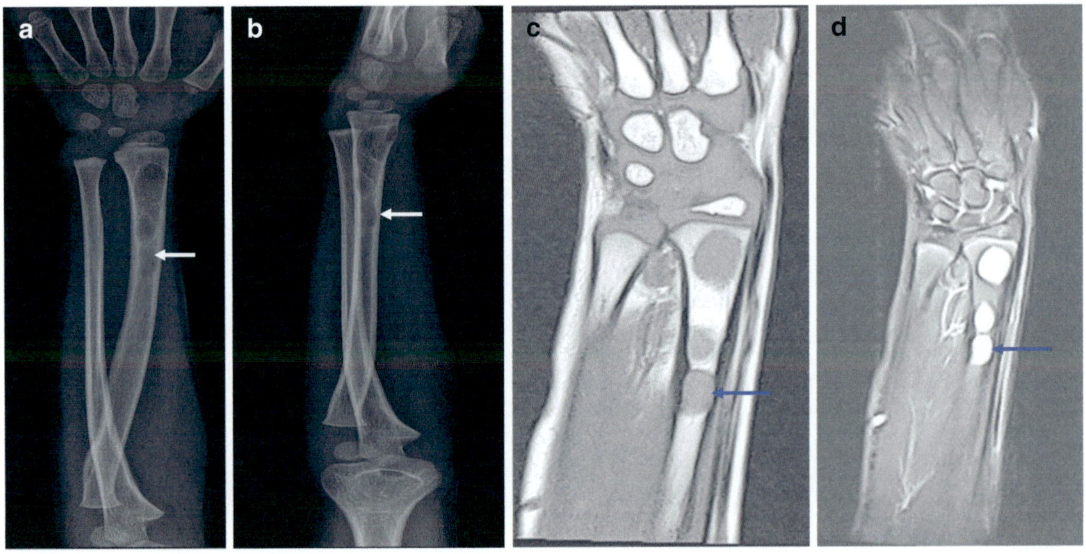

Fig. 19.4 AP and lateral radiographs of the right forearm (**a** and **b**) showing few radiolucent lesions without significant bone expansion in the distal radius (white arrows). Coronal T1W (**c**) and STIR (**d**) MR images showing cystic lesions in the distal radius consistent with simple bone cysts (blue arrows)

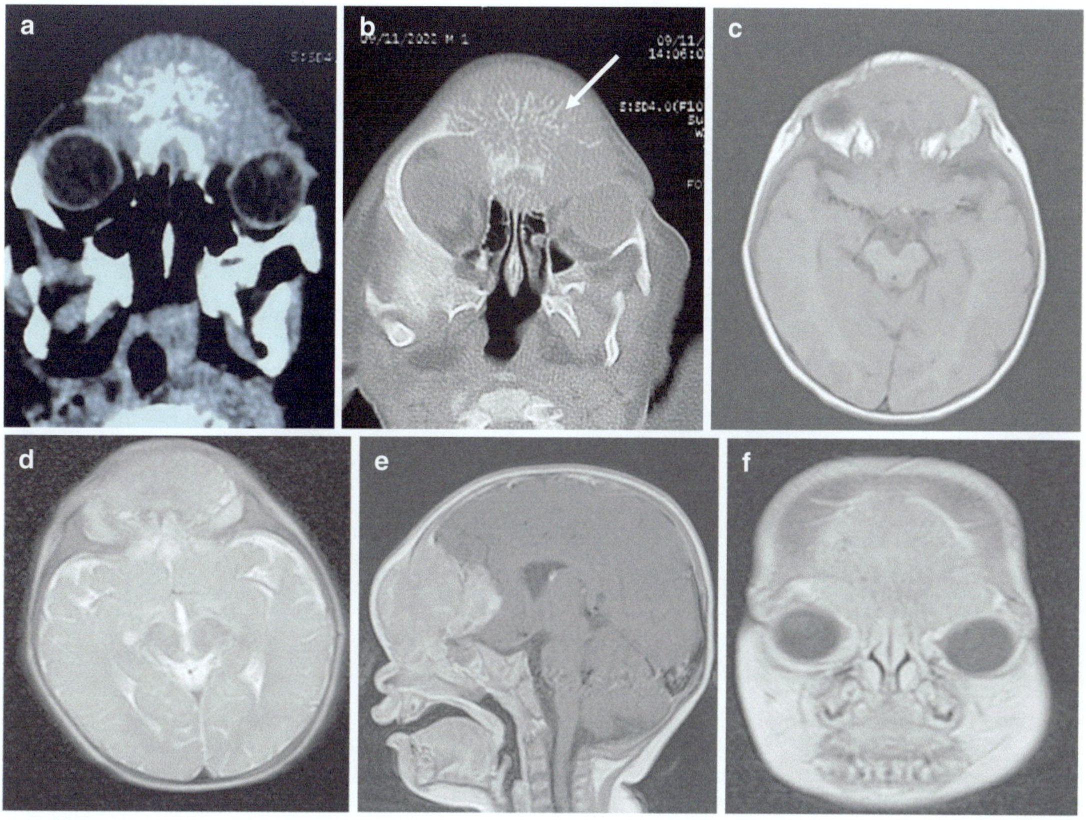

Fig. 19.5 Axial CT images (**a** and **b**), done at outside Institution, in a child with rapidly growing forehead swelling showing an aggressive mass lesion causing bone destruction in the ethmoid bone with spiculated periosteal reaction (white arrow). Axial T1W and T2W MR images (**c** and **d**) and post-contrast sagittal and coronal T1W MR images (**e** and **f**) showing the heterogeneously enhancing mass lesion causing bone destruction with intra-cranial and intra-orbital extension. Histopathology findings were consistent with Ewing's sarcoma

19.5 Post-treatment Imaging

With improved diagnosis and treatment strategies, children with benign and even malignant tumors have good survival rates. This requires prolonged periods of follow-up of children sometimes up to the adulthood. Post-treatment imaging in children is challenging since anatomical changes in children are quite different from those in adults. A thorough knowledge of imaging appearance of the expected post-treatment changes and complications is necessary for optimal post-treatment care in children treated for osseous tumors.

Radiographs are still the first-line imaging modality for routine follow-up evaluation of patients treated for bone tumors. Routine MRI plays an integral role in structural evaluation like the extent of marrow and soft tissue involvement and to a certain extent, tumor characterization. However, in case of tumor recurrence, or to evaluate the treatment response, the exact extent of tumor necrosis and the presence of tumor viability are essential rather than the tumor size alone.

Functional magnetic resonance imaging like dynamic contrast MRI, diffusion MRI, and in-phase/opposed-phase MRI are helpful problem-solving tools in this scenario. Diffusion MRI can be used to assess cellularity and cell-membrane integrity in tumor tissue both qualitatively and quantitatively [20]. Areas of high signal intensity in diffusion and low ADC values (1.1×10^{-3} mm^2/s) indicate high cellularity hence malignant tumor or recurrence (Fig. 19.6a–c).

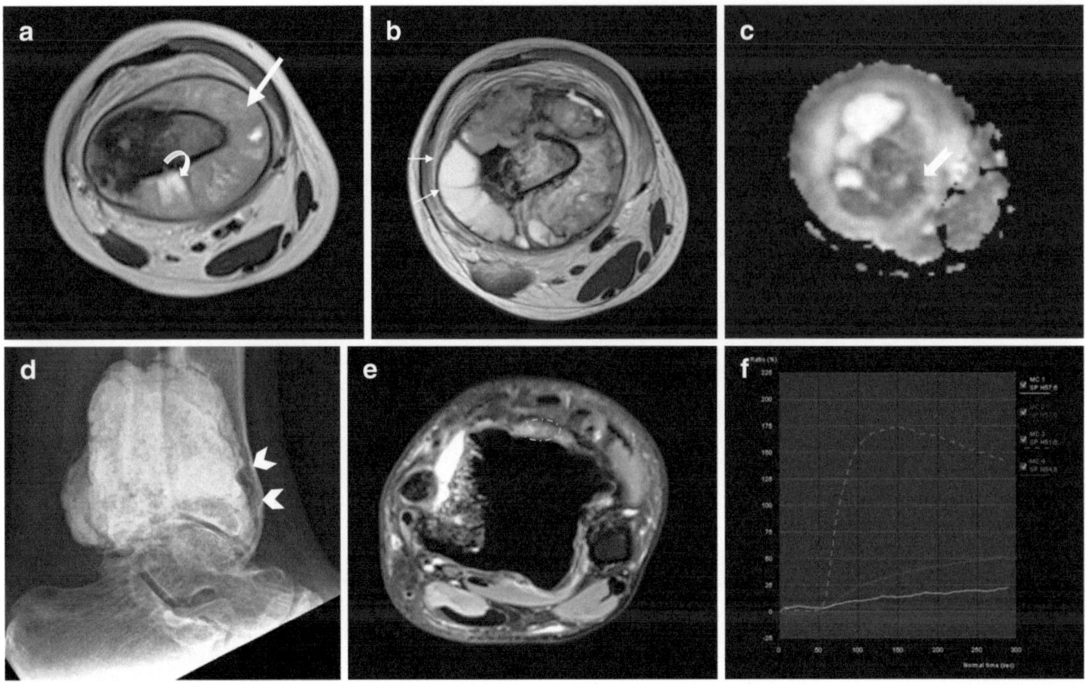

Fig. 19.6 Tumor response following chemotherapy for osteosarcoma in the distal femur. T2 W axial image (**a**) shows hypointense tumor mass in the bone and periosteal soft tissue {arrow}indicating high cellularity with a small focus of necrosis in the soft tissue component {curved arrow}. Post-chemotherapy T2W image (**b**) shows extensive heterogeneity {asterisk} due to tumor necrosis which poses a challenge in identifying the residual lesion. There was also an increase in fluid pockets {small arrows} suggesting areas of necrosis as a result of partial treatment response. Diffusion-weighted image (**c**) shows significantly reduced ADC within this area {notched arrow} indicating persistent tumor. *Dynamic contrast study for tumor recurrence* (**d**–**f**) The distal tibial aneurysmal bone cyst was treated with curettage and cement placement. The follow-up radiograph showed suspicious irregular lucency {chevron} around the anterior aspect of the graft (**d**). Axial fat-suppressed T2W image (**e**) showed nonspecific hyperintensity around the anterior aspect of the graft {orange circle}. A dynamic contrast of this area (**f**) shows rapid contrast uptake and gradual increased enhancement suggesting tumor recurrence {orange curve, as compared to fibrosis and aorta, yellow and purple curve respectively}

Post-treatment tumor necrosis causes loss of cell wall integrity and hence increases in the ADC value [20]. Dynamic contrast MRI or perfusion MRI is a technique wherein the early (within 5 min of injection in the region of interest of the tumor, adjacent artery, and healthy muscle) enhancement pattern of the tumor is monitored after bolus injection of intravenous gadolinium. This provides information about the perfusion, capillary permeability, and interstitial compartment volume which help to identify the viable tumor areas [21].

The time-intensity curves provide the clue for tumor perfusion. Typically, five types of curves are described.

- Type I is no enhancement (benign avascular tumors like lipoma or hematoma).
- Type II shows mild and slow enhancement indicating benign myxoid tumors like schwannoma.
- Type III shows early peak enhancement which plateaus which is the grey area with overlap between certain benign/malignant lesions, and even abscesses.
- Type IV curve has rapid early enhancement followed by washout. Several vascular malignant tumors and a few benign tumors like giant cell tumors, and osteoid osteoma nidus show this pattern of enhancement.
- Type V curve has rapid early enhancement followed by slow gradual enhancement. This pattern is typically seen in tumors following chemo or radiotherapy and myxoid tumors.

  Less than a 90% decrease in slope value or no change as compared to pretherapy value indicates poor responders (Fig. 19.6d–f). Changes in the time-intensity curve with at least a 60% decrease in the slope value indicate more than 90% of tumor necrosis, which defines a good treatment response with accuracy ranging from 85.7% to 100% [21]. Details about tumor response following chemotherapy are in Table 19.4.

Chemical shift imaging and recently Dixon sequence is another tool that detects marrow infiltration by tumor cells by quantifying the fat and water content in the marrow. Fat fraction values can be computed using in-phase and opposed-phase images and a cut-off value of more than 0.8 indicates a tumor [22].

MR spectroscopy may provide detailed insights into the metabolic profiles of lesions, facilitating earlier detection and improved differentiation between benign and malignant conditions. Choline concentration detected by spectroscopy is an indirect estimate for tumor cellularity, and rate of proliferation since it's a component of phospholipid metabolism of cell membranes [23–25].

19.6 Expected Post-treatment Changes

Treatment of the benign pediatric tumor can be either by complete excision or by minimally invasive image-guided procedures. Image-guided procedures are safe alternatives especially when the tumor is small, difficult to surgical access, or proximity to the growth plate. Details of minimally invasive procedures for benign lesions are enumerated in Table 19.5 [26–29].

Table 19.4 Imaging characteristics of malignant bone tumors following chemotherapy

Imaging modality	Osteosarcoma	Ewing sarcoma
Radiographs/CT	Increased tumor ossification, peripheral ossification	Disappearance of soft-tissue mass; cortical, medullary sclerosis
MRI: T1W sequences	No change	No change Increased marrow signal
T2W sequences	Increased signal suggests necrosis	Disappearance of soft tissue
Contrast	No enhancement in necrotic regions	No soft-tissue enhancement
Dynamic contrast	1. Decreased time-intensity curve slopes (>60% reduction in slope) 2. Persistent/increasing delayed enhancement without washout	1. Decreased slope of residual mass (>60% reduction in slope) 2. Persistent/increasing delayed enhancement without washout
Diffusion values	Increased ADC values indicate tumor response	An increase in ADC values indicates tumor necrosis

Table 19.5 Treatment modalities for benign bone lesions with expected imaging outcome

Benign bone lesion	Preferred treatment modalities	Expected imaging outcome
Osteoidosteoma	RFA Microwave ablation Laser ablation HIFU ablation	*MRI:* Immediate decrease (6 months) in tumor and peritumoral edema, reduction in joint effusion, and synovial thickening; progressive consolidation of lytic lesion *CT:* Avoid up to 1 year to monitor bone remodeling *Follow-up:* Persistent edema and pain may need repeat procedures or surgery
Osteoblastoma	RFA Cryoablation Laser ablation HIFU ablation	*MRI:* Follow-up at 6 and 12 months showing absence of reactive inflammatory processes and contrast enhancement *CT:* At 12 months for ossification assessment *Outcome:* Gradual bone reshaping over 2 years
Chondroblastoma	RFA Cryoablation	*MRI:* Decrease in tumor size and peritumoral edema; progressive consolidation of the lytic lesion *Risk:* Articular collapse for lesions >2.5 cm; curettage and bone substitutes preferred
Simple bone cyst	Intralesional steroid injection Bone marrow condensate Allograft	*MRI:* Decrease in size, with progressive ground glass to dense ossification of the cavity; cortical thickening *Follow-up:* Every 60–90 days; after 1 year, radiographs every 6 months or 1 year *Recurrence:* Persistent expanding lytic areas indicate possible recurrence
Aneurysmal bone cyst	Intralesional sclerotherapy (polidocanol, doxycycline) Cryoablation RFA Microwave ablation Embolization (adjunct)	*MRI:* Follow-up at 3 months, 6 months, half-yearly for the first 2 years, and yearly for the third to fifth year *Outcome:* Absence of pain, ossification, and fracture; complete healing defined as consolidation with newly formed bones, with thickened borders and small radiolucent areas <1 cm in size (Neer classification) *Recurrence:* Osteolysis or cyst >50% of bone diameter indicates residual tumor

19.6.1 Surgical Treatment of Benign Osseous Lesions

For large tumors not suitable for minimally invasive techniques or requiring structural support post-excision, surgical management is necessary. The primary goal is to remove the tumor completely while preserving bone growth and joint function. In children, bone grafts—autografts, allografts, or synthetic substitutes—are used to restore bone strength and morphology (Fig. 19.7). Cement is avoided due to its potential to cause early osteoarthritic changes [30].

Bone grafts serve as scaffolds for new bone formation and adapt to mechanical stress. For large defects, strut or on-lay grafts with internal fixation provide enhanced stability [31, 32]. Incorporation of allografts, influenced by factors like particle size and graft type, can take over 27 weeks, while autografts show similar incorporation rates in smaller defects (Fig. 19.8).

Radiographic follow-up is crucial. Autografts appear as normal cortical bone on CT and radiographs, while MRI shows early T1 hypointensity and T2 hyperintensity due to granulation tissue, eventually resembling host bone. Allografts, lacking viable marrow, initially show T1 hypointensity and T2 hyperintensity but blend with the host bone post-incorporation, with CT revealing density similar to cortical bone and a disappearing radiolucent boundary ceramic graft substitutes, often used in children and adolescents, are radiodense and composed of materials like hydroxyapatite and tricalcium phosphate. They appear dense with a radiolucent border initially

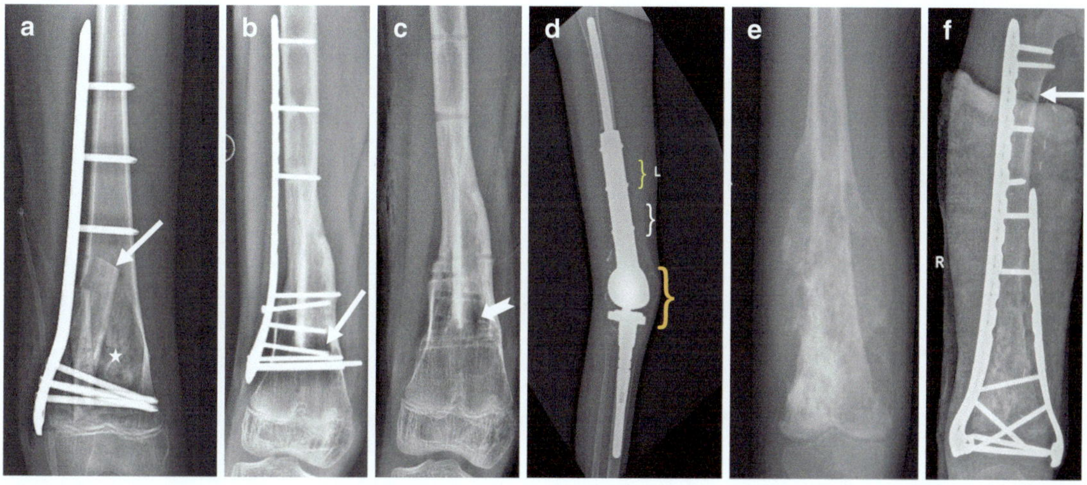

Fig. 19.7 Bone graft materials, substitutes, and stabilizing techniques in children and adolescents. (**a**) Radiographs of distal femoral recurrent aneurysmal bone cyst in a 13-year-old boy who had undergone internal fixation following curettage, bone grafting with allograft struts and chips. Struts {arrow} show similar density as the cortical bone and allograft chips {asterisk} are heterogeneously dense than native bone in the early postoperative period which will be incorporated by 21 months in this case due to the large size of the cavity. (**b**, **c**) Intercalary allograft placement and internal fixation with medial plate and screws in a patient with recurrent large aneurysmal bone cyst. Allografts were fixed by screws on either end of the host bone-graft junction visualized as radiolucent zone {arrow}. The growth plate and epiphysis are spared during the reconstruction. Good incorporation was seen in 15 months as evidenced by the complete disappearance of lucency between the host bone and graft junction {notched arrow}. (**d**) Modular endoprosthesis placement in a 10-year-old girl with osteosarcoma. The radiograph shows a tibial stem and femoral components. There is a distal femoral rotating hinge component {orange bracket} with one module {white bracket} and a modular femoral stem {yellow bracket}. (**e**, **f**) Extracorporeal radiotherapy and reimplantation of the irradiated bone with internal fixation in a 12-year-old boy with osteosarcoma. The replanted bone is of the same size and shape and hence acts as a perfect fit prosthesis. Most of the periosteal component is cleared off before irradiation and the density of the bone is slightly reduced in the immediate post-irradiation period. The plate and screws are seen placed just beyond the replanted bone-normal bone junction seen as the lucent line in radiograph {arrow}

but show reduced radiodensity and loss of the border as they incorporate into the host bone [33–36].

Complications Following curettage and bone graft placement for benign tumors, complications can include fractures, infections, tumor recurrence, and autograft resorption or mild rejection in allografts (Fig. 19.9). Donor site issues for autografts may involve chronic pain, scarring, and occasionally nerve damage. Allografts carry a risk of disease transmission. Persistent radiolucency often signals inadequate graft incorporation. Smooth, progressive lucency at the graft-host interface suggests resorption, while rapid growth or irregular lucency, particularly after initial incorporation, may indicate tumor recurrence. CT can reveal trabecular bone configuration of the graft, indicating non-incorporation if lucency is present. MRI typically shows tumor characteristics similar to pre-treatment scans. Additionally, fractures of on-lay or strut grafts, if not supported by internal plates and screws, are a potential complication [31].

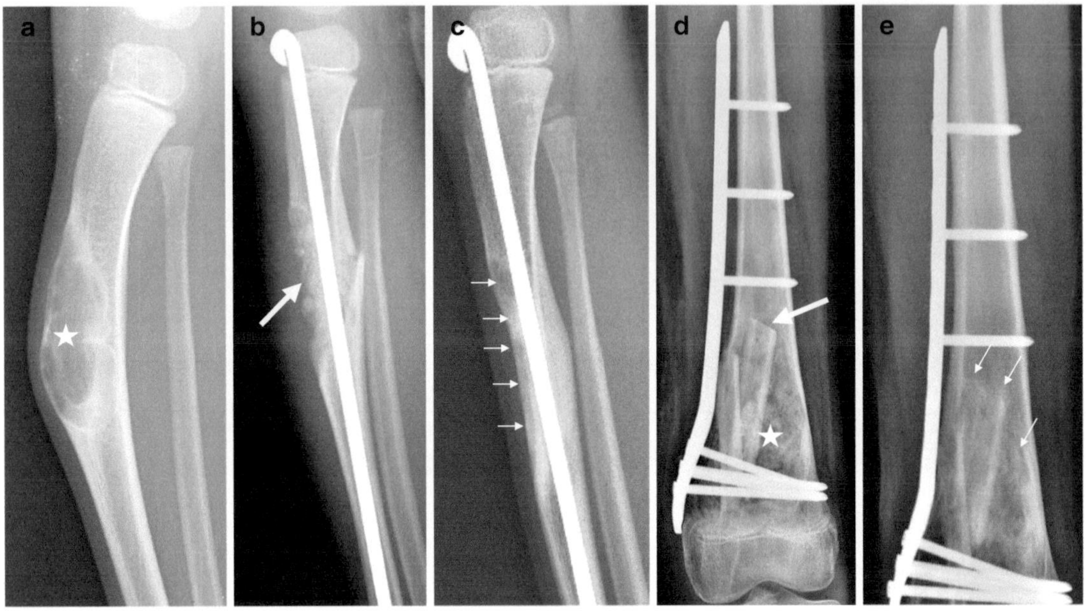

Fig. 19.8 Expected patterns of graft incorporation into the host bone. (**a–c**) Allograft chips packing of the tumor cavity with good incorporation by 20 months. The large lesion {asterisk} in the anterior tibial cortex of the proximal tibia resulted in anterior bowing in a 10-year-old boy which was curetted and packed with allograft chips. Additionally, osteotomy was performed for deformity correction, with rush nailing of the tibia sparing the growth plate for stability. The multiple dense discrete bone chips {arrow} show a reduction in density with complete homogenization {small arrows} indicating good fusion in follow-up radiograph. (**d**, **e**) Good incorporation of strut graft and allograft chips in postoperative case of recurrent aneurysmal bone cyst. Struts {arrow} show similar density as the cortical bone and allograft chips {asterisk} are heterogeneously dense than native bone in the early postoperative period. There is a gradual loss of density of both strut graft and chips which is similar to the density of the medullary cavity following the incorporation by 21 months of duration

19.6.2 Surgical Treatment of Malignant Osseous Lesions

Limb salvage surgery is preferred for tumors with complete excision, adequate margins, and preserved function. Contraindications include neurovascular invasion, pathological fractures, and inappropriate biopsy tracts. While limb salvage and amputation offer similar survival rates, limb salvage is now standard for many bone sarcomas to preserve function [37, 38].

In children, surgical decisions often depend on limb length discrepancy. Discrepancies under 3 cm may be addressed with prophylactic lengthening of 1–2 cm during surgery, while those over 3 cm usually require surgical correction. Rotationplasty, using the ankle as a knee after femur or tibia resection, has functional benefits but notable cosmetic and psychological impacts. Reconstruction options include:

- *Endoprosthetic:* Conventional implants are modular and customizable, with cement or porous stems. Expandable prostheses allow limb lengthening using invasive worm screws or non-invasive electromagnetic methods, limited to 10 mm at a time.
- *Biological:* Includes intercalary or osteoarticular allografts, often combined with vascular-

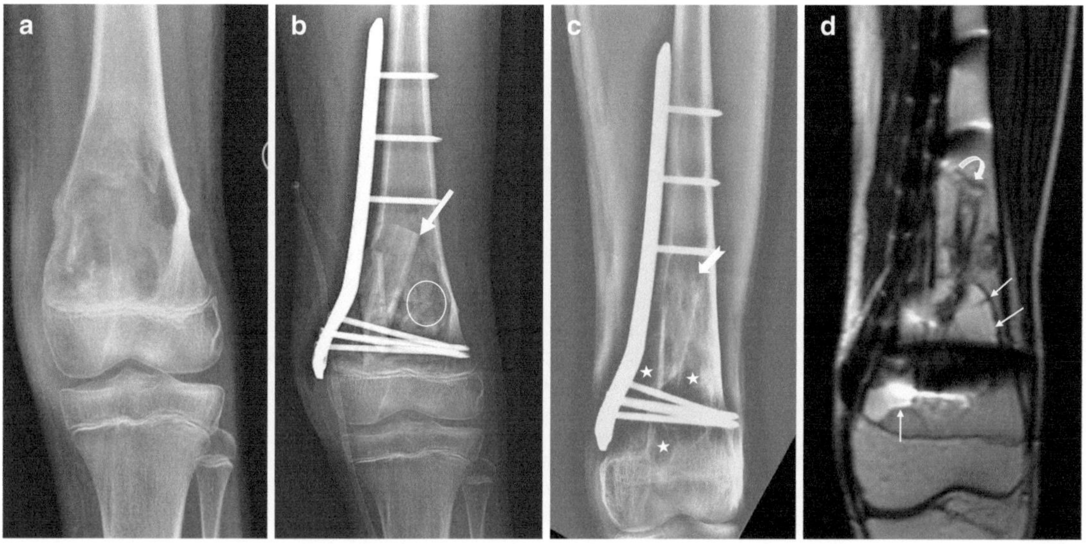

Fig. 19.9 Lesion recurrence in an 11-year-old boy. (**a**) Image obtained at the time of the initial biopsy shows an expansile lytic lesion at the distal femoral metadiaphysis. (**b**) Radiograph obtained immediately following curettage and bone grafting shows allograft strut grafts {arrow} and also bone chips {circled} filling the cavity. Internal fixation plates and screws were used for stabilization. (**c**) A radiograph obtained 9 months ago shows the development of widespread radiolucency and increased expansion, involving both strut grafts and bone chips at the distal end {asterisks}, findings that are indicative of recurrence. However proximal aspect shows good incorporation into the host bone without any destruction {notched arrow}. (**d**) Coronal T2W MR image confirms a recurrent aneurysmal bone cyst with multiple fluid levels {small arrows}. There is hyperintensity within the entire strut graft in the MRI indicating lesion involvement up to the proximal aspect {curved arrow} which was not evident on the radiograph. The recurrent lesion characteristic will be the same as in the preoperative scan as seen in this patient

ized fibular autografts. Radiographs show dense allografts initially, with decreasing density and integration over time. MRI reveals persistent marrow signal with speckled heterogeneous T1 hypointense/T2 hyperintense area and persistent contrast enhancement in these areas for up to 2 years, likely due to vascular ingrowth and new bone formation (Fig. 19.8).

Extracorporeal irradiated tumor (ECRT) bone is an emerging option, sterilized with 50Gy radiation, providing a size-matched graft but unsuitable for weak or fractured bones. Complications include non-union, fracture, and infection. For detailed bone substitutes, see Table 19.6 [39–47].

Table 19.6 Bone substitutes commonly used following tumor excision

Type of bone substitute	Indications	Expected healing pattern and imaging appearance	Advantages	Disadvantages and complications
Autografts: Bone obtained from the same patient				
Bone chips: Smaller bone fragments from the iliac crest, tibia, rib, fibula	Small resected cavities; adjunct to other grafts	*Radiograph/CT:* Appears isodense to bone. Complete incorporation matches normal bone density. *MRI:* Initial hypointense T1 and hyperintense T2 due to granulation; normal marrow signal upon incorporation	Preferred over cement in children; good mechanical support for small cavities	Donor site morbidity; limited to small defects; resorption may mimic tumor recurrence on X-ray
Free vascularized fibular grafts	Large constructs; can be combined with allografts	*Three patterns:* 1. Decreased density due to stress shielding, followed by cancellous appearance 2. Hypertrophy with preserved vascularity but fracture 3. Gradual resorption	Minimizes chemotherapy-related complications; maintains biomechanical integrity	May not match the shape of the bone; large defects can be challenging
Allografts: Deep-frozen fresh cadaver bone				
Intercalary grafts	Large tumors with preserved joint and epiphysis	*Healing:* Periosteal reaction and callus formation by 40 weeks. Density peaks at 15 weeks, normalizes by 100 weeks *Imaging:* Decreasing density over time	Provides good stability and anatomical match; can be enhanced with vascular grafts	High rates of fracture, non-union, and infection within 3 years
Osteoarticular grafts	Tumors involving one joint side; no prosthesis available	*Healing:* Callus formation by 60–80 weeks, with density changes observed over 2 years *Imaging:* Periosteal reaction, increasing density initially, then normalization	Anatomical match offers good functional outcomes	Risks include delayed union, non-union, fractures, infection, cartilage degeneration, and joint instability
Graft-prosthesis composites: Also called composite biologic implant	Used when grafts do not match the defect	*Imaging:* Similar to joint replacement; typically uses internal fixation plates or screws	Allows use of mismatched allografts; provides tendon attachment	Risks include infection, fracture, and non-union
Endoprostheses	Expandable prostheses for extensive bone and joint loss	*Imaging:* Similar to joint replacement *Radiographs:* Assess limb length discrepancy	Maintains limb length in growing children; non-invasive expansion options available	Complications include infection, dislocation, mechanical failure, aseptic loosening, and tumor progression
Extracorporeal radiation (ECRT):	Limb salvage for large tumors	*Healing:* Similar to intercalary grafts *Imaging:* Matches intercalary fusion appearance	Size-matched graft; can be used with other biological materials	Risks of non-union, fracture, and infection; not suitable for structurally weak or fractured bones

19.7 Complications of Surgery

Endoprosthetic reconstruction can lead to several complications, including infection, aseptic or septic loosening, implant failure, periprosthetic fracture, and local disease recurrence (Fig. 19.10) [37, 48].

Radiographic and MRI Findings [49–54]:

- *Aseptic Loosening:* Typically presents as thigh or leg pain that intensifies with weight-bearing and subsides with rest. Radiographically, a well-defined radiolucent zone around the stem, less than 2 mm with a thin sclerotic margin, is generally normal. Progressive radiolucency, cortical thickening, or stem migration may indicate loosening. MRI may show similar findings with increasing radiolucent areas.
- *Infection:* Characterized by persistent pain. Imaging often reveals well-defined radiolucent areas at the cement-bone or component-bone interface, suggesting infection or particle disease.
- *Bone Scintigraphy:* Effective for differentiating infection from non-septic loosening. A negative scan virtually rules out infection. Combined leukocyte-marrow scintigraphy is highly precise (over 90%) for diagnosing infection, while PET scans, with about 90.4% accuracy, are particularly valuable if activity is observed around the bone-prosthesis interface.
- *Implant Failure:* May result from excessive stress on the implant, unexpected limb length changes, or infection risks associated with percutaneous lengthening.
- *Biologic Reconstruction:* Nonunion is indicated by persistent gaps at the bone-graft interface beyond 1 year, with an incidence of

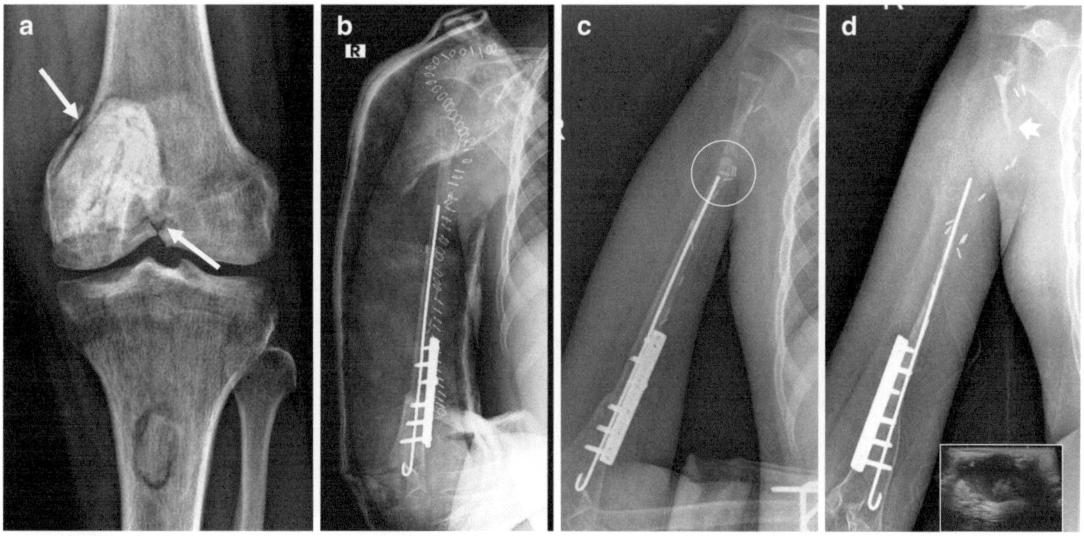

Fig. 19.10 Complications in the postoperative period following bone tumor resection. (**a**) Perigraft fracture in a 20-year-old male who was treated for distal femoral aneurysmal bone cyst with transphyseal extension 6 years back. There is radiodense graft material in the postoperative cavity, with a fracture extending from the medial cortex adjacent to graft material which was seen extending to the intercondylar notch {arrows}. There is uniform thickness lucency around the graft which on MRI showed fluid around the graft communicating into the joint through fracture. Also seen in the image is the graft harvest site in the proximal tibia {asterisk}. (**b**–**d**) Infected intercalary graft in a 13-year-old girl. A fibular intercalary strut graft was placed following the resection of Ewing's sarcoma in the mid-shaft of the right humerus. An intramedullary rush nail with an internal plate and screws in the distal end was used for stabilization. 8 weeks following the surgery, the patient presented with new-onset pain, and radiographs showed a small break {circled} in the host bone at the proximal tip of the intramedullary rush nail. There was rapid destruction of the proximal shaft of the host humerus {notched arrow} and also part of the bone around the proximal aspect of the intramedullary nail in the next 1 week. There was also soft tissue thickening around the bone destruction which revealed collection on ultrasound {inserted image}

11–12%. Non-union rates increase in patients undergoing adjuvant chemotherapy (27–32%). Persistent bone resorption and prolonged soft tissue swelling beyond 6 months may signal infection [41–45].

Ongoing radiographic monitoring is crucial for detecting and managing these complications.

MRI findings in postoperative complications are given in Table 19.7.

Children diagnosed with bone tumors require prolonged imaging follow-up. Multimodality imaging and a multidisciplinary approach are key to the optimal management of children with complications. Thorough knowledge of various prostheses, grafts, instrumentation, and surgical techniques used for treatment along with normal and complicating imaging findings are essential for reporting radiologists and referring clinicians.

19.8 Conclusion

A wide spectrum of bone tumors is seen in children which includes both aggressive and non-aggressive lesions. It is important for the radiologist to reach a differential diagnosis based on a practical checklist-based approach. Establishing the correct diagnosis followed by appropriate management and follow-up will spare undue agony to the child as well as family.

Table 19.7 Postoperative complications

Complication	MRI findings	Role of advanced imaging	Pitfalls and precautions
Hematoma/ seroma	*Hematoma:* Variable signal intensity with age. *Seroma:* T1 hypointense, T2 hyperintense, homogeneous with low-intensity rim	*Gradient-echo:* Blooming artifact *DWI:* High ADC compared to tumors	Hemorrhage in tumors may mimic recurrence. Myxomas may appear similar
Post-surgical hypertrophic scar/ pseudotumor	T1 and T2 hypointense, irregular mass Little or no enhancement	*DWI:* High ADC *DCE:* Rare arterial phase enhancement	Early inflammatory changes may mimic tumors
Pseudo-progression	Heterogeneous signal intensity Enlarged central non-enhancing area with reduced enhancement	*Residual tumor:* Persistent enhancement and diffusion restriction *Pseudo-progression:* Blooming artifact, no diffusion restriction	Avoid imaging for 4–6 weeks post-therapy
Post radiation changes in soft tissue, flaps, and bone	*Soft tissue:* Edema with preserved architecture T1: Muscle texture sign or feathering sign *Radiation Osteitis:* T2/ STIR hyperintense *Radiation osteonecrosis:* Heterogeneous, T1 hyperintense, T2 intermediate	*DWI:* Low signal on DWI and high signal on ADC *DCE:* Delayed enhancement	Monitor for atrophy and fat overgrowth. Distinguish from new masses (e.g., sarcoma: shows heterogenous signal intensity with matrix calcification)
Tumor recurrence bone/soft tissue	Focal, heterogeneous mass T1 hypointense, T2 hyperintense Matches primary tumor	*DCE:* Early enhancement with washout or plateau *DWI:* Increased restriction, low ADC(<1.0 × 10–3 mm^2/s) Diffusion quantification (tumor ADC histograms)	Ossified or fibrous tumors may remain T2 hypointense. No standard ADC cut-off Certain densely

References

1. Shah JN, Cohen HL, Choudhri AF, Gupta S, Miller SF. Pediatric benign bone tumors: what does the radiologist need to know?: pediatric imaging. Radiographics. 2017;37(3):1001–2. https://doi.org/10.1148/rg.2017160143. PMID: 28493806.
2. Al-Qassab S, Lalam R, Botchu R, Bazzocchi A. Imaging of pediatric bone tumors and tumor-like lesions. Semin Musculoskelet Radiol. 2021;25(1):57–67. https://doi.org/10.1055/s--0041-1723965. Epub 2021 May 21. PMID: 34020468.
3. Lalam R, Bloem JL, Noebauer-Huhmann IM, Wörtler K, Tagliafico A, Vanhoenacker F, Nikodinovska VV, Sanal HT, Woude HV, Papakonstantinou O, Åström G, Davies M, Isaac A, Weber MA. ESSR consensus document for detection, characterization, and referral pathway for tumors and tumorlike lesions of bone. Semin Musculoskelet Radiol. 2017;21(5):630–47. https://doi.org/10.1055/s-0037-1606130. Epub 2017 Oct 12. PMID: 29025191.
4. Expert Panel on Musculoskeletal Imaging, Bestic JM, Wessell DE, Beaman FD, Cassidy RC, Czuczman GJ, Demertzis JL, Lenchik L, Motamedi K, Pierce JL, Sharma A, Sloan AE, Than K, Walker EA, Ying-Kou Yung E, Kransdorf MJ. ACR Appropriateness Criteria® primary bone tumors. J Am Coll Radiol. 2020;17(5S):S226–38. https://doi.org/10.1016/j.jacr.2020.01.038. PMID: 32370967.
5. Cederberg KB, Iyer RS, Chaturvedi A, McCarville MB, McDaniel JD, Sandberg JK, Shammas A, Sharp SE, Nadel HR. Imaging of pediatric bone tumors: A COG Diagnostic Imaging Committee/SPR Oncology Committee White Paper. Pediatr Blood Cancer. 2023;70(Suppl 4(Suppl 4)):e30000. https://doi.org/10.1002/pbc.30000. Epub 2022 Oct 17. PMID: 36250990; PMCID: PMC10661611.
6. González-Huete A, Salgado-Parente A, Suevos-Ballesteros C, Antolinos-Macho E, Ventura-Díaz S, Michael-Fernández A, Blázquez-Sánchez J, Acosta-Batlle J. Radiographic evaluation of bone tumors. Radiographics. 2023;43(11):e230048. https://doi.org/10.1148/rg.230048. PMID: 37824409.
7. Gemescu IN, Thierfelder KM, Rehnitz C, Weber MA. Imaging features of bone tumors: conventional radiographs and MR imaging correlation. Magn Reson Imaging Clin N Am. 2019;27(4):753–67. https://doi.org/10.1016/j.mric.2019.07.008. PMID: 31575404.
8. Chotel F, Franck F, Solla F, Dijoud F, Kohler R, Berard J, Abelin Genevois K, French Sarcoma Group – Bone Tumour Study Group. Osteoid osteoma transformation into osteoblastoma: fact or fiction? Orthop Traumatol Surg Res. 2012;98(6 Suppl):S98–104. https://doi.org/10.1016/j.otsr.2012.03.017. Epub 2012 Sept 13. PMID: 22981644.
9. Caracciolo JT, Temple HT, Letson GD, Kransdorf MJ. A modified Lodwick-Madewell grading system for the evaluation of lytic bone lesions. AJR Am J Roentgenol. 2016;207(1):150–6. https://doi.org/10.2214/AJR.15.14368. Epub 2016 Apr 12. PMID: 27070373.
10. Sweet DE, Madewell JE, Ragsdale BD. Radiologic and pathologic analysis of solitary bone lesions. Part III: matrix patterns. Radiol Clin North Am. 1981;19(4):785–814. PMID: 7323292.
11. Costelloe CM, Madewell JE. Radiography in the initial diagnosis of primary bone tumors. AJR Am J Roentgenol. 2013;200(1):3–7. https://doi.org/10.2214/AJR.12.8488. PMID: 23255735.
12. Silva FD, Pinheiro L, Cristofano C, et al. Magnetic resonance imaging in pediatric bone tumors. Curr Radiol Rep. 2014;2:77. https://doi.org/10.1007/s40134-014-0077-5.
13. Van Dyck P, Vanhoenacker FM, Vogel J, Venstermans C, Kroon HM, Gielen J, Parizel PM, Bloem JL, De Schepper AM. Prevalence, extension and characteristics of fluid-fluid levels in bone and soft tissue tumors. Eur Radiol. 2006;16(12):2644–51. https://doi.org/10.1007/s00330-006-0250-1. Epub 2006 Apr 13. PMID: 16612549.
14. Chaib B, Malhotra K, Khoo M, Saifuddin A. Pathological fracture in paediatric bone tumours and tumour-like lesions: a predictor of benign lesions? Br J Radiol. 2021;94(1125):20201341. https://doi.org/10.1259/bjr.20201341. Epub 2021 July 28. PMID: 34319796; PMCID: PMC9327763.
15. James SL, Panicek DM, Davies AM. Bone marrow oedema associated with benign and malignant bone tumours. Eur J Radiol. 2008;67(1):11–21. https://doi.org/10.1016/j.ejrad.2008.01.052. Epub 2008 Mar 20. PMID: 18358660.
16. Nascimento D, Suchard G, Hatem M, de Abreu A. The role of magnetic resonance imaging in the evaluation of bone tumours and tumour-like lesions. Insights Imaging. 2014;5(4):419–40. https://doi.org/10.1007/s13244-014-0339-z. Epub 2014 July 9. PMID: 25005774; PMCID: PMC4141345.
17. Sajadi KR, Heck RK, Neel MD, Rao BN, Daw N, Rodriguez-Galindo C, Hoffer FA, Stacy GS, Peabody TD, Simon MA. The incidence and prognosis of osteosarcoma skip metastases. Clin Orthop Relat Res. 2004;426:92–6. https://doi.org/10.1097/01.blo.0000141493.52166.69. PMID: 15346057.
18. Wang T, Wu X, Cui Y, Chu C, Ren G, Li W. Role of apparent diffusion coefficients with diffusion-weighted magnetic resonance imaging in differentiating between benign and malignant bone tumors. World J Surg Oncol. 2014;12:365. https://doi.org/10.1186/1477-7819-12-365. PMID: 25432796; PMCID: PMC4265400.
19. Chan BY, Gill KG, Rebsamen SL, Nguyen JC. MR imaging of pediatric bone marrow. Radiographics. 2016;36(6):1911–30. https://doi.org/10.1148/rg.2016160056. PMID: 27726743.
20. Costa FM, Ferreira EC, Vianna EM. Diffusion-weighted magnetic resonance imaging for the evaluation of musculoskeletal tumors. Magn Reson Imaging Clin N Am. 2011;19(1):159–80. https://doi.org/10.1016/j.mric.2010.10.007. PMID: 21129640.

21. Verstraete KL, Lang P. Bone and soft tissue tumors: the role of contrast agents for MR imaging. Eur J Radiol. 2000;34(3):229–46. https://doi.org/10.1016/s0720-048x(00)00202-3. PMID: 10927164.
22. Zajick DC Jr, Morrison WB, Schweitzer ME, Parellada JA, Carrino JA. Benign and malignant processes: normal values and differentiation with chemical shift MR imaging in vertebral marrow. Radiology. 2005;237(2):590–6. https://doi.org/10.1148/radiol.2372040990. PMID: 16244268.
23. Wang CK, Li CW, Hsieh TJ, Chien SH, Liu GC, Tsai KB. Characterization of bone and soft-tissue tumors with in vivo 1H MR spectroscopy: initial results. Radiology. 2004;232(2):599–605. https://doi.org/10.1148/radiol.2322031441. PMID: 15286325.
24. Qi ZH, Li CF, Li ZF, Zhang K, Wang Q, Yu DX. Preliminary study of 3T 1H MR spectroscopy in bone and soft tissue tumors. Chin Med J. 2009;122(1):39–43.
25. Hsieh TJ, Li CW, Chuang HY, Liu GC, Wang CK. Longitudinally monitoring chemotherapy effect of malignant musculoskeletal tumors with in vivo proton magnetic resonance spectroscopy: an initial experience. J Comput Assist Tomogr. 2008;32(6):987–94.
26. Tomasian A, Cazzato RL, Sharma K, Gangi A, Jennings JW. Benign bone tumors: state of the art in minimally invasive percutaneous interventions. Radiographics. 2023;43(2):e220041. https://doi.org/10.1148/rg.220041. PMID: 36563097.
27. Acanfora C, Grassi E, Giacobbe G, Ferrante M, Granata V, Barile A, Cappabianca S. Post-procedural follow-up of the interventional radiology's management of osteoid osteomas and osteoblastomas. J Clin Med. 2022;11(7):1987. https://doi.org/10.3390/jcm11071987. PMID: 35407593; PMCID: PMC8999856.
28. Fernbach SK, Blumenthal DH, Poznanski AK, Dias LS, Tachdjian MO. Radiographic changes in unicameral bone cysts following direct injection of steroids: a report on 14 cases. Radiology. 1981;140(3):689–95. https://doi.org/10.1148/radiology.140.3.7280236. PMID: 7280236.
29. Capanna R, Dal Monte A, Gitelis S, Campanacci M. The natural history of unicameral bone cyst after steroid injection. Clin Orthop Relat Res. 1982;166:204–11.
30. Schindler OS, Cannon SR, Briggs TW, Blunn GW. Composite ceramic bone graft substitute in the treatment of locally aggressive benign bone tumors. J Orthop Surg (Hong Kong). 2008;16(1):66–74.
31. Beaman FD, Bancroft LW, Peterson JJ, Kransdorf MJ, Menke DM, DeOrio JK. Imaging characteristics of bone graft materials. Radiographics. 2006;26(2):373–88.
32. Glancy GL, Brugioni DJ, Eilert RE, Chang FM. Autograft versus allograft for benign lesions in children. Clin Orthop Relat Res. 1991;262:28–33.
33. Malinin TI, Carpenter EM, Temple HT. Particulate bone allograft incorporation in regeneration of osseous defects: importance of particle sizes. Open Orthop J. 2007;1:19–24. 7.
34. Temple HT, Malinin TI. Microparticulate cortical allograft: an alternative to autograft in the treatment of osseous defects. Open Orthop J. 2008;2:91–6.
35. Jelinek JS, Kransdorf MJ, Moser RP, Temple HT, Lenhart MK, Berrey BH. MR imaging findings in patients with bone-chip allografts. AJR Am J Roentgenol. 1990;155(6):1257–60.
36. Yamamoto T, Onga T, Marui T, Mizuno K. Use of hydroxyapatite to fill cavities after excision of benign bone tumours: clinical results. J Bone Joint Surg Br. 2000;82(8):1117–20.
37. Abed R, Grimer R. Surgical modalities in the treatment of bone sarcoma in children. Cancer Treat Rev. 2010;36(4):342–7.
38. Nystrom LM, Morcuende JA. Expanding endoprosthesis for pediatric musculoskeletal malignancy: current concepts and results. Iowa Orthop J. 2010;30:141–9.
39. Nelson CL, Gioe TJ, Cheng EY, Thompson RC Jr. Implant selection in revision total knee arthroplasty. J Bone Joint Surg Am. 2003;85-A((suppl 1):S43–51. 15.
40. Taljanovic MS, Jones MD, Hunter TB, et al. Joint arthroplasties and prostheses. Radiographics. 2003;23(5):1295–314. 16.
41. Yang JH, Yoon JR, Oh CH, Kim TS. Primary total knee arthroplasty using rotating-hinge prosthesis in severely affected knees. Knee Surg Sports Traumatol Arthrosc. 2012;20(3):517–23.
42. Abdel-Aal AM. Ilizarov bone transport for massive tibial bone defects. Orthopedics. 2006;29(1):70–4.
43. Stoffelen D, Lammens J, Fabry G. Resection of a periosteal osteosarcoma and reconstruction using the Ilizarov technique of segmental transport. J Hand Surg Br. 1993;18(2):144–6.
44. Kattapuram SV, Phillips WC, Mankin HJ. Giant cell tumor of bone: radiographic changes following local excision and allograft replacement. Radiology. 1986;161(2):493–8.
45. Kattapuram SV, Phillips WC, Mankin HJ. Intercalary bone allografts: radiographic evaluation. Radiology. 1989;170(1 pt 1):137–41.
46. Kattapuram SV, Rosol MS, Rosenthal DI, Palmer WE, Mankin HJ. Magnetic resonance imaging features of allografts. Skeletal Radiol. 1999;28(7):383–9.
47. Puri A, Gulia A, Agarwal M, Jambhekar N, Laskar S. Extracorporeal irradiated tumor bone: a reconstruction option in diaphyseal Ewing's sarcomas. Indian J Orthop. 2010;44(4):390–6. https://doi.org/10.4103/0019-5413.69310. PMID: 20924479; PMCID: PMC2947725.
48. Jeys LM, Kulkarni A, Grimer RJ, Carter SR, Tillman RM, Abudu A. Endoprosthetic reconstruction for the treatment of musculoskeletal tumors of the appendicular skeleton and pelvis. J Bone Joint Surg Am. 2008;90(6):1265–71.

49. Pluot E, Davis ET, Revell M, Davies AM, James SL, Hip arthroplasty. II. Normal and abnormal radiographic findings. Clin Radiol. 2009;64(10):961–71.
50. Zbojniewicz AM, Sorger JI. Posttreatment imaging of pediatric musculoskeletal tumors. Radiographics. 2014;34(3):724–40. https://doi.org/10.1148/rg.342135069. PMID: 24819791.
51. Manaster BJ. Total hip arthroplasty: radiographic evaluation. Radiographics. 1996;16(3):645–60.
52. Love C, Tomas MB, Marwin SE, Pugliese PV, Palestro CJ. Role of nuclear medicine in diagnosis of the infected joint replacement. Radiographics. 2001;21(5):1229–38. 34.
53. Zhuang H, Yang H, Alavi A. Critical role of 18F-labeled fluorodeoxyglucose PET in the management of patients with arthroplasty. Radiol Clin North Am. 2007;45(4):711–8. vii.
54. Jeys LM, Grimer RJ, Carter SR, Tillman RM. Periprosthetic infection in patients treated for an orthopaedic oncological condition. J Bone Joint Surg Am. 2005;87(4):842–9.

20 Pediatric Musculoskeletal Soft Tissue Tumors

Praveen Kumar Chinniah

20.1 Introduction

Structures that constitute soft tissue are muscle, tendon, nerve, blood vessel and fibrous tissues like fascia, capsule and ligament, fat, and synovium (Fig. 20.1). World Health Organization (WHO) subsumes these structures as "connective, subcutaneous, and other non-parenchymatous-organ soft tissues, as well as the peripheral and autonomic nervous system". Tumors arising from these soft tissue structures are rare in children [1]. Most of the musculoskeletal soft tissue mass lesions in children are tumor mimic lesions such as ganglion cysts, vascular malformations, and benign lesions. Soft tissue sarcomas (STS) comprise only approximately 6% of all childhood malignant tumors, and rhabdomyosarcoma (RMS) is the most common STS in children [2, 3].

20.1.1 WHO Classification

As per the latest WHO musculoskeletal soft tissue tumors classification (2020), there are 12 groups of tumors based on the cell origin of the tumor with 121 subtypes which are further categorized according to their biological potential (aggressiveness or pathological grade of the lesions) into benign, intermediate (locally aggressive), intermediate (rarely metastasizing), and malignant tumors [1]. Some of these tumors occur exclusively in adults and can occur occasionally in children as well. Excluding the gastrointestinal stromal tumor and chondro osseous tumor (which usually occurs in adults), pediatric musculoskeletal STS can be divided into 9 groups based on the cell origin of the tumor with 54 subtypes (Table 20.1).

P. K. Chinniah (✉)
Department of Radiology, Christian Medical College Hospital, Vellore, Tamil Nadu, India

I. Kumar et al. (eds.), *Practical Approach to Imaging in Pediatric Oncology*,
https://doi.org/10.1007/978-981-96-8158-7_20

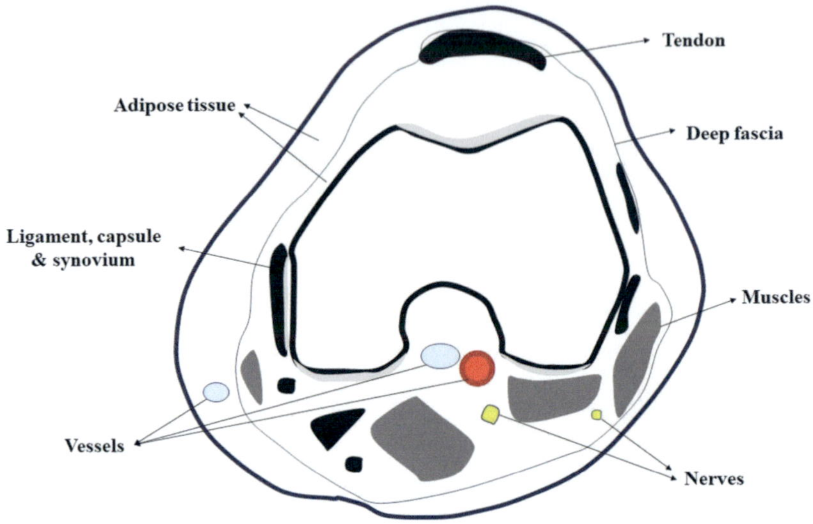

Fig. 20.1 Axial schematic representation at the level of left distal femur shows various structures that constitute soft tissue

20.1.2 Imaging Modalities

Children with extremity soft tissue mass must undergo ultrasound as the initial imaging modality which is a radiation-free and easily available modality with the ability to characterize cystic lesions and tumor mimics like ganglion cysts and vascular malformations. Nevertheless, the exquisite soft tissue contrast resolution of magnetic resonance imaging (MRI) makes MRI with intravenous (IV) gadolinium as the modality of choice to characterize and locally stage soft-tissue tumors. Diffusion-weighted imaging may not be always contributory to the diagnosis. Radiographs will help in identifying periosteal reaction, calcifications, and any bony involvement. CT is not employed in the evaluation of the pediatric musculoskeletal soft tissue tumors due to poor soft tissue resolution and radiation exposure. PET-CT helps in identifying distant metastasis and also can predict malignant transformation of neurofibromas in neurofibromatosis (NF1) patients. Although PET-CT can differentiate few low-grade from high-grade sarcomas, reliability of this modality is poor as it cannot distinguish low-grade tumors from benign lesions [2–4].

Table 20.1 WHO classification of soft tissue tumors (2020)—showing pediatric musculoskeletal soft tissue tumors

Cell type of origin	Benign	Indeterminate (locally aggressive)	Indeterminate (rarely metastasizing)	Malignant
Adipocytic tumors	Lipoma Lipomatosis Lipoblastoma Lipoblastomatosis Familial lipomas			Liposarcoma Well-differentiated Dedifferentiated Myxoid Pleomorphic Myxoid pleomorphic
Fibroblastic and myofibroblastic tumors	Nodular fasciitis Proliferative fasciitis Proliferative myositis Myositis ossificans Fibrous hamartoma of infancy fibromatosis coli Juvenile hyaline fibromatosis Inclusion body fibromatosis Calcifying aponeurotic fibroma Gardner fibroma	Fibromatosis palmar/plantar desmoid type lipofibromatosis Giant cell fibroblastoma	Dermatofibrosarcoma protuberans Inflammatory myofibroblastic tumor Infantile fibrosarcoma	Low-grade fibromyxoid sarcoma
So-called fibrohistiocytic tumors		Plexiform fibrohistiocytic tumor		
Vascular tumors	Hemangioma Infantile Congenital Epithelioid hemangioma Acquired tufted hemangioma	Kaposiform Hemangioendothelioma	Retiform Hemangioendothelioma, papillary Intralymphatic Angioendothelioma, composite Hemangioendothelioma, Kaposi sarcoma, Pseudomyxogenic Hemangioendothelioma	Epithelioid Hemangioendothelioma, epithelioid Hemangioendothelioma with Yap1- Tfe3 fusion Angiosarcoma

(continued)

Table 20.1 (continued)

Cell type of origin	Benign	Indeterminate (locally aggressive)	Indeterminate (rarely metastasizing)	Malignant
Pericytic tumors	Myopericytoma Myofibroma			
Skeletal muscle tumors	Rhabdomyoma			Rhabdomyosarcoma Embryonal Alveolar Pleomorphic Spindle cell Ectomesenchymoma
Smooth muscle tumors	Not commonly seen in children			
Gastrointestinal stromal tumor	Not a common musculoskeletal tumor			
Chondro-osseous tumors	Not commonly seen in children			
Peripheral nerve sheath tumors	Schwannoma Neurofibroma Benign triton tumor/ neuromuscular choristoma			Malignant peripheral sheath tumor
Tumors of uncertain differentiation		Epithelioid Angiomyolipoma Hemosiderotic Fibrolipomatous tumor	Angiomatoid fibrous histiocytoma	NTRK rearranged spindle cell neoplasm Synovial sarcoma Epithelioid sarcoma Alveolar soft part sarcoma Desmoplastic small round cell tumor Extra-renal rhabdoid tumor
Undifferentiated small round cell sarcoma of bone and soft tissues				Extra skeletal Ewing's sarcoma Sarcoma with BCOR genetic alterations

20.2 Consensus Guideline(s) for Imaging

Timely diagnosis and treatment of pediatric musculoskeletal soft tissue tumor, especially STS, are done by a team of expert professionals that usually includes treating physician (Orthopedician, Radiation oncologist & Medical oncologist), Pathologist and Radiologist, which is also called a Multi-Disciplinary Team (MDT). Imaging plays a crucial and central role not only in the diagnosis & staging but also in treatment response assessment and surveillance of STS. As the MDT involves various inter-departmental experts with limited expertise in other fields of medicine, it is essential that internationally standardized common terminology and criteria are used in the diagnosis, treatment, and response assessment to ensure ideal management of children with STS and also to promote clinical research and advancements globally (Fig. 20.2).

In order to develop such a common international consensus on STS, the INternational Soft Tissue saRcoma Consortium (INSTRuCT) was established in 2017, which integrates clinical data from three large cooperative clinical trial organizations: Children's Oncology Group (COG), European paediatric Soft Tissue Sarcoma Study Group (EpSSG), and Cooperative Weichteilsarkom Studiengruppe. In the year 2021, the INSTRuCT Diagnostic Imaging Working Group was created, which consisted of pediatric radiologists, nuclear medicine physicians, and oncologists to develop consensus standardization of imaging acquisition, terminology, and response assessment methods to evaluate pediatric soft-tissue sarcomas.

As rhabdomyosarcoma (RMS) and non-rhabdomyosarcoma soft tissue sarcoma (NRSTS) tumors in children differ considerably in clinical behavior, the latest INSTRuCT consensus statement (2023) on RMS and NRSTS has been published separately (Tables 20.2 and 20.3), which consists of guidelines for imaging at diagnosis (primary tumor & metastatic workup), follow-up imaging, tumor response assessment and surveillance [5, 6]. Primary tumor site and loco-regional nodal imaging should occur before core-needle

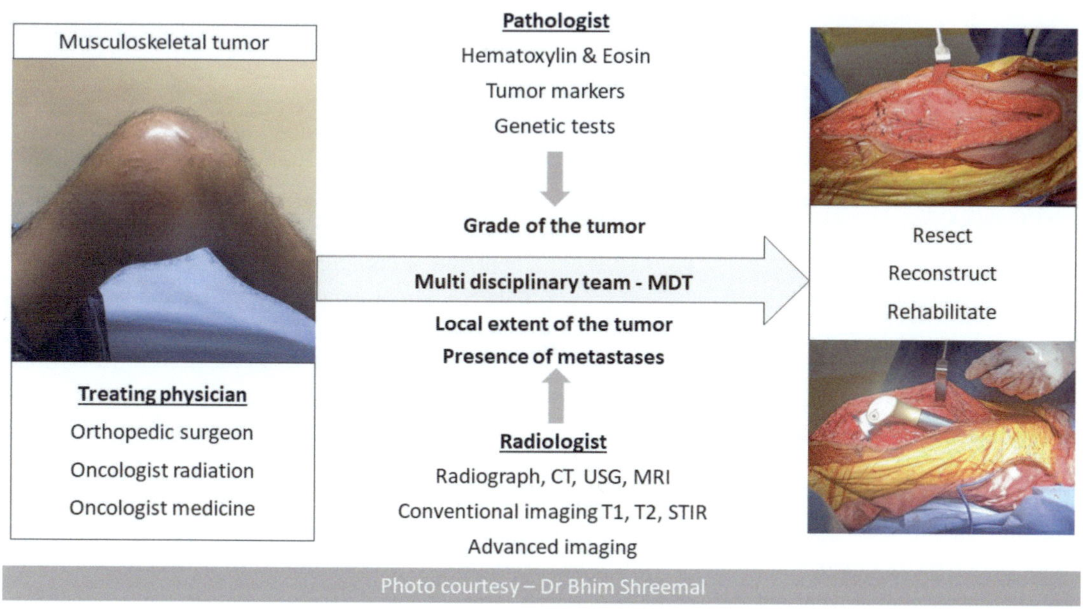

Fig. 20.2 Shows a schematic representation of multi-disciplinary team approach in the management of musculoskeletal tumors

Table 20.2 INSTRuCT consensus guidelines for imaging of rhabdomyosarcoma (RMS)

Disease	Screening (within 28 days before treatment)	Induction therapy	Maintenance therapy	Off therapy surveillance
Localized disease				
Primary tumor and locoregional lymph nodes, preferably with MRI	Yes	Yes	Yes	Yes
Chest—CT/X-ray	Yes	Yes	Yes	Yes
Distant lymph nodes and potential extra-pulmonary metastatic sites, FDG PET-CT/MRI	Yes	–	–	–
Metastatic disease				
Primary tumor and locoregional lymph nodes, preferably with MRI	Yes	Yes	Yes	Yes
Pulmonary metastases, CT chest/chest x-ray	Yes	Yes	Yes	Yes
Distant lymph nodes and extra-pulmonary metastases, FDG PET-CT/MRI at screening, follow-up as per local practice	Yes	Yes	Yes	Case by case

Table 20.3 INSTRuCT consensus guidelines for imaging of non-rhabdomyosarcoma soft tissue sarcoma (NRSTS)

Disease	Staging (within 28 days)	During treatment	Off therapy surveillance
Primary tumor with MRI	Yes	Yes	Yes
Locoregional lymph nodes	Yes	–	–
Pulmonary metastases, chest CT/chest x-ray	Yes	Yes	Yes
Distant lymph nodes and extra-pulmonary metastases, 18FDG-PET CT/MRI	Yes	Yes	Yes
Whole-body MRI	Yes	Yes	Yes
Brain MRI	Yes	–	–

or excisional biopsy because invasive procedures may result in local inflammatory changes and reactive lymph nodes, complicating interpretation of the findings. Furthermore, pre-treatment imaging should be obtained no more than 1 month before treatment initiation to reduce the possibility of changes in tumor size and extent that could impact clinical grouping.

20.2.1 Imaging Guidelines in Rhabdomyosarcoma (RMS) [5]

MRI is recommended as the modality of choice for evaluation of the primary tumor and the same mode of investigation of tumor sites must be used throughout the treatment and follow-up. It is recommended that imaging of suspected tumors should be done on a high-field system (minimum 1.0 Tesla). Frequency of the imaging depends on the treatment protocol, at least before local treatment and at completion of induction and maintenance treatment (approximately every 3–4 months).

Evaluation of pulmonary lesions must be done with chest CT if positive in screening chest radiograph. Interval of assessment during treatment depends according to treatment protocol, at least before local treatment and at completion of induction and maintenance treatment (approximately every 3–4 months). If chest CT is negative or there are indeterminate nodules at diagnosis and no metastatic lesions elsewhere, chest CT could be replaced by chest XR.

For evaluation of extra-pulmonary metastases at diagnosis, FDG PET-CT or FDG PET-MRI is recommended.

20.2.2 Imaging Guidelines in Non-rhabdomyosarcoma Soft Tissue Sarcoma (NRSTS) [6]

MRI is recommended as the modality of choice for evaluation of the primary tumor, and the same mode of investigation of tumor sites must be used throughout the treatment and follow-up. Frequency of the imaging depends on the treatment protocol, at least before local treatment and at completion of induction treatment (approximately every 3–4 months).

Evaluation of locoregional lymph node involvement is recommended for patients with epithelioid sarcoma, angiosarcoma, alveolar soft part sarcoma, clear-cell sarcoma, or extracranial malignant rhabdoid tumor. Timing of locoregional lymph node assessment will depend on local practice and can be done either at the same time with primary tumor imaging (while the histologic diagnosis may not yet be known) or later in the diagnostic process with additional imaging. There is no evidence advocating for ultrasound, MRI, or 18F-FDG-PET CT. In case of uncertainty or inconsistent findings, core biopsy or lymph node resection for pathologic evaluation is recommended. Follow-up with the same imaging technique is recommended for involved nodes at similar intervals of primary tumor evaluation. For patients without lymph node involvement, imaging of locoregional lymph nodes at the completion of therapy is encouraged for these selected histotypes and will determine the need to image during surveillance.

Chest CT is the most commonly used technique for the detection of pulmonary metastases and the imaging depends on the Fédération Nationale des Centres de Lutte Contre le Cancer (FNCLCC) grade of the tumor. In patients with low risk NRSTS (i.e., FNCLCC grade 1 or 2), small tumor size (<5 cm) and/or completely resected at diagnosis, workup by chest CT could be replaced by chest x-ray (in two orthogonal planes).

18F-FDG-PET CT at screening is recommended for all NRSTS patients with lung metastases (any grade) for the detection of extra-pulmonary disease. For patients with FNCLCC grade 3 NRSTS (including without lung metastases) staging with 18F-FDG-PET CT could be considered by the multidisciplinary team.

For patients with myxoid liposarcomas, staging and follow-up with whole-body MRI is recommended. In patients with extremity primaries, follow-up with physical examination with or without ultrasound may suffice. For patients with alveolar soft part sarcoma and myxoid liposarcomas, longer follow-up is recommended for the detection of late relapses: every 6 months during the third, fourth, and fifth year and then once yearly up to 10 years after diagnosis. For patients with alveolar soft part sarcoma, clear-cell sarcoma, and angiosarcoma, brain MRI is recommended at staging.

20.3 Imaging Algorithm for Interpretation and Approach to Diagnosis

When a child presents with a musculoskeletal tumor, Radiologist must exclude vascular malformations, tumor mimics, and benign typical lipoma, mostly by using ultrasound and MRI (Fig. 20.3). The only soft tissue tumor a Radiologist can diagnose with 100% accuracy is benign typical lipoma and surgical excision of typical lipoma is decided according to the cosmetic needs of the patients [4]. Vascular malformations are managed by Interventional Radiology team and some of the common treatment options include sclerotherapy for slow-flow vascular malformation and trans-arterial embolization for high-flow vascular malformation. Tumor mimics like ganglion cyst and parameniscal cysts can be

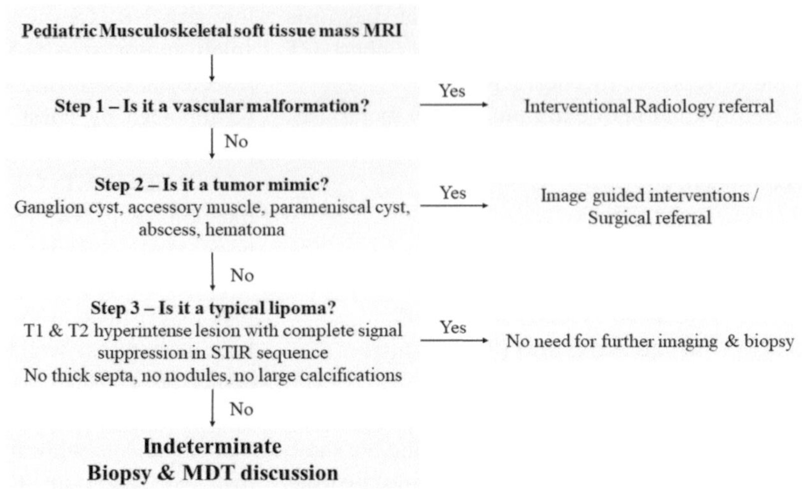

Fig. 20.3 Shows step-wise MRI approach to pediatric musculoskeletal soft tissue mass lesions

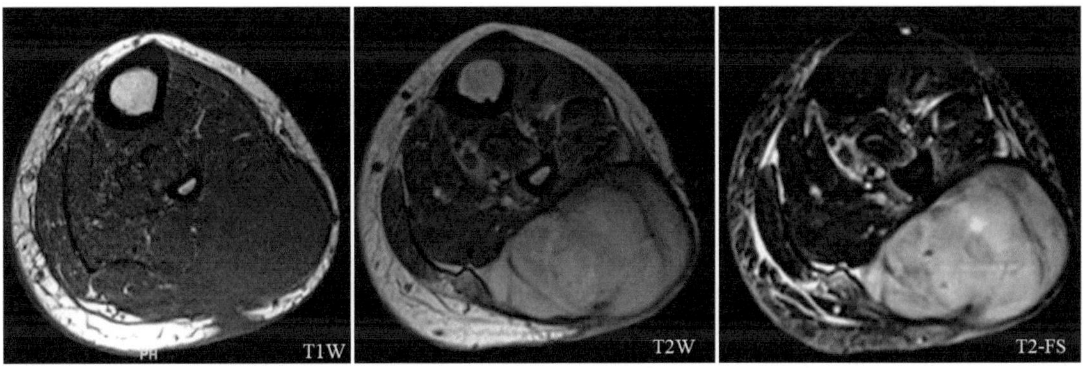

Fig. 20.4 Shows a well-defined T1 hypointense, T2 & T2-FS hyperintense mass lesion in left leg, deep to deep fascia. This is an indeterminate lesion and diagnosis cannot be obtained by imaging alone. This is a biopsy-proven case of intermediate-grade spindle cell sarcoma

managed by using ultrasound-guided interventions or surgical methods.

Accurate imaging-based diagnosis in rest of the soft tissue tumors is not always possible (not required either) by the Radiologist as most of the lesions enlisted in Table 20.1 (50 subtypes) share non-specific imaging features (Fig. 20.4) and usually appear T1 iso to hypointense, T2/STIR heterogenous signal, predominantly hyperintense with varying degrees of contrast enhancement in MRI. Hence lesions, which are not tumor mimics, vascular malformation, and typical lipoma, have to be labeled as indeterminate and biopsy must be performed which should be followed by MDT discussion for further management. Once the lesion is confirmed to be STS by pathologist, three questions have to be answered before definite surgery: grade of the tumor (by the pathologist), local extent of the tumor, and presence of metastases (by the Radiologist) [5, 6].

20.4 Structured Radiological Reporting and Interpretation

20.4.1 Protocol

MRI is the imaging modality of choice in the evaluation of STS (Fig. 20.5). MRI protocol usually consists of a large FOV STIR coronal and T1

What does the clinician needs to know from imaging ?

- Initial tumor characterization
- Tumor extent & staging
- Treatment planning
- Response to therapy
- Postoperative surveillance

Points to remember

- Not all well-defined soft tissue tumors are benign and not all infiltrative lesions are malignant
- Look for T1 hyperintense signal, T2 hypointense signal, fat, hemorrhage & blood-fluid levels, hemosiderin rim
- Synovial sarcoma rarely occurs at synovium

Pediatric MSK soft tissue tumors - reporting template of MRI MSK

- Demographics, history, comparison studies
- Non-contrast multisequence multiplanar imaging

FINDINGS

▪ MR signal	characteristic or not, fat, blood, fluid levels
▪ Local infiltration	with reference to anatomic landmarks
▪ Neurovascular involved	yes/no
▪ Joint involved	yes/no
▪ Skip lesions & nodes	yes/no
▪ Radiograph	bone involvement and aggressive features
▪ Ultrasound	cyst & compressibility

IMPRESSION

- Tumor or tumor mimic
- Diagnosis / differentials & what next?

FINAL DIAGNOSIS & MANAGEMENT

@ MDT discussion

Fig. 20.5 Shows MRI reporting template for pediatric musculoskeletal soft tissue mass lesions

coronal imaging of the affected limb, axial (T1, T2 & T2-FS) and T2-FS sagittal imaging through the lesion.

Post-contrast imaging and diffusion-weighted imaging can be reserved for cases of diagnostic dilemma such as post op surveillance to differentiate between recurrence and post-treatment changes. Imaging with intravenous Gadolinium contrast is not used universally and is considered of value in cases of uncertainty if a lesion is myxomatous or purely cystic, hemorrhage where an underlying soft tissue tumor may be suspected and in cases with equivocal findings. Myxomatous tumors are often misinterpreted as benign findings due to their similarity to cysts. Intravenous Gadolinium contrast medium helps clarify this issue. Malignant soft tissue tumors are often the reason for hemorrhage in unusual locations and may be difficult to identify even with Gadolinium contrast medium. The imaging protocol should in these cases consist of as a minimum of axial spin echo T1-weighted sequence, with identical imaging parameters as a pre-contrast sequence. If fat saturation is used, a pre-contrast fat-saturated sequence is thus needed. If needed for further anatomic evaluation, a sagittal spin echo T1-weighted sequence with fat saturation may be performed. It is recommended to abstain from further imaging with Gadolinium contrast medium in cases of purely lipomatous tumors—low signal on STIR sequence, high signal on T1-weighted sequence without fat saturation and in cases where no tumor is identified on the initial three scan sequences [5, 6].

20.4.2 Reporting

Radiographs must always be evaluated while reporting MRI as it will help in identifying calcifications and periosteal reactions, which may otherwise be missed in MRI. While reporting the MRI the lesion has to be characterized based on its T1, T2, and T2-FS signal, also presence of fat, blood, and blood-fluid levels must be actively looked for, as this will help narrow down the diagnosis. Though most of the lesions are T1 hypointense and T2 hyperintense in nature, some lesions have characteristic MRI signal (Fig. 20.6) such as T1 hyperintensity (fat, blood, melanin), some lesions have T2 hypointensity (fibrous tissue, pigmented villonodular synovitis, giant cell tumor of tendon sheath, amyloid, gout, blood and melanin). Identification of such characteristic

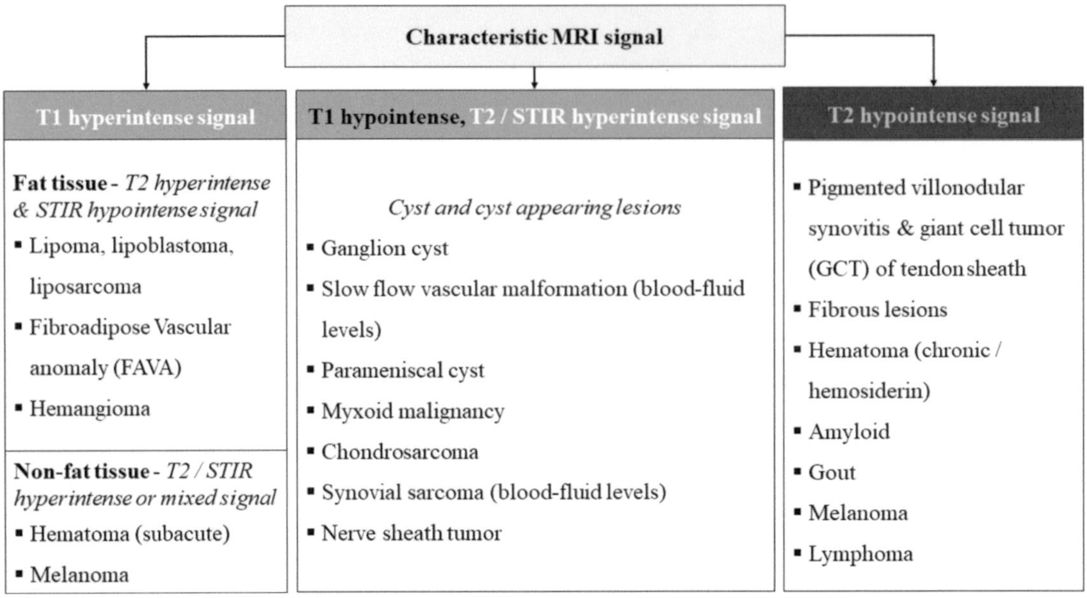

Fig. 20.6 Shows characteristic MRI signal of various soft tissue mass lesions

Table 20.4 Reporting template

Size	---x—x—cm
Location	
Tumor matrix	<T1 and T2 characteristics> <fluid-fluid levels> <homogenous/heterogenous> <ADC value > <solid/cystic/mixed/ calcification/ macroscopic fat/ fibrosis> <necrosis: % of necrosis within the mass>
Post contrast	<absent/ mild/ marked enhancement> < homogenous/heterogenous/ peripheral (thin/ thick rim)>
Time intensity curve (DCE MR)	<Type I/II/III/IV/IV> <Slope> <mixed curves: describe>
Transition zone	<sharp/ narrow/ wide > <edema>
Extent	<compartments: intracompartment/ extracompartment> <muscular involvement/ intermuscular plane/ tendons> < subcutaneous plane>
Neurovascular involvement	<present/absent> <specific nerve involvement>
Bone involvement	<Present/ absent> <periosteal reaction: none/ present> <intraarticular involvement>
Lymph nodes	<present/absent>
Coexisting lesion	<metastatic> <incidental>
Normal structure	<if the lesion can be a normal structure: accessory/supernumerary/anomalous muscle> <hematoma/strain>

signal will not only help in arriving at an accurate pre op diagnosis but also help in guiding biopsy. Care must be taken to describe the tumor's location, size, characteristics (margins, solid and necrotic components, vascularity, and cellularity), relation to surrounding anatomic structures, including bone and the neurovascular bundles, and assessment of the loco-regional lymph node basin. A structured reporting template is shown in Table 20.4.

20.4.3 Role of Radiologist

The primary role of a Radiologist in the evaluation of pediatric soft tissue tumors is to character-

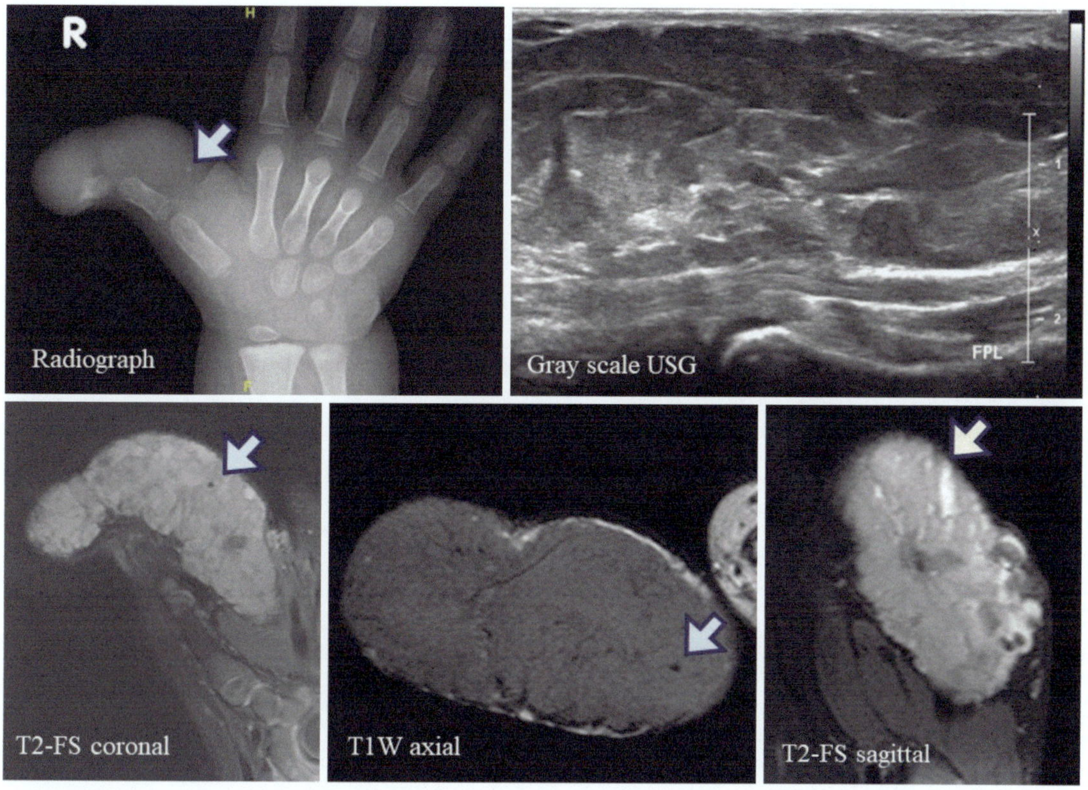

Fig. 20.7 Shows soft tissue thickening in subcutaneous plane of right thumb in a 3-year-old child with tiny calcification (blue arrow) that appears STIR hyperintense & T1 hypointense with blood-fluid levels (yellow arrow) in MRI and corresponding heterogeneous appearance in the gray scale ultrasonography. This was a proven case of veno-lymphatic (slow flow) vascular malformation and the patient was successfully treated with sclerotherapy by the interventional Radiology team

ize the lesion by using multiple modalities (predominantly ultrasound and MRI) and ascertain whether they are vascular malformation (Fig. 20.7), tumor mimics such as abscess (Fig. 20.8), or lipoma (Fig. 20.9). The rest of the lesions quite mimic each other in imaging appearance, making the accurate diagnosis impossible in the majority of cases (unless they have characteristic MRI signal as discussed above). Such lesions with non-specific imaging appearance must be labelled as indeterminate and be subjected to biopsy and MDT discussion. Malignant lesions are broadly classified into (Rhabdomyosarcoma) RMS (Fig. 20.10) and non-rhabdomyosarcoma (NRSTS) tumors to facilitate optimal chemotherapy and follow-up.

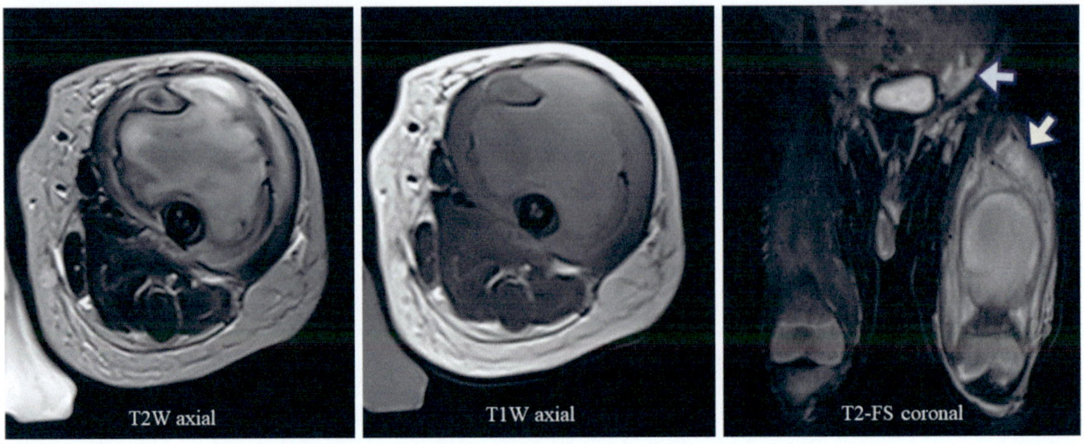

Fig. 20.8 Shows an irregular lesion in the anterior muscular compartment of the left thigh in a 2-year-old child with T1 iso to hyperintense signal and T2/T2-FS predominantly hyperintense signal. Also, perilesional inflammatory changes are evident in the form of feathery edema in quadriceps (yellow arrow) and enlarged left inguino femoral lymph nodes (blue arrow). This was a proven case of intramuscular abscess in left anterior thigh

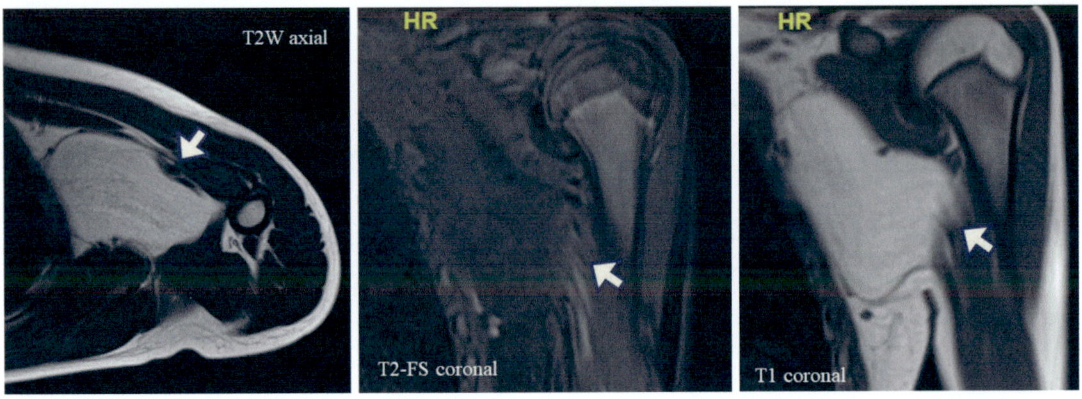

Fig. 20.9 Shows well-defined encapsulated lesion with fat containing lesion (T1 and T2 hyperintense signal and complete signal suppression in T2 fat suppressed sequence) that displaces the axillary neurovascular bundle (yellow arrow). This was a proven case of typical lipoma

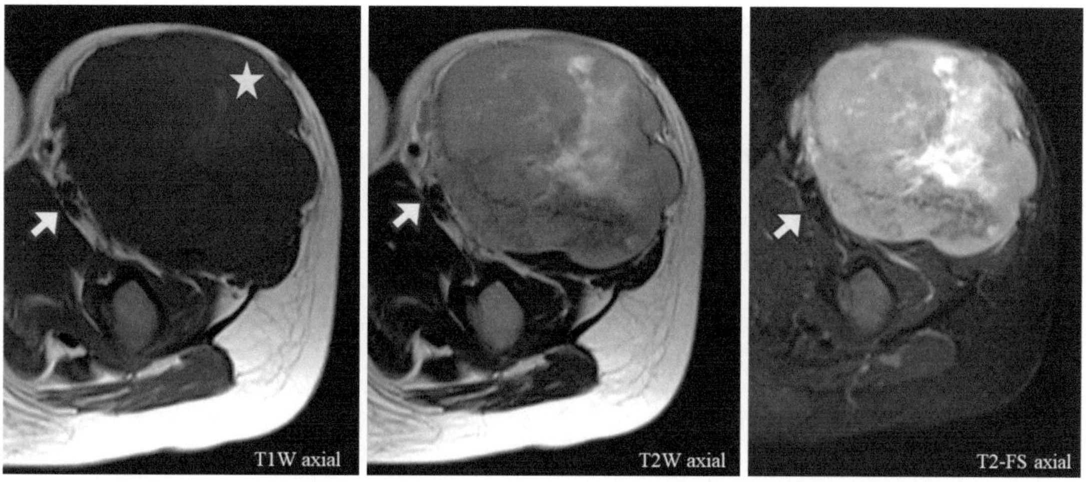

Fig. 20.10 Shows a multi-lobulated T1 hypointense, T2 & T2-FS predominant hyperintense signal lesion with subtle central T1 hyperintense signal, representing areas of hemorrhage (star) in the anterior muscular compartment of the left proximal thigh that displaces femoral vessels medially (yellow arrow). This lesion was a proven case of rhabdomyosarcoma (RMS)

20.5 Post-treatment Imaging

For both RMS and NRSTS, MRI with IV gadolinium of the affected extremity is recommended to assess tumor response to treatment. MRI should be performed using similar technical parameters and the same field-of-view as at the time of diagnosis. Children's Oncology Group (COG) white paper (August 2022) recommends using 1-D measurements per Response Assessment Criteria in Solid Tumors (RECIST) 1.1 criteria for the primary tumor and metastatic disease response assessment. As pediatric sarcomas are irregular accurate measurement using longest diameter in any plane as per the RECIST version 1.1 may not be feasible in all cases. Some authors suggest 3D volumetric measurements, however this also has not been a reliable marker. The method of tumor measurement may ultimately depend on treatment protocols or institutional practice patterns [5, 6].

20.5.1 Post-treatment Imaging Guidelines in Rhabdomyosarcoma (RMS) [5]

During off-therapy surveillance, imaging of the primary site must be done with the same modality used at baseline, at 4-month intervals for the first 2 years off therapy and only obtaining imaging when clinically indicated thereafter.

For evaluation of pulmonary metastasis post treatment, assessment with a chest radiograph at 4-month intervals is recommended for the first 2 years off therapy and only obtaining imaging when clinically indicated thereafter. A CT chest is recommended for better characterization of suspicious lesions found on chest radiograph.

Post-treatment follow-up of extra-pulmonary metastases is only recommended in patients with metastatic disease and should be performed as per local practice; there is currently insufficient evidence to recommend routine follow-up with FDG PET-CT/MRI.

20.5.2 Post-treatment Imaging Guidelines in Non-rhabdomyosarcoma Soft Tissue Sarcoma (NRSTS) [6].

During off-therapy surveillance, imaging of the primary site is recommended every 3–4 months, with the same modality and technical settings used at baseline for the first 2 years off therapy. Thereafter, individual characteristics should be considered. In patients with extremity primaries, physical examination with or without ultrasound may suffice. For patients with alveolar soft part sarcoma and myxoid liposarcomas, longer follow-up is recommended for the detection of late relapses: every 6 months during the third, fourth, and fifth year and then once yearly up to 10 years after diagnosis.

Pulmonary nodules should be monitored with chest CT. In patients with localized disease and low-grade NRSTS (i.e., FNCLCC grade 1 or 2), a follow-up chest CT could be replaced by chest x-ray. After completion of treatment, follow-up with chest x-ray at 3–4 months interval is recommended for the first 2 years. Longer follow-up (up to 5 years) with chest x-ray could be considered: every 6 months in the third year and once yearly in the fourth and fifth year. In patients treated for metastatic NRSTS, treating physicians could choose for chest CT for surveillance.

Non-pulmonary metastases should be monitored during treatment. Most commonly used techniques are whole-body MRI. It is recommended to use the same technique as used at staging.

20.6 Future Directions

Most of the research aim to predict the prognostic factors by imaging and accurate pre-operative diagnosis of the tumors. Multi-parametric MRI variables such as apparent diffusion coefficient (ADC) and dynamic contrast enhancement (DCE) are widely used to predict the biological nature of the tumors.

20.6.1 Dynamic Contrast-Enhanced (DCE) MRI

DCE MRI is preferred to assess perfusion within tumors to identify necrosis, viability, granulation tissue, or fibrosis. DCE-MRI relies on acquiring images after injection of IV contrast material using a time-resolved MR angiography technique. Some authors have proposed the use of quantitative DCE-MRI to better reflect tumor biology and have shown its feasibility for early prediction of pathological response of soft-tissue sarcomas to neoadjuvant therapy [7].

20.6.2 Radiomics

Radiomics analysis refers to the conversion and extraction of quantitative data contained in medical digital images with the purpose of creating models that can predict outcomes and this can be done with a variety of imaging modalities. Integrating demographic, clinical, genomic, and comorbidity data can expand this analysis. This has been particularly studied in RMS in children. Banerjee et al. could classify histopathological subtypes of RMS using radiomics framework by assessing the fusion of diffusion-weighted imaging and contrast-enhanced T1-weighted images [8].

Acknowledgments Dr. Madhavi K and Dr. Kirthi S, Christian Medical College, Vellore.

References

1. Bansal A, Goyal S, Goyal A, Jana M. WHO classification of soft tissue tumours 2020: an update and simplified approach for radiologists. Eur J Radiol. 2021;143:109937.
2. Porrino J, Al-Dasuqi K, Irshaid L, Wang A, Kani K, Haims A, Maloney E. Update of pediatric soft tissue tumors with review of conventional MRI appearance-part 1: tumor-like lesions, adipocytic tumors, fibro-

blastic and myofibroblastic tumors, and perivascular tumors. Skeletal Radiol. 2022;51(3):477–504.
3. Maloney E, Al-Dasuqi K, Irshaid L, Wang A, Kani K, Haims A, Porrino J. Update of pediatric soft tissue tumors with review of conventional MRI appearance-part 2: vascular lesions, fibrohistiocytic tumors, muscle tumors, peripheral nerve sheath tumors, tumors of uncertain differentiation, and undifferentiated small round cell sarcomas. Skeletal Radiol. 2022;51(4):701–25.
4. Reid C, Saifuddin A. A review of paediatric soft tissues masses referred to a tertiary musculoskeletal sarcoma centre. Br J Radiol. 2021;94(1117):20200790.
5. Schoot RA, van Ewijk R, von Witzleben AA, Kao SC, Merks JHMH, Morosi C, Pace E, Shulkin BL, Ferrari A, von Kalle T, van Rijn RR, Weiss AR, Sparber-Sauer M, Ter Horst SAJ, McCarville MB. INternational soft tissue saRcoma ConsorTium (INSTRuCT) consensus statement: imaging recommendations for the management of rhabdomyosarcoma. Eur J Radiol. 2023;166:111012.
6. Schoot RA, Ferrari A, von Kalle T, Khalatbari H, McCarville MB, Morosi C, van Rijn RR, von Witzleben AA, Weiss AR, Kao SC. Imaging recommendations for the management of pediatric non-rhabdomyosarcoma soft tissue sarcoma (NRSTS): consensus statement of the International Soft Tissue Sarcoma Consortium (INSTRuCT). EJC Paediatr Oncol. 2023;1:100008.
7. Acord MR, Pace E, El-Ali A, Chaturvedi A, Iyer RS, Navarro OM, Pandit-Taskar N, Parikh K, A, Schechter A, Shaikh R, McCarville MB. Imaging of pediatric extremity soft tissue tumors: a COG diagnostic imaging committee/SPR Oncology Committee white paper. Pediatr Blood Cancer. 2023;70(Suppl 4(Suppl 4)):e29944. https://doi.org/10.1002/pbc.29944.
8. Banerjee I, Crawley A, Bhethanabotla M, Daldrup-Link HE, Rubin DL. Transfer learning on fused multiparametric MR images for classifying histopathological subtypes of rhabdomyosarcoma. Comput Med Imaging Graph. 2018 Apr;65:167–75.

Part IV

Abdominal

21 Neuroblastoma and Renal Tumors

Nikshita Jain, Anurima Patra, and Sridhar Gibikote

In a child presenting with a palpable abdominal mass or other abdominal symptoms such as hematuria, pain, or distention, the first line of investigation is ultrasound abdomen. Pediatric ultrasound is an incredibly useful tool, due to easy availability, lack of radiation, and high sensitivity in detecting abnormalities in pediatric abdomen, attributed to the minimal abdominal wall fat in this population.

Ultrasound assesses several key aspects:

- Confirming the presence of mass.
- Identifying the organ of origin (e.g., renal, suprarenal, or others).
- Assessing morphology, including whether the mass is solid or cystic, presence of internal hemorrhage, necrosis, vascularity, and regional infiltration.
- Evaluating complications—tumor rupture, ascites, hemoperitoneum.
- Abdominal metastases.

Once a preliminary diagnosis is made on ultrasound, further cross-sectional imaging is planned to accurately stage the mass and guide subsequent management. In this chapter, we will separately discuss neuroblastoma and renal masses.

21.1 Neuroblastoma

Neuroblastoma is part of the spectrum of neurogenic tumors which also includes ganglioneuroma and ganglioneuroblastoma, that arise from embryonic cells of the sympathetic chain, including adrenal medulla [1]. About 46% of neuroblastomas originate from the adrenal gland, 18% from extra-adrenal abdomen, 14% from the posterior mediastinum, and the remainder from the neck, pelvis, and other locations [1]. Typically diagnosed in children under 5 years old, neuroblastoma is the most common extracranial solid neoplasm in this age group. It has a rather unpredictable course, with some tumors spontaneously regressing, while others result in fatal outcomes despite treatment.

To provide the optimal treatment to the diverse biological behavior of neuroblastoma, risk groups have been defined. This risk stratification is based on patient's age, disease stage, histopathology, MYCN oncogene status, DNA ploidy, and chromosome aberrations [2]. Of note, tumors with MYCN amplification are categorized as high risk, regardless of localization [2].

Clinical presentation of neuroblastoma varies depending upon site of origin and presence of paraneoplastic syndromes. Common

N. Jain (✉) · S. Gibikote
Christian Medical College, Vellore, Tamil Nadu, India

A. Patra
Tata Medical Centra, Kolkata, India

I. Kumar et al. (eds.), *Practical Approach to Imaging in Pediatric Oncology*,
https://doi.org/10.1007/978-981-96-8158-7_21

presentations are localized disease, disseminated disease, and 4S/MS disease [2]. Among the paraneoplastic syndromes, opsoclonus-myoclonus syndrome is most often (2–4% cases) encountered [2]. It is characterized by rapid, multidirectional eye movements, ataxia, and quick, involuntary muscle jerks. These children usually have localized disease, and although they have good prognosis regarding their tumor, the majority will have long-term neurological deficit, as removal of the tumor does not reverse the symptoms completely [2]. Neuroblastoma presents with metastatic disease almost 50% of the time. When there is widespread bone marrow disease, children often present with bone pain, limping, or irritability (Hutchinson syndrome). Stage MS/4S is reserved for patients younger than 18 months with metastases to liver, skin, and bone marrow and a relatively small primary tumor with widespread metastatic disease [2].

Imaging findings in neuroblastoma typically show a heterogenous mass with internal calcifications and increased vascularity, often encasing the adjacent vessels (typically described as lifting aorta from prevertebral plane). When in suprarenal location, differentials to consider are adrenal cortical carcinoma (larger in size more than 4 cm, less common in pediatric age) and benign neurogenic tumors (lesser diffusion restriction on MRI, lack of metastases). When the mass infiltrates the kidney, Wilms' becomes a close differential and certain pointers to differentiate the two have been subsequently listed in the Wilms' section. Lymphoma is a consideration, especially with high nodal burden, but shows a more homogenous hypoenhancing morphology, and more commonly involves anterior mediastinum unlike neuroblastoma that involves posterior mediastinum.

21.1.1 Consensus Guideline(s) for Imaging

In 2004, investigators from the Children's Oncology Group (COG) from North America and Australia–New Zealand, the German Pediatric Oncology and Hematology Group (GPOH), the Japanese Neuroblastoma Study Group (JNBSG), and the International Society of Pediatric Oncology Europe Neuroblastoma (SIOPEN) Group—and China formed the International Neuroblastoma Risk Group (INRG) Task Force, which developed the INRG Staging System (INRGSS) and the INRG Risk Classification System for neuroblastoma [3].

The INRGSS (Fig. 21.1) was published in 2009 and is meant for staging the tumor prior to any treatment, including surgery. It accounts for stage, age, histologic category, grade of tumor differentiation, status of MYCN oncogene, chromosome 11q status, and DNA ploidy [4]. On imaging, this staging system utilizes IDRF—which are image-defined risk factors based on the SIOPEN surgical risk factors, that help define surgical resectability at the time of presentation and distant metastases to guide management and thereby predict event-free survival [4].

There are two key concepts that must be emphasized when reporting any imaging for a child with suspected or proven neuroblastoma—identification of primary tumor site (sympathetic chain in abdomen, pelvis, paravertebral, posterior mediastinum, or neck) and the description of IDRFs with respect to primary site. The reason to identify primary tumor site is because post chemotherapy, while the residual tumor may be functionally inactive, removal of primary tumor is imperative for completion of treatment.

Fig. 21.1 International Neuroblastoma Risk Group Staging system [4]

- **L1** : Localised tumour limited to one body compartment with no IDRFs
- **L2** : Locoregional tumor with one or more IDRFs
- **M**: Distant metastatic disease (except stage MS)
- **MS**: Metastatic disease in children younger than 18 months with metastases confined to skin, liver and/or bone marrow

Due to diverse clinical presentations of neuroblastoma, establishing a standard protocol for diagnosis and staging work-up is challenging (Figs. 21.2a and 21.2b). On imaging, staging of neuroblastoma requires both anatomical and functional detail. Anatomical imaging entails contrast-enhanced CT (CECT) or MRI, MRI being preferred due to its superior assessment of marrow involvement, chest wall invasion, and spinal canal involvement. MRI protocol includes conventional sequences, and high b value diffusion-weighted imaging (DWI) (as neuroblastoma strongly restricts) which helps in detection of even small distant metastases, guiding appropriate biopsy sites, and differentiating between malignant neuroblastoma/ganglioneuroblastoma and benign ganglioneuroma, as recommended by the COG diagnostic committee/SPR Oncology Committee white paper [2, 4]. Ganglioneuroma shows significant higher apparent diffusion coefficient values when compared to poorly differentiated neuroblastoma. CT is superior for post-chemotherapy surgical planning due to better evaluation of tumor morphology (post-treatment fibrosis and calcifications render the lesion T1 and T2 dark on MRI) and vascular anatomy, particularly in the identification of artery of Adamkiewicz for posterior mediastinal lesions.

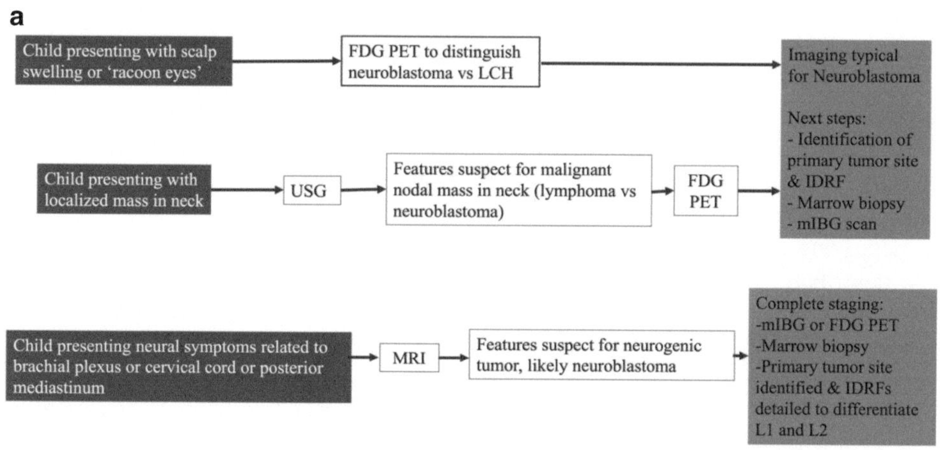

Fig. 21.2a Approach to imaging in a child with various clinical presentations of neuroblastoma

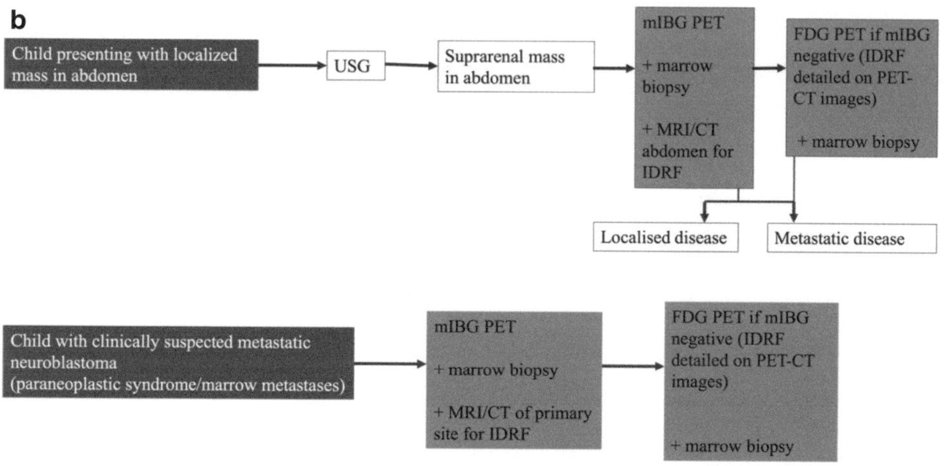

Fig. 21.2b Approach to imaging in a child with various clinical presentations of neuroblastoma

Functional imaging options include ^{123}I-mIBG planar and SPECT/CT or 18Fluorine-Fluorodeoxyglucose positron emission tomography/CT (18F-FDG PET). More than 90% of (primary) neuroblastoma are MIBG-avid [2]. ^{123}I-mIBG provides prognostic information and is used to select patients appropriate for ^{131}I-mIBG therapy [4]. For non-MIBG avid tumors, 18 F-FDG PET-CT is recommended [5]. FDG PET offers advantage of providing both anatomical and functional information in a single examination, and also ruling out differentials such as hematological malignancies. Hence if a single investigation is chosen for both anatomical and functional imaging, 18F-FDG PET is recommended.

Reporting for primary staging of neuroblastoma primarily depends on defining the IDRFs for primary tumor and each metastatic site. In the defining of IDRFs, certain terms must be used judiciously, and are depicted in Figs. 21.3a and 21.3b [3]. IDRF for each possible primary tumor location has been listed in Fig. 21.4.

After identifying the primary tumor, its local extent is described as vascular involvement (Fig. 21.5), infiltration of adjacent organs (mainly the kidneys and liver) (Fig. 21.7), and infiltration of the neural foramina and epidural space of the spinal canal (Fig. 21.8) in cases where the primary tumor arises from a paraspinal sympathetic chain [3]. Next is the identification of regional nodes adjacent to the primary tumor as well as distant metastasis (Fig. 21.6). Multifocal primary neuroblastomas are rare and may be familial, and manifest as either synchronous or metachronous non-contiguous tumors [3]. Each tumor requires separate staging, and multifocality is not regarded as an IDRF.

Differentials for neuroblastoma include adrenal cortical neoplasm (Fig. 21.9) which are more common in older children and predominantly show peripheral calcifications. These tumors are also often metastatic at the time of presentation.

21.1.2 Post-treatment Imaging

In evaluation of anatomic response, the same imaging modality used at diagnosis is recommended at all follow-up time points [4]. For evaluation of bone disease, extramedullary soft tissue component is measured and compared using same criteria as soft tissue lesions elsewhere. Bone lesions lacking a soft tissue mass are deemed non-measurable, and anatomic imaging is not used for their evaluation, either by CT or MRI. Therapeutic response is assessed with functional imaging, at both primary tumor site,

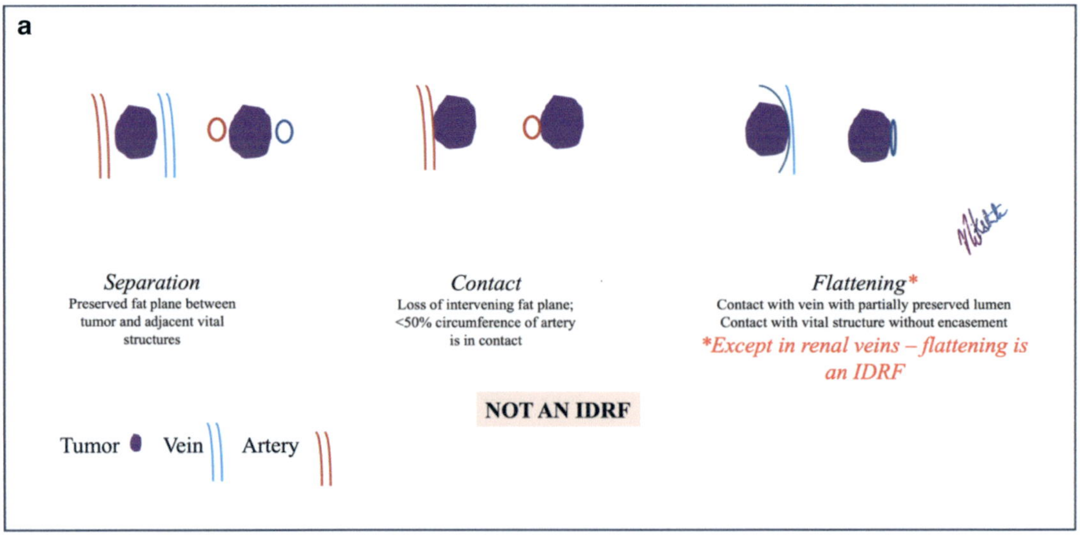

Fig. 21.3a Vascular relations that do not qualify as an image-defined risk factor

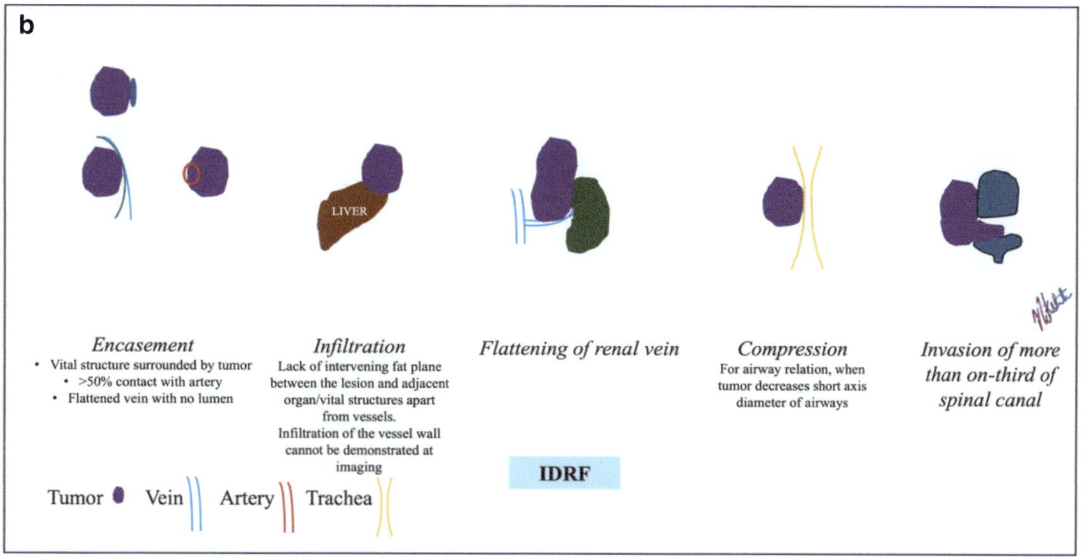

Fig. 21.3b Vascular, airway, and spinal canal relations that qualify as image-defined risk factors

Anatomic region	IDRF
Neck	➢ Tumor encasing carotid artery, vertebral artery, and/or internal jugular vein ➢ Tumor extending to skull base ➢ Tumor compressing trachea
Cervicothoracic junction	➢ Tumor encasing brachial plexus roots ➢ Tumor encasing subclavian vessels, vertebral artery, and/or carotid artery ➢ Tumor compressing trachea
Thorax	➢ Tumor encasing aorta and/or major branches ➢ Tumor compressing trachea and/or principal bronchi ➢ Lower mediastinal tumor infiltrating costovertebral junction between T9 and T12 vertebral levels
Thoraco-abdominal junction	Tumor encasing aorta and/or vena cava
Abdomen and pelvis	➢ Tumor infiltrating porta hepatis and/or hepatoduodenal ligament ➢ Tumor encasing branches of superior mesenteric artery at mesenteric root ➢ Tumor encasing origin of celiac axis and/or origin of superior mesenteric artery ➢ Tumor invading one or both renal pedicles ➢ Tumor encasing aorta and/or vena cava ➢ Tumor encasing iliac vessels ➢ Pelvic tumor crossing sciatic notch
Intraspinal tumor extension	Intraspinal tumor extension (whatever the location) provided that more than one-third of spinal canal in axial plane is invaded, the perimedullary leptomeningeal spaces are not visible, or the spinal cord signal intensity is abnormal
Infiltration of adjacent organs and structures	Pericardium, diaphragm, kidney, liver, duodenopancreatic block, and mesentery
Multiple body compartments	Ipsilateral tumor extension within two body compartments (ie, neck and chest, chest and abdomen, or abdomen and pelvis)

Fig. 21.4 Image-defined risk factors, adapted from Brisse et al. [3]

and metastatic sites (including bone involvement), to differentiate postoperative changes from residual tumor at resection sites.

Timing of surveillance imaging is based on risk group, with no uniform consensus yet available. In the setting of remission, surveillance is initiated 3 years from the start of treatment, and subsequently stratified according to the risk category [4]. For low-risk, congenital, or localized abdominal or pelvic neuroblastoma, without the risk of epidural extension, ultrasound is recommended every 1–2 months for 1 year and then yearly for 3 years [6, 7]. Similarly, intermediate-risk neuroblastomas with favorable biology and lacking risk of epidural extension can be followed with ultrasound every 3 months for the first year,

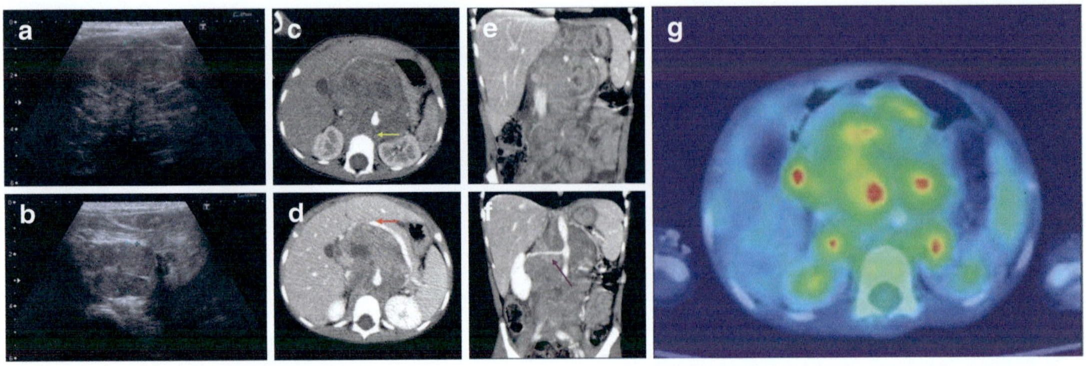

Fig. 21.5 A 4-year-old girl with 10 days history of fever, chills, and abdominal tenderness. Ultrasound showed a heterogenous retroperitoneal mass (**a**) and matted para-iliac nodes (**b**) raising suspicion of neuroblastoma and lymphoma. PET-CT was ordered. Axial CT from the PET (**c** and **d**) showed a retroperitoneal mass originating from left adrenal gland, encasing the aorta and lifting it from anterior vertebral margin (yellow arrow), flattening the portal vein (red arrow), and encasing right renal artery (purple arrow) (**f**). FDG PET shows diffuse uptake in the retroperitoneal mass (**g**). Histopathology confirmed the diagnosis of poorly differentiated neuroblastoma

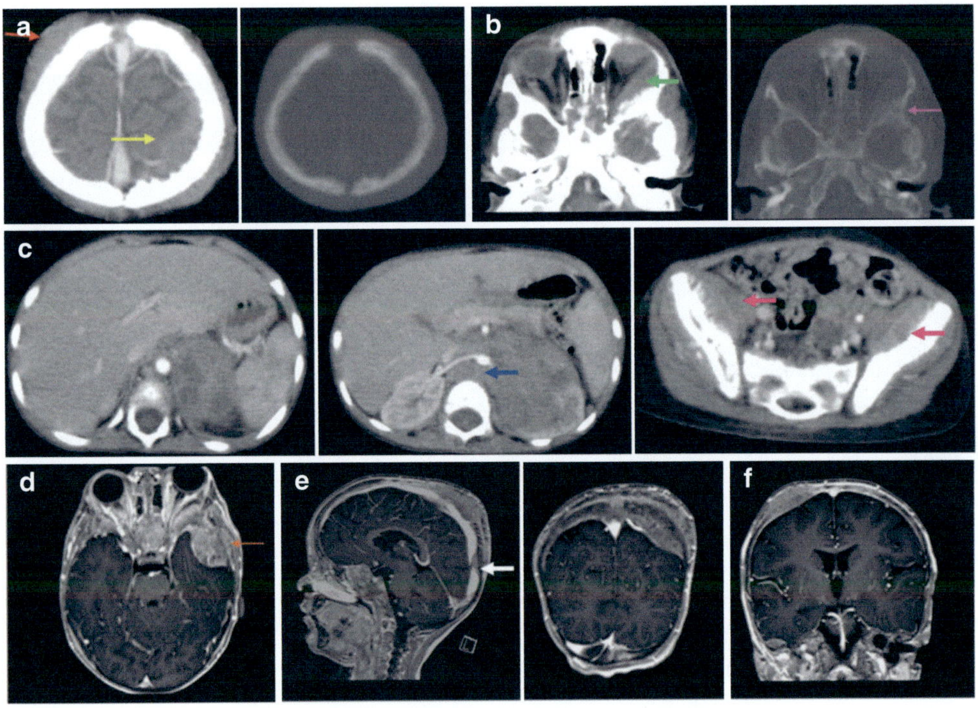

Fig. 21.6 A 4-yr-old boy presenting with scalp swellings and difficulty in weight bearing. FDG PET-CT was directly ordered due to high clinical suspicion of metastatic pathology. Axial CT of skull (**a**) in soft tissue (right) and bone window (left) shows diffuse lytic sclerotic lesions involving the bilateral frontoparietal bones, associated with both intracranial (yellow arrow) and extracranial soft tissue (red arrow). Axial CT at the level of the orbit (**b**) in soft tissue window (right) and bone window (left) shows lytic sclerotic lesion involving the lateral wall of left orbit (purple arrow) with associated intraorbital soft tissue (green arrow). Axial CT abdomen (**c**) shows a heterogenous left suprarenal mass crossing the midline (blue arrow) and lifting aorta from prevertebral space. It encases aorta and right renal artery. Axial sections at the level of pelvic inlet show bilateral iliac lesions with sunburst periosteal reaction and soft tissue component (pink arrow). MRI with contrast was done to delineate the intracranial soft tissue and relation with dural sinuses and shows left temporal soft tissue (orange arrow in image **d**), extradural soft tissue in bilateral parietal regions (image **f**), with thrombus within the superior sagittal sinus (white arrow in image **e**). Final histopathology revealed metastatic neuroblastoma

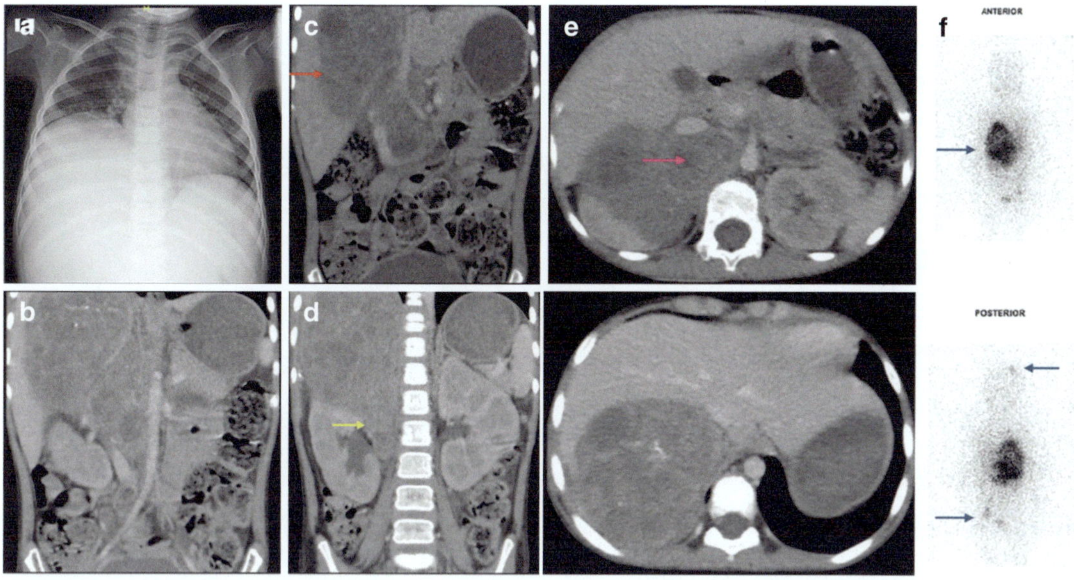

Fig. 21.7 A 5-yr—old girl presented with fever and myalgia since 4 months & abdominal distention since 1 month. On chest radiograph (**a**), elevated right hemidiaphragm likely secondary to intra-abdominal mass (possibly hepatic) is suspected. CT abdomen (axial **e** and coronal **b**,**c**,**d**) was subsequently ordered and revealed a heterogenous right suprarenal mass originating from right adrenal extending inferiorly to renal hilum (yellow arrow) with resulting right renal pelvic dilatation. It infiltrates the liver (red arrow) and pushes IVC forward (pink arrow). On mIBG scan (**f**), increased tracer activity is noted in the right side of the skull, right upper abdomen, and left pelvic bone (blue arrows). On histopathology: neuroblastoma, positive for amplification of MYCN gene

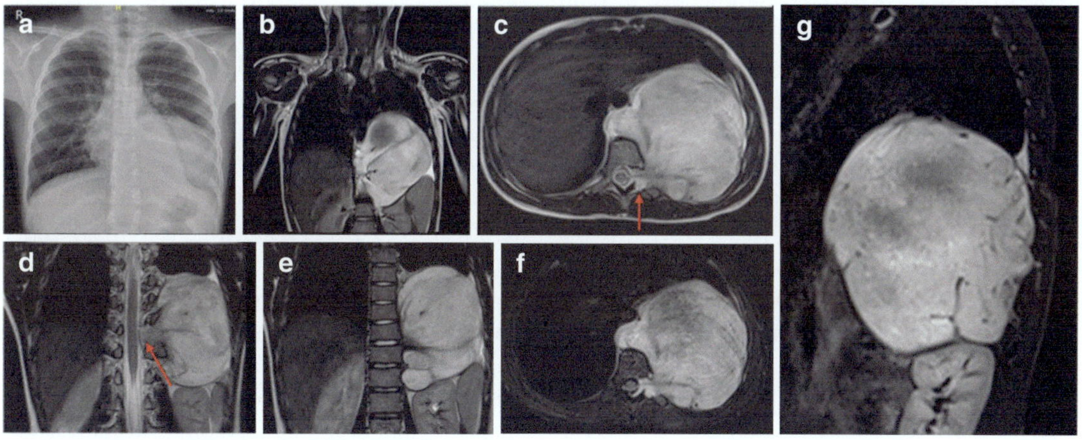

Fig. 21.8 A 8-yr-old girl with incidentally detected posterior mediastinal mass on chest radiograph (**a**) showing widened posterior intercostal spaces. MRI thorax shows a well-defined lobulated homogenously T2 hyperintense mass (coronal T2, **b**) with neural foraminal invasion on T2-weighted axial and coronal images (red arrow on images **c** and **d**) occupying less than one-third of the spinal canal (axial T2, **c**, and **f**). The left adrenal was not seen separately and left suprarenal origin was suspected as left kidney was inferiorly displaced (coronal T2, **e**, and sagittal T2 fat sat, **g**)

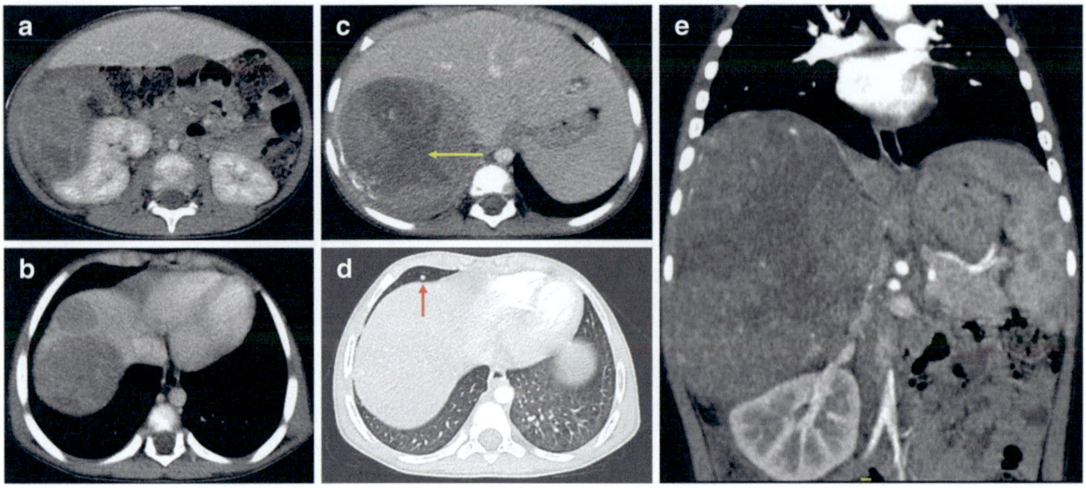

Fig. 21.9 A 4-yr-old boy with abdominal distention and fever since 1 month. On clinical evaluation, there were features of precocious puberty and right hypochondriac mass. On axial CECT (**a**–**c**), a heterogenous well-defined right suprarenal mass with adrenal origin, showing necrotic changes and peripheral calcifications. The right kidney is displaced inferiorly, as seen on the coronal CT image E. Indeterminate right lung subpleural nodule on HRCT reconstruction (**d**). Biopsy of right suprarenal mass revealed adrenal cortical neoplasm with oncocytic morphology

every 4 months for one year, then yearly for 3 years [6]. For intermediate-risk neuroblastoma with unfavorable biology, or with risk for epidural extension, MRI is recommended [4]. In such cases, MR and CT should be performed in conjunction with scintigraphic studies every 3 months for 1 year, every 6 months for 1 year, then yearly for 3 years [6]. In high-risk patients, anatomic and functional imaging should be performed every 3 months for 2 years, every 4 months for a year, then yearly for 3 years. Whole-body 99mTc-MDP bone scan is not recommended for routine surveillance due to its lower sensitivity for detecting relapse compared to ^{123}I-mIBG [4].

21.2 Renal Masses

21.2.1 Consensus Guideline(s) for Imaging

Often, a child will present with an abdominal mass/mass-associated distention. Occasionally, hematuria can be a presenting complaint, or presentation secondary to tumor rupture, however these are uncommon. The claw sign (sharp angles with the renal parenchyma on either side of the mass) is of particular use in determining renal origin.

Ultrasound is the modality for initial evaluation, due to availability and ease of performing. It helps to confirm the renal origin, detect presence of renal vein or IVC thrombus, and differentiate between bland and tumor thrombus. It is also the investigation of choice for surveillance of children with genetic predisposition to Wilms' tumor [8].

CECT or MRI abdomen is used to characterize renal masses and for baseline locoregional staging. When performing CT, only a portal venous phase (55–60 s post-contrast injection) is adequate, and oral contrast administration is not required. If MRI is performed, the sequences include conventional, DWI, and contrast imaging. MRI is preferred over CT due to superior soft tissue resolution, better differentiation between hemorrhage, necrosis, solid vs. cystic components within the mass and detection of multifocality. DWI helps in mapping for diagnosis, preoperative risk classification, post neoadjuvant chemotherapy response assessment (particularly among Wilms' tumor with large necrotic components, in which post-treatment size may not be significantly reduced).

CECT thorax is necessary for detection of pulmonary metastasis, evaluating the superior extent of tumor thrombus into the right atrium, any pathological mediastinal nodes, and pulmonary thromboembolism.

While combining CT thorax with MRI abdomen, CT should be done prior to giving anesthesia, to avoid obscuration of nodules by anesthesia-related atelectasis.

21.2.2 Structured Radiological Reporting and Interpretation

The radiological report must include the following information:

Mass size	[*X*] cm; Previously [x] cm on [most relevant comparison date] (Number and location (side) of renal masses (each mass to be separately described)
Parenchyma	<solid> < cystic: Septated> <mixed> <calcification> < macroscopic fat> < central/ crescentic rim necrosis> < subcapsular/ intraparenchymal hemorrhage>
MRI	<ADC value> < signal drop on out-of phase> < cystic component> <hemorrhage>
Enhancement	<none> <minimal > <marked> < enhancement type: Entire mass/septal/mural/nodular/no enhancement>
Location	<upper pole/ interpolar/lower pole> < anterior /posterior/ both> < perilobar/ intralobar>
Margin	<circumscribed> <irregular>
Pelvicalyceal involvement	<sinus fat invasion> < pelvicalyceal involvement> < not involved: Distance from sinus fat>
Tumor rupture	<retroperitoneal hemorrhage: Present/ absent> < indistinct margin> < ascites/ ipsilateral pleural effusion>
Local invasion	< psoas> < posterior/lateral abdominal wall> < colon/ bowel> <peritoneal> <adrenal> < whether crossing midline> < encasement of aorta/ its branches>
Tumor thrombus	<extent: Renal vein/ IVC (infrahepatic/hepatic) > <length: Renal vein/ IVC > <caval wall invasion>
Bland thrombus	<present> <absent>
Lymph nodes	<suprahilar> <hilar> <infrahilar> <paraaortic> <aortocaval> <paracaval> <others>
Metastasis	< none> <possible> <definite>
Ascites	<mild> < moderate/severe>
Relevant anatomy	<ipsilateral renal artery anatomy> < ipsilateral renal vein anatomy> < renal anatomy>
Contralateral kidney	<size> <enhancement> <pathology>
Follow-up recommendation	<CR/MRI/USG > in [x] months

There are 2 staging systems in practice for Wilms'-National Wilms' tumor study group (NWTSG) and the Societe internationale D'oncologie pediatrique (SIOP) system, and both of these are based on post-surgical criteria. The role of imaging is to determine disease extent, surgical resectability at presentation (lesions without venous invasion can go for upfront resection, without neoadjuvant chemotherapy), and for response to chemotherapy.

21.2.3 Imaging Algorithm for Interpretation and Approach to Diagnosis

Age is the most important consideration in formulating a differential diagnosis for a renal mass in children [9] and an imaging algorithm has been proposed in Fig. 21.10. This is because solid renal masses are largely indistinguishable on imaging, and biopsy/surgical excision provides

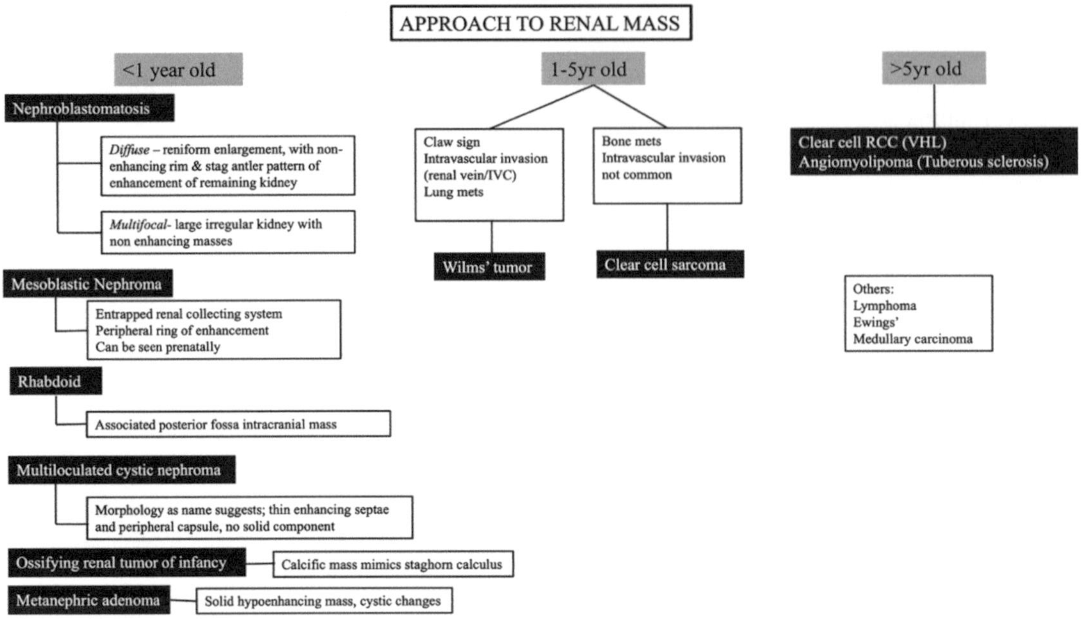

Fig. 21.10 Age-based imaging algorithm for interpretation and approach to diagnosis of pediatric renal masses

definitive histopathology. When imaging favors a malignant etiology, pre-surgical biopsy may be imperative to properly guide management, and image-guided biopsy must be done from lateral/posterolateral approach (so as to not breach peritoneum).

This section will cover the spectrum of renal neoplasms in children, with emphasis on lesions that predominate in the first decade of life. Commonest renal mass in children older than 10 yrs. of age include renal cell carcinoma that has imaging morphology similar to adults.

21.3 Wilms' Tumor

This comprises of more than 90% of pediatric renal tumors [9]. Majority of cases are seen in children less than 5 years of age, with peak incidence at 2–3 years [9]. On ultrasound, presence of heterogeneity, due to internal necrosis and hemorrhage, favors its diagnosis. Echogenic calcifications with shadowing can be seen in 9% of patients on ultrasound, and almost 15% of patients on CT [9]. Due to intrarenal location, the masses depict the 'claw sign' on CT characterized by a rind of normal renal parenchyma around the edge of the lesion (Fig. 21.11). Whether the SIOP or NWTSG system of staging is being followed (depends on the treating team's protocol), imaging descriptors remain the same (checklist above). Reiterating the complete evaluation of contralateral kidney, to not miss any synchronous bilateral lesions that significantly impact management and prognosis. Genetically predisposed Wilms' is seen in younger age group (12–15 months) and is generally bilateral. Genetic causes for Wilms' have been enumerated under the nephroblastomatosis section.

MRI is the preferred imaging modality for known bilateral Wilms' tumors or known bilateral tumor predisposition [10]. For the detection of small Wilms' tumors and nephrogenic rests, high-spatial-resolution post-contrast images of the renal parenchyma in the nephrographic phase are needed [10]. Diffusion-weighted images can aid in the detection of small synchronous tumors/multifocal tumors [10]. There is as yet no data to

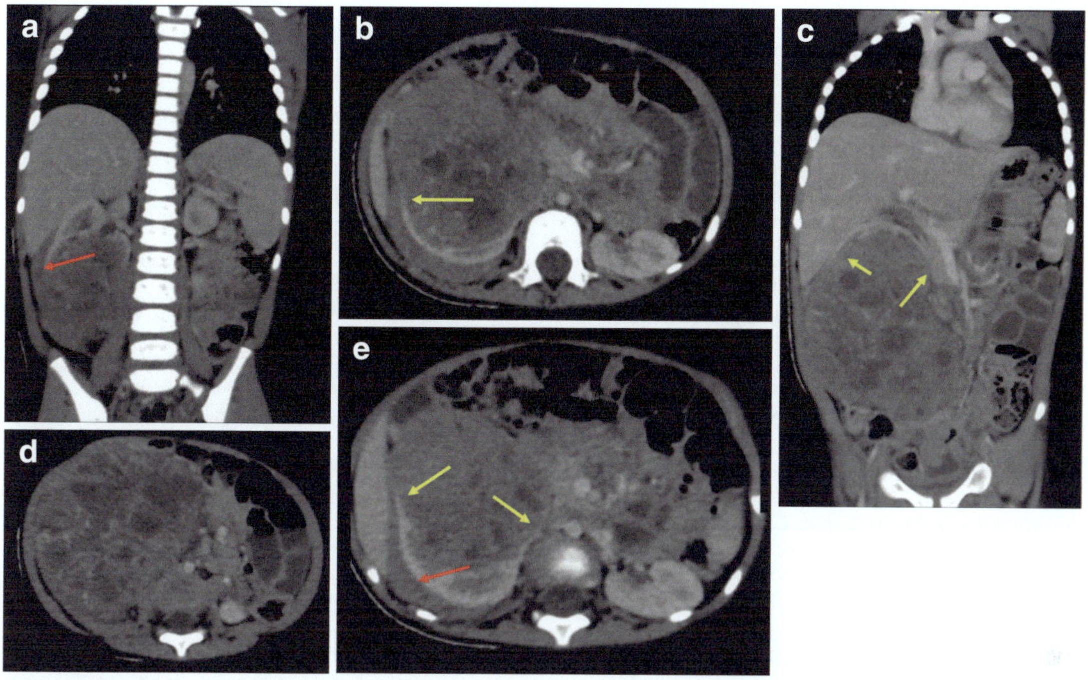

Fig. 21.11 A 1-yr-old child presented with fullness and mass in right side of abdomen, noticed by the mother. CECT shows a large heterogenous right renal mass, showing the characteristic claw sign (yellow arrows). A peripheral rind of similar heterogenous soft tissue is noted, possibly suggesting contained tumor rupture or perinephric extension. Histopathology: Mixed type Wilms' (25% blastemal component, 35% epithelial component, 40% stromal component)

suggest that ADC values can aid in differentiating small Wilms' tumor from nephrogenic rests [10].

Occasionally, a child may present acutely, and tumor rupture needs to be ruled out (also favored if there is coexisting drop in hemoglobin levels). Imaging features that favor tumor rupture include indistinct tumor margins, retroperitoneal fluid as well as ascites, perinephric fat stranding, and ipsilateral pleural effusion on CT [9]. Metastases are most commonly to lung (almost 85%), other sites include liver (20%) (Figs. 21.12a and 21.12b) and rarely, bone [9].

Imaging differentials include (Table 21.1):

1. Neuroblastoma
2. Clear cell sarcoma—similar imaging morphology with Wilms', bone metastases more common with clear cell sarcoma.
3. Rhabdoid—similar imaging morphology with Wilms' except for subcapsular hemorrhage being typical for rhabdoids (comparatively, since Wilms' is far more common, therefore, even with the presence of subcapsular hemorrhage, Wilms' will be more likely [9], synchronous intracranial tumors
4. Focal bacterial nephritis & associated abscess—similar imaging morphology, clinical history (fever, pain, urinary symptoms) will help make the distinction (Wilms' is painless).

The Children's Oncology Group staging system is used for the management of Wilms' and relies on surgical/histopathological findings for locoregional disease. On imaging, the pertinent findings to be evaluated for are:

- Intravascular extension of tumor—renal vein, intrahepatic IVC, right atrium

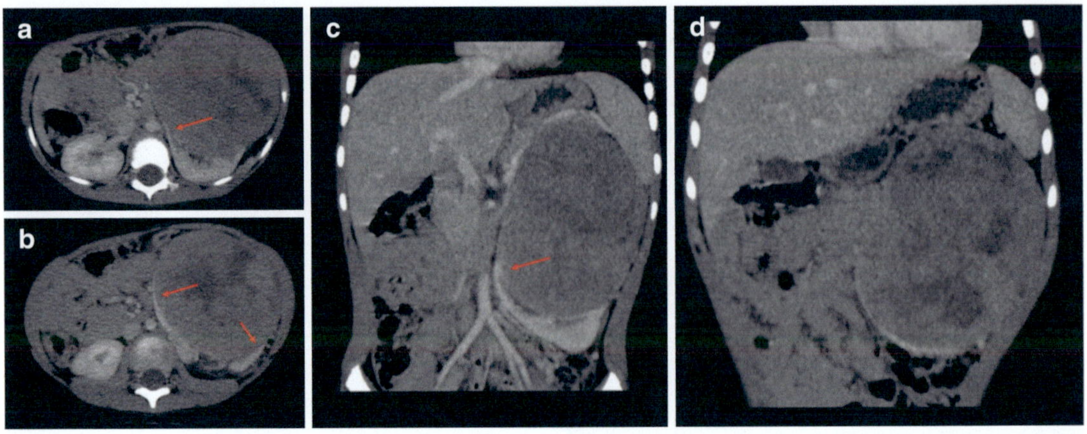

Fig. 21.12a A 5-yr-old child with increased frequency of urine and no fever. Axial (images **a** and **b**) and coronal (images **c** and **d**) contrast-enhanced CT shows heterogenous left renal mass with areas of necrosis and well-defined margins. Claw sign is evident (red arrows). Underwent nephrectomy and histopathology: Wilms' with WT1 mutation

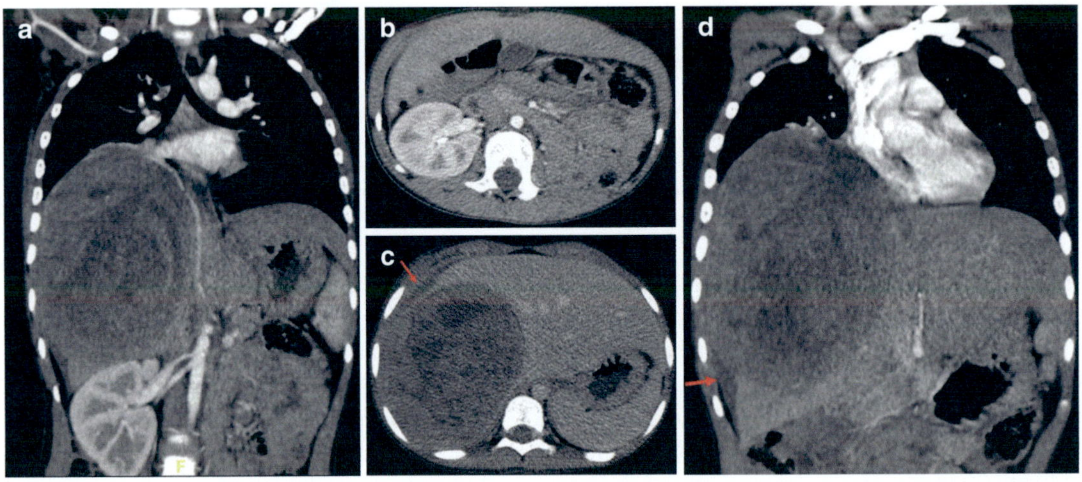

Fig. 21.12b Same child returned 3 years after treatment completion (image B showing post left nephrectomy status), with a solitary right hepatic mass with morphology similar to the primary left renal mass. Coronal CT sections (**a** and **d**) show the liver lesion with associated exophytic component. Red arrows on images **c** and **d** show minimal perihepatic fluid. Underwent right hepatectomy and histopathology suggestive of Wilms' metastases

- Ureteral involvement
- Infiltration of adjacent structures (apart from adrenals)
- Synchronous contralateral lesions
- Peritoneal metastases
- Features of tumor rupture
- Hepatic or lung metastases

Table 21.1 Key differentiating features between neuroblastoma and Wilms'

	Neuroblastoma	Wilms'
Age	Younger (<2 years of age)	Slightly older (3–4 years)
Metastasis	Bone	Liver, lung
Retroperitoneal adenopathy	More common, bulky	Less common
Extension into spinal canal	Present	Absent
Crosses midline	Yes, commonly behind the aorta	Usually not
Vessels	Encasement	Invasion
Cystic component	Present	Rare
Calcification	Very common: 90%	Uncommon: 10–15%
Organ of origin	Renal, claw sign	Extrarenal, displaces kidney
Clinical presentation	Abdominal distension	Irritability

21.4 COG Staging [10]

Stage I	Tumor limited to kidney and completely resected with no residual microscopic disease	Tumor capsule intact Renal sinus not involved Lymph nodes sampled and negative No preoperative biopsy
Stage II	Tumor completely resected with no evidence of tumor at or beyond margins	Regional extension of the tumor: Renal sinus invasion at pathological evaluation Breach of capsule at pathological evaluation Lymph nodes sampled and negative
Stage III	Residual non-hematogenous tumor in abdomen following surgery	Positive lymph nodes Tumor is removed in more than one piece Contiguous tumor extension into adjacent organs resulting in incomplete resection Intraoperative tumor spill Preoperative tumor rupture into retroperitoneum or peritoneal cavity Preoperative tumor biopsy
Stage IV	Distant metastases	Lungs, liver, bone, brain, etc. Lymph node metastases outside the abdomen/pelvis
Stage V	Bilateral renal involvement at diagnosis	

Detection of capsular infiltration to distinguish between Stage I and Stage II tumors has been shown to be limited by cross-sectional imaging because capsular invasion is often microscopic, and detection on imaging is further compounded by lack of perinephric fat in small children [10].

Pre-operative tumor rupture is seen on imaging as ascites beyond cul-de-sac (irrespective of Hounsfield units), retroperitoneal fluid, and peritumoral fat stranding. Intratumoral hemorrhage or subcapsular fluid does not equate to tumor rupture [10]. Small amount of free fluid should not be regarded as a sign of rupture, as this may be reactive or secondary to mass effect on IVC. Though imaging findings of rupture have high specificity (88%), the diagnosis of rupture has to be confirmed at surgery in the COG's current staging guidelines [10].

For nodal metastases, size and morphology criteria have shown limited accuracy for determining involvement and surgical sampling remains the standard protocol. No definite size criteria for lung nodules are established to differentiate benign vs malignant nodules, however suggested features to support metastases include a non-calcified pulmonary nodule that is sharply marginated (not fuzzy) and is not located in a fissure (latter favors intra-fissural lymph node) [10].

21.5 Nephroblastomatosis

After 36 weeks of gestation, persistent embryonal renal tissue (metanephric blastema) are called nephrogenic rests. Nephroblastomatosis implies multiple discrete or diffuse nephrogenic rests, and is a precursor for Wilms', seen in almost 40% of kidneys resected for Wilms' and all bilateral Wilms' [9]. Essentially, these are associated with the genetic causes that predispose to Wilms', such as [9]:

- Wilms' Tumor (WT1) gene 1, also shows genitourinary abnormalities and renal dysfunction.
- WAGR syndrome (Wilms' tumor, aniridia, genitourinary abnormalities including ambiguous genitalia in males, and mental retardation).
- Denys-Drash syndrome (Wilms' tumor, male pseudohermaphroditism, and progressive glomerulonephritis).
- Wilms' tumor gene 2 (WT2)—this is associated with overgrowth syndromes:
  1. Beckwith-Wiedemann syndrome (macroglossia, omphalocele, organomegaly, genitourinary anomalies, and increased risk for abdominal tumors).
  2. Hemihypertrophy with or without associated BWS.
  3. Perlman syndrome (visceromegaly, gigantism, renal dysplasia, genitourinary anomalies, and characteristic facies).
  4. Sotos syndrome (cerebral gigantism, renal anomalies, cardiac anomalies, Wilms' tumor).
- WTX domain on the X chromosome.
- β-catenin (CTNNB1) gene,
- Tumor suppressor gene TP53 on chromosome 17—strong association with anaplastic tumor histology and poor prognosis.

Renal development is centrifugal, and hence depending on the time of development, nephrogenic rests can be intralobar (earlier, centrally located) or perilobar (peripherally located in the column of Bertin, more common). Perilobar rests are more commonly seen with overgrowth syndromes (hemihypertrophy with or without BWS carries highest risk of Wilms' at 3%) and trisomy 18 [9]. Intralobar rests are seen with WT1 mutations, and all children with sporadic aniridia [9]. Intralobar rests have a higher risk of neoplastic transformation, and children with sporadic aniridia with or without WAGR syndrome have maximum risk of developing Wilms' tumor at 33% [9].

On imaging, nephrogenic rests can be seen as focal or diffuse lesions. Focal lesions are seen as poorly enhancing foci surrounded by normal renal parenchyma. Diffuse lesions are seen as circumferential soft tissue compressing the normal renal tissue toward the center of the kidney. On ultrasound focal lesions may be hypo or hyperechoic compared with renal echogenicity, and diffuse nephroblastomatosis is seen as diffusely hyperechoic kidney with poor corticomedullary differentiation. These ultrasound features have poor sensitivity and specificity, and CT or MRI is required for characterization. CT shows focal hypoenhancing lesions or thick peripheral rind of soft tissue with striated enhancement pattern [9]. On MR, these rests are hypointense to renal parenchyma on T1W images, with homogenous post-contrast enhancement.

It is challenging to distinguish between nephrogenic rests and small Wilms' with both CT (Fig. 21.13) and MRI. Features favoring interlobar rests over Wilms' are peripheral subcapsular location, ovoid/elliptical shape, and homogenous morphology [8]. Continued screening is warranted (with ultrasound or MRI if feasible), and features concerning for neoplastic transformation (Wilms') are increasing size or heterogenous morphology or spherical configuration on follow-up. Due to the central intrarenal location and heterogenous morphology of intralobar rests, these are far more difficult to differentiate from Wilms' [8].

The detection of nephroblastomatosis entails syndromic/genetic work-up. Management strategy remains controversial and depends on the treating team. In those children with predisposing syndromes, screening for Wilms' should start at 6 months, with serial ultrasound every 3 months up to 8 years of age, after which incidence of Wilms' declines [9].

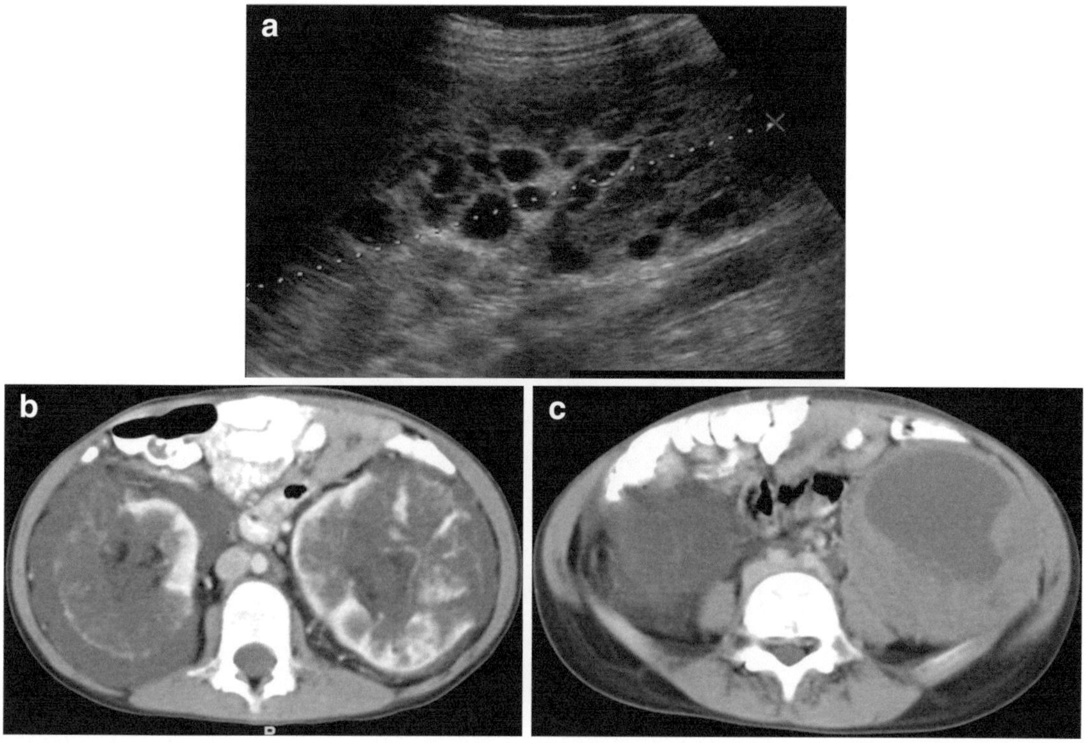

Fig. 21.13 Ultrasound (**a**) of a 4-year-old girl shows enlarged right kidney with diffusely altered echogenicity and cystic areas. Axial contrast-enhanced CT (**b**) shows bilateral subcapsular, diffuse, and extensive, low-attenuation non-enhancing masses with nephromegaly causing compression of the renal parenchyma and the pelvicalyceal system. Left lower renal pole mass with necrosis within is suggestive of Wilms' (**c**)

21.6 Congenital Mesoblastic Nephroma (CMN)

This is the most common renal neoplasm of neonates, but overall represents only 3–6% of pediatric renal tumors [9]. While most are diagnosed up to 3 months of age, 90% are diagnosed by age 1 year [9]. These tumors can be diagnosed as early as mid-second trimester and are often found on antenatal scans [9]. After age 2, diagnosis of mesoblastic nephroma is unlikely and must be challenged. Slight male predilection exists, with a male: female ratio of 1.5:1 [9]. Presentation is with a palpable abdominal mass. However, some of the lesions can complicate antenatal period with polyhydramnios, hydrops fetalis, and preterm delivery [9]. Uncommonly, paraneoplastic syndromes such as hypertension and hypercalcemia are seen.

Histologically, there are 2 subtypes, namely classic and cellular or a mixed pattern. Cellular type lesions are larger, occur in children >3 months of age, and unencapsulated, with hemorrhagic and necrotic areas within [9]. Chromosomal abnormalities, namely polysomy of chromosome 11 and chromosomal translocation t(12;15)(p12;q25), resulting ETV6-NTRK3 gene fusion, are only seen with the cellular type [9].

On imaging, classic CMN is typically seen as a solid homogenous mass, involving the renal hilum, but not invading the vessels (Fig. 21.14). A peripheral vascular ring on ultrasound Doppler, appearing as a concentric hyperechoic and hypoechoic rim on grey-scale, is seen, probably secondary to peripherally dilated blood vessels seen on microscopy. This is also reflected in the typical peripheral enhancement seen on CECT/MR. MR signal char-

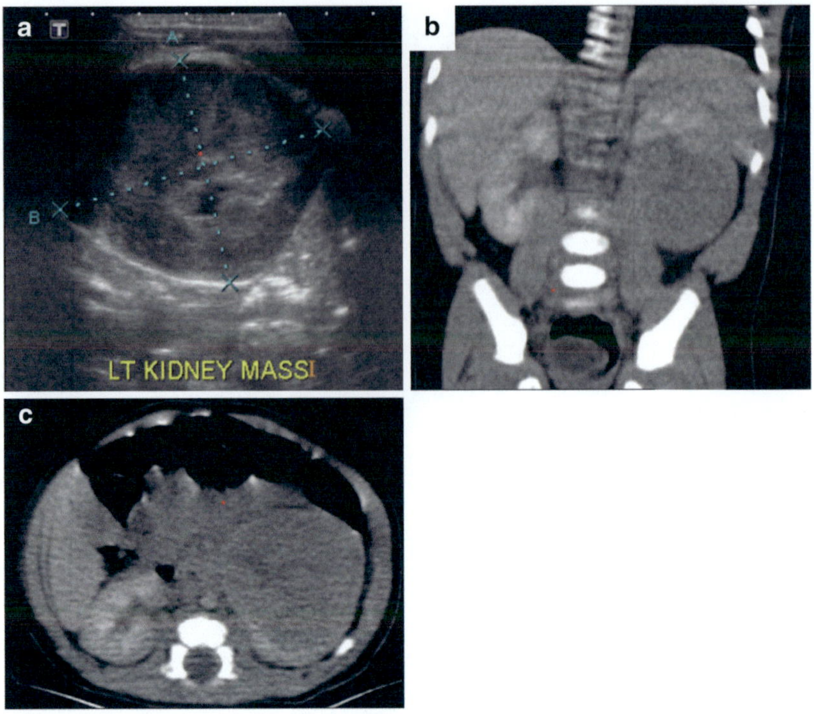

Fig. 21.14 An 11-month-old child with mass in abdomen. Ultrasound of left kidney (**a**) shows a well-defined heteroechoic mass in lower pole of left kidney. On axial (**c**) and coronal (**b**) CT, a well-defined hypoenhancing mass is seen in the lower pole of left kidney with no significant internal necrosis/hemorrhage. Histopathology: Mesoblastic nephroma

acteristics are variable. On the contrary, cellular type of CMN is heterogenous with hemorrhagic and necrotic changes within. Post-contrast enhancement in only the solid component, with CT and MR characteristics in keeping with mixed hemorrhagic and cystic/necrotic content is typical. As these tumors are larger, they may cross the midline, and also result in encasement of vessels or invade adjacent organs [9].

Ossifying renal tumor of infancy (ORTI) and rhabdoid tumors can be differentiated by the typical osteoid matrix in ORTI (calcification is uncommon in CMN) and associated posterior fossa tumor in rhabdoids [9]. Neuroblastoma is a close differential with respect to imaging features, such as crossing the midline, vascular encasement, and spinal canal invasion, all which can be seen with cellular CMN [9]. The one differentiating feature is calcifications, more commonly seen with neuroblastoma. Wilms' and clear cell sarcoma are indistinguishable on imaging with cellular CMN, but are rarely seen in infancy. In older infants, multilocular cystic renal tumors can be considered a differential for cystic cellular CMN, however presence of a solid enhancing component favors CMN.

CMN is a tumor of variable biological behavior, majority being benign, with 5–10% showing local recurrence and metastases (these are mostly the cellular subtype) [9]. Treatment is mostly with nephrectomy, and prognosis is best if tumor is resected before the age of 6 months [9]. Recommended close ultrasound follow-up for the cellular subtype, at least for a year since most recurrences are discovered within one year of initial presentation [9].

21.7 Rhabdoid Tumor

First described as sarcomatous type of Wilms' (due to the histological resemblance to muscle), rhabdoid tumor is now a distinct and rare entity, accounting for less than 2% of pediatric renal neoplasms, with 80% diagnosed before the age of 2 years. In up to 15% of cases, it is associated with brain metastases or synchronous primary intracranial neoplasms (primitive neuroectodermal tumor, ependymoma, medulloblastoma, astrocytoma) [9].

Presenting symptoms include hematuria (secondary to renal collecting system invasion) and occasionally hypercalcemia (secondary to parathormone elevation). Tumors are often metastatic (lung, brain, or bones) at the time of presentation due to fairly aggressive tumor behavior. Definitive diagnosis is aided with molecular genetic evaluation showing loss of function of the INI-1 tumor suppressor gene on chromosome 22q.

Imaging morphology is similar to Wilms' tumor. However, certain features such as subcapsular hemorrhage, crescentic rim of necrosis, or curvilinear calcification are said to be characteristic of rhabdoid tumor that may help in differentiating them from Wilms' tumor. Another differential is clear cell sarcoma which is distinguished by early metastases to bone in the later.

For complete evaluation, MRI brain and spine is recommended pre-operatively if neurological symptoms are present, or postoperatively after diagnosis is confirmed. Treatment strategy includes surgery (radical nephrectomy and nodal dissection), chemotherapy, and radiation. Overall, prognosis remains poor, particularly for those with high-stage disease, children less than 1 year of age and with synchronous intracranial tumor [9].

21.8 Multilocular Cystic Nephroma

On imaging, it is a well-circumscribed large (~5-10 cm in size) multiseptated cystic mass with no solid components. The capsule and septa may enhance after intravenous contrast administration. Occasionally, the locules may be small and mimic solid morphology. Ultrasound is most sensitive to identify the septa [9]. It characteristically shows herniation into the collecting system (also resulting in hematuria). The cystic component has attenuation similar to or slightly higher than that of water on CT (Fig. 21.15a), is of fluid intensity on T2-weighted MRI (Fig. 21.15b), and has variable signal intensity on T1-weighted images, depending on the amount of protein or blood products in the cyst.

Differentials include nonneoplastic cystic lesions such as severe hydronephrosis (cysts communicate with each other) and multicystic dysplastic kidney (diagnosed prenatally or at birth, renal parenchyma replaced with multiple non-communicating cysts of various sizes). Among the neoplastic differentials, Wilms', mesoblastic nephroma, and clear cell sarcoma are considered when they have a predominant cystic component. The small locules in cystic nephroma

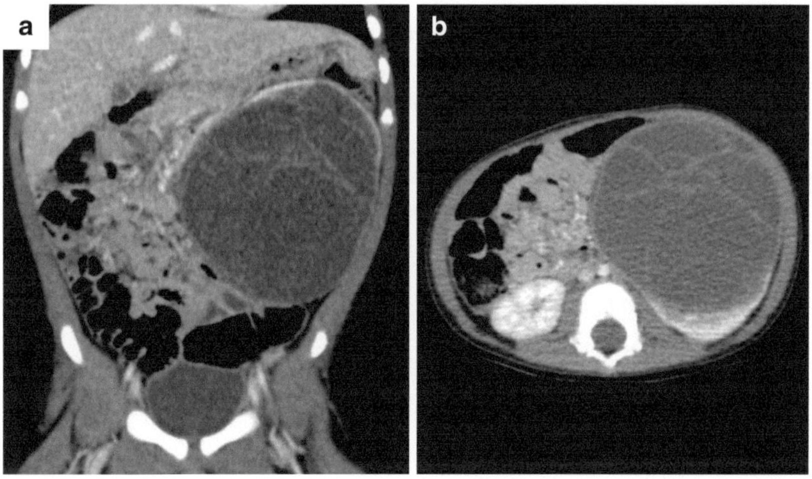

Fig. 21.15a A 12-month-old baby with axial (B) and coronal contrast enhanced CT (A) showing a well-circumscribed, encapsulated, multiseptated cystic mass with enhancement of capsule and septa involving the mid and lower poles of the left kidney with mass effect on adjacent structures; no nodular solid component/calcifications; Left renal vein (not shown) and IVC is normal. Claw sign is seen on image B. Diagnosis—multilocular cystic tumor

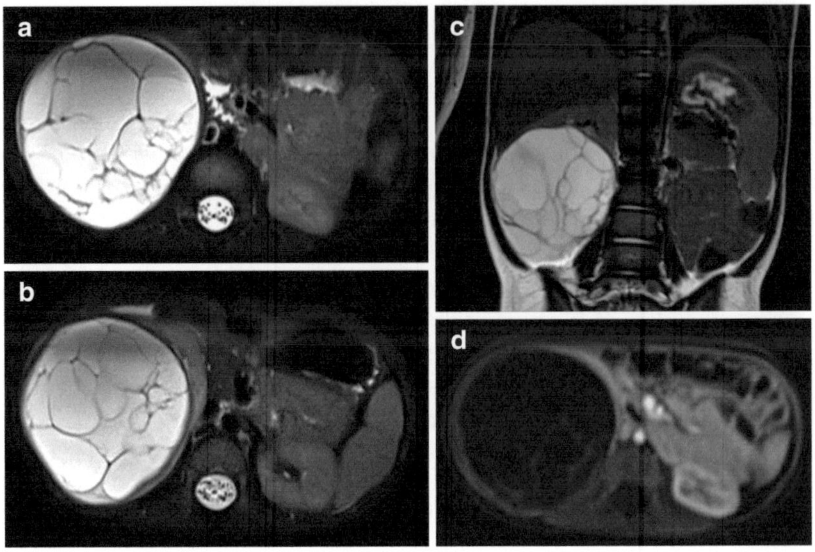

Fig. 21.15b A 22-month-old baby presenting with right renal mass that shows multiloculated cystic morphology (image **a**) and claw sign (axial T2, image **b**; Coronal T2, image **c**), with thin enhancing septae on the post-contrast images (image **d**). Diagnosis: multilocular cystic renal tumor

may mimic solid component and need biopsy for proper differentiation. Otherwise presence of enhancing solid component favors Wilms'.

21.9 Ossifying Renal Tumor of Infancy

As the name suggests this is a rare tumor showing osteoid matrix and presenting in infancy. The etiology is uncertain (possibly nephrogenic rests) and histopathologically this mass shows osteoid core, osteoblasts, and spindle cells [11]. It is attached to the renal papilla and grows into the collecting system [9]. On imaging this mass shows calcification and hence appears as an echogenic heterogenous intrarenal mass with posterior acoustic shadowing on ultrasound and calcified non-enhancing mass on CT. It may cause obstruction of the collecting system, and mimics a staghorn calculus [11]. Treatment is with renal preserving surgical excision. Chemotherapy or nephrectomy is not required.

21.10 Clear Cell Sarcoma

This is the second most common malignant tumor of the kidney after Wilms' tumor in the first decade of life. Its peak incidence occurs at 1–4 years of age, predominantly affecting boys in a ratio of 2:1. There are no imaging findings to differentiate clear cell sarcoma from Wilms' tumor (Fig. 21.16). Distinction can be made if bone or node metastases are present. Being a sarcoma, it typically shows metastasis to bones and nodes at initial diagnosis due to hematogenous spread, in up to 5–18% of patients. Bone lesions can be lytic/sclerotic/mixed and bone scintigraphy is routinely recommended once diagnosis of clear cell sarcoma is established.

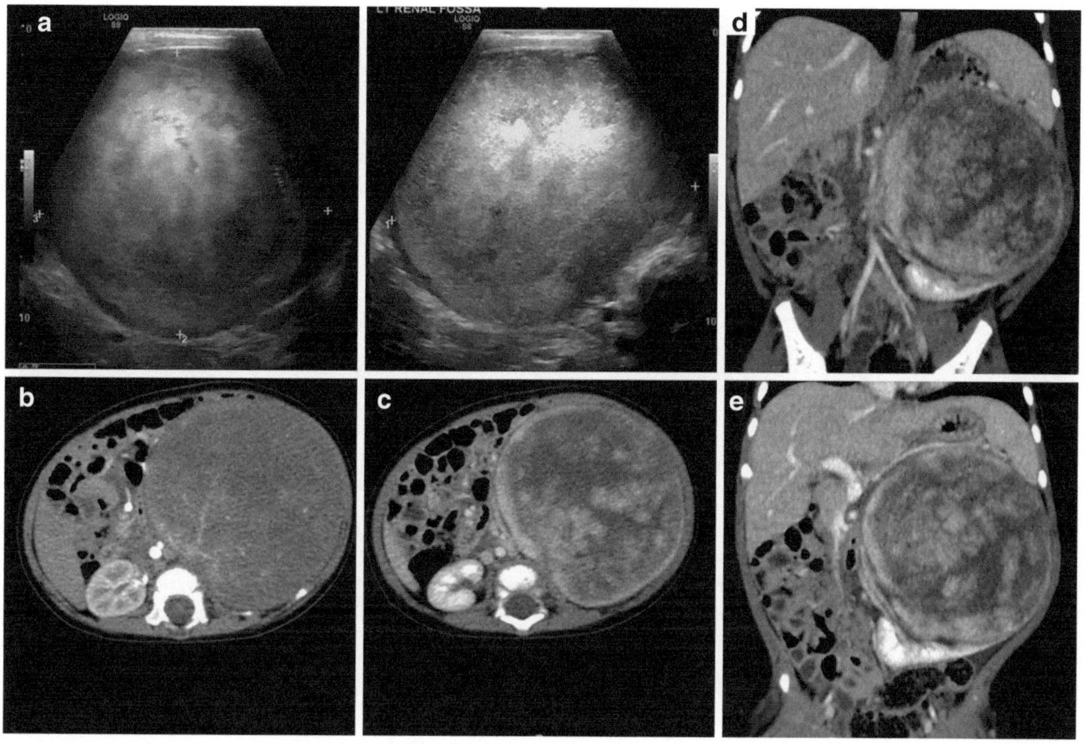

Fig. 21.16 A 7-month-old baby, with left-sided abdominal mass noticed by mother since 3 months. History of hematuria. Ultrasound (**a**) shows a *large* predominantly echogenic mass arising from left kidney. On arterial phase (**b**), mild vascularity is noted within, however on venous phase (**c**), there is significant heterogenous post-contrast enhancement. Coronal images (**d** and **e**) show the left renal origin clearly. Diagnosis- Clear cell sarcoma

21.11 Renal Cell Carcinoma (RCC)

In children, the imaging morphology of RCC (Fig. 21.17) is similar to adults and shows a heterogenous mass with a well-defined capsule. The histological spectrum however is different.

- Xp11.2 translocation RCC—most common subtype in children that typically appears hyperdense on non-contrast CT and is associated with retroperitoneal adenopathy [12]. Prior administration of chemotherapy is a predisposing factor.
- Papillary RCC—less enhancing than renal parenchyma, shows calcifications.
- Clear cell RCC—in children with von Hippel-Lindau disease, presents earlier, hypervascular.

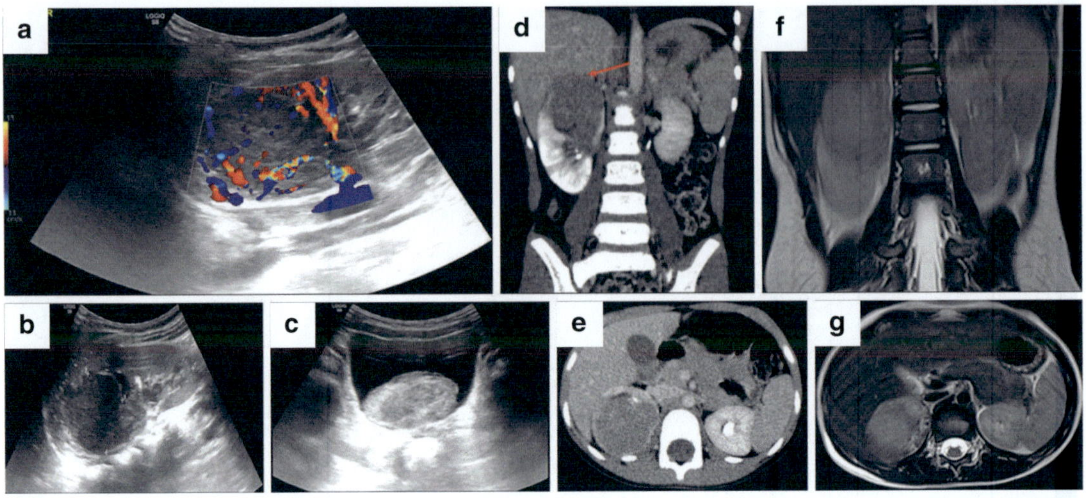

Fig. 21.17 A 5-yr-old with painless hematuria since 1 week. Ultrasound showed a well-defined right renal upper pole mass with internal vascularity (**a** and **b**) and urinary bladder clot (**c**). Coronal (**d**) and axial contrast-enhanced CT (**e**) showed heterogeneous hypodense upper pole renal mass. There was suspicion of liver infiltration (red arrow). Axial and coronal T2 MRI abdomen showed well-defined non-infiltrative margins (**f** and **g**). Histopathology: TFE3 rearranged renal cell carcinoma

21.12 Angiomyolipoma

Angiomyolipoma (AML) is a benign solid tumor, continuing a disordered arrangement of blood vessels, smooth muscle, and fatty elements. They usually occur only with underlying tuberous sclerosis and present by 10 years of age. Radiologically, AML may be classified as 'Fat rich,' 'Fat poor,' or 'Fat invisible.' The imaging appearance is variable and depends upon the fat content. CT and MR are superior and more accurate than ultrasound in the detection of fat. Ultrasound demonstrates highly echogenic foci (more echogenic than the renal sinus fat) that correlates with the macroscopic fat. 'Fat poor' lesions will have variable echogenicity, may be iso-echoic to the renal parenchyma and hence can be missed on ultrasound. MRI with capability of chemical shift imaging is superior to CT, for detection of microscopic fat in 'fat poor' AML. Diagnosis is confirmed by characteristic imaging features and biopsy is contraindicated in view of the risk of life-threatening hemorrhage.

21.13 Others

Besides Wilms' tumor, a wide variety of primary renal tumors can affect the pediatric kidneys, although uncommon. Their key imaging appearances have been enumerated in Table 21.2.

21.13.1 Post-treatment Imaging

For post-neoadjuvant chemotherapy, CT or MRI is done for response assessment, to delineate vascular anatomy and extent of tumor for surgical planning. Ultrasound abdomen is recommended for surveillance, after curative surgery. Cross-sectional imaging is done for any suspicious findings detected on ultrasound, and single kidney is not a contraindication for intravenous contrast if renal function is normal [8]. Tumor biology and initial staging will dictate the surveillance guidelines.

Table 21.2 Summary of uncommon pediatric renal masses

Tumor	Age at presentation	Associated conditions	Imaging features
Angiomyolipoma	Usually less than 10 yrs.	TSC, HF, VHL	Macroscopic fat, hypervascular, multiple expansile masses
Lymphoma	Children and adolescents >5 yrs	NHL	Unifocal or multifocal solid hypoenhancing masses, restricted diffusion on MRI, adenopathy outside the kidney
Ossifying renal tumor of infancy	0-1 yr	–	
Clear cell sarcoma	1-4 yrs	–	Solid well-defined mass, bone metastasis
Renal cell carcinoma	Older children (9-10ys)	VHL	Solid or cystic renal mass, calcifications, hemorrhage
Medullary carcinoma	Adolescent	Sickle cell trait	Infiltrative growth pattern, reniform shape preserved, extends into collecting system, metastatic at presentation
Metanephric tumors	Any, no age group		Well-defined expansile mass, centered in the medulla, calcification
Ewing's sarcoma (previously PNET)	–	–	Large complex mass replacing the kidney Metastasis to lungs, liver, bone is common at presentation

21.13.2 Recent Updates and Future Directions

Newer PET agents such as ^{18}F Fluorodihydroxyphenylalanine (18F-FDOPA), Meta [^{18} F] Fluorobenzylguanidine (^{18} F-mFBG), ^{124}I-mIBG may provide several advantages to ^{123}I-mIBG planar and SPECT/CT imaging including higher spatial resolution, improved tumor-to-background ratios, same day administration and imaging, quantification of tracer uptake, and shorter imaging times. The increased sensitivity afforded by their use may more accurately quantify disease burden, leading to improvements in staging, prognostication, and treatment management [4]. Another area of ongoing research is CT signatures for mycn amplification.

References

1. Swift CC, Eklund MJ, Kraveka JM, Alazraki AL. Updates in diagnosis, management, and treatment of Neuroblastoma. Radiographics. 2018;38(2):566–80.
2. Littooij AS, De Keizer B. Imaging in neuroblastoma. Pediatr Radiol. 2022;53(4):783–7.
3. Brisse HJ, McCarville MB, Granata C, Krug KB, Wootton-Gorges SL, Kanegawa K, et al. Guidelines for imaging and staging of Neuroblastic tumors: consensus report from the international Neuroblastoma risk group project. Radiology. 2011;261(1):243–57.
4. Lai HA, Sharp SE, Bhatia A, Dietz KR, McCarville B, Rajderkar D, et al. Imaging of pediatric neuroblastoma: a COG diagnostic imaging committee/SPR oncology committee white paper. Pediatr Blood Cancer. 2023;70(S4):e29974.
5. Bar-Sever Z, Biassoni L, Shulkin B, Kong G, Hofman MS, Lopci E, et al. Guidelines on nuclear medicine imaging in neuroblastoma. Eur J Nucl Med Mol Imaging. 2018;45(11):2009–24.
6. Kushner BH. Neuroblastoma: A disease requiring a multitude of imaging studies.
7. Papaioannou G. Neuroblastoma in childhood: review and radiological findings. Cancer Imaging. 2005;5(1):116–27.
8. Artunduaga M, Eklund M, Van Der Beek JN, Hammer M, Littooij AS, Sandberg JK, et al. Imaging of pediatric renal tumors: a COG diagnostic imaging committee/SPR oncology committee white paper focused on Wilms tumor and nephrogenic rests. Pediatr Blood Cancer. 2023;70(S4):e30004.
9. Chung EM, Graeber AR, Conran RM. Renal tumors of childhood: radiologic-pathologic correlation part 1. The 1st decade: *from the radiologic pathology archives*. Radiographics. 2016;36(2):499–522.
10. Servaes SE, Hoffer FA, Smith EA, Khanna G. Imaging of Wilms tumor: an update. Pediatr Radiol. 2019;49(11):1441–52.
11. Son J, Lee EY, Restrepo R, Eisenberg RL. Focal renal lesions in pediatric patients. Am J Roentgenol. 2012;199(6):W668–82.
12. Chung EM, Lattin GE, Fagen KE, Kim AM, Pavio MA, Fehringer AJ, et al. Renal tumors of childhood: radiologic-pathologic correlation part 2. The 2nd decade: from the radiologic pathology archives. Radiographics. 2017;37(5):1538–58.

22 Hepatic Tumors

Nikshita Jain and Seema Kembhavi

22.1 Hepatic Tumors

22.1.1 Introduction

Primary liver tumors comprise of benign and malignant liver lesions which account for 5–6% of intra-abdominal masses in children [1]. Many of these tumors have unique imaging characteristics and in combination with clinical factors such as age, tumor markers, a prompt diagnosis can be established based on imaging. Thus, the knowledge of their imaging characteristics is crucial for a pediatric radiologist.

22.1.2 Consensus Guidelines for Imaging

Initial evaluation is with ultrasound, which will help identify the organ of origin and further appropriately protocol the subsequent cross-sectional study. When in doubt about liver origin, there are 2 clues that can help; one is that a liver mass will move with the liver, while the liver will slip over retroperitoneal masses. The other clue is that liver masses are associated with dilated regional intrahepatic vessels, both hepatic arteries and veins [2]. Once liver origin is confirmed, vascular evaluation, namely portal vein and its primary branches, hepatic veins, and IVC must also be evaluated for on ultrasound. It can show subtle vascular invasion that may not be identified on CT/MRI, and it can also be used as problem-solving tool after cross-sectional imaging.

Both CT and MRI can help in the effective staging of pediatric liver lesions, however given its superior soft tissue resolution and lack of ionizing radiation, MRI (with contrast) is the modality of choice [1]. Figure 22.1 shows a sample MRI protocol recommended by the pediatric LI-RADS working group.

Proper acquisition of post-contrast sequences at the appropriate times is essential for characterization of the liver lesion and the relevant vascular anatomy for staging and surgical planning. There are two ways to optimally acquire optimal post-contrast image times—either with the bolus tracking method (sequential scanning of the abdominal aorta at one level and triggering start of arterial phase) or the 'best guess' method (timings mentioned are appropriate for pediatric population), that is, arterial phase at 18–20 s after initiation of contrast agent injection, portal venous phase at 55–60 s and delayed venous phase between 2 and 3 min [1]. The T1-weighted fast spin-echo (FSE) fat-saturated sequence can be acquired after the dynamic postcontrast

N. Jain (✉)
Christian Medical College, Vellore, India

S. Kembhavi
Mackay Hospital and Health Services,
Mackay, Australia

I. Kumar et al. (eds.), *Practical Approach to Imaging in Pediatric Oncology*,
https://doi.org/10.1007/978-981-96-8158-7_22

Pre-contrast:

- Coronal single-shot T2-weighted
- Axial in-phase and out-of-phase
- Axial 3D T1-weighted gradient echo precontrast

Inject contrast:

- Dynamic axial 3D T1-weighted gradient echo in the hepatic arterial phase, portal venous phase, and delayed phase (timings elaborated in text)
- Coronal 3D T1-weighted gradient echo
- Axial T1-weighted FSE with fat saturation
- Axial 3D T1-weighted gradient echo delayed
- Axial T2-weighted fast spin-echo (FSE) with fat saturation Axial diffusion (*b* values = 0, 100, 800 sec/mm2)

At 20 min (with gadoxetate) and at 45 min (with gadobenate) from start of injection

- Hepatobiliary phase: axial and coronal 3D T1-weighted gradient echo

Fig. 22.1 Sample MRI protocol. (Adapted from Reference (1))

sequences and is helpful for lesion demarcation and its adjacent relations, especially in smaller children [1].

MRI Contrast: both extracellular (macrocyclic agents preferred—gadobutrol, gadoterate meglumine) and hepatobiliary specific agents (gadobenate dimeglumine and gadoxetate disodium) can be used. Gadoxetate is the preferred HBA of the two as it provides an earlier hepatobiliary phase than does gadobenate (20 minutes vs 45–60 min for gadobenate dimeglumine), and this is an important consideration in children undergoing MRI under anesthesia [1]. The utility of hepatobiliary agents is essentially due to a portion of the injected amount of the HBA being taken up by hepatocytes and excreted through bile which helps differentiates between liver lesions with and without functioning hepatocytes.

In the evaluation of pediatric liver lesions, multiphasic CT entails 2 phases only—a late arterial phase (antegrade filling of the hepatic artery and portal vein with no contrast agent in the hepatic veins) covering the dome of diaphragm to the lower pole of the kidneys and a portal venous phase covering the entire chest, abdomen and pelvis [1]. A third delayed venous phase between 3 and 5 min covering the liver is recommended only in patients undergoing screening for HCC (can be avoided if there is no lesion on the arterial phase by checking the image in real time); namely those children with chronic liver disease and in children older than 10 years [1].

At present, no role for PET-CT/bone scan/MRI brain is defined for pediatric liver lesions, as hepatoblastomas mainly metastasize to lungs.

22.2 Structured Radiological Reporting and Interpretation

The detailed discussion about PRETEXT stages and the annotation factors has been discussed subsequently (Table 22.1).

Note:

1. The same staging system is used after chemo and called PosText instead of PreText.
2. Even in non-hepatoblastoma Liver Tumors, it is useful to describe all the above-mentioned features.
3. Same reporting format to be used for MR imaging.

Important considerations when evaluating a child with a liver lesion are the age of the patient, laboratory findings (specifically serum AFP lev-

Table 22.1 Reporting template for hepatic mass in a child

Focality	One or more (F_0/F_1)
Size	[---]x[---]x[---] cm
Segments involved	<segments I/II/III/Iva/IVb/V/VI/VII/VIII>; sections involved: left lateral/left medial/right anterior/right posterior>
Caudate lobe	Yes/no
Parenchyma	<Homogenous/heterogenous> <intratumoral septation/bleed/calcification/ fat> <rupture (R)> <central scar: with/without calcification>
Margin	<Well defined/ill-defined/smooth/irregular/lobulated> <adjacent parenchyma>
MRI	<T1/T2 signal intensity> <scar/bleed/septation> <fibrous pseudo capsule>
Enhancement	<mild/marked> <homogenous/heterogenous/peripheral> <enhancement of scar: present/ absent>
Venous invasion	Hepatic vein <V_0/V positive: IVC/RHV/MHV/LHV>; Portal vein <P_0:P positive: PV Main/ Right branch/Left Branch>
Biliary system	<Involved/not involved> <segmental duct/CHD/CBD/GB> <IHBRD: present/absent>
Extrahepatic spread	<diaphragm> <adjacent organs> <omental/peritoneal nodule> <others>
Ascites	<absent/mild/moderate/gross> <peritoneal hemorrhage> <enhancing peritoneal lining>
Nodal status	<present/absent: N0/N1> <Periportal/retroperitoneal/others>
Distant metastasis	<present/absent>
Other organs	<other findings>
Impression	Likely diagnosis: PreText Stage: I/II/III/IV Additional factors F R E N C H P M

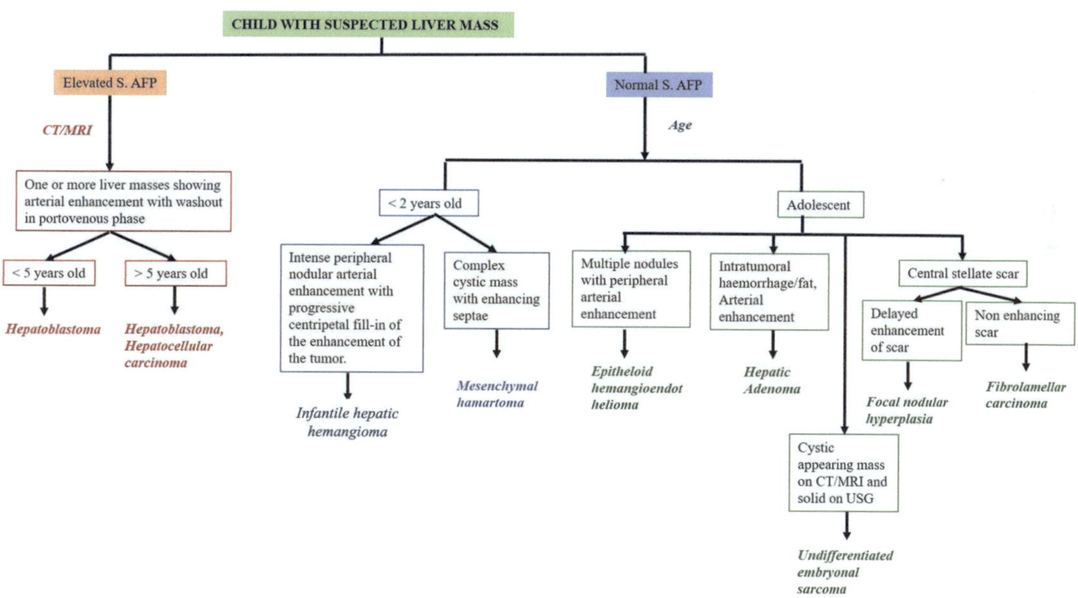

Fig. 22.2 Algorithmic approach to pediatric liver lesions

els), and imaging features. An algorithmic approach is suggested in Fig. 22.2.

It is pertinent to remember that serum AFP levels are normally elevated at birth, measuring 25,000–50,000 ng/mL, and do not reach the normal adult level of less than 25 ng/mL until 6 months of age. From birth till 6 months of age, the reference values are not yet standardized, however, Bader et al. [3] conducted a large literature review and suggested that the reference interval for AFP concentrations at birth was 15.7–146.5 Ag/mL, which was based on a 95% confidence interval (CI).

The neoplastic lesions of the liver in the pediatric population can be classified into benign and malignant types and the common such tumors are listed in Figs. 22.3a, 22.3b, 22.3c, 22.3d, and 22.3e, in the order of decreasing occurrence (Table 22.2). The most common primary malignant hepatic tumor in the pediatric population is hepatoblastoma and it occurs exclusively in patients younger than 5 years having no history of liver disease [4].

While some lesions seen in the pediatric liver are also found in adults, others are found exclusively in children, namely infantile and congenital hemangioma, hepatoblastoma, and mesenchymal hamartoma [1]. Like in adults, the most common neoplasm involving the liver in children is metastatic disease, usually from neuroblastoma, Wilms' tumor, or lymphoma.

Two-thirds of primary liver tumors in the pediatric population are malignant, and malignant primary hepatic tumors account for 1–2% of all childhood cancers [4]. Primary malignant hepatic neoplasms in children include epithelial (hepatocyte-derived) tumors, which are more common and include hepatoblastoma, HCC, and FLC, and tumors of mesenchymal derivation, which include UES, rhabdomyosarcoma, and malignant vascular tumors [4].

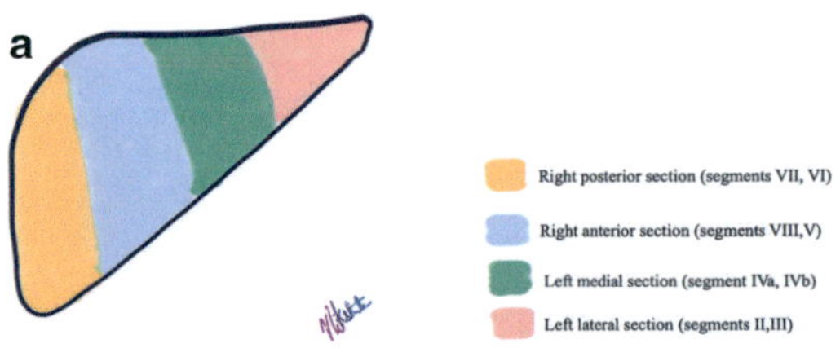

Fig. 22.3a PRETEXT groups have been schematically represented in (**a**)

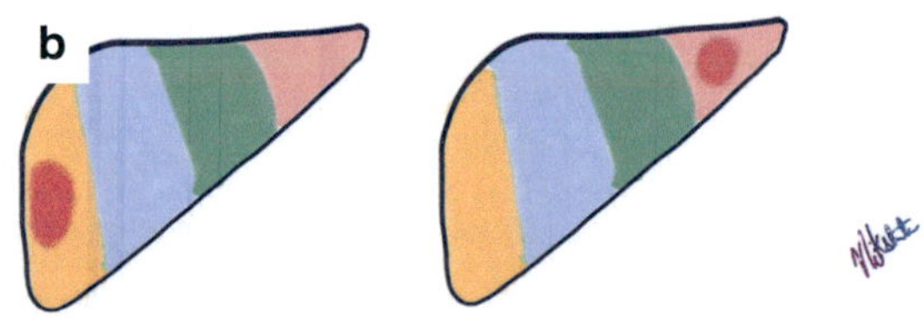

Fig. 22.3b Pretext I has been schematically represented in all possible presentations that can be categorized as Pretext I

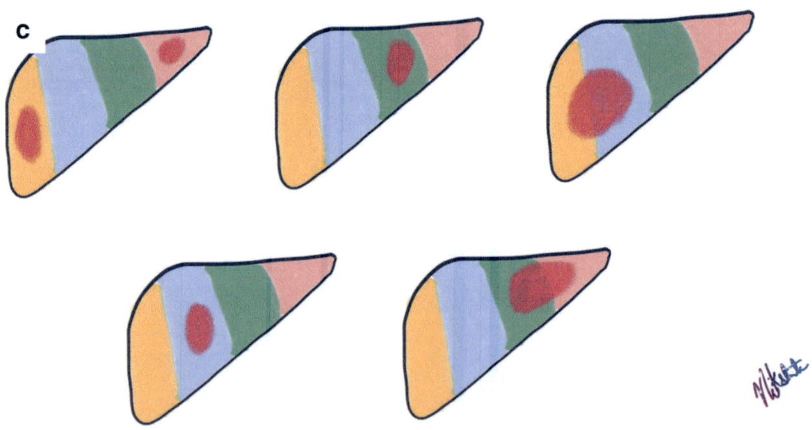

Fig. 22.3c Pretext II has been schematically represented in all possible presentations that can be categorized as Pretext II. Note how in Pretext II, only when 2 contiguous sections are free, it accounts for Pretext II, whether it is a unifocal or multifocal mass

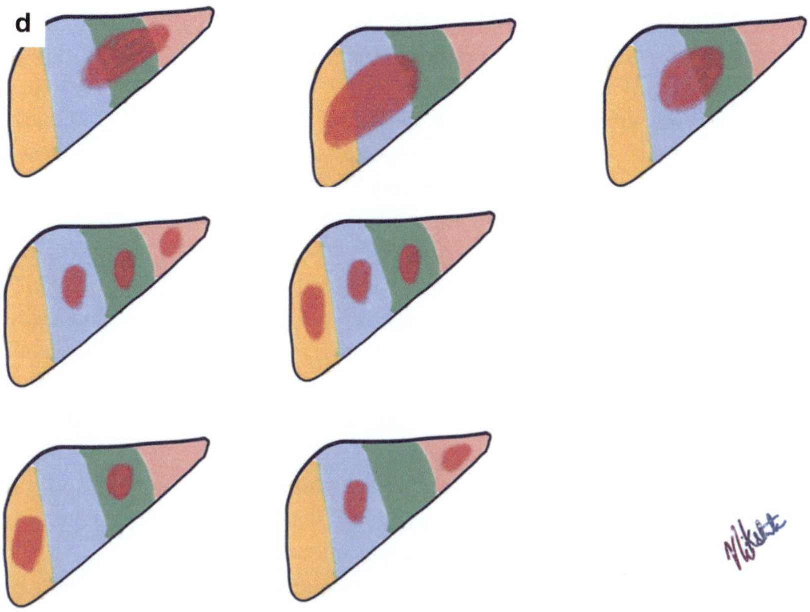

Fig. 22.3d Schematic representation of all possible presentations for Pretext III. Note that single large mass occupying three sections or single tumor occupying right anterior and left medial sections is Pretext III (first row) as well as multifocal tumors (3 lesions) occupying three contiguous sections (second row) or multifocal tumors (2 lesions) occupying two non-contiguous sections (third row) is also Pretext III

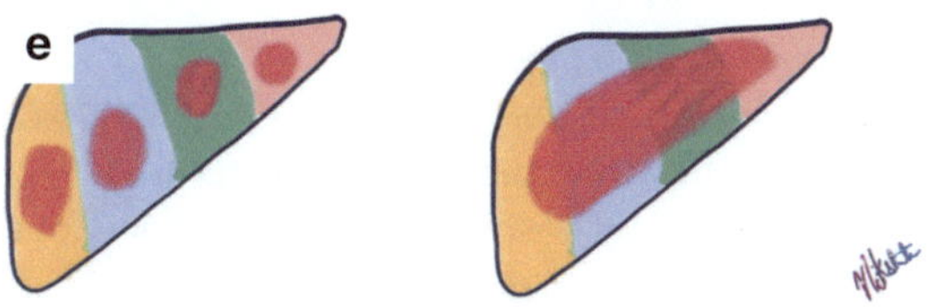

Fig. 22.3e Schematic representation of Pretext IV

Table 22.2 Liver lesions in children

Benign tumors	Malignant tumors
Infantile hepatic hemangioma (IHH)	Hepatoblastoma
Focal nodular hyperplasia (FNH)	Hepatocellular carcinoma (HCC)
Mesenchymal hamartoma	Fibrolamellar carcinoma (FLC)
Nodular regenerative hyperplasia (NRH)	Undifferentiated (embryonal) sarcoma (UES)
Hepatocellular adenoma	Angiosarcoma
	Embryonal rhabdomyosarcoma
	Epithelioid hemangioendothelioma (EHE)

22.3 Hepatoblastoma

A malignant neoplasm whose cells resemble embryonic liver, hepatoblastoma is the most common primary hepatic tumor in children, with 68% of cases manifesting in the first 2 years of life and 90% seen in patients younger than 5 years of age. A slight male-to-female predominance of 1.5:1 to 2:1 is seen.

At least 90% of patients with hepatoblastoma show abnormal elevation of AFP level. In patients with hepatoblastoma and elevated AFP level, serum AFP levels serve as a marker to monitor therapy and detect recurrence. In those children without raised AFP levels, also termed as low AFP hepatoblastoma, it is considered a high-risk feature, and predicts poor prognosis, with tumors often being metastatic at presentation.

Metastatic disease most frequently involves the lungs, with pulmonary metastases seen in 10–20% of cases. Other common sites of metastasis include the bone, brain, lymph nodes, eye, and ovary.

On imaging, the tumor is well circumscribed and may appear lobulated with septa. Epithelial hepatoblastomas typically demonstrate a homogeneous appearance, while mixed epithelial and mesenchymal tumors appear more heterogeneous due to osteoid, cartilaginous, and fibrous components. Like HCC, hepatoblastoma can invade the portal or hepatic veins. The appearance of hepatoblastoma at CT reflects a sharply circumscribed mass that is slightly hypoattenuating relative to the adjacent liver parenchyma on unenhanced and contrast-enhanced images. Speckled or amorphous calcification is seen in more than 50% of lesions. The tumor enhances slightly, but less than adjacent liver. About one-half of hepatoblastomas appear lobulated or septated, especially on contrast-enhanced images. In the arterial phase, enhancement of the periphery of the mass or of septa may be observed.

Differentials: IHH occurs almost exclusively in children under 1 year of age and may also contain calcifications, but the calcifications in IHH are generally fine and granular compared with the coarse, chunky calcifications in hepatoblastoma. Furthermore, IHH is a vascular tumor and enhances much more than adjacent liver, while hepatoblastoma typically enhances much less than adjacent liver. Occasionally, the peripheral rim enhancement on arterial phase images seen in hepatoblastoma may suggest IHH, but IHH is distinguished by intense nodular or corrugated peripheral enhancement with centripetal fill-in on delayed phase images. Finally, IHH is rarely associated with elevated serum AFP level, while AFP levels are elevated in most patients with hepatoblastoma.

Mesenchymal hamartoma of liver (MHL) can usually be distinguished by normal serum AFP levels in MHL and the fact that MHL is usually predominantly cystic.

HCC does occur in children and also causes elevation in serum AFP levels; however, it generally manifests after age 5 years often in children with underlying liver disease, while hepatoblastoma is rarely diagnosed after age 5 years and arises in normal liver.

22.4 Staging of Pediatric Liver Tumors

The staging of hepatoblastoma is done by using the PRETEXT system. The PRETEXT system was designed by the International Childhood Liver Tumor Strategy Group (SIOPEL—**S**ociété **I**nternationale d'**O**ncologie **P**édiatrique—**E**pithelial **L**iver Tumor Study Group) [2]. PRETEXT is used to describe tumor extent before any therapy, thus allowing more effective comparison between studies conducted by different groups. The system has good inter-observer reproducibility and good prognostic value in children with hepatoblastoma and is the basis of risk stratification [2]. After neo-adjuvant chemotherapy, the annotation is changed to POST-TEXT.

PRETEXT staging is based on Couinaud's system of segmentation of the liver.

In the pretext system, the liver segments are grouped into four sections as follows (Fig. 22.3a):

- Segments 2 and 3 (left lateral section).
- Segments 4a and 4b (left medial section).
- Segments 5 and 8 (right anterior section).
- Segments 6 and 7 (right posterior section).

The term section is used (where other authors use segment or sector) to avoid terminological confusion. Any disease that involves the caudate lobe is at least stage II.

The PRETEXT number is derived by subtracting the highest number of contiguous liver sections that are not involved by tumor from four. *Alternatively, the PRETEXT group (I, II, III, or IV) is based on determining the number of contiguous tumor-free liver sections, that is, the number of contiguous sections that would have to be resected to completely remove the tumor* [2].

This number is an estimate of the difficulty of the expected surgical procedure and also the residual liver tissue that is likely to be left after resection. Pedunculated tumors are considered to be confined to the liver and to occupy only the section(s) from which they originate. In addition to describing the intrahepatic extent of the primary tumor(s), the PRETEXT system includes certain other criteria. These assess multifocality, involvement of the inferior vena cava (IVC) or hepatic veins (designated V), involvement of the portal veins (P), extrahepatic abdominal disease (E), hemoperitoneum (H), nodal status (N), and distant metastases (M). Based on the presence of these imaging features, the pre-treatment risk stratification is done as mentioned in Table 22.3. The acronym FRENCH PM can be used to remember the additional criteria:

Table 22.3 PRETEXT additional criteria

Caudate lobe involvement (C): If the caudate lobe is involved, the tumor is said to be at least PRETEXT II by convention. (as the caudate lobe can be resected with either a right or a left hepatectomy)
Tumor focality (F): Two or more discrete hepatic tumors with normal intervening liver tissue is defined as multifocal disease Children presenting with multifocal disease tend to have a poorer prognosis compared to those with a single tumor focus With tumor shrinkage following neoadjuvant chemotherapy, it is possible for a unifocal tumor to transition into a multifocal presentation. In such cases, the PRETEXT classification may initially indicate a unifocal tumor, while the POST-TEXT classification may show it as multifocal
Portal vein status Positive: Any of the following: 1. The tumor obliterates the lumen (non-visualized) of both first-order portal veins or the main portal vein 2. The tumor encases over 50% or 180° of either both first-order portal veins or the main portal vein 3. Tumor thrombus in the right, left, or main portal veins First-order portal vein: Segment between the main portal vein bifurcation and its first major branch Any thrombus in the right, left, or main portal vein, including cavernous transformation is considered tumor thrombus
Hepatic vein /IVC involvement: V Positive: Any of the following: 1. Tumor obliterates the lumen of all three first-order hepatic veins or the intrahepatic IVC 2. Tumor encases over 50% or 180° of all three first-order hepatic veins or the intrahepatic IVC 3. Tumor thrombus in any first-order hepatic vein or the intrahepatic inferior vena cava Inability to visualize the lumen does not imply functional obstruction of the IVC. No need for collateral venous pathways or clinical signs for confirmation **First-order hepatic vein:** Segment between its junction with the IVC and its central branch **Intrahepatic inferior vena cava:** Portion surrounded by liver tissue by more than 50% or 180° **Tumor thrombus:** Any thrombus in a first-order hepatic vein or IVC is classified as a tumor thrombus, appearing as an enhancing mass on imaging
Extra-hepatic abdominal disease (E): Any one of the following: **Positive:** Any of the following: 1. Tumor crosses boundaries/tissue planes, appearing both above and below the diaphragm or extending through the abdominal wall 2. Tumor is surrounded by normal tissue by over 180° (not applicable to intrahepatic tumors surrounded by normal liver) 3. Presence of peritoneal nodules: at least one nodule $\geq$10 mm or two or more nodules $\geq$5 mm Simple ascites is not considered extrahepatic disease Biopsy tracks: tumor should not be considered as present unless there is a discrete tumor nodule Coronal or sagittal planes should be used to assess for diaphragmatic disease and other extra-hepatic disease
Tumor rupture or intraperitoneal hemorrhage: R positive: (any one of the following) 1. Internal complexity/septations within fluid 2. High-density fluid on CT (>25 Hounsfield units) 3. Imaging characteristics of blood or blood degradation products on MRI 4. Heterogeneous fluid on ultrasound with echogenic debris 5. Visible rupture/hepatic capsular defect on imaging Non-hemorrhagic or simple ascites, hemorrhage resulting from a tumor biopsy, surgical rupture, subcapsular fluid collections are not considered tumor rupture
Nodal metastases: N positive: 1. Lymph node with a short-axis diameter of >1 cm or a portocaval lymph node with short-axis diameter >1.5 cm OR; 2.Spherical lymph node shape with loss of fatty hilum Nodal metastases in hepatoblastoma are much less common than in hepatocellular carcinoma

(continued)

Table 22.3 (continued)

Distant metastases: M positive: 1. At least one non-calcified pulmonary nodule ≥5 mm; OR 2. Two or more non-calcified pulmonary nodules, each ≥3 mm Hepatoblastoma is common in premature infants, often linked to chronic lung disease and potential atelectasis due to anesthesia **Imaging strategies:** 1. Perform chest CT before abdominal imaging for sedated children 2. Use positive pressure for lung inflation if intubated 3. Prone imaging can improve lung base clarity in persistent atelectasis Bone and brain metastases are uncommon; routine imaging beyond chest CT is unnecessary unless symptoms or increased serum alpha-fetoprotein levels occur. Bone pain may result from fractures or paraneoplastic osteopenia rather than metastasis, and a biopsy is recommended to confirm bone metastases

1. **C**audate lobe involvement
2. Tumor **F**ocality
3. **P**ortal vein involvement
4. **H**epatic vein/IVC involvement
5. **E**xtrahepatic disease
6. Tumor **R**upture/hemoperitoneum
7. **N**odal metastases
8. Distant **M**etastases

Although the PRETEXT system is principally used for hepatoblastoma, it is intended to be applicable to all primary malignant liver tumors of childhood, including hepatocellular carcinoma and epithelioid hemangioendothelioma. Figures 22.4a, 22.4b, 22.5, 22.6, 22.7, 22.8a, 22.8b, 22.9, 22.10, 22.11, 22.12, 22.13, and 22.14 showcase examples for various Pretext groups (Figs. 22.15, 22.16, 22.17, 22.18, 22.19, 22.20, 22.21, 22.22, and 22.23).

PRETEXT grouping (Figs. 22.3a, 22.3b, 22.3c, 22.3d, and 22.3e).

PRETEXT I (Fig. 22.3b): Includes a small proportion of childhood liver tumors localized to the left lateral or right posterior section.

PRETEXT II (Fig. 22.3c): Tumors are limited to the right or left lobe, including left medial or right anterior sections. Multifocal tumors involving only the left lateral and right posterior sections are rare.

PRETEXT III (Fig. 22.3d): Unifocal tumors spare either the left lateral or right posterior section and are common. Distinguishing invasion from compression is vital for risk assessment in hepatoblastoma. Anterior central tumors involve segment 4 and either or both segments 5 and 8. Multifocal PRETEXT III tumors may spare the right anterior or left medial sections, or involve two noncontiguous sections, which are rare.

PRETEXT IV (Fig. 22.3e): Involves all liver sections, often as multifocal tumors or a large solitary tumor encompassing all four sections.

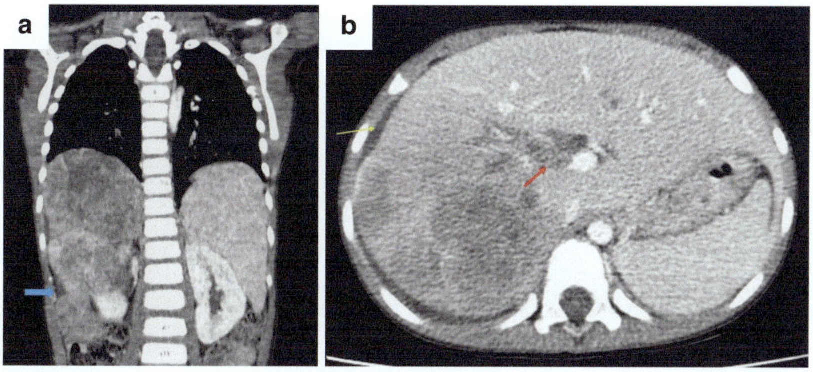

Fig. 22.4a Coronal reformatted contrast-enhanced CT section of a 4-year-old boy with hepatoblastoma depicting extrahepatic extension of tumor (blue arrow). Axial post-contrast CT section depicting thrombosis of the right branch of the portal vein (red arrow) and perihepatic fluid (yellow arrow). Since left lobe is free of tumor, staged as Pretext II

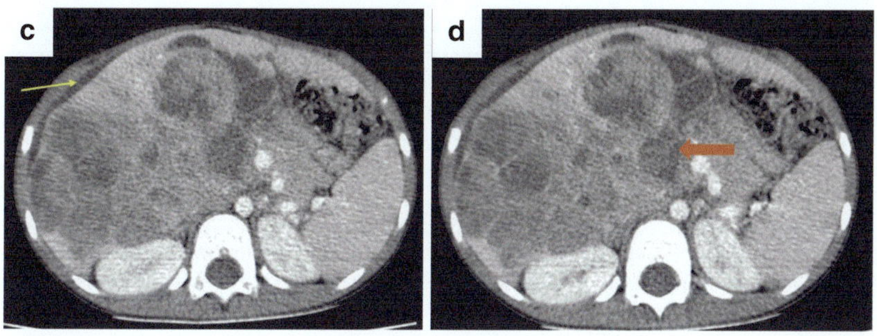

Fig. 22.4b Axial contrast-enhanced sections of the same patient with multifocality (F1) seen on the image on the right. An enlarged periportal node (orange arrow) (N1) is seen in the image on the left. Thin rim of ascites/perihepatic fluid (yellow arrow) is also notedHence, final staging: Pretext II F1 N1 P1

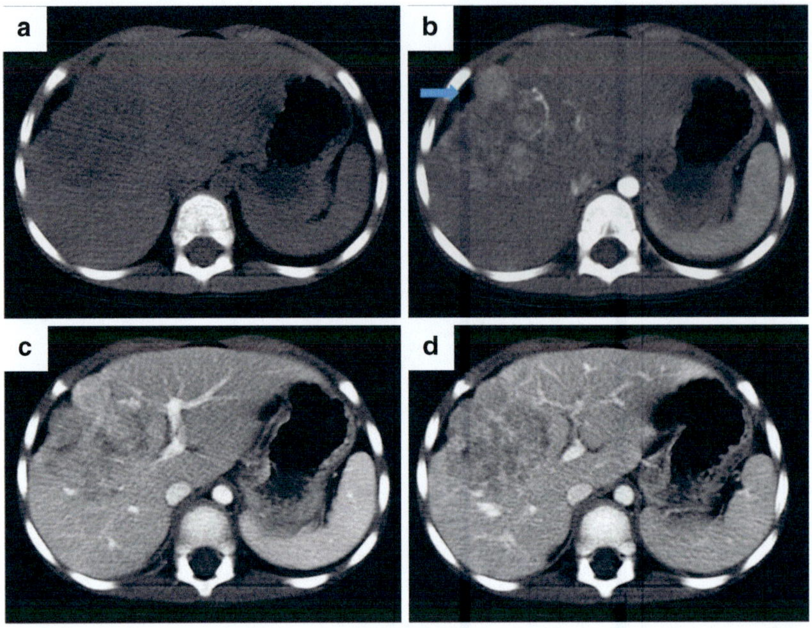

Fig. 22.5 Axial CT sections at the same level taken in different phases: plain (**a**, top right), arterial phase (**b**, top left), portal phase (**c**, bottom right), and delayed venous phase (**d**, bottom left). The patient is a 3-year-old male child with raised AFP levels, diagnosed to be hepatoblastoma
An ill-defined lesion showing arterial phase enhancement (**b**) with washout in the portovenous phase (**c, d**) is seen limited to the right anterior section. Since the left medial and lateral sections (contiguous) are free of tumor, this patient is staged as PRETEXT II. The blue arrow shows the surface irregularity and capsular retraction that was considered as extrahepatic extension in the earlier Pretext grouping but not in the 2017 update
Final stage: Pretext II E0

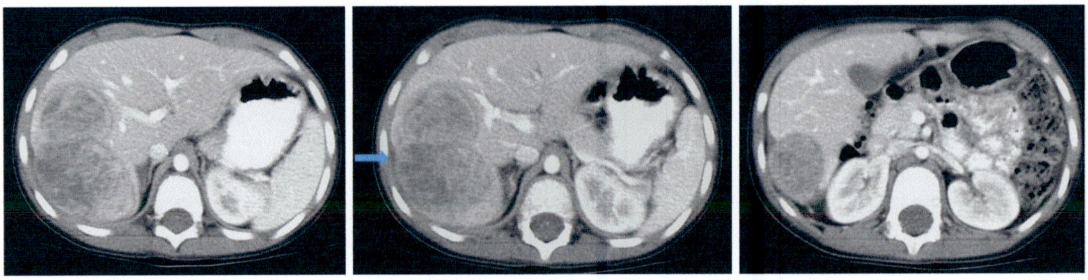

Fig. 22.6 Axial post-contrast CT sections of a 3y/M with hepatoblastoma (elevated AFP), depicting a heterogeneously enhancing well-marginated lesion occupying the right anterior and posterior sections, with the left medial and lateral sections free of tumor, hence staged as PRETEXT II. A separate lesion is noted in segment VI, thus making it multifocal
Final staging: Pretext II F1

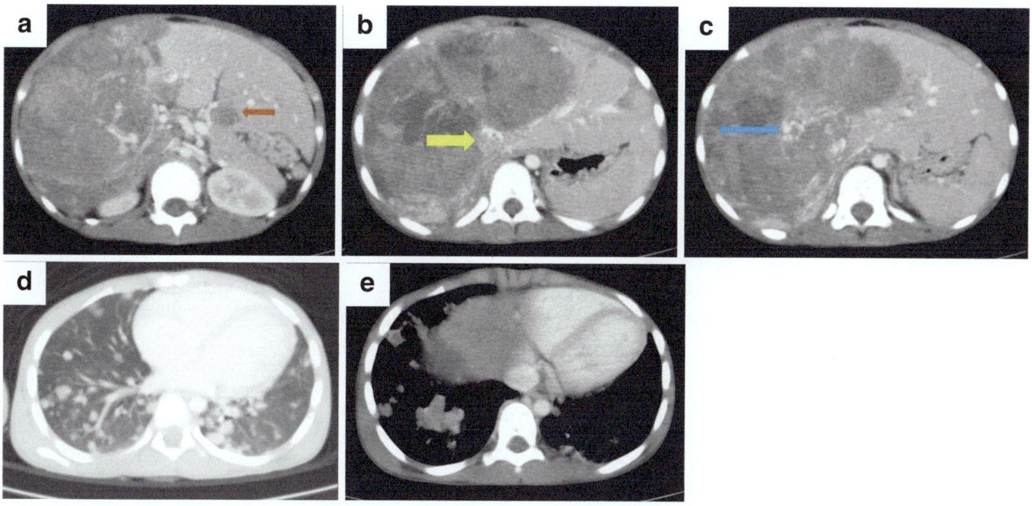

Fig. 22.7 A 9-year-old girl with raised AFP and large liver mass, diagnosed as hepatoblastoma. Post-contrast axial CT sections depict a large heterogeneously enhancing lesion, occupying all sections. Multiple separate lesions (orange arrow in image **a**) were noted in left lobe. Hence, no section free of tumor seen. The right branch of portal vein was thrombosed (blue arrow in image **c**)
Involvement of IVC also noted (yellow arrow in image **b**)
Axial CT in lung window (**d**) and soft tissue window (**e**) of same patient showing metastatic lung lesions
Hence final staging: Pretext IV F1 P1 V3 M1

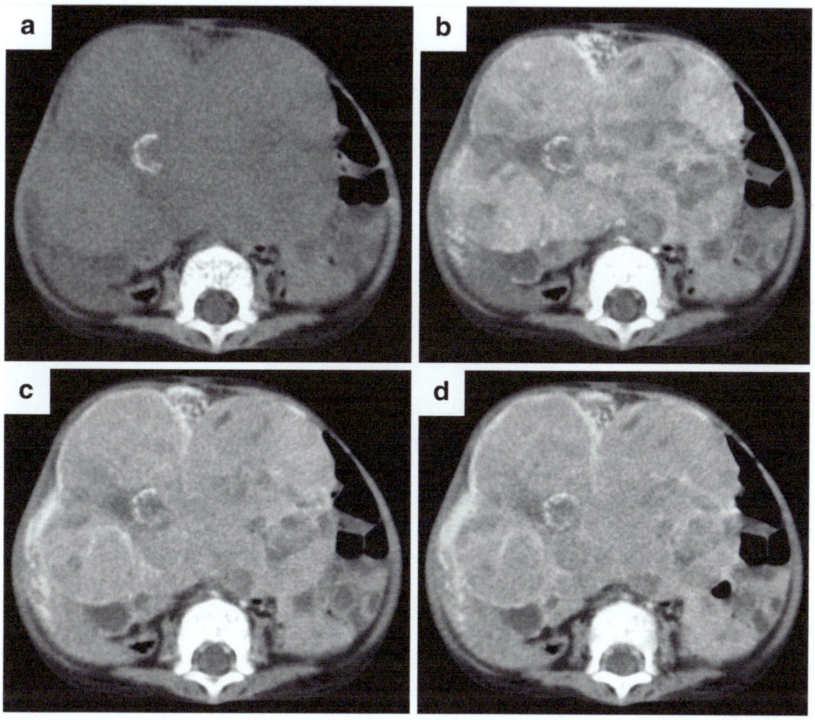

Fig. 22.8a 2y/M with a lobulated capsulated mass histopathologically proven hepatoblastoma. Pretext III (only right posterior section is free)
Triphasic CT done and demonstrates the following:
Plain axial CT section shows calcifications within the mass (top left)
There is intense enhancement of the mass in the arterial phase (top right), with washout in the portovenous phase (bottom right and left). The mass appears almost isodense to liver in the delayed venous phase (bottom right)
Note made of persistent enhancement of the capsule

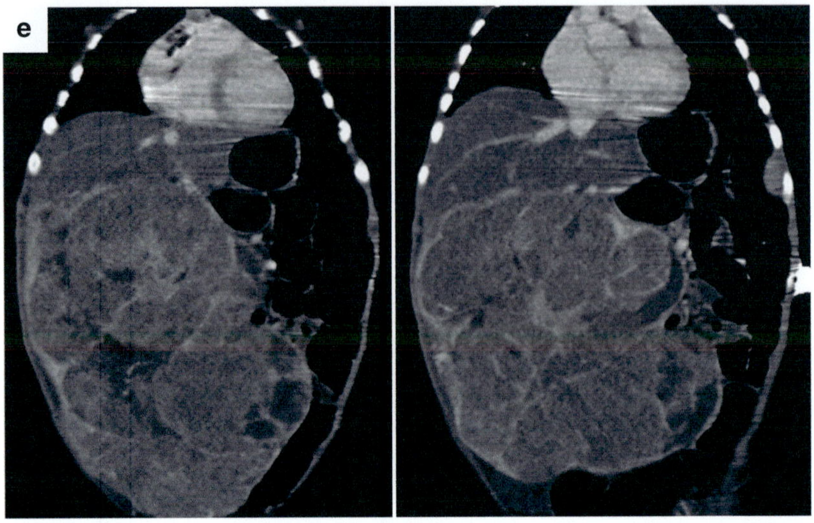

Fig. 22.8b Coronal reformatted images of the same patient showing the mass limited by a well-defined capsule, hence favoring exophytic nature of the mass, as opposed to extrahepatic spread. Since this patient had no other high-risk factors, it is vital to definitively comment on extrahepatic spread of tumor for decision on management

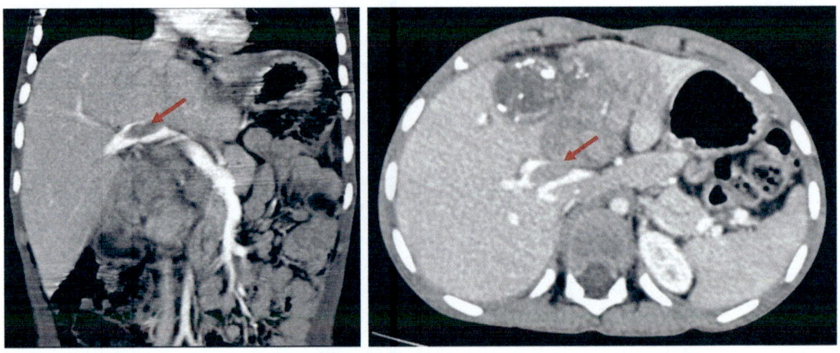

Fig. 22.9 Coronal and axial post-contrast CT images of a 4-year-old boy with Pretext III hepatoblastoma, depicting main portal vein thrombosis (red arrow)

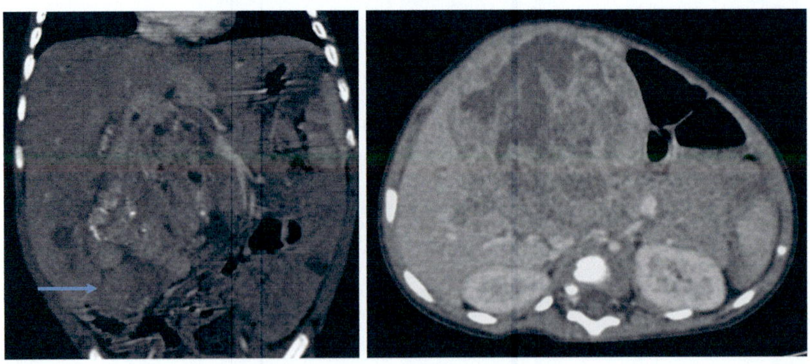

Fig. 22.10 Coronal and axial post-contrast CT sections of a 7-month-old male child with a heterogeneously enhancing mass occupying 3 sections of the liver and with foci of calcifications within proven hepatoblastoma (Pretext III) demonstrating a separate peritoneal nodule in the right subhepatic space (blue arrow)
Final stage: Pretext III E2

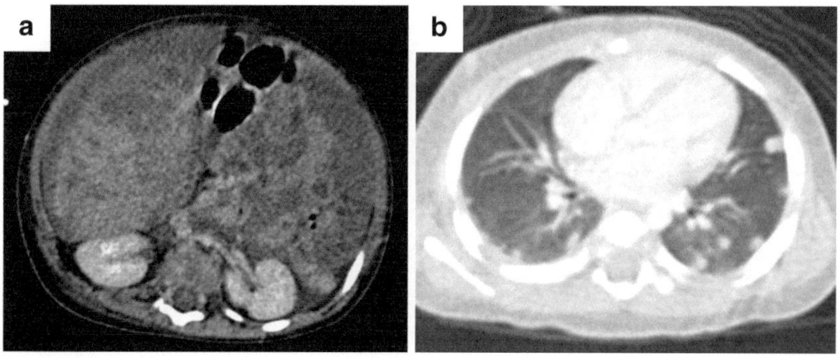

Fig. 22.11 A 1-year-old male child presenting with hepatoblastoma presenting with tumor rupture and lung metastases. Image (**a**) depicts a heterogeneously enhancing liver mass with hemoperitoneum (attenuation of 40–50HU). Image (**b**) is axial CT section in lung window revealing multiple soft tissue nodules suggestive of metastases. Final diagnosis: Pretext I H1 M1

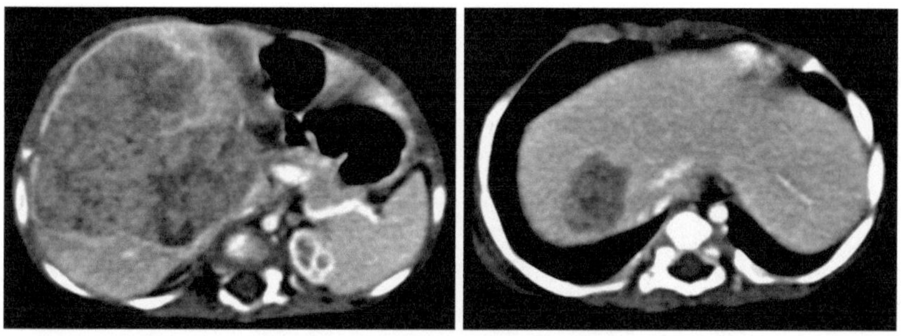

Fig. 22.12 Post-contrast axial CT sections in a 6-month-old male child with hepatoblastoma, revealing a large lobulated mass limited by compressed liver tissue forming a pseudocapsule. Another separate lesion is noted in the right posterior section, making it multifocal disease. Final stage: Pretext II F1

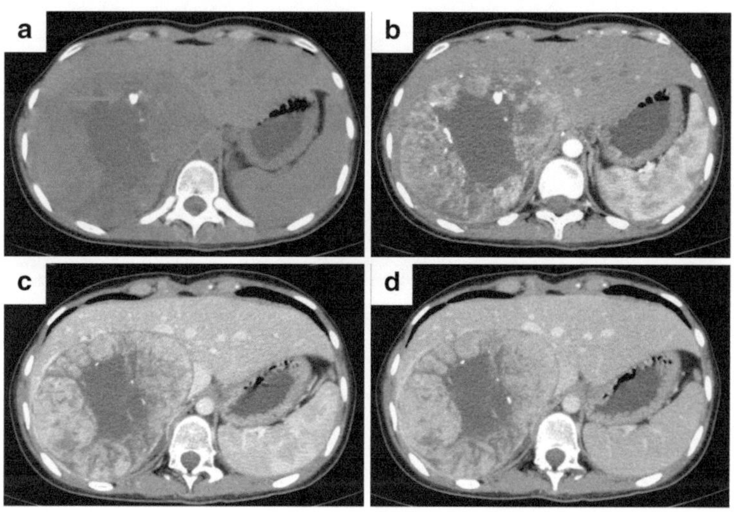

Fig. 22.13 Case of hepatoblastoma in a 14-year-old female child. Hepatoblastoma is unusual in children >5 years old. This case also depicts atypical imaging features. Plain and post-contrast triphasic axial CT sections reveal a well-circumscribed predominantly peripherally enhancing mass with central necrotic changes and foci of calcifications (blue arrow in image **a**) within. The enhancing portion is hyperenhancing in the arterial phase (image **b**) with washout in the portovenous phase (image **c**) appears almost isodense to liver in the delayed venous phase (image **d**). Portal vein and IVC are uninvolved. Pretext I E0 V0 P0

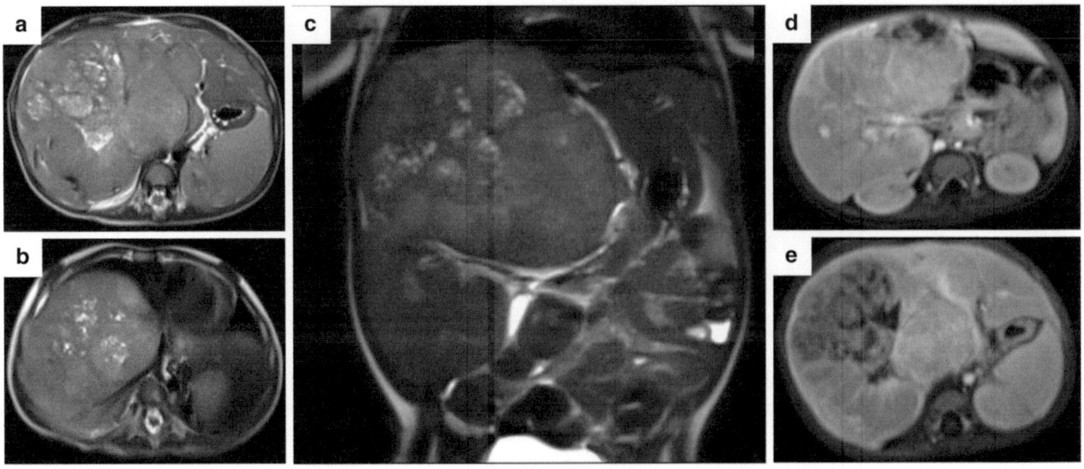

Fig. 22.14 2-year old with elevated serum AFP and well-defined liver mass (image **a**) sparing only segments II and III (left lateral section) suggesting PRETEXT III hepatoblastoma. Segment VII is involved, and hence right posterior section is involved. The mass shows heterogenous internal morphology with intermediate to T2 signal hyperintensity (images **b** and **c**). On post-contrast images (**d** and **e**) shows heterogenous post contrast enhancement with necrotic non-enhancing areas within

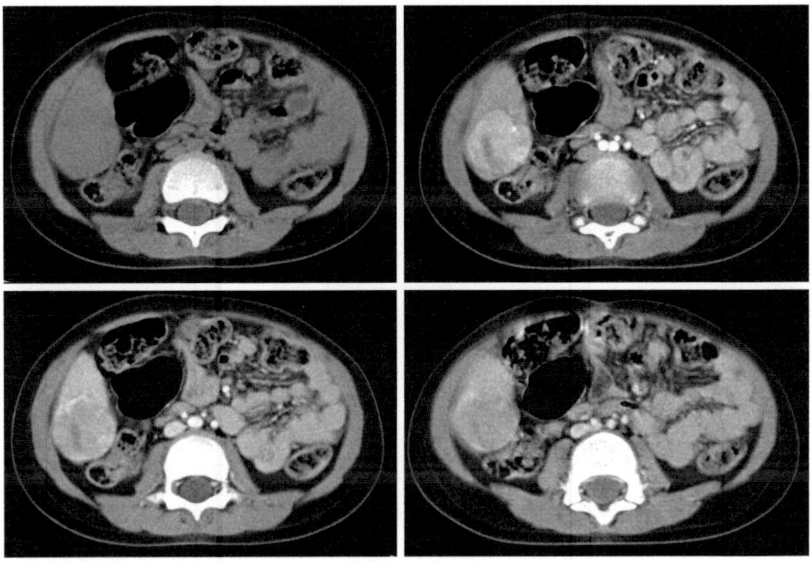

Fig. 22.15 Plain and post-contrast triphasic axial CT sections reveal a well capsulated mass in segment VI of liver, appearing isodense to liver on plain scan (top right), with intense arterial enhancement (top left) and washout on the portovenous images, appearing almost isodense to liver on the delayed phase (bottom left). Typical imaging features of HCC in an adolescent male child

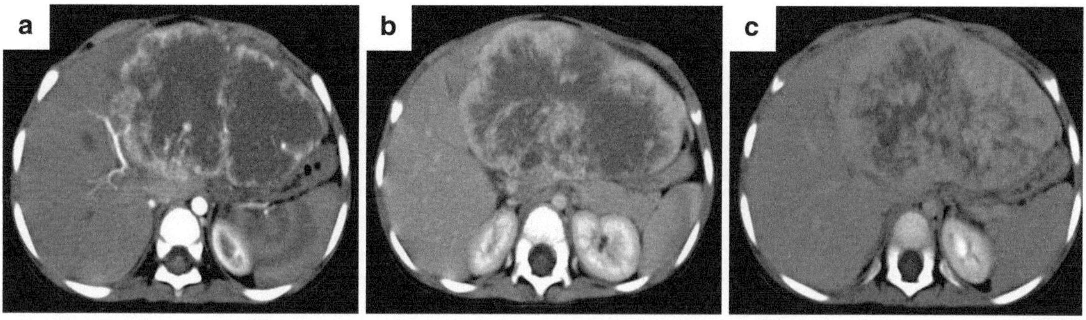

Fig. 22.16 Axial post-contrast CT depicting a well circumscribed liver mass showing peripheral nodular enhancement in the arterial phase (**a**), with progressive centripetal fill-in of enhancement in the portal phase (**b**), appearing almost isodense to liver in the delayed phase (**c**), suggestive of infantile hemangioma

Fig. 22.17 Axial post-contrast CT in a 11-month-old female with normal AFP, depicting multiple lesions with nodular peripheral enhancement. Morphologically the lesion is typical for infantile hemangiomas. Due to the absence of any section free of tumor, this is PRETEXT IV
M ultifocality noted
Final staging: Pretext IV F1

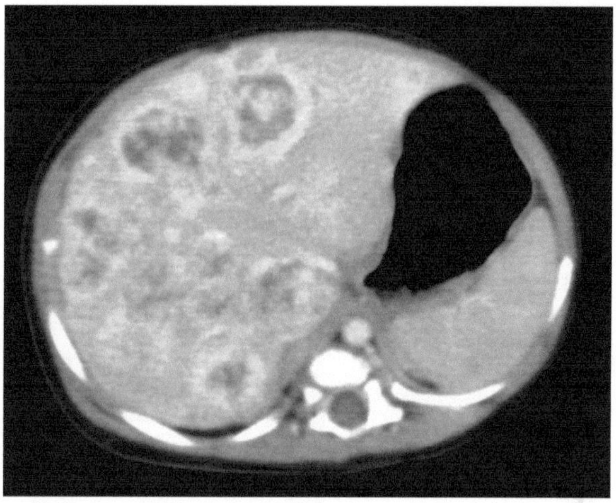

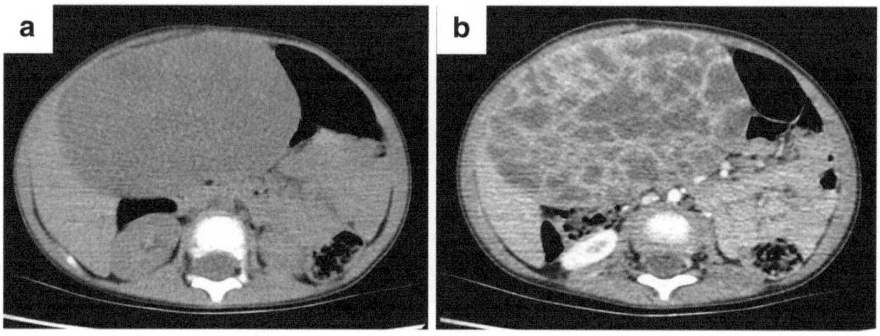

Fig. 22.18 Pre (image **a**) and post-contrast (image **b**) axial CT sections in an 18-month-old male with normal AFP levels, showing a complex cystic mass with enhancing septae. The normal AFP levels rules out possibility of hepatoblastoma. The pattern of enhancement is not typical for infantile hemangioma, known to occur in this age group and also showing normal AFP levels. Hence, a final diagnosis of mesenchymal hamartoma was made based on the imaging morphology and tumor marker levels

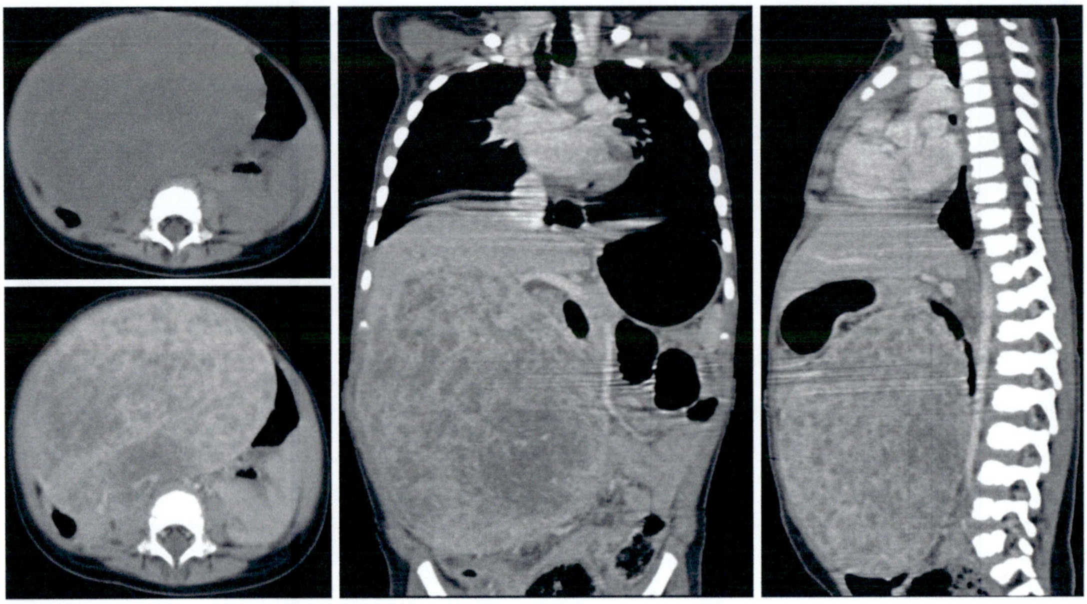

Fig. 22.19 Plain and post-contrast axial and reformatted sagittal and coronal images depicting a large heterogeneously enhancing mass with multiple cystic spaces within and exophytic component, in a 16-month-old female child. Diagnosis-mesenchymal hamartoma

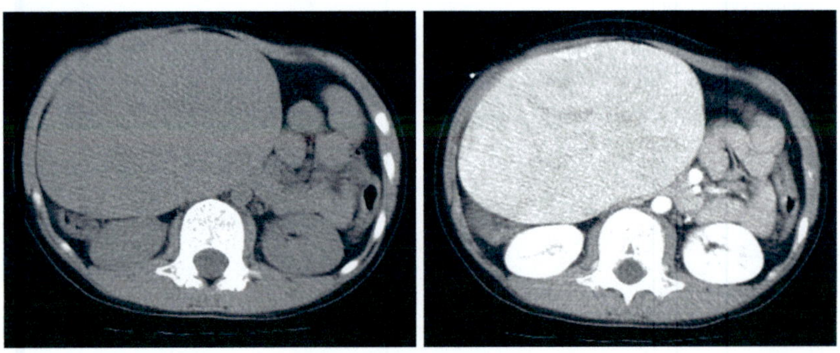

Fig. 22.20 An 11-year-old male child with plain and post-contrast axial CT sections demonstrating an inhomogenously enhancing mass arising from left lobe of liver. Histopathological diagnosis: hepatic adenoma

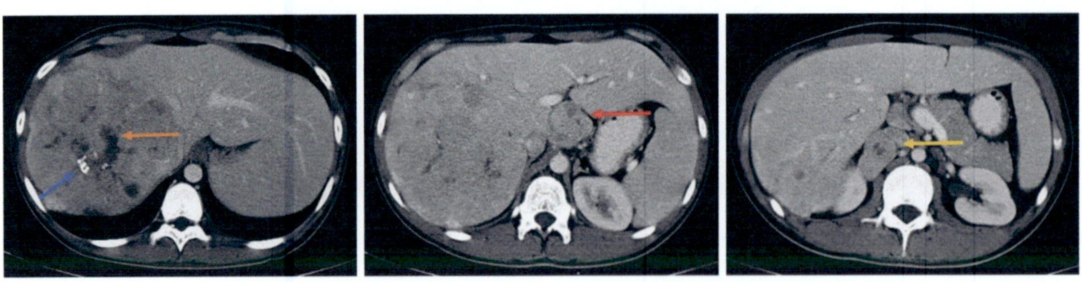

Fig. 22.21 A 15-year-old male with contrast-enhanced axial CT sections revealing a heterogeneously enhancing mass with central non-enhancing scar (orange arrow) and foci of calcifications (blue arrow) within. Enlarged nodal metastases are also noted in the celiac (red arrow) and paracaval region (yellow arrow). Pretext II N1. Final histopathological diagnosis-fibrolamellar carcinoma

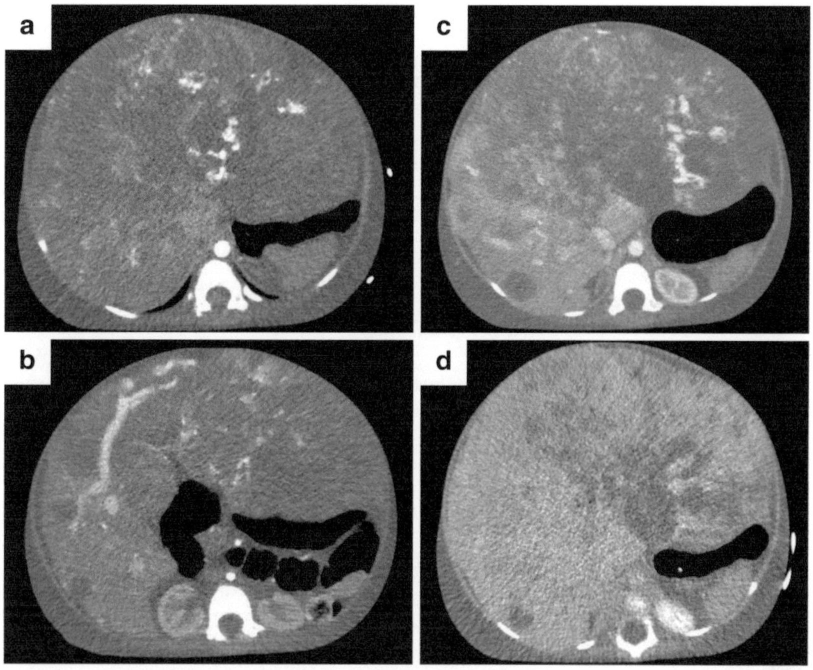

Fig. 22.22 A 4-year-old presented with bleeding and low platelet count. Arterial phase (images **a** and **b**) shows intense focal areas of puddling of contrast, particularly in the periphery as well as a hypertrophied vessel within. On the portovenous phase (**c**) there is further filling in of contrast which is further evident in the delayed phase (**d**). Serum AFP levels were normal. While imaging characteristics are fairly similar to that of a hemangioma, histopathology revealed hepatic angiosarcoma with Kasabach-Merrit syndrome

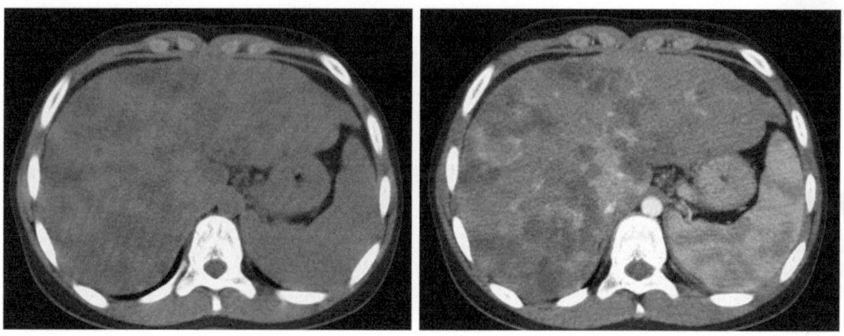

Fig. 22.23 Multiple hypoattenuating liver nodules on plain axial CT, showing predominant peripheral rim enhancement on post-contrast images, in a case of epithelioid hemangioendothelioma in a 10-year-old male child

22.5 Children's Oncology Group (COG) Staging

In the continent of North America, upfront surgery is often offered to patients with liver tumors. In such cases, the COG staging system is used (Table 22.4) and for hepatoblastoma it is defined by the extent of tumor resection and tumor histology before initiation of chemotherapy (Table 22.5).

22.5.1 Hepatocellular Carcinoma (HCC)

HCC is a malignant tumor of cells of hepatocyte differentiation and the second most common pediatric primary hepatic malignancy. In the pediatric age group, HCC usually occurs in children 10–14 years of age with a male-to-female ratio of 1.8:1 to 2.2:1.

Table 22.4 Children's Oncology Group (COG) staging for hepatoblastoma

Stage I	Complete surgical resection with negative margins
Stage II	Gross total resection with microscopic residual disease at surgical margins; or preoperative or intraoperative tumor rupture
Stage III	Unresectable tumors; or partially resected tumors with residual measurable tumor; or patients with abdominal lymph node involvement
Stage IV	Metastatic disease with complete or incomplete tumor resection

At unenhanced CT, HCC usually appears as a solitary mass or as multiple well or poorly defined, slightly hypoattenuating masses. A mosaic appearance is more commonly seen in larger lesions owing to components of hemorrhage, necrosis, fat, and calcification. HCC is predominantly supplied by the hepatic artery and typically appears hyperattenuating in the hepatic arterial phase. The appearance during the portal venous phase is variable and may or may not demonstrate rapid washout of contrast material. If present, a tumor capsule may be seen as a

Table 22.5 Summary of diagnostic pearls for pediatric hepatic masses

	Age	S. AFP	Imaging	D/D
Infantile hepatic hemangioma (IHH)	<6 months	Normal	Arterial phase: intense peripheral nodular or corrugated enhancement Portal venous and delayed phase: Progressive centripetal fill-in of the enhancement of the tumor 50% show stippled calcifications	Hepatoblastoma Mesenchymal hamartoma Metastatic neuroblastoma Angiosarcoma
Focal nodular hyperplasia	Adolescent	Normal	Central stellate scar that shows delayed enhancement	Hepatoblastoma HCC FLC Hepatic adenoma
Mesenchymal hamartoma	<2 years	Normal	Complex cystic mass with enhancing septae	Hepatoblastoma Infantile hemangioendothelioma UES
Nodular regenerative hyperplasia		Normal	Hypodense, non-enhancing	
Hepatic adenoma	>10 years, girls	Normal	Intratumoral hemorrhage, arterial enhancement	HCC FNH FLC
Hepatoblastoma	<2 years	Elevated	Coarse, chunky calcifications Hypoenhancing as compared to normal liver	Infantile hemangioendothelioma Mesenchymal hamartoma HCC
Hepatocellular carcinoma	10–14 years	Elevated	Arterial phase enhancement with washout in portovenous phase	FLC Hepatic adenoma FNH Metastases
Fibrolamellar carcinoma	Young adults	Slightly increased	Well demarcated, non-enhancing scar	FNH HCC Hepatic adenoma Focal nodular hyperplasia

hypoattenuating rim on unenhanced images and may enhance in the delayed phase. Portal and hepatic venous invasion may be identified. Rarely, tumor rupture may be seen with intra- or extrahepatic hemorrhage.

22.5.2 Infantile Hepatic Hemangioma

Hepatic hemangioma (HH) is a vascular neoplasm and the most common benign hepatic tumor of infancy. Based on the International Society for the Study of Vascular Anomalies (ISSVA), HHs are classified into three different subtypes: focal HH, multiple infantile HH (IHH), and diffuse IHH [5]. Focal HH, also known as congenital HH (CHH), is the hepatic form of the congenital hemangioma of the skin and is fully formed at birth [5]. CH may demonstrate three distinct patterns—tumors may rapidly involute in infancy—rapidly involuting congenital hemangioma (RICH), do not involute — non-involuting congenital hemangioma (NICH), or partially involute—involuting congenital hemangioma (PICH) [6]. In contrast, IHH shares the same proliferation and regression phases as cutaneous infantile hemangioma (IH) [5]. Nearly 90% of hepatic hemangioma are diagnosed in the first 6 months of life, and one-third are diagnosed within the first month. There is a slight female predominance and an increased prevalence in patients with hemihypertrophy and Beckwith-Wiedemann syndrome.

Serum α-fetoprotein (AFP) levels are rarely elevated and if elevated, it is much lower than hepatoblastoma. Some IHHs can result in severe complications, including congestive heart failure, hypothyroidism, and abdominal compartment syndrome [5]. Thrombocytopenia, coagulopathy, and anemia may possibly co-exist in patients with IHH which may overlap with the Kasabach–Merritt phenomenon (KMP) that is exclusively associated with Kaposiform hemangioendothelioma and tufted angioma [5].

Hepatic hemangiomas are high-flow vascular tumors. Central hemorrhage, necrosis, fibrosis, and calcification are often seen in large lesions. In diffuse disease, the liver is massively enlarged and replaced by multiple large masses, causing mass effect on adjacent organs and compression of the inferior vena cava. Evidence of high flow is manifested by enlargement of the hepatic arteries and veins and tapering of the abdominal aorta below the origin of the celiac axis. Due to the risk of bleeding, biopsy of these masses is avoided, and the diagnosis is made on the basis of typical imaging findings and the demonstration of involution at follow-up [7, 8].

On dynamic contrast-enhanced CT, precontrast images show well-defined mass or masses that are hypoattenuating to the adjacent uninvolved liver. Speckled calcifications are noted in up to 50% of cases, usually in the large focal tumors. On arterial phase images, there is generally intense peripheral nodular or corrugated enhancement. On portal venous and delayed phase images, there is progressive centripetal fill-in of the enhancement of the tumor. Small multifocal tumors enhance intensely and uniformly, whereas large focal tumors with central hemorrhage, necrosis, or fibrosis enhance centripetally and may never completely enhance in the center. Patients with diffuse disease demonstrate near total replacement of the liver by innumerable lesions with centripetal enhancement [8, 9].

22.5.3 Focal Nodular Hyperplasia

Focal nodular hyperplasia (FNH) is a benign hepatic lesion very rarely described in the pediatric population. FNH has been reported in all pediatric age groups with prevalence in 7–8-year-old children [8, 10, 11].

Vascular malformations, such as hypoplasia or agenesis of the portal vein, vascular dysplasia, Budd-Chiari syndrome, hereditary hemorrhagic telangiectasia, and vascular injuries, such as thrombosis, vasculitis, intimal hyperplasia, high sinusoidal pressure, or increased flow after pediatric oncological therapy, have all been suggested as the underlying mechanism. It has been reported more frequently in patients treated for pediatric cancers with chemotherapy or hematopoietic stem cell transplantation. The use of high dosage of alkylating agents, the occurrence of venous occlusive disease, graft-versus-host disease, and other variables linked to the hematopoietic stem cell transplantation procedure can represent risk factors for the development of FNH in the pediatric age [10, 11].

It arises from a polyclonal proliferation of hepatocytes, Kupffer cells, vascular structures, and biliary ductules. The lesion demonstrates a complex architecture, with well-differentiated hepatocytes forming nodules subdivided by fibrous septa, which coalesce to form a characteristic central vascular stellate scar [8, 9].

Reflecting its pathological features, it appears similar to normal liver, and the lesion may be inapparent except for mass effect on adjacent structures. Pediatric patients with a history of malignancy are more likely to have multiple FNH nodules and less likely to have central scars, while pediatric patients without a history of malignant lesions are more likely to have FNH lesions with central scars [11, 9].

At unenhanced CT, FNH is typically well circumscribed and iso to slightly hypoattenuating to uninvolved liver, and the scar is hypoattenuating. It has a typical homogeneous appearance, which is a very helpful feature for distinguishing FNH from malignant tumors, which are more likely to appear heterogeneous due to hemorrhage, necrosis, and calcifications. It typically demonstrates early, uniform enhancement after intravenous administration of contrast. The mass enhances more than the adjacent liver in the arterial and early portal venous phases due to vascular supply from the hepatic artery, and becomes isoattenuating to the liver in the late portal venous and delayed phases. Enlarged feeding arteries may be apparent on arterial phase images. The stellate scar typically enhances on delayed images.

22.5.4 Mesenchymal Hamartoma

Mesenchymal hamartoma of the liver is the second most common benign liver mass in children. Most commonly seen in children younger than 2 years of age, with nearly all lesions (95%) discovered by age 5 years. There is a slight male predominance. Serum AFP levels are typically normal [12, 13].

The imaging spectrum ranges from a predominantly cystic mass with thin or thick septa to a predominantly solid mass containing a few small cysts. On CT, mesenchymal hamartoma appears as a complex cystic mass. The cystic components show water attenuation, whereas the stromal components are hypoattenuating to surrounding liver. The septa and solid (stromal) elements enhance [12, 14].

22.5.5 Nodular Regenerative Hyperplasia

Nodular regenerative hyperplasia (NRH) is a rare benign process of the liver which consists of multiple monoacinar regenerative nodules in the absence of fibrous septa and is frequently associated with various nonhepatic chronic diseases, including myeloproliferative disorders (leukemia, polycythemia vera), lymphoproliferative disorders (lymphoma, plasma cell dyscrasia), and collagen diseases (rheumatoid arthritis, polyarteritisnodosa, lupus erythematosus). Rare pediatric cases are mostly in association with the congenital absence of the portal vein [15–17].

They usually appear hypodense to surrounding liver parenchyma, with no significant enhancement in arterial and portovenous phases. This is a differentiating feature from hepatic adenoma and focal nodular hyperplasia.

22.5.6 Hepatocellular Adenoma

Hepatocellular adenoma, also known as hepatic adenoma, is rare and pediatric patients mainly consist of girls over 10 years old. Androgenic steroid therapy is also associated with an increased prevalence of hepatic adenoma and is hence seen in those with Fanconi anemia. It is seen in association with glycogen storage disease types I and III, galactosemia, and familial diabetes mellitus. There is also an association with congenital and acquired abnormalities of the hepatic vasculature, such as portal vein absence or occlusion, and other hypervascular hepatic neoplasms, including adult hemangioma and FNH [9]. The main clinical concern is intratumoral hemorrhage, which occurs in approximately 10% of patients. Results of liver function tests are usually normal with no elevation of AFP level.

The typical imaging appearance is due to the presence of intratumoral hemorrhage and intracellular fat. Those without hemorrhage are homogeneous and similar in appearance to adjacent normal liver. Hepatocellular adenomas are sharply marginated lesions, with a pseudocapsule seen in 25%–30% of cases. On unenhanced images, areas of hyperattenuation are seen due to recent hemorrhage, as well as fat attenuation due to lipid content [9].

Smaller lesions, less than 4 cm, are typically homogeneously enhancing, whereas larger lesions heterogeneously enhance because of necrosis, fat, hemorrhage, and calcification. Hepatocellular adenomas demonstrate hepatic arterial enhancement, being hyperattenuating compared with the normal liver in the arterial phase and isoattenuating in the portal venous and delayed phases [9].

22.5.7 Fibrolamellar Carcinoma

Fibrolamellar carcinoma develops in normal livers in young adults, with no clear sex predilection. It is a slow-growing malignant tumor made up of eosinophilic neoplastic hepatocytes separated into cords by lamellar fibrous strands [7, 9]. Tumor markers are usually not elevated, although alpha-fetoprotein may be slightly increased.

Most cases are discovered when the tumor becomes massive (>10 cm); it is solitary, well demarcated, and lobulated. Necrosis and hemorrhage are seen in the center. On nonenhanced CT, a hypodense, solitary mass is seen. In about half of cases, central calcification is present. On dynamic CT inhomogeneous enhancement is observed during the arterial phase. A poorly enhanced, hypodense area generally reflects necrosis. In the equilibrium (or delayed) phase, delayed enhancement of the central scar is seen in about 25% of cases.

22.5.8 Undifferentiated (Embryonal) Sarcoma (UES)

Undifferentiated embryonal sarcoma is a rare malignant neoplasm that occurs in childhood and adolescence. It grows rapidly and cystic degeneration, intratumoral hemorrhage, or necrosis frequently occurs. Serum alpha-fetoprotein is not elevated. The histological resemblance to mesenchymal hamartoma suggests that undifferentiated embryonal sarcoma is its malignant counterpart.

On nonenhanced CT the tumor appears as a large, well-circumscribed cystic mass. A diagnosis of UES is strongly suggested by the presence of a large hepatic lesion that has a seemingly cystic appearance on CT and MR images and a largely solid appearance on US images. The use of delayed phase contrast-enhanced CT and MR imaging is also useful because these techniques demonstrate tumoral enhancement and help exclude purely cystic lesions from the differential diagnosis [8, 9].

22.5.9 Angiosarcoma

Angiosarcoma is a rare malignant hepatic tumor but is the most frequently encountered malignant mesenchymal tumor of the liver. Most patients are older men who have a history of exposure to toxins such as vinyl chloride monomer, Thorotrast, arsenic, or anabolic steroids. Intrahepatic tumors range from solitary to diffuse.

On nonenhanced CT, angiosarcomas are seen as heterogeneous hypodense masses. Because of hemorrhage, the center may appear hyperdense. In cases with associated intraperitoneal bleeding, a hyperdense area may be noted owing to acute clot adjacent to the tumor. On dynamic CT, these tumors are well-enhanced in the arterial phase, occasionally showing peripheral nodular enhancement and progressive and delayed filling enhancement on the delayed phase [9].

22.5.10 Epithelioid Hemangioendothelioma

Epithelioid hemangioendothelioma (EHE) is a rare soft-tissue tumor of vascular origin that may occur in the liver. Hepatic EHE is a tumor of intermediate malignant potential, between that of benign IHE and the highly aggressive angiosarcoma. Most cases are diagnosed in young to middle-aged adults, but a small number of pediatric cases have been reported. There is a female predominance, with a female-to-male ratio of 3:2. AFP levels are usually normal [9].

Two patterns are demonstrated at imaging: multifocal and diffuse. The multifocal form consists of multiple, predominantly peripheral nodules and corresponds to the early stage of the disease. As nodules enlarge, they tend to coalesce into confluent masses, producing the diffuse pattern seen in the advanced stages. Individual masses frequently demonstrate a target-like appearance, which corresponds to the zonal architecture observed pathologically. Adjacent capsular flattening or retraction due to fibrosis is an unusual and distinctive finding of EHE that may be detected at cross-sectional imaging. At unenhanced CT, the predominantly peripheral nodules are hypoattenuating relative to normal liver. Calcifications are noted in 20% of cases. Compensatory enlargement of unaffected portions of the liver may be noted. At contrast-enhanced CT, the central, relatively hypocellular portion does not enhance. Peripheral rim enhancement is typically seen, which correlates with the hyperemia demonstrated at pathologic evaluation. A more peripheral concentric hypoattenuating rim may also be observed, which likely corresponds to the thin avascular rim seen at macroscopic examination. Multiphase CT demonstrates peripheral and progressive centripetal enhancement in larger lesions with incomplete fill-in on delayed phase images. Smaller lesions may show central enhancement with centrifugal progression at dynamic imaging.

22.6 Post-treatment Imaging

Children with hepatoblastoma and hepatocellular carcinoma will need to be imaged during their neoadjuvant chemotherapy with a CT or MRI (preferred, with hepatocyte-specific agent) [2]. If a CT is performed, imaging is only needed during the portal venous phase for hepatoblastoma [2]. In children with hepatocellular carcinoma, both arterial-phase and portal venous phase imaging are recommended [2]. During routine follow-up, chest CT is only required if the child had pulmonary metastases at diagnosis [2]. However, if there is a rising serum alpha-fetoprotein level, or suspected infection, chest CT is an important tool used to diagnose new metastases or pneumonia [2].

The PRETEXT group (I, II, III, and IV) and all PRETEXT annotation factors (V, P, E, F, R, C, N, M) should be reassessed during each imaging time point [2]. After diagnosis, these are referred to as POST-TEXT (POST-Treatment EXTent of disease) factors. After the tumor has been surgically resected, the POST-TEXT factors no longer apply [2].

22.7 Recent Updates and Future Directions

Contrast-enhanced ultrasound is radiation-free and can be done even without sedation in infants.

Contrast-enhanced ultrasound can be used for evaluation of a newly discovered focal liver lesion as per the recommendations of the American College of Radiology Pediatric LI-RADS Working Group. CEUS should not be performed if there are more than two liver lesions that may represent different types of lesions such as in a patient who has undergone a Fontan procedure, multiple different types of benign and malignant lesions may be present simultaneously [18, 19].

Interpretation of CEUS is based on the lesion's pattern of enhancement in the arterial phase combined with the appearance of the lesion in the portal venous and delayed phases of enhancement. The degree and timing of washout are important. Contrast retention on delayed imaging indicates a lesion is benign, in which case the arterial enhancement pattern is important for definitive characterization. Contrast washout, or hypoenhancement compared with adjacent liver parenchyma, is suspicious for malignancy.

Quantitative multiparametric MRI mapping techniques have been well explored and their utility established in adults. Quantitative multiparametric mapping sequences allow for assessment of intrinsic characteristics of tissues and include measurements such as T1- (either with or without intravenous contrast), T2-, and diffusion-weighted imaging (DWI) or intravoxel incoherent motion imaging [20]. In the pediatric population, this is still being studied and can have a potential role in differentiation of various hepatic masses in the future. For example, the use of the mono-exponential model DWI is better than T2-weighted images for the detection of focal liver lesions and facilitates differentiation of benign and malignant lesions [21]. In neonates and young infants, hepatic lesions with decreased signal intensity on an ADC map could lead to the diagnosis of hepatoblastoma [21]. In addition, the differentiation of hepatic adenoma or hepatocellular carcinoma could be aided by DWI as it is in adults [21].

Artificial intelligence (AI)-based research efforts are active in both automated or semi-automated lesion detection and segmentation as well as lesion classification and prediction of treatment-response [20].

References

1. Chavhan GB, Schooler GR, Tang ER, Squires JH, Rees MA, Nguyen HN, et al. Optimizing imaging of pediatric liver lesions: guidelines from the pediatric LI-RADS Working Group. Radiographics. 2023;43(1):e220043.
2. Towbin AJ, Meyers RL, Woodley H, Miyazaki O, Weldon CB, Morland B, et al. 2017 PRETEXT: radiologic staging system for primary hepatic malignancies of childhood revised for the Paediatric Hepatic International Tumour Trial (PHITT). Pediatr Radiol. 2018;48(4):536–54.
3. Bader D, Riskin A, Vafsi O, Tamir A, Peskin B, Israel N, et al. Alpha-fetoprotein in the early neonatal period – a large study and review of the literature. Clin Chim Acta. 2004;349(1–2):15–23. https://doi.org/10.1016/j.cccn.2004.06.020.
4. Chung EM, Lattin GE, Cube R, Lewis RB, Marichal-Hernández C, Shawhan R, et al. From the archives of the AFIP: pediatric liver masses: radiologic-pathologic correlation part 2. Malignant tumors. RadioGraphics. 2011;31(2):483–507.
5. Gong X, Li Y, Yang K, Chen S, Ji Y. Infantile hepatic hemangiomas: looking backwards and forwards. Precis Clin Med. 2022;5(1):pbac006. https://doi.org/10.1093/pcmedi/pbac006.
6. Berenguer B, Mulliken JB, Enjolras O, Boon LM, Wassef M, Josset P, Burrows PE, Perez-Atayde AR, Kozakewich HP. Rapidly involuting congenital hemangioma: clinical and histopathologic features. Pediatr Dev Pathol. 2003;6(6):495–510.
7. Stocker JT. Hepatic tumors in children. Clin Liver Dis. 2001;5:259–81, viii–ix
8. Chung EM, Cube R, Lewis RB, et al. Paediatric liver masses: radiologic-pathologic correlation part 1. Benign tumors. RadioGraphics. 2010;30:801–26.
9. Chiorean L, Cui X-W, Tannapfel A, et al. Benign liver tumors in pediatric patients – review with emphasis on imaging features. World J Gastroenterol. 2015;21(28):8541–61.
10. Bouyn CI, Leclere J, Raimondo G, et al. Hepatic focal nodular hyperplasia in children previously treated for a solid tumor. incidence, risk factors, and outcome. Cancer. 2003;97:3107–13.
11. Towbin AJ, Luo GG, Yin H, et al. Focal nodular hyperplasia in children, adolescents, and young adults. Pediatr Radiol. 2011;41:341–9.
12. Ishak KG, Goodman ZD, Stocker JT. Benign mesenchymal tumors and pseudotumors. In: Rosai J, Sobin L, editors. Atlas of tumor pathology: tumors of the liver and intrahepatic bile ducts. Washington, DC: Armed Forces Institute of Pathology; 2001. p. 71–157.

13. Stocker JT, Ishak KG. Mesenchymal hamartoma of the liver: report of 30 cases and review of the literature. Pediatr Pathol. 1983;1(3):245–67.
14. Edmondson HA. Tumors of the liver and intrahepatic bile ducts. In: Edmondson HA, editor. Atlas of tumor pathology. Washington, DC: Armed Forces Institute of Pathology; 1958.
15. Mahamid J, Miselevich I, Attias D, et al. Nodular regenerative hyperplasia associated with idiopathic thrombocytopenic purpura in a young girl: a case report and review of the literature. J Pediatr Gastroenterol Nutr. 2005;41:251–5.
16. Reshamwala PA, Kleiner DE, Heller T. Nodular regenerative hyperplasia: not all nodules are created equal. Hepatology. 2006;44:7–14.
17. Devarbhavi H, Abraham S, Kamath PS. Significance of nodular regenerative hyperplasia occurring de novo following liver transplantation. Liver Transpl. 2007;13:1552–6.
18. Fang C, Anupindi SA, Back SJ, Franke D, Green TG, Harkanyi Z, Jüngert J, Kwon JK, Paltiel HJ, Squires JH, Zefov VN, McCarville MB. Contrast-enhanced ultrasound of benign and malignant liver lesions in children. Pediatr Radiol. 2021;51(12):2181–97. https://doi.org/10.1007/s00247-021-04976-2. Epub 2021 May 12. PMID: 33978801; PMCID: PMC8566652
19. Squires JH, Beth McCarville M. Contrast-enhanced ultrasound in children: implementation and key diagnostic applications. Am J Roentgenol. 2021;217(5):1217–31.
20. Schooler GR, Infante JC, Acord M, Alazraki A, Chavhan GB, Davis JC, Khanna G, Morani AC, Morin CE, Nguyen HN, Rees MA, Shaikh R, Srinivasan A, Squires JH, Tang E, Thacker PG, Towbin AJ. Imaging of pediatric liver tumors: a COG diagnostic imaging committee/SPR oncology committee white paper. Pediatr Blood Cancer. 2023;70(Suppl 4(Suppl 4)):e29965. https://doi.org/10.1002/pbc.29965.
21. Yoon H, Shin HJ, Kim MJ, Lee MJ. Quantitative imaging in pediatric hepatobiliary disease. Korean J Radiol. 2019;20(9):1342–57. https://doi.org/10.3348/kjr.2019.0002.
22. Siegel MJ, Chung EM, Conran RM. Pediatric liver: focal masses. Magn Reson Imaging Clin N Am. 2008;16(3):437–52. https://doi.org/10.1016/j.mric.2008.04.001.

23 Gastrointestinal Tract (GIT) Tumors

Ishan Kumar, Pramod Kumar Singh,
and Ashish Verma

23.1 Introduction

Tumors of the gastrointestinal (GI) tract are rare in children with less than 5% of childhood tumors arising from the GI tract [1]. Due to non-specific presentation and low degree of clinical suspicion, the diagnosis is often delayed. The most common GI tumors of childhood are lymphoma, gastrointestinal stromal tumor (GIST), carcinoma, carcinoid, and other benign tumors [2]. Both malignant and benign tumors of GIT in the pediatric age group may have an underlying genetic disorder, and it is essential for a radiologists to be familiar with the imaging findings as well as the associations.

Ultrasound (US) is usually the first modality a child is subjected to for abdominal complaints, however it is operator-dependent and not sensitive for diagnosis. CT and MRI are the primary modalities used for the evaluation of GIT masses. Radiologically, there are two predominant patterns of presentation, i.e., (i) diffuse or eccentric wall thickening and (ii) as polypoidal mass lesion with variable degree of luminal and/or extraluminal involvement. In this chapter, we discuss the structured approach to the evaluation of GI masses [3–5].

23.2 Structured Reporting Format

Table 23.1 shows a suggested structured reporting format for gastrointestinal mass.

- ***Anatomical location:*** Esophageal tumors are rarely seen in pediatric age group. Esophageal cancers are reported in patients who had either Barret esophagus or other predisposing factors for gastroesophageal reflux such as spinal palsy, hiatus hernia, or esophageal atresia. In stomach, most of the reported tumors have mesenchymal origin and are benign, such as leiomyoma, benign teratoma, hemangioma, adenoma, schwannoma, fibroma, and neurofibroma [6]. Tumors with borderline malignant potential include IMT and epitheliomesenchymal biphasic tumor. Primary malignant tumors of stomach are rare but include adenocarcinoma, leiomyosarcoma, malignant germ cell tumor, rhabdomyosarcoma, lymphoma, and peripheral primitive neuroectodermal tumor [7]. In colon, commonest reported benign tumors are polyps, with or without hereditary polypoidal syndromes. Others include lipomas, leiomyomas, and neurofibromas [8]. Malignant tumors of colon include adenocarcinoma, carcinoid, and lymphoma. Table 23.2

I. Kumar (✉) · P. K. Singh · A. Verma
Department of Radiodiagnosis and Imaging, Institute of Medical Sciences, Banaras Hindu University, Varanasi, Uttar Pradesh, India

I. Kumar et al. (eds.), *Practical Approach to Imaging in Pediatric Oncology*,
https://doi.org/10.1007/978-981-96-8158-7_23

Table 23.1 Structured reporting format for GI masses

Anatomical location	<Stomach> <duodenum> <jejunum> <ilium> < caecum/ colon> <rectal> < anal canal>
Extent of involvement	
Gross appearance	<wall thickening> < polypoidal mass lesion > <mixed>
Length of involvement	< focal involvement> < segmental involvement (6–40 cm) < diffuse involvement> (> 40 cm).
Circumferential location	<circumferential involvement> < incomplete involvement: % circumference; clock position>
Distance from anatomical landmark	<anal verge/ anorectal junction/ ileocecal junction / pyloroduodenal junction/ gastroesophageal junction>
Degree of thickening	<mild (3–4 mm) > < moderate (5–9 mm) > <marked (≥10 mm) > <size of mass –x–x—cm >
Shape	<round> < lobulated> <irregular>
Location in bowel wall	<mucosal> <subepithelial> <Serosal>
Mucosal surface	<maintained> <involved> < irregular/ulcerated>
Growth pattern	< endoluminal> <mixed> <exophytic>
Bowel lumen	<luminal narrowing> < luminal dilatation> < proximal obstruction> < non-obstructive>
Tumor parenchyma	
Characteristics	<predominant T1/T2 signal> <hemorrhage> < cyst> <calcification> <necrosis>
Mural enhancement pattern	<target appearance> < homogeneous enhancement> < heterogeneous enhancement> < diminished enhancement>
Degree of enhancement	< poor> <mild> <strong> < homogenous/ heterogeneous enhancement>
Dynamic enhancement pattern	< homogeneous arterial and persistent enhancement> < peripheral to central progressive enhancement> < heterogeneous gradual enhancement>
Diffusion	<restricted> <facilitated> < ADC value >
PET scan	<homogenous tracer uptake> < heterogenous tracer uptake> < no uptake> SUV:
Adjacent structures	
Mesentery	<mesenteric involvement> < mesenteric fat stranding> < prominent vascularity> < mesenteric kink> <calcification>
Vessels	< vascular encasement> <thrombosis> <other>
Lymphadenopathy	<present> <absent>
Metastasis:	Anatomic location
Other findings/associated complication:	<perforation> <fistula> <intussusception> <others>

summarizes the location-wise distribution of common GI tumors in pediatric age group.

- ***Growth pattern:*** Polypoidal lesions can grow in an intraluminal, extraluminal, or mixed (dumbbell-shaped) pattern. The intraluminal growth pattern occurs when a tumor is entirely confined to the bowel lumen without bulging into the extraluminal space. The extraluminal growth pattern occurs when a mass is confined to the extraluminal (bowel wall and mesentery) space without bulging into the bowel lumen. A mixed growth pattern is seen when a tumor combines features of both intraluminal and extraluminal growth.
- ***Location in bowel wall:*** A distinction between epithelial (mucosal layer origin) and subepithelial mass (submucosal origin) should be made by careful evaluation of the mucosal layer. Epithelial masses, such as carcinoma, include focal, eccentric, and asymmetric wall thickening with overlying mucosal destruction or irregularity as well as abnormal (hypo-, hyper-, or mixed) enhancement compared to the adjacent normal GI wall. In contrast, subepithelial masses (GIST, carcinoid tumor) show smooth mucosal surface with intraluminal or extraluminal growth; the overlying mucosal layer is generally intact, with

Table 23.2 Location-wise distribution of common GI tumors in pediatric age group

Stomach	Polyps Inflammatory pseudotumor.	Lymphoma, GIST, Leiomyosarcoma, Teratoma
Duodenum	Brunner gland hyperplasia, Polyp, inflammatory pseudotumor	Neuroendocrine tumor
Small bowel	Polyp, hemangiomas Neurofibromas, fibromas, Leiomyomas, lipomas, inflammatory pseudotumor	GIST, lymphoma, neuroendocrine tumor
Colon	Polyp, lipoma, leiomyoma, Neurofibroma	Adenocarcinoma, carcinoid Lymphoma

the exception of the focal ulcerated area [9]. It is sometimes difficult to distinguish between a large bowel wall mass with exophytic growth and extramural mass. Preservation of the fat plane between a mass and the displaced GI wall may be a clue to the extramural origin of the mass. Mass with mural origin shows irregular contact surface with the wall and often deforms the edge of the wall into a beak shape. Assessment using multiplanar reformats may be helpful in determining the origin of the mass [9].

- ***Length, thickness, size, and shape:*** A wall thickness of >3 mm for an adequately distended loop is considered abnormal in pediatric age group. Bowel wall thickening may be related to several entities, including normal variants, inflammatory/infective conditions, and neoplastic thickening. The CT findings that need to be analyzed when assessing thickened bowel include length and degree of thickening; symmetric versus asymmetric thickening, mural pattern; and associated peri-enteric abnormalities.
  - *Length:* Pathologic thickenings tend to cause focal involvement (≤ 5 cm), segmental involvement (6–40 cm), or diffuse involvement (> 40 cm) [5]. Conditions that cause focal bowel abnormalities include neoplasms, Crohn's disease, tuberculosis, and ulcer disease. Among neoplasms, GIST, carcinoid, and carcinoma may present as focal wall thickening. Segmental or diffuse thickening is usually suggestive of benign pathologies such as Crohn's disease, ischemic bowel disease, infective enteritis, however marked segmental thickening with homogenous enhancement is suggestive of bowel lymphoma.
  - *Degree of wall thickening*: Neoplastic pathologies usually present with marked thickening of the bowel wall (> 2 cm) which can be differentiated with benign infectious/inflammatory thickening which usually show mild to moderate thickening (< 1 cm). Lymphoma usually shows thickening >4 cm. Occasionally, adenocarcinoma and some lymphoma may present with moderate thickening [10].
- ***Bowel lumen:*** Carcinoma, tuberculosis, and IBD usually cause narrowing of the bowel lumen and are associated with intestinal obstruction. Lymphomas, despite their large soft-tissue components and marked bowel wall thickening, are associated with preservation of the lumen and often with dilatation of the lumen (aneurysmal dilatation), typically without obstruction. This is secondary to complete replacement of the muscle fibers with lymphoid tissue [11, 12]. GIST, due to their submucosal location, also usually do not cause obstructive symptoms even with significant intraluminal component. Intratumoral gas in the GIST is suggestive of ulceration and communication with lumen [13]. Carcinoid of small bowel may be associated with direct tumoral luminal narrowing or more commonly kinking of bowel lumen due to desmoplastic reaction and mass in the adjoining mesentery [14].
- ***Symmetry***: Asymmetrical thickening is the hallmark of malignancies such as carcinoma, GIST, and carcinoid tumors. Long-standing Crohn's disease may uncommonly show asymmetrically thickened bowel. Lymphoma

may present with symmetric or asymmetrical thickening [5].

- ***Tumor parenchyma:*** If the thickened segment of bowel displays a stratified target appearance with mucosal and serosal enhancement and a low-attenuation submucosal layer, a benign non-neoplastic process should be considered. Homogenous enhancement can be associated with tumors such as lymphoma or active phase of Crohn's disease. Heterogeneous enhancement is typical of tumors such as carcinoma, or malignant GIST. Infective pathology such as tuberculosis also usually shows heterogeneous enhancement.
- A study in adult GIST has shown that almost all high-risk GIST seem to have a heterogeneous enhancement and avascular areas independent of their size and that low-risk GIST tend to show a homogenous enhancement. GIST are usually hypervascular on arterial phase and are hypoenhancing on portal venous phase [15–17].
- Colorectal carcinomas can appear as focal, irregular wall thickening, pericolonic fat tissue infiltration, serosal irregularity, and with lymphadenopathy on CT. On MRI they are seen as T1 hypointense, T2 hyperintense lesions with heterogenous enhancement. Calcification is seen in mucinous adenocarcinoma (MAC) with a majority of area showing hypoattenuation whereas the solid portion also shows lesser degree of enhancement. On MRI, these lesions typically show T2 signal (higher or similar to mesorectal fascia) due to mucin pools. Dynamic contrast-enhanced sequences have been shown to be helpful in the early diagnosis of inconspicuous masses with heterogenous enhancement of cellular component [18]. Sometimes dark T2 rim is observed helping in identification of tumor contour.
- Carcinoid tumors show marked arterial phase contrast enhancement and decreased enhancement in later phases. On MRI they show low signal on T1 and a heterogeneously high signal on T2 sequences, and positive gadolinium enhancement. In small tumors, arterial contrast enhancement might be the only imaging finding [19].
- Inflammatory myofibroblastic tumor appears as hypoechoic or hyperechoic solid masses with variable vascularity on Doppler imaging. They are homogeneous or heterogeneous lesions with variable enhancement on delayed acquisitions. On MRI they appear as hypointense masses on both T1- and T2-weighted images, representing the fibrotic tissue. On dynamic post-contrast sequences, they show minimal to absent enhancement in the arterial phase, with progressive-variable enhancement in the delayed phase [20].
- *Mesentery:* Mesenteric fat stranding with bowel wall thickening is usually associated with Crohn's disease or infective conditions (tuberculosis). Uncommonly, fat stranding in the surrounding mesentery can be seen in locally advanced carcinoma or lymphoma. Mesenteric calcification associated with bowel mass can be seen in treated lymphoma, carcinoid, or mucinous carcinoma [18].

Figure 23.1 highlights a generalized approach to radiological diagnosis of pediatric GI masses.

23.2.1 Gastrointestinal Stromal Tumor (GIST)

GIST are the mesenchymal tumor of GI tract, arising from the interstitial cell of Cajal in muscularis propria. Pediatric GIST is a rare occurrence and although it resembles adult GIST on imaging, the histology, clinical course, and thus imaging approach are different [21]. In children they may occur with other tumor syndromes, such as Neurofibromatosis Type-1 (NF1), Carney Triad (GIST, pulmonary chondroma, and extraadrenal paraganglioma), and Carney-Stratakis Syndrome (GIST with familial paraganglioma). Unlike in adults, the KIT or PDGFRA mutations occur in only 11% of pediatric GIST and the Wild-type GIST (lacking these mutations) is more common (Fig. 23.2). Majority of the pediatric GIST show mutations in succinate dehydrogenase (SDH) protein complex [21–24].

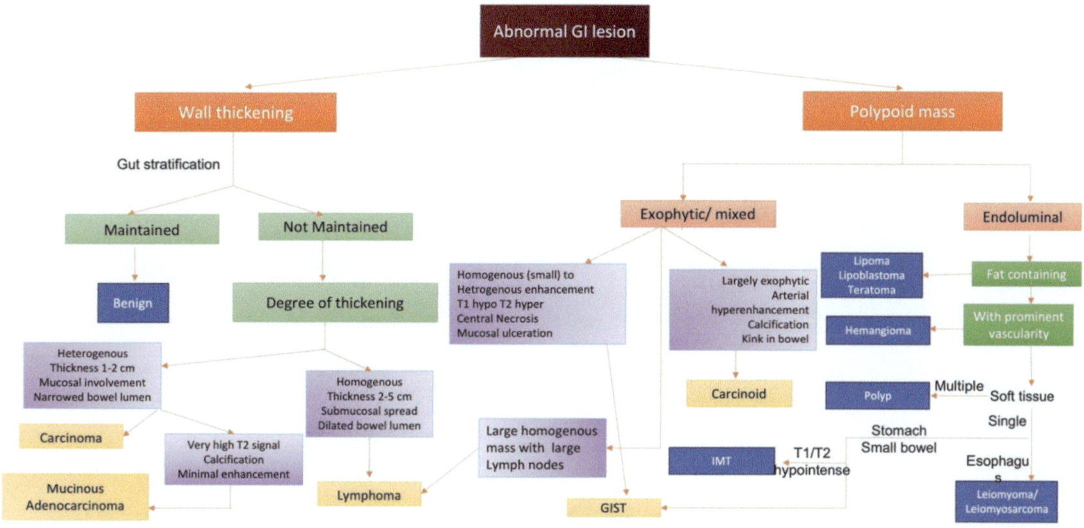

Fig. 23.1 Approach to diagnosis and further evaluation and management

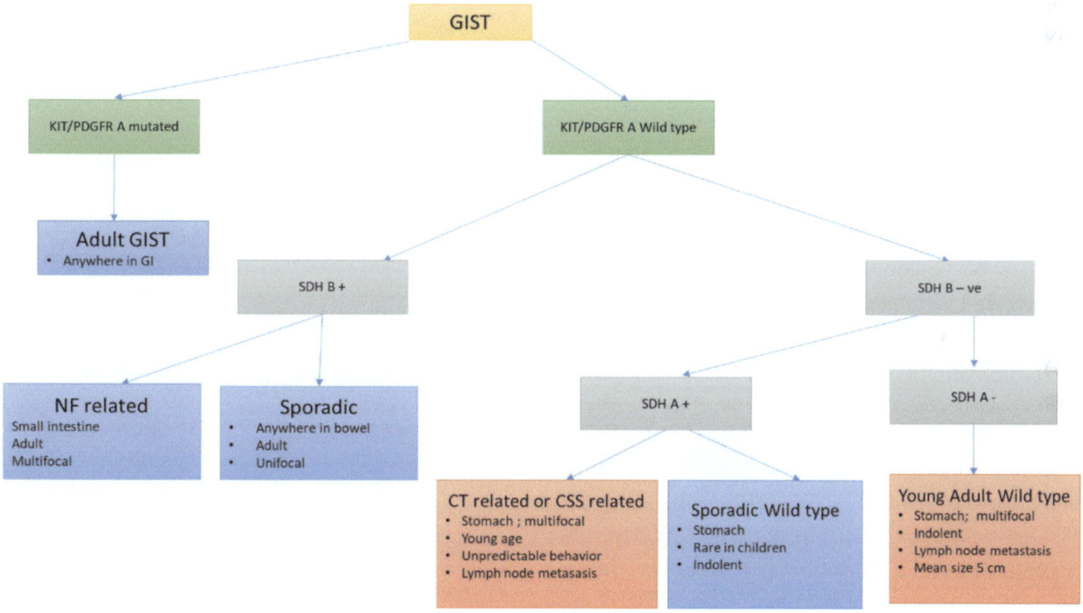

Fig. 23.2 Types of gastrointestinal stromal tumor

23.2.1.1 Imaging Features

The most common location of GIST is stomach followed by small intestine. They can be completely endoluminal or exophytic/mixed. On CT, they are large (> 5 cm), exophytic, hypervascular tumors with a heterogeneous enhancement on contrast-enhanced CT (Fig. 23.3). The heterogeneity observed is caused by necrosis, cystic degeneration, and hemorrhage. Calcification is rare. Cavitation and overlying mucosal ulceration can be seen and intratumoral air/air-fluid level (Torricelli-Bernoulli sign) suggests communication with the gastrointestinal lumen and should not be misinterpreted as a superimposed infection [25]. On MRI, Small tumors (< 5 cm) appear as round tumors with intense, homogeneous arterial

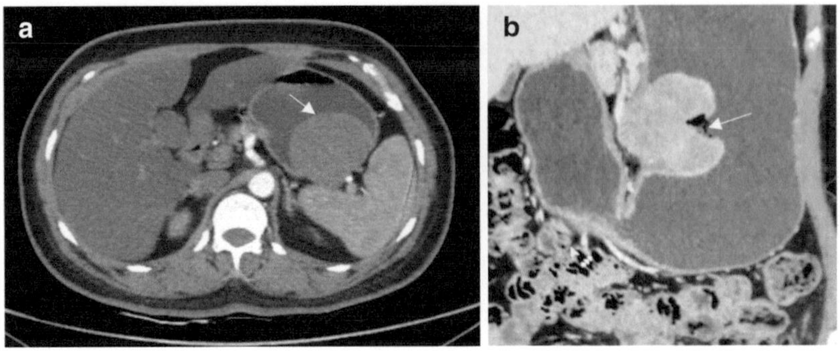

Fig. 23.3 (**a**) CECT of gastrointestinal stromal tumor (arrow) showing a well-defined endoluminal mass arising from greater curvature of the stomach. (**b**) Another well-defined mass showing both endoluminal and exophytic component with inner ulcerated margin (arrow)

postcontrast enhancement. Large tumors (> 5 cm) more often are irregular lobulated, have a mild gradual and heterogeneous contrast enhancement, and they frequently exhibit intratumoral cysts. Presence of cysts or a low ADC value is suggestive of a high-risk/malignant GIST [26].

Treatment is primarily surgery. Wild-type pediatric GIST do not respond to adjuvant Imatinib therapy and second-generation kinase inhibitors (TKI) such as Sunitinib©, Nilotinib©, etc. can be considered in those with metastatic disease. In cases where complete resection is performed, MRI is recommended for postoperative scan whereas ultrasound and chest x ray are performed 6 monthly. In cases of incomplete resection or metastatic disease, MRI is performed after resection, MRI with CEUS is done at 6 months and ultrasound with Chest X ray is done at 1 year. For patients with TKI inhibitor MRI is done on seventh day or CEUS can be performed on day 7, 14, and 2 months [27]. On CEUS, GIST are hypervascular on arterial phase and are hypo-enhancing on portal venous phase. High-risk GIST shows a heterogeneous enhancement and avascular areas independent of their size. PET-CT can also be used to assess distant metastasis and response to therapy. GIST typically shows a homogenous intense tracer uptake with increased standardized uptake value (SUV). 18FDG-PET response is characterized by a marked decrease in uptake after therapy. For response assessment, purely size-based criteria such as RECIST have been largely replaced by Choi criteria (CT scan) or PERCIST criteria (PET-CT) [27, 28] (Table 23.3).

Table 23.3 Response assessment in GIST

	Response	Progressive disease/ non-response:
CT	Decrease in tumor size ≥10% or Decrease in density (in HU) by ≥15%	Increase in tumor size by ≥10% No decrease in density (in HU) by ≥15%. New detectable nodule in the nodule (secondary resistance) Magnification of already known nodules
MRI	T2-hyperintense and T1-hypointense lesions with minimal to no post-contrast enhancement. Cystic appearance TKI may lead to tumoral bleed with temporary increase in tumor size. Increase in ADC > 30% is seen in responders after one week	Persistent enhancement No significant change Metastatic nodule T2 hyperintense with post-contrast enhancement

23.2.2 Carcinoma

Carcinoma is rare in children and most commonly affects colon and rectum. Abdominal pain and vomiting are the most common presenting symptoms which are non-specific for pediatric age group and often lead to diagnostic delays. 10–30% of the pediatric colorectal carcinoma are associated with predisposing conditions such as familial adenomatous polyposis (FAP), ulcerative colitis, Crohn disease, and Peutz-Jegher syndrome. High microsatellite instability (MSI) is the most common associated genetic mutation. The majority are mucinous adenocarcinoma (50%) followed by poorly differentiated adenocarcinoma (32%) [29–31]. The usual age of diagnosis is second decade.

Evaluation should be done using colonoscopy and cross-sectional imaging studies (CT/MRI) for local/distal extension of the tumor, lymph nodes, and/or metastasis. MRI is the preferred modality on which carcinomas can appear as focal, irregular wall thickening, which are T1 hypointense and hyperintense-heterogeneous masses on T2-weighted images. In the early stage of small tumors without wall thickening, arterial contrast enhancement might be the only imaging finding. Penetration and invasion of bowel wall layers are best demonstrated on T2-weighted sequence. Distance from anal verge should be recorded to identify low lying cancers. Circumferential resection margin (CRM) corresponds to mesorectal fascia which is a T2 hypointense fascial layer that surrounds the rectum and mesorectal fat. Tumor in vicinity (<1 mm) of mesorectal fascia is considered CRM positive and is non-resectable. Mesorectal fat should be assessed for lymph nodes, and tumor deposits on CT calcification can be seen in mucinous carcinoma [18]. Calcification is seen in mucinous adenocarcinoma (MAC) with a majority of area showing hypoattenuation whereas the solid portion also shows lesser degree of enhancement. On MRI, these lesions typically show T2 signal (higher or similar to mesorectal fascia) due to mucin pools [29–32]. Lymph nodes should be assessed for their size as well as morphology as half of the metastatic lymph nodes are <5 mm in short axis. Internal heterogeneity, irregular outer border, attenuation values >100 Hounsfield units (HU), and cluster of three or more normal-sized nodes suggest malignant nodes. Low-density lymph nodes can also be present in mucinous adenocarcinoma. Presence of ascites, peritoneal nodules suggests peritoneal spread. Inflammatory bowel disease, intestinal tuberculosis, and bowel lymphoma are the differential diagnosis. The management of colorectal cancer in children is similar to adults.

23.2.3 Carcinoids and Neuroendocrine Tumors

Neuroendocrine tumors (NETs) are epithelial neoplasms with predominant neuroendocrine differentiation and can involve various parts of the body such as lungs, pancreas, and GI tract. Tumors of the embryological gut are called gastroenteropancreatic neuroendocrine tumors [33, 34] and are rare in pediatric age group with varying malignant potential. Carcinoid tumors are well-differentiated neuroendocrine tumors that are mostly benign, even though they can show infiltration of the mesentry and surrounding tissues, and lymph nodal spread. Appendix is the most common site of NET in children followed by duodenum and small bowel. Pediatric appendiceal tumors are mostly benign and all extra-appendiceal NET, well-differentiated (carcinoid) or poorly differentiated (neuroendocrine carcinoma), show high risk of metastasis. NETs can either be sporadic or can be associated with familial syndromes such as multiple endocrine neoplasia (MEN) I and II, Von Hippel-Lindau (VHL) syndrome, and neurofibromatosis type I (NF-I) [34].

Both CT and MRI can be done to study the anatomy of the lesion, involvement of surrounding tissues and lymph node, vascular infiltration, and the presence of metastases. CT/MR enterography with arterial phase imaging on CT/MR are optimal techniques for small bowel lesions (Fig. 23.4). Carcinoid tumors in the small bowel may be polypoid or intramural, and show arterial phase hyperenhancement and decreased enhancement on subsequent phases. They frequently show calcification and fibrosis with focal kinking of the intestine, especially if there is contiguous mesenteric involvement [18, 34]. Clinically, the kink in the bowel can

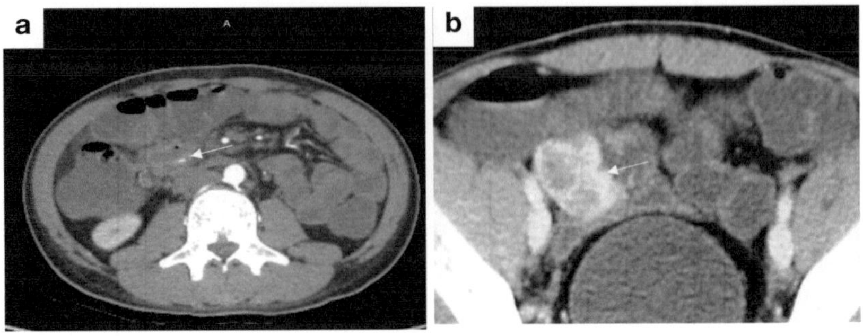

Fig. 23.4 (**a**) Carcinoid tumor (arrow) along the serosal margin of ileal loop showing arterial phase vascularity. (**b**) Hypervascular mass in right iliac fossa along ileal loop (arrow)

manifest as recurrent subacute intestinal obstruction. Duodenal carcinoids may invade pancreas. CT or preferably MRI can easily detect liver metastasis which are arterial phase enhancing and T2 hyperintense nodules. EUS can aid in the identification of gastric, duodenal, pancreatic, or rectal carcinoid tumors. Bronchial and pancreatic NETs will be discussed with their corresponding chapters. Functional imaging is mostly indicated in extra-appendiceal NET as they have a higher malignant potential. SPECT-CT allows both functional and anatomic imaging and recommended for initial staging. PET with Ga-DOTATOC(1,4,7,10-tetraazacyclododecane-1,4,7,10-tetraacetic acid (DOTA)-D-Phe1- Tyr3-octreotide (TOC) is being increasingly used nowadays with higher detection rate of metastases [34].

Treatment is surgical resection of the tumor with adequate lymph nodal resection. EUS, and MRI are recommended both for follow-up to limit the radiation exposure to pediatric patients. (NCCN). Also laboratory tests should be done for follow up such as chromogranine A (CgA) for estimation of tumor burden and 5-hydroxyindoleacetic acid (5 HIAA) for tumors with hepatic metastasis. Table 23.4 summarizes the various protocols for follow-up [33–37].

Table 23.4 Protocols for follow-up of neuroendocrine tumor

NCCN	ESMO	ENETS
CgA and urine 5-HIAA, and multiphasic CT or MRI at 3 and 12 months after resection, and then once a year up to 10 years from surgery	CT or MRI and CgA and urine 5-HIAA every 3–6 months; somatostatin receptor imaging, either Octreoscan or PET CT with 68Ga-DOTATOC, at 18 to 24 months from resection (if expression of SSTR2a has been proven on the tumor cells)	CT scan, somatostatine receptor scintigraphy, and CgA levels at 6 and 12 months, then once a year for at least 3 years

NCCN National Comprehensive Cancer Network; *ESMO* European Society for Medical Oncology; *ENETS* European NeuroEndocrine Tumor Society; *SSTR2A* synaptophysin and somatostatin receptor type 2A

23.2.4 Lymphoma

Lymphoma is the most common pediatric GI malignancy. Contrary to adult lymphoma which mostly involves stomach, small and large bowel, especially terminal ileum and ileocecal junction, are the most common locations of pediatric lymphoma [38]. Also, GI tract is the most common extranodal site of non-Hodgkin lymphoma. Burkitt lymphoma is the predominant histological subtype at small and large bowel whereas diffuse large B-cell lymphoma (DLBCL), extra nodal marginal zone lymphoma (EMZL), and other types are more common in stomach [20]. Primary gastrointestinal lymphoma shows presence of a predominant gastrointestinal lesion (GI component >75% of tumor volume), with or without expansion to regional lymph nodes and absence of involvement of the spleen, liver, mediastinal nodes, and normal total and differential white blood cell count [39, 40].

The most common CT/MR patterns of involvement of small bowel lymphoma (Fig. 23.5) are [39–42].

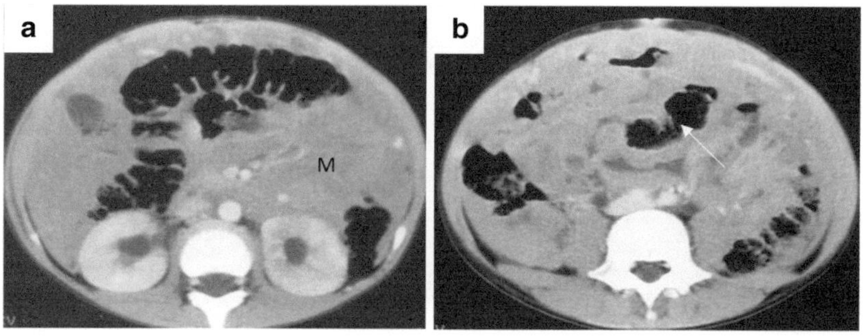

Fig. 23.5 CECT images (**a, b**) of a 12-year-old boy with Burkitt lymphoma show a mass arising from small bowel causing its aneurysmal dilatation (arrow) with a large associated exophytic mesenteric mass (m)

- Polypoidal pattern: subepithelial polyp protruding into bowel lumen. This may be associated with intussusception.
- Infiltrative pattern: symmetrical/ asymmetrical, segmental thickening of bowel loop, with median thickness of 1.5–2 cm, showing mostly homogenous post-contrast enhancement.
- Aneurysmal pattern: segmental bowel thickening (coexisting with infiltrative form) with dilated bowel lumen, due to destruction of muscle layer and myenteric plexus (Fig. 23.5).
- Exophytic/mesenteric mass: large exophytic masses (often >5 cm) with secondary involvement of mesentery and surrounding tissues (Fig. 23.5). Larger masses may be associated with ulceration, perforation, and entero-enteric fistula.
- Stenosing mass is a rare form and causes bowel lumen narrowing with minimal pre-stenotic dilatation. This is more common in Hodgkin's lymphoma with higher fibrotic content.

The imaging pattern of gastric lymphoma is diffuse or segmental wall thickening with low contrast enhancement and extensive lateral extension of the tumor due to submucosal spread and contiguous lymphadenopathy. Polypoidal mass, ulcerative lesions, or mucosal nodularity are less common patterns (Fig. 23.5). The involvement of large bowel is similar to small bowel lesions, manifesting as bulky polypoidal mass, focal infiltrative tumor, and aneurismal dilatation. The usual site is caecum with extension into terminal ileum (Fig. 23.6).

Due to its functional capability, FDG PET CT has gradually replaced CT scan as the initial staging modality for lymphoma and for follow-up of these tumors after therapy. However, normal peristaltic activity, normal GI lymphoid tissue, and inflammatory conditions may present a potential pitfall in PET interpretation. Involvement of various parts of GIT presents with variable picture on PET. Gastric lymphoma presents with diffuse gastric uptake, higher than liver. Small bowel lymphoma presents as multiple foci of FDG uptake in curvilinear pattern and large bowel lymphoma shows focal, nodular, or diffuse hypermetabolic activity [43].

23.2.5 Inflammatory Myofibroblastic Tumor

These are inflammatory pseudotumors of the GI tract caused possibly by chronic infection, previous surgery, or trauma. IMT mainly involves the stomach, followed by small and large intestines. On US, they appear like hypoechoic or hyperechoic solid masses. CT shows well-defined, hypodense, heterogeneous mass lesions with variable enhancement on delayed acquisitions (due to the presence of fibrous tissue formed by the accumulation of myofibroblasts and fibroblast). MRI shows hypointense masses on both T1- and T2-weighted images, representing the fibrotic tissue. Their characteristic post-contrast enhancement pattern is hypointense lesion in the arterial phase, with progressive-variable enhancement in the delayed phase [2, 20].

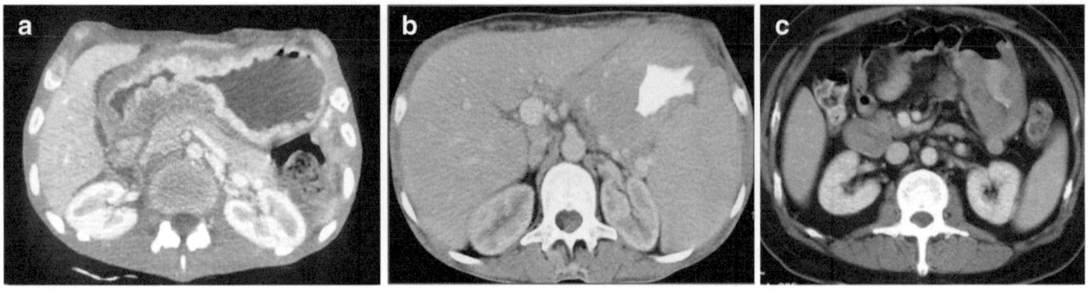

Fig. 23.6 Patterns of gastric lymphoma. (**a**) Submucosal thickening (arrow) in antropyloric region, (**b**) diffuse wall thickening (arrow), (**c**) thickening with aneurysmal dilatation of lumen

23.2.6 Polyps and Polyposis Syndromes

Polyps are distinct intraluminal projections of mucosal or submucosal tissue. GI polyps are rare findings in pediatric age group, and polyps found in pediatric age group are not usually precancerous, except in inherited polyposis syndromes [44, 45].

Syndrome	Gene mutation	Polyps	Association	Malignant risk	Other malignancies
Gardner syndrome/ familial adenomatous polyposis (FAP)	Adenomatous polyposis coli gene (5q21)	Adenomatous intestinal polyps in stomach, colon	Multiple osteomas in the skull, maxillae, and mandible; and multiple epidermoids and desmoids	All polyps undergo malignant transformation	Thyroid, medulloblastoma, hepatoblastoma, Desmoid tumor
Juvenile polyposis syndrome:	*SMAD4* and *BMPR1A*	>5 juvenile hamartomatous polyps in colon Any number with family history or if present in both upper and lower GI endoscopy	Hereditary hemorrhagic telangiectasia	Stomach/colon cancer (median age 35 years; occasional presentation in childhood	Pancreatic cancer
Peutz-Jeghers syndrome (Fig. 23.7)	STK11	Pedunculated polyps in small and large bowel (most common in jejunum)	Perioral freckling/ hyperpigmentation, Precocious puberty	Colorectal carcinoma (presents in adulthood)	Sertoli cell tumors testis, breast, pancreatic, and lung cancers

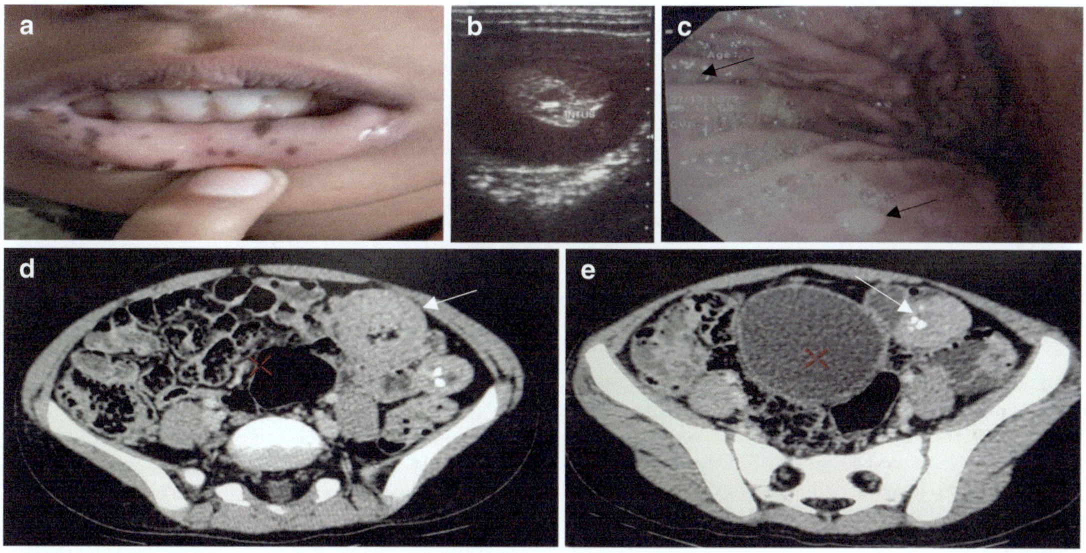

Fig. 23.7 Peutz-Jeghers syndrome. 12-year-old girl with recurrent abdominal pain, melena, and anemia shows (**a**) perioral hyperpigmentation, (**b**) ultrasound shows bowel in bowel appearance suggestive of intussusception involving jejunal loop. (**c**) Colonoscopy shows multiple polyps in descending colon (arrows) (**d, e**) CECT images showing intussusception involving jejunal loops in left lumbar region associated with a polypoidal mass acting as lead point (arrows) showing calcification

Syndrome	Gene mutation	Polyps	Association	Malignant risk	Other malignancies
Bannayan-Riley-Ruvalcaba syndrome (*PTEN* hamartoma tumor syndrome/ Cowden syndrome)	*PTEN*	Mixed polyps. (juvenile, hamatomas, inflammatory, ganglioneuromatous, lipomatous, and others)	Macrocephaly and autism spectrum disorder.	None	Thyroid cancer (pediatric) and other adult-onset cancers
Constitutional mismatch repair deficiency		Infancy with polyposis	Café-au-lait hyperpigmented lesions, agenesis of the corpus callosum, immunoglobulin deficiency	Colorectal cancers (early onset in childhood)	Brain tumors and leukemia/ lymphoma

A variety of polyps such as juvenile, hamartomatous, andenomatous, inflammatory, and lipomatous can be seen. It should be noted that the term 'juvenile' is referred to the histopathological type and not the age of patient. Colonoscopy and fiber optic endoscopy is the primary modality for diagnosis and surveillance. The role of radiology is to evaluate complications such as obstruction or intussusception, and to evaluate the extent of GI and other system malignancies associated with the syndrome. Recently, US has been suggested as a sensitive modality to evaluate polyps with graded compression and application of color Doppler [46]. On US, juvenile polyps appear as solid hypoechoic nodules with small cystic areas within bowel lumen. Color Doppler shows a vascular pedicle coursing through the stalk of the polyp. This appearance is maintained even when the polyp presents as the lead point of intussusception. In adenomatous polyp there is no internal blood flow or well-defined cystic spaces. Inflammatory pseudopolyps are more echogenic, lack a stalk with a vascular pedicle, and are found in association with areas of bowel wall thickening with inflammatory bowel disease [46].

References

1. Ladd AP, Grosfeld JL. Gastrointestinal tumors in children and adolescents. Semin Pediatr Surg. 2006;15:37–47.
2. Özcan HN, Yavuz ÖÖ, Ekinci S, Oguz B, Kutluk T, Haliloglu M. Imaging findings of gastrointestinal tract tumors in children and adolescents. Insights Imaging. 2022;13(1):51.
3. Mazzei MA, Bagnacci G, Gentili F, Capitoni I, Mura G, Marrelli D, Petrioli R, Brunese L, Cappabianca S, Catarci M, Degiuli M, De Manzoni G, De Prizio M, Donini A, Romario UF, Funicelli L, Laghi A, Minetti G, Morgagni P, Petrella E, Pittiani F, Rausei S, Romanini L, Rosati R, Ianora AAS, Tiberio GAM, Volterrani L, Roviello F, Grassi R. Structured and shared CT radiological report of gastric cancer: a consensus proposal by the Italian research Group for Gastric Cancer (GIRCG) and the Italian Society of Medical and Interventional Radiology (SIRM). Eur Radiol. 2022;32(2):938–49.
4. KSAR Study Group for Rectal Cancer. Essential items for structured reporting of rectal cancer MRI: 2016 consensus recommendation from the Korean Society of Abdominal Radiology. Korean J Radiol. 2017;18(1):132–51.
5. Macari M, Megibow AJ, Balthazar EJ. A pattern approach to the abnormal small bowel: observations at MDCT and CT enterography. AJR Am J Roentgenol. 2007;188(5):1344–55.
6. Wang LM, Chetty R. Selected unusual tumors of the gastric: a review. Int J Surg Pathol. 2012;20:5–14.
7. Curtis JL, Burns RC, Wang L, Mahour GH, Ford HR. Primary gastric tumors of infancy and childhood: 54-year experience at a single institution. J Pediatr Surg. 2008;43:1487–93.
8. Caffey Pediatric Diagnostic Imaging, 12th ed. B Coley, M Hernanz-Schulman, A Panigraphy eds. Philadelphia, PA.
9. Lee NK, Kim S, Kim GH, Jeon TY, Kim DH, Jang HJ, Park DY. Hypervascular subepithelial gastrointestinal masses: CT-pathologic correlation. Radiographics. 2010;30(7):1915–34.
10. Balthazar EJ, Noordhoorn M, Megibow AJ, Gordon RB. CT of small-bowel lymphoma in immunocompetent patients and patients with AIDS: comparison of findings. AJR. 1997;168:675–80.
11. Herrmann R, Panahon AM, Barcos MP, Walsh D, Stutzman L. Gastrointestinal involvement in non-Hodgkin's lymphoma. Cancer. 1980;46(1):215–22.
12. Jasti R, Carucci LR. Small bowel neoplasms: a pictorial review. Radiographics. 2020;40(4):1020–38.
13. Inoue A, Ota S, Yamasaki M, Batsaikhan B, Furukawa A, Watanabe Y. Gastrointestinal stromal tumors: a comprehensive radiological review. Jpn J Radiol. 2022;40(11):1105–20.
14. Ramachar SM, Hegde N. Small bowel carcinoids: a single surgeon's experience in southern India. J Clin Diagn Res. 2015 Nov;9(11):PC04–8.
15. Shah P, Gao F, Edmundowicz SA, et al. Predicting malignant potential of gastrointestinal stromal tumors using endoscopic ultrasound. Dig Dis Sci. 2009;54:1265–9.
16. Dietrich CF, Jenssen C, Hocke M, Cui XW, Woenckhaus M, Ignee A. Imaging of gastrointestinal stromal tumours with modern ultrasound techniques – a pictorial essay. Z Gastroenterol. 2012;50(5):457–67.
17. Quiroz HJ, Willobee BA, Sussman MS, et al. Pediatric gastrointestinal stromal tumors-a review of diagnostic modalities. Transl Gastroenterol Hepatol. 2018;3:54.
18. Muccillo A, Marchiori E, Penna CR, Guimarães RR, Zanetti G, Abdalla G, Ventura N, Constantino CL, Pereira ML, Brandão V, Martins P, Canellas R, Varella de Oliveira R. Colon mucinous adenocarcinoma in childhood: a case report with emphasis on image findings. Case Rep Med. 2010;2010:327634.
19. Degnan AJ, Tadros SS, Tocchio S. Pediatric neuroendocrine carcinoid tumors: review of diagnostic Imaging findings and recent advances. AJR Am J Roentgenol. 2017;208(4):868–77.
20. Sanders BM, West KW, Gingalewski C, Engum S, Davis M, Grosfeld JL. Inflammatory pseudotumour of the alimentary tract: clinical and surgical experience. J Pediatr Surg. 2001;36:169–73.
21. Herzberg M, Beer M, Anupindi S, Vollert K, Kröncke T. Imaging pediatric gastrointestinal stromal tumor (GIST). J Pediatr Surg. 2018;53(9):1862–70.
22. Nannini M, Biasco G, Astolfi A, Pantaleo MA. An overview on molecular biology of KIT/PDGFRA wild type (WT) gastrointestinal stromal tumours (GIST). J Med Genet. 2013;50:653–61.
23. Prakash S, Sarran L, Socci N, DeMatteo RP, Eisenstat J, Greco AM, et al. Gastrointestinal stromal tumors in children and young adults. J Pediatr Hematol Oncol. 2005;27:179–87.
24. Janeway KA, Liegl B, Harlow A, Le C, Perez-Atayde A, Kozakewich H, et al. Pediatric KIT wildtype and platelet-derived growth factor receptor alpha-wildtype gastrointestinal stromal tumors share KIT activation but not mechanisms of genetic progression with adult gastrointestinal stromal tumors. Cancer Res. 2007;67:9084–8.
25. Monterubbiano L, Cereser L, D'Alì L, Girometti R, Zuiani C. I saw the Torricelli-Bernoulli sign: when physics provides imaging insights. Clin Imaging. 2024;107:110095.

26. Yu MH, Lee JM, Baek JH, Han JK, Choi B-I. MRI features of gastrointestinal stromal tumors. AJR Am J Roentgenol. 2014;203:980–91.
27. Choi H, Charnsangavej C, Faria SC, Macapinlac HA, Burgess MA, Patel SR, et al. Correlation of computed tomography and positron emission tomography in patients with metastatic gastrointestinal stromal tumor treated at a single institution with imatinib mesylate: proposal of new computed tomography response criteria. J Clin Oncol. 2007;25:1753–9.
28. Tirkes T, Hollar MA, Tann M, Kohli MD, Akisik F, Sandrasegaran K. Response criteria in oncologic imaging: review of traditional and new criteria. Radiographics. 2013;33:1323–41.
29. Koh KJ, Lin LH, Huang SH, Wong JU. CARE–pediatric colon adenocarcinoma: a case report and literature review comparing differences in clinical features between children and adult patients. Medicine (Baltimore). 2015;94(6):e503.
30. Blumer SL, Anupindi SA, Adamson PC, et al. Sporadic adenocarcinoma of the colon in children: case series and review of the literature. J Pediatr Hematol Oncol. 2012;34:e137–41.
31. Sultan I, Rodriguez-Galindo C, El-Taani H, et al. Distinct features of colorectal cancer in children and adolescents: a population-based study of 159 cases. Cancer. 2010;116:758–65.
32. Leung YCL, Chung LA, Liu CSW, et al. Metastatic small bowel adenocarcinoma in a 10-year-old Chinese girl. J Ped Surg Case Reports. 2015;3:38e40.
33. Oberg K, Knigge U, Kwekkeboom D, et al. Neuroendocrine gastroentero- pancreatic tumors: ESMO clinical practice guidelines for diagnosis, treatment and follow-up. Ann Oncol. 2012;23(suppl 7):vii124–30.
34. Gaiani F, de Angelis N, Minelli R, Kayali S, Carra MC, de Angelis GL. Pediatric gastroenteropancreatic neuroendocrine tumor: a case report and review of the literature. Medicine (Baltimore). 2019;98(37):e17154.
35. Cernaianu G, Tannapfel A, Nounla J, et al. Appendiceal carcinoid tumor with lymph node metastasis in a child: case report and review of the literature. J Pediatr Surg. 2010;45:e1–5.
36. Clark OH, Benson AB III, Berlin JD, et al. NCCN clinical practice guidelines in oncology: neuroendocrine tumors. J Natl Compr Cancer Netw. 2009;7:712–47.
37. Delle Fave G, Kwekkeboom DJ, Van Cutsem E, et al. ENETS consensus guidelines for the management of patients with gastroduodenal neoplasms. Neuroendocrinology. 2012;95:74–87.
38. Veerabhadra R, Kumar GK, Bibekanand J, Kumar NB, Kumaravel S, Bhawana B, Biswajit D. Bowel lymphoma in children: management and outcome. Indian J Med Paediatr Oncol. 2018;39(02):184–7.
39. Qadri SK, Shah A, Hamdani NH, Baba KM. Primary gastrointestinal lymphomas in children: an experience of 12 years from a tertiary care center of North India. Indian J Cancer. 2016;53(2):300–3.
40. Dawson IM, Cornes JS, Morson BC. Primary malignant lymphoid tumours of the intestinal tract. Report of 37 cases with a study of factors influencing prognosis. Br J Surg. 1961;49:80–9.
41. Lo Re G, Federica V, Midiri F, Picone D, La Tona G, Galia M, Lo Casto A, Lagalla R, Midiri M. Radiological features of gastrointestinal lymphoma. Gastroenterol Res Pract. 2016;2016:2498143.
42. Granata V, Pradella S, Cozzi D, Fusco R, Faggioni L, Coppola F, Grassi R, Maggialetti N, Buccicardi D, Lacasella GV, Montella M, Ciaghi E, Bellifemine F, De Filippo M, Rengo M, Bortolotto C, Prost R, Barresi C, Cappabianca S, Brunese L, Neri E, Grassi R, Miele V. Computed tomography structured reporting in the staging of lymphoma: a Delphi consensus proposal. J Clin Med. 2021;10(17):4007.
43. Paes FM, Kalkanis DG, Sideras PA, Serafini AN. FDG PET/CT of extranodal involvement in non-Hodgkin lymphoma and Hodgkin disease. Radiographics. 2010;30(1):269–91.
44. MacFarland SP, Zelley K, Katona BW, Wilkins BJ, Brodeur GM, Mamula P. Gastrointestinal polyposis in pediatric patients. J Pediatr Gastroenterol Nutr. 2019;69(3):273–80.
45. Katabathina VS, Menias CO, Khanna L, Murphy L, Dasyam AK, Lubner MG, Prasad SR. Hereditary gastrointestinal cancer syndromes: role of Imaging in screening, diagnosis, and management. Radiographics. 2019;39(5):1280–301.
46. Zhang Y, Li SX, Xie LM, et al. Sonographic diagnosis of juvenile polyps in children. Ultrasound Med Biol. 2012;38(9):1529–33.

24 Tumors of the Peritoneum, Omentum, Mesentery, and Retroperitoneum

Pallavi Sinha and Devasenathipathy Kandsamy

24.1 Definitions and Anatomy

The peritoneum is a thin serous membrane that consists of a single layer of simple cuboidal epithelium called a mesothelium [1]. The peritoneum that lines the abdominal wall is called the parietal peritoneum, while that lining the viscera is called the visceral peritoneum. Folds of the peritoneum constitute ligaments and support the various structures within the abdominal cavity.

A mesentery is a ligament composed of a double layer of peritoneum [2]. It covers the small bowel and parts of the colon and fixes them to the posterior abdominal wall. The root of the [3] small bowel mesentery extends from the duodeno-jejunal flexure in the left upper quadrant to the ileocecal junction in the right lower quadrant [4]. The transverse mesocolon connects the second part of the duodenum and the head of the pancreas to the transverse colon [5].

An omentum is a ligament that fixes the stomach to other structures [2]. The lesser omentum connects the lesser curvature of the stomach to the left lobe of the liver as well as the duodenum to the liver [1]. The greater omentum connects the greater curvature of the stomach to the transverse colon [6]. Primary abnormalities of the peritoneum are rare in children [7]. However, there is frequent secondary involvement of the peritoneal cavity and its specialized folds, the mesentery and omentum by infectious, neoplastic, and traumatic conditions originating at other sites in the abdomen or pelvis [8]. However, in contrast to adults where the most common masses are adenocarcinoma in origin, the tumors in children are either sarcomas or tumors of other origins. Primary tumors of the peritoneum in children are usually mesenchymal in origin [8].

Common tumors affecting the peritoneum, omentum, mesentery, and retroperitoneum will be discussed in this chapter. The adrenal neuroblastoma and the tumors involving the kidneys will be covered elsewhere in the book.

24.2 Imaging Modalities

Ultrasound (USG) is the initial and preferred imaging modality used to evaluate peritoneal diseases in children due to the absence of ionizing radiation [9], and easy availability. It is particularly useful for characterizing the solid and cystic nature of the mass as well as the vascularity of the mass using Doppler [10]. A major drawback of USG is that it does not provide a global assessment of the abdominal and pelvic anatomy and is limited by bowel gases, the inability of children to understand commands, and excessive crying

P. Sinha (✉)
Radiodiagnosis, Vallabhbhai Patel Chest Institute, Delhi, India

D. Kandsamy
Radiodiagnosis and Interventional Radiology, AIIMS, New Delhi, India

I. Kumar et al. (eds.), *Practical Approach to Imaging in Pediatric Oncology*,
https://doi.org/10.1007/978-981-96-8158-7_24

[11]. Cross-sectional imaging is, therefore, necessary to evaluate the complete extent of disease. USG is usually the modality of choice for sampling the peritoneal, omental, and mesenteric lesions in children [12].

Computed tomography (CT) enables a much better evaluation of the peritoneal cavity and allows clearer differentiation and compartmentalization of the masses in intra, retro, and extraperitoneal compartments. The main advantages of CT are the lack of operator dependency and the short duration of the examination. However, the main concern is ionizing radiation, especially in cases that need follow-up imaging [13]. The staging system used for primary peritoneal surface malignancy is the same as ovarian cancer and fallopian tube malignancies. Peritoneal cancer index (PCI) comprehensively estimates tumor volume within the peritoneal cavity. Imaging however underestimates PCI. CECT is still an excellent tool for identifying those who may not benefit from cytoreductive surgery and HIPEC [3].

MR imaging in general is considered more sensitive for the evaluation of peritoneal diseases than CT. The lack of ionizing radiation is a big advantage over CT. The main disadvantages of MRI are the duration of the examination, the need for sedation, motion artifacts, and the relatively low availability (particularly in the emergency setting outside normal working hours). MRI has lower spatial resolution than CT and the need for a gadolinium (Gd) contrast agent may be a limiting factor as well, because of the concern of deposition of Gd chelates in body tissues in children. [13, 14] MRI of the peritoneum has emerged as a promising alternative for staging and surveillance. It provides excellent soft tissue contrast [15].

PET/CT is an excellent technique for ruling out nodal and extraperitoneal disease and detecting recurrences that may be missed on CT. However, it may be false-negative in small peritoneal deposits, mucinous tumors, or signet ring cancers, and may be false-positive in nonmalignant inflammatory lesions.

24.3 Approach to Tumors of the Peritoneum, Omentum, Mesentery, and Retroperitoneum

Mesenteric, peritoneal, omental, and retroperitoneal masses in children may be initially classified as solid or cystic. If the mass is cystic it is further categorized into multilocular and unilocular. The solid lesions are further characterized based on the number of lesions, margins of the lesion, and contents like fat and calcification. A useful approach to characterize these masses is depicted in Chart 24.1.

Chart 24.1 Imaging approach to tumors of the peritoneum, omentum, mesentery, and retroperitoneum

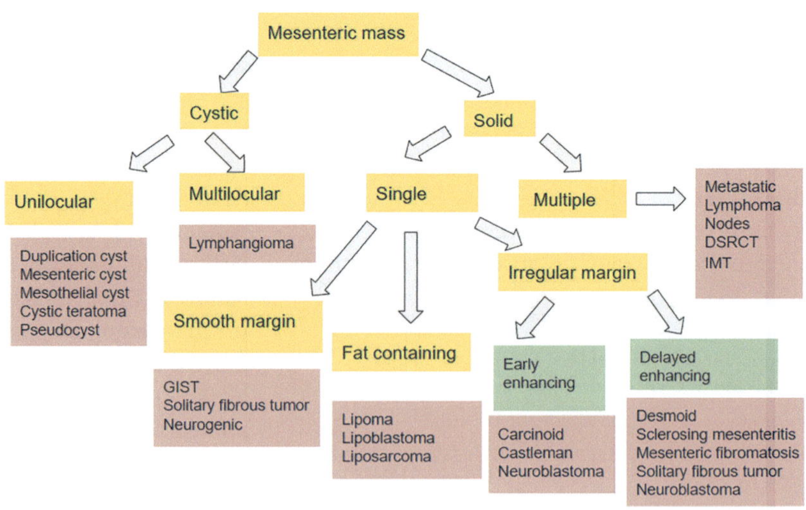

24.4 Cystic Tumors of the Mesentery, Omentum, and Retroperitoneum (Table 24.1)

24.4.1 Cystic Teratoma

On imaging, cystic teratomas can range from being a purely cystic mass to a complex cystic mass with solid components. Cross-sectional imaging has excellent sensitivity for diagnosing this entity due to the presence of macroscopic fat (Fig. 24.1). In addition to the detection of fat, other clues such as the fat-fluid level, floating ball sign, palm tree-like protrusion, and reversed chemical shift artifacts may be seen. Minute quantities of fat can also be detected with chemical shift imaging (in/opposed phase) on MRI.

24.4.2 Cystic Lymphangioma

Lymphangiomas are benign lesions of vascular origin that show lymphatic differentiation or may result from embryonic sequestration of lymphatic tissue [16]. They consist of endothelium-lined spaces surrounded by a connective tissue stroma of varying thickness containing lymphoid tissue and occasionally smooth muscles [15]. These lesions have been currently classified as slow-flow vascular malformations. On USG, lymphangiomas are unilocular or multilocular cystic masses that are anechoic or contain echogenic debris. On CT these appear as hypodense, insinuating masses with little or no mass effect on adjacent structures. On CECT, they may show thin enhancement of the cyst wall and septa (Fig. 24.2). The fluid component is typically homogeneous with low attenuation values unless complicated by hemorrhage. Occasionally, negative attenuation values may be seen due to the presence of chyle. Calcification may occur rarely. The signal pattern of lymphangiomas on MRI resembles that of fluid. The presence of hemorrhage or infection in the lesion may alter the MRI signal pattern.

24.4.3 Duplication Cyst

Enteric duplication cysts (EDC) are rare developmental anomalies, originating anywhere along the alimentary tract from the tongue to the anus. The abdominal cavity (75%) is the most common site, followed by thoracic (20%) and thoracoabdominal (5%) locations. Ileal lesions are the most common (53%), followed by mediastinal (18%) lesions. Duplication cysts may be spherical (80%) or tubu-

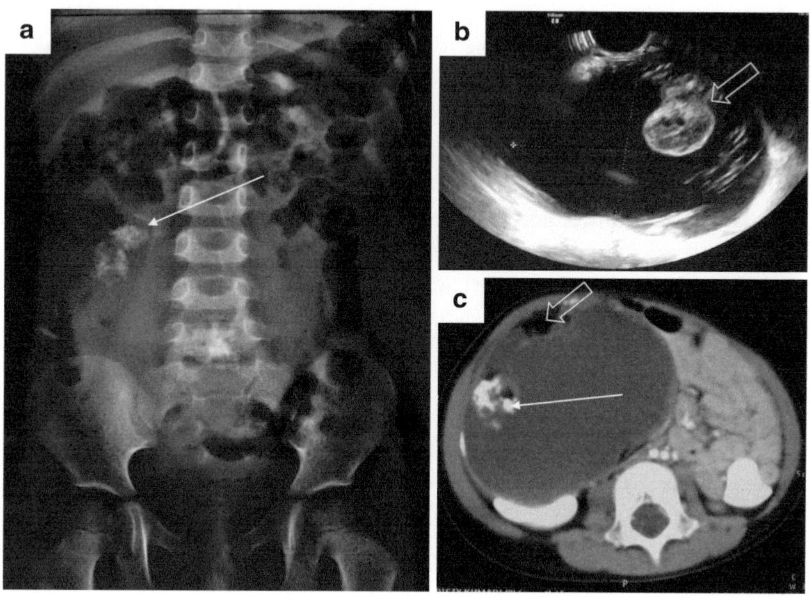

Fig. 24.1 (**a**, **b**): Abdominal radiograph (**a**) of a child shows increased soft tissue opacity in the right side of the abdomen with areas of calcification (arrow). USG (**b**) and CECT (**c**) images show a well defined, predominantly cystic lesion in the right anterior pararenal space with areas of fat (outlined arrows) and calcification (arrow) suggestive of retroperitoneal mature cystic teratoma

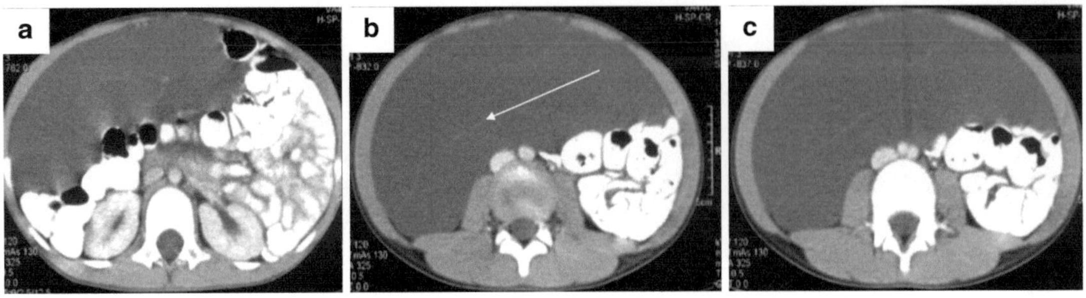

Fig. 24.2 (**a–c**): Axial CECT abdomen show a cystic attenuation mass with thin enhancing septae in the peritoneal cavity (arrow). The mass is displacing the ascending colon and small bowel loops to the left side and is also abutting the retroperitoneal structures like psoas, aorta and inferior vena cava. These features are suggestive of retroperitoneal lymphatic malformation

lar (20%). Spherical cysts typically do not communicate with the bowel. The tubular duplication cysts are parallel to the bowel lumen, and more often have communication with the gut, and peristalsis is more commonly identified in them. Atypical EDC is a non-communicating isolated duplication cyst that is completely separated from the bowel due to a vascular insult. USG is the imaging method of choice for the diagnosis of EDCs; it is only suboptimal for the evaluation of esophageal EDCs for which transoesophageal USG might be useful. A typical uncomplicated EDC on USG is seen as a cystic lesion abutting the gut with a double-wall or muscular rim sign (gut signature sign). The gut signature results from the inner hyperechoic mucosa and outer hypoechoic smooth muscle layer (muscularis propria). Rarely all five layers are identified (Fig. 24.3). However, the double-wall sign may be seen in other cystic lesions (mesenteric cyst, Meckel's diverticulum, or torsioned ovarian cyst). An EDC shares a wall with the adjacent bowel and may demonstrate the "Y" sonographic configuration of the muscle layer caused by the splitting of the shared muscularis propria between the cyst and the adjacent loop and is pathognomonic for EDC.

24.4.4 Chylolymphatic Mesenteric Cyst

Chylolymphatic mesenteric cysts are rare lesions that are lined by endothelial cells and lack the disorganized smooth muscle layer seen in cystic lymphangioma [17]. They contain chylous fluid and originate from the small bowel mesentery. These are mainly seen in older children and young adults with female preponderance. On USG and CT, it is difficult to differentiate it from unilocular cystic lymphangiomas. However, on MRI, the fat content of the chyle is T1 and T2 hyperintense, with loss of signal intensity on T1-weighted out-of-phase and/or fat-suppressed images. [18, 19] Occasionally, these cysts may show a fluid-fluid level composed of nondependent chyle.

24.4.5 Adrenal Cyst

Adrenal cysts are rare retroperitoneal lesions that account for only 4% of all adrenal masses. Adrenal cysts are mostly benign and have malignant potential in only 7% of cases [19]. Most of the adrenal cysts are unilateral but around 8%–15% can present bilaterally. Symptoms vary in presentation according to the size and location of the cyst. Smaller cysts are often asymptomatic, nonfunctional, and discovered incidentally on imaging. Larger cysts (>10 cm) are symptomatic. These lesions are extremely uncommon before second decade of life but sometimes may have syndromic associations and are present in children. These are often associated with polycystic renal disease, Klippel-Trenaunay-Weber syndrome, Beckwith-Wiedemann syndrome, schwannomas, and aortic aneurysms. Infrequently, metastasis can present as cystic

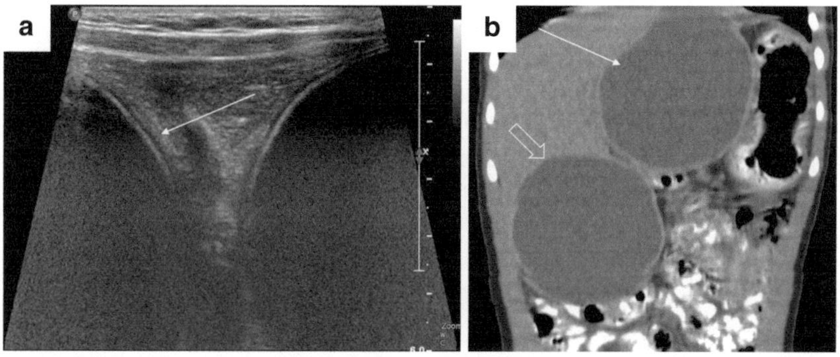

Fig. 24.3 (**a**, **b**): USG (**a**) shows a thin walled cystic lesion with typical gut signature sign depicted by 3 layers (arrow). Coronal CECT abdomen (**b**) shows two well defined cystic attenuation mass, one of them closely abutting the stomach (arrow) and the other one abutting the colon (outlined arrow). No fat, calcification, septa, or enhancing soft tissue component noted within the lesion. These features are suggestive of enteric duplication cysts

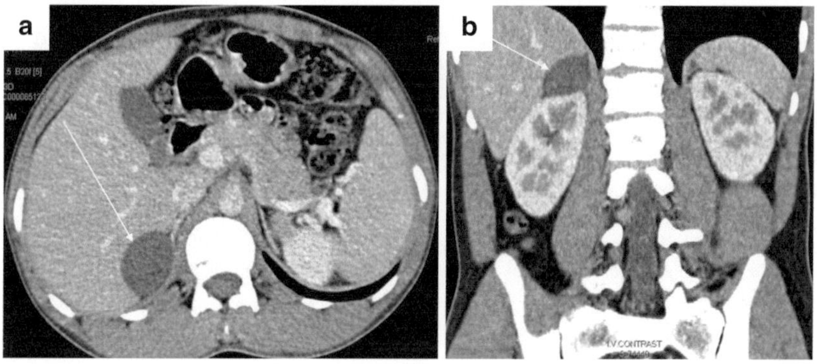

Fig. 24.4 (**a**, **b**): Axial and coronal CECT abdomen images show a well defined, fluid attenuation mass in the right adrenal gland without any contrast enhancement. No fat or calcification noted within the lesion. USG (not shown here) showed a cystic lesion. The above features are typical for adrenal cyst

adrenal lesions. Simple adrenal cysts are thin-walled lesions that appear anechoic on USG, and non-enhancing well-defined cystic attenuation lesions on CT (Fig. 24.4). Adrenal Pseudocyst.

Pseudocysts are complex cysts, resulting from hemorrhage into the adrenal parenchyma due to birth injury, asphyxia, trauma, toxins, or infections. Other causes include uremia, Waterhouse-Friderichsen syndrome, burns, adrenal vein thrombosis, syphilis, leukemia, and incompatible blood transfusions [19]. They are usually unilocular, encapsulated, and devoid of inner wall lining, and may show calcification of the fibrous capsule. The cyst cavity usually contains blood clots and proteinaceous materials. Rarely, these pseudocysts may be associated with neoplastic lesions including adenomas, hemangiomas, pheochromocytomas, or malignant hemangioendothelioma [19]. Adrenal hemorrhage may appear as a heterogeneous, thick-walled cystic lesion with thin septations and internal echoes on CT/USG (Fig. 24.5) However, MRI usually is diagnostic in these cases. Similarly, adrenal abscess may also present as a complex lesion on USG but diagnostic aspiration/MRI can clinch the diagnosis.

24.4.6 Peritoneal Simple Mesothelial Cyst (PSMC)

PSMC is a congenital cyst that can occur in the small bowel, mesentery, mesocolon, or omentum. It is formed due to the failure of the mesothelium-lined peritoneal surfaces to coalesce. Children may present with acute abdominal pain due to rupture, inflammation, infection, torsion, or hemorrhage within the cyst. CT, MRI, or USG reveals a simple appearing thin-walled unilocular cyst without internal septa. The imaging features are non-specific and histopathological evaluation is the gold standard for diagnosis. The mesothelial cells lining the cyst can be further characterized with immunohistochemistry [20].

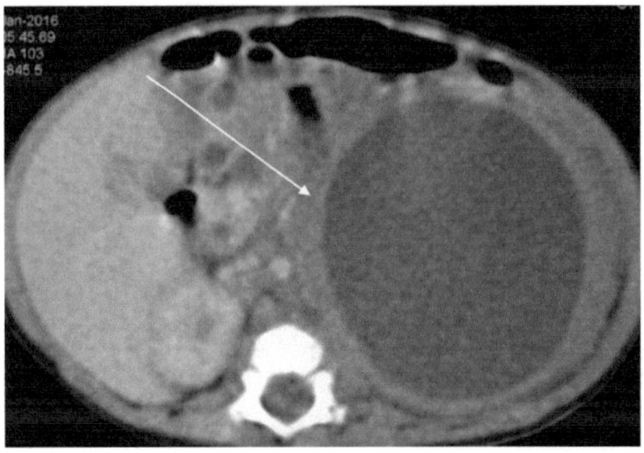

Fig. 24.5 Axial CECT abdomen image shows a well defined thick walled, cystic attenuation lesion (arrow) in the region of left adrenal gland without post contrast enhancement. No fat or calcification noted within the lesion. These features are suggestive of adrenal pseudocyst in a child with a history of adrenal hemorrhage

24.5 Solid Tumors of the Mesentery, Omentum, and Retroperitoneum (Table 24.1)

24.5.1 Rhabdomyosarcoma

Rhabdomyosarcoma (RMS) is the most common soft-tissue sarcoma in children, accounting for 5–8% of childhood cancers. The tumors have a wide variety of histological types and patterns of spread. Rhabdomyosarcomas can be divided into embryonic, botryoid, alveolar, and undifferentiated subtypes. The margins of the tumor may be infiltrative or well-defined. RMS may infiltrate locally, and metastasize by lymphatic and hematogenous routes to the lungs, and bone marrow which are common at the time of diagnosis. Retroperitoneal RMS are usually large at the time

Table 24.1 Tumors of the peritoneum, omentum, mesentery, and retroperitoneum in pediatric patients with their salient imaging features

Cystic lesions	Cystic teratoma	Maybe mature or immature Macroscopic Fat/calcification/tooth or bone-like structures help in clinching diagnosis
	Lymphangioma	A cystic, pliable lesion that insinuates between the structures Maybe microcystic or macrocystic Absent or minimal enhancement
	Duplication cyst	Spherical/tubular Anechoic cystic lesion closely abutting bowel loops Gut signature on USG
	Chylolymphatic mesenteric cyst	Content is T1 and T2 hyperintense, with signal drop on T1-weighted out-of-phase and/or fat-suppressed images A fat-fluid level may be seen
	Adrenal cyst	Thin-walled lesions Anechoic on USG A non-enhancing well-defined lesion with cystic attenuation lesion on CT
	Adrenal pseudocyst	Unilocular/multilocular Thin-walled/thick-walled Usually anechoic with variable amounts of debris It may show calcification of the fibrous capsule
	Peritoneal simple mesothelial cyst	Thin-walled unilocular cyst without internal septations

(continued)

Table 24.1 (continued)

Solid lesions	Rhabdomyosarcoma	Margin-infiltrative or well-defined Bulky mass with heterogeneous attenuation Necrosis common Calcifications are rare
	Lymphoma	Sandwich sign Lymphadenopathy especially below the renal hilum Homogeneous enhancement similar to the muscles Absent calcification Burkitt's lymphoma is one of the fastest-growing tumors that can present with a solid mass usually in the right lower quadrant
	Liposarcoma	Rare in children less than 10 years Fat attenuation It may have solid enhancing components or enhancing septae Large retroperitoneal tumors even when they appear completely fatty on imaging should be considered malignant
	Lipoblastoma	Well-defined Fat-containing mass in a child less than 4 years of age
	Germ cell tumors	Mature/immature Solid/cystic/mixed Fat/calcification
	Ganglioneuroma	Homogenous mass with calcification
	Ganglioneuroblastoma	Solid, well-marginated, oblong paraspinous mass with homogeneous enhancement An irregular, cystic, poorly marginated, locally invasive mass.
	Carcinoid tumor	Ileal location is common Arterial hyperenhancement Desmoplastic reaction and retraction of adjacent small bowel loops Calcification may be present
	Inflammatory myofibroblastic tumors	Well-defined focal lesions Can have calcifications Ascites absent
	Castleman disease	Unicentric (benign) or multicentric (aggressive) Homogeneously enhancing masses May show calcification Poor avidity in FDG
	Mesenteric fibromatosis	Solid, multiple No calcification No ascites Association with familial adenomatous polyposis
	Desmoplastic small round cell tumors	Multiple lesions Lobulated, heterogeneous masses with increased vascularity Arterial enhancement without prolonged enhancement or washout is seen on portal venous and delayed phase images Intralesional fluid-fluid levels suggesting hemorrhagic necrosis
	Nerve sheath tumor	Fascicle sign T2 central hypointensity Split fat sign Orientation along nerve Rim sign These signs are rare in retroperitoneal and omental nerve sheath tumors
	Solitary fibrous tumor	T2 hypointensity Delayed progressive enhancement
	Primary peritoneal mesothelioma	Sheet-like or nodular peritoneal thickening Ascites Mesenteric involvement, and omental soft tissue masses

(continued)

Table 24.1 (continued)

	Adrenal adenoma	Solid lesion HU < 10 is diagnostic APW > 60 RPW > 40
	Myelolipoma	Well-defined fat-containing mass Signal drop on CSI and fat-sat images. Intra-tumoral aneurysms may be seen Calcification in 20–30% cases Hemorrhage
	Pheochromocytoma	Solid, mixed solid-cystic, or cystic Classical "light-bulb" bright appearance on T2W MRI Calcification—10% cases Extraadrenal location—Paraganglioma (well-defined, solid, soft tissue mass which lack calcification in 90% cases)
	Adrenal cortical carcinoma	Large, heterogeneous, irregular mass with variable enhancement, calcifications, and hemorrhage
	Metastases	Signal characteristics similar to primary and metastasis elsewhere Multiple lesions Peritoneal thickening Omental masses Ascites

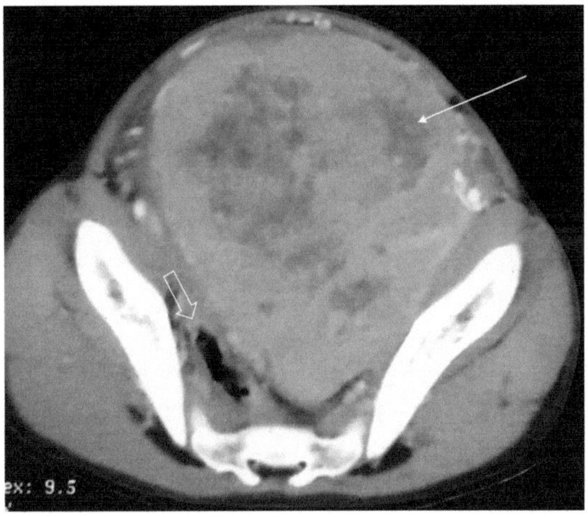

Fig. 24.6 Axial CECT image depicts a large, heterogeneously enhancing solid mass with few central areas of non enhancing cystic/necrotic component (arrow) noted in the pelvis arising from the left lateral pelvic wall abutting the rectum (outlined arrow). No calcification or fat noted in the mass. Biopsy came out to be rhabdomyosarcoma

of diagnosis and appear as a bulky mass with heterogeneous attenuation equal to or slightly less than muscle on CT. Areas of low attenuation representing necrosis are common, and calcifications are rare (Figs. 24.6 and 24.7). The precise origin of the tumor is often difficult to determine because of the infiltration of adjacent organs. The tumor shows heterogeneous enhancement on contrast-enhanced scans. The appearance on MRI is that of a heterogeneous mass with areas of necrosis and bleed. They are usually T2 hyperintense, the magnitude of which depends on the histopathological type of RMS.

24.5.2 Lymphoma

Common presenting symptoms of lymphoma are pain in the abdomen, palpable mass, intestinal obstruction due to bowel compression or intussusception, and acute appendicitis. Weight loss, fever, and other systemic features are seen more in patients with disseminated disease. Initial presentation with a retroperitoneal mass is uncommon. Non-Hodgkin's lymphomas are more common than Hodgkin's Lymphoma in children younger than 5 years of age. They might be seen as single central or symmetrical bilateral masses along the abdominal great vessels. Homogeneous, moderate enhancement, and restricted diffusion are characteristically seen. Enhancement similar to muscles is one of the typical features of lymphoma on CECT scans. Necrosis is uncommon but can occur in aggressive types of lymphoma and calcifications are extremely rare (Figs. 24.8 and 24.9).

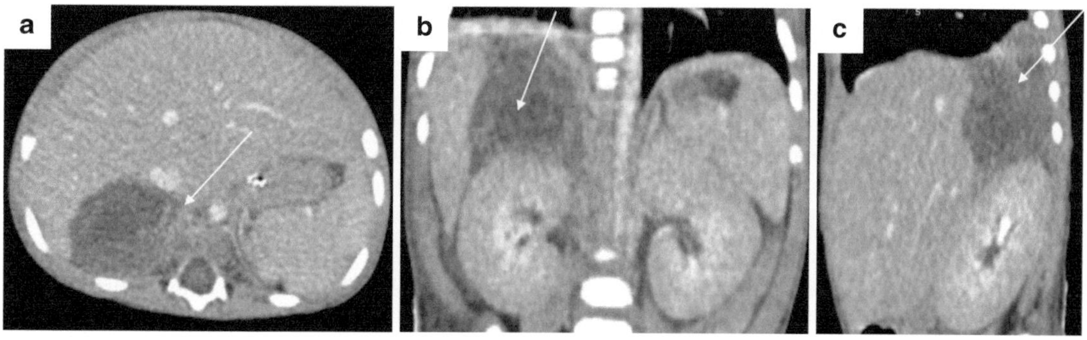

Fig. 24.7 (**a–c**): There is a well defined, heterogenous, solid lesion in the right adrenal region (arrow) which showing heterogeneous enhancement on post-contrast images. Biopsy of the lesion proved this lesion to be adrenal rhabdomyosarcoma

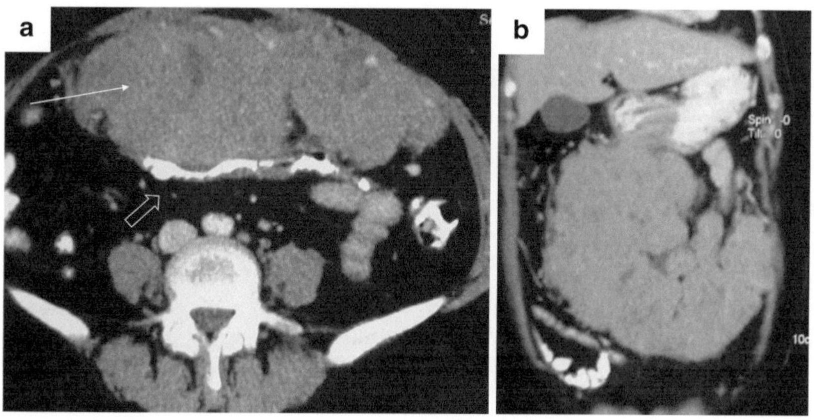

Fig. 24.8 (**a**, **b**): Axial and coronal CECT images show a large, lobulated, homogeneously enhancing omental mass without any calcification (arrow). The mass is closely abutting the anterior wall of the transverse colon (outlined arrow). Visualised bowel loops do not show any feature of obstruction. Biopsy of the mass showed omental lymphoma

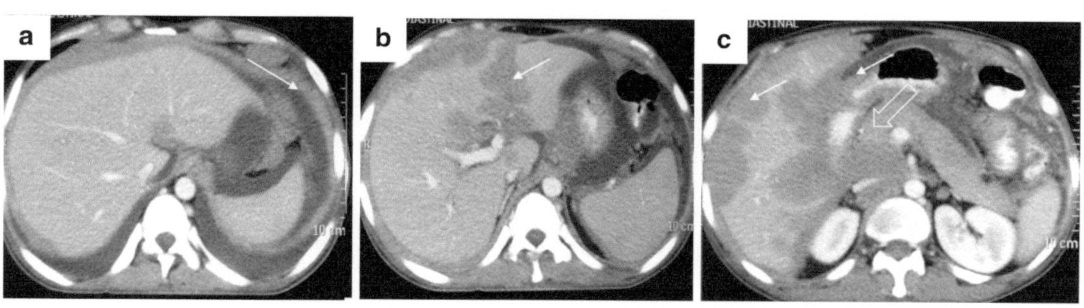

Fig. 24.9 (**a–c**): Axial CECT images show diffuse, homogeneously enhancing nodular peritoneal thickening (arrow). Multiple, hypodense, hypoenhancing ill defined lesions are also noted along the hepatic fissure and in the subdiaphragmatic location. Enlarged peripancreatic nodes are also seen (outlined arrow). There is mild bilateral pleural effusion with nodular thickening of pleura at places. These features are suggestive of peritoneal spread in a patient with lymphoma

24.5.3 Lipomatous Tumors

Tumors of fatty origin include lipoma, lipoblastoma, lipoblastomatosis, and liposarcoma. Lipoma and lipoblastoma are well-delineated tumors. Lipoblastomatosis is usually extensive and locally invasive. Liposarcoma is a malignant tumor that is locally invasive and can metastasize to distant sites. In children under 4 years, lipoblastoma is the most common lipomatous tumor of the retroperitoneum. On CT, retroperitoneal lipoblastoma shows characteristic fat within the lesion. However, some may demonstrate areas of relatively increased attenuation due to the presence of myxoid tissue [21, 22]. Depending on the cellular composition and the presence of myxoid material, the percentage of visible fat in tumors varies [23, 24]. Calcifications are rare in these tumors (Fig. 24.10).

24.5.4 Germ Cell Tumors (GCT)

These are benign or malignant tumors derived from the primordial germinal epithelial layer cells in gonadal or extragonadal sites. GCTs are classified into seminomatous, nonseminomatous GCTs (embryonal carcinomas, yolk sac tumors, and choriocarcinomas), and teratomas. Primary retroperitoneal extragonadal germ cell tumors (EGCTs) are rarely encountered neoplasms, accounting for only 1–2.5% of all germ cell tumors [25].

The majority of retroperitoneal germ cell tumors represent metastatic tumors from a gonadal primary lesion (Fig. 24.11). Benign teratomas are the most common retroperitoneal tumor in children after neuroblastoma and Wilm's tumor [26, 27]. Mature teratomas contain histologically well-developed tissues, such as soft tissue, fat, fluid, or calcium. Immature teratomas contain at least 10% undifferentiated tissue and are devoid of malignant components or metastases (Fig. 24.12). These tumors may be cystic, solid, or a combination of both. Retroperitoneal teratoma typically appears as a large complex mass containing fluid, fat, fat-fluid level, and calcifications. Large areas of hemorrhage, necrosis, and infiltration into adjacent tissue are pointers toward malignant lesions [28]. Radiologically, benign germ cell tumors appear as cystic masses with fat/ calcification or complex masses with Rokitansky protuberance. Calcification in mature teratomas is usually coarse and located within the lesion. Malignant germ cell tumors more commonly demonstrate enhancing solid components and peripheral rim calcification. Infiltration into surrounding structures lymphadenopathy, and ascites are other features that are pointers toward malignant germ cell tumors. The criteria favoring

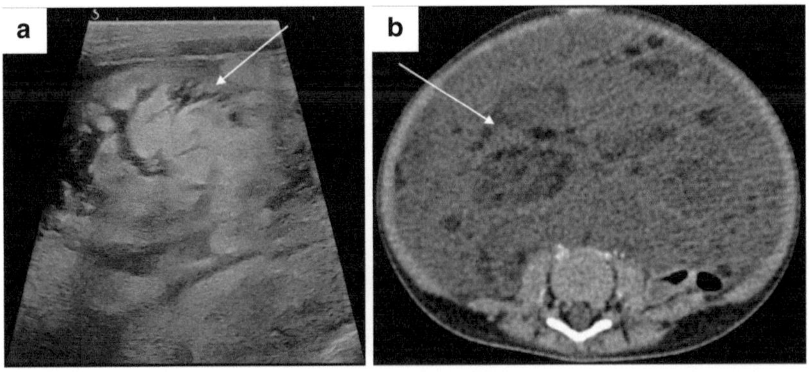

Fig. 24.10 (**a**, **b**): USG image of a 10 month old child presenting with abdominal distension since birth shows a large mass with multifocal areas of hyperechogenicity within. CECT axial image shows a poorly enhancing, fat containing mass in the abdominopelvic region. The mass is insinuating between the structures and encasing mesenteric vessels as well as bowel loops (not shown here). No calcification was seen within the mass. No bowel obstruction, nodal spread or ascites was found. These imaging features are suggestive of lipoblastoma

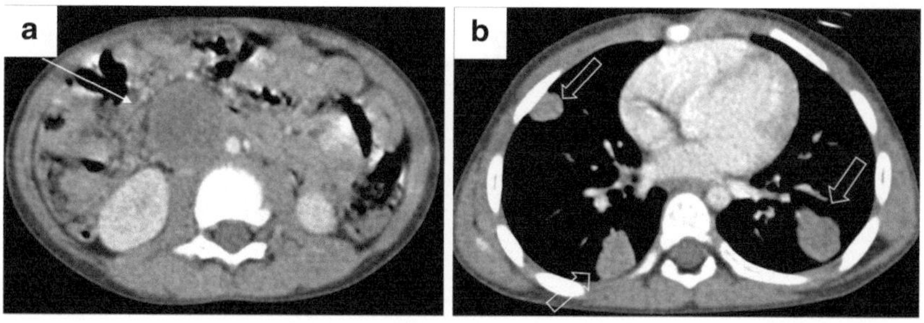

Fig. 24.11 (**a**, **b**): Axial CECT image at the level of right renal hilum shows a well defined, rounded, soft tissue attenuation mass showing homogenous post contrast enhancement (arrow). Axial CECT image of thorax shows multiple, variable sized, homogeneously enhancing lung parenchymal masses (outlined arrows). These features are consistent with a disseminated disease in a patient who was operated for testicular germ cell tumor in the past

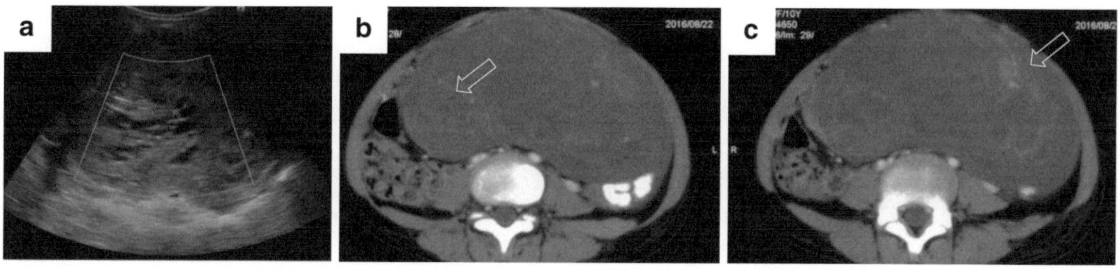

Fig. 24.12 (**a**–**c**): USG image (**a**) and CECT images (**b**, **c**) show a large, solid, heterogenous mass with enhancing soft tissue component (outlined arrow) in the retroperitoneum. The germ cell markers were elevated in this child. The imaging and biochemical feature are suggestive of immature germ cell tumor which was confirmed on post-operative histopathology

immature teratomas in prepubertal patients are the young age of the child, larger tumor size, and increased AFP level, with a cut-off of 8 months, 2.5 cm, and 23 ng/mL, respectively [28].

24.5.5 Ganglioneuroma and Ganglioneuroblastoma

Ganglioneuroma arises from the autonomic nervous system, most commonly from the peripheral sympathetic system [29]. On CT, they appear as well-circumscribed, solid, encapsulated paravertebral masses with a longitudinal orientation. They appear iso to hypoattenuating to muscle on CT. Approximately 10–25% of cases of ganglioneuroma demonstrate calcification. Scattered spotty, fine, or grain-like calcification indicates benign lesions, while large patchy or irregular, coarse calcification is usually seen in malignant lesions [30]. They appear as a homogeneously low or intermediate signal mass on T1 and appear as a heterogeneously intermediate or high signal mass on T2 which shows none to heterogeneous enhancement. (Figure 13) The apparent diffusion coefficient (ADC) values derived from diffusion-weighted imaging tend to be higher than that of a neuroblastoma [31].

Ganglioneuroblastoma is a transitional tumor of the sympathetic nervous system that lies on the intermediate spectrum of disease between a well-differentiated, low-grade, ganglioneuroma and an undifferentiated, high-grade, neuroblastoma. They appear as solid, well-marginated, oblong paraspinal masses with homogeneous enhancement or as irregular, cystic, poorly-marginated, locally invasive masses (Fig. 24.13).

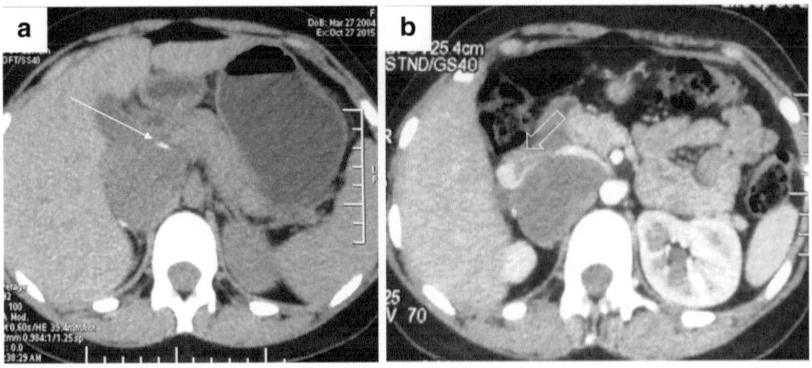

Fig. 24.13 (**a**, **b**): Axial NCCT (**a**) and CECT (**b**) images of abdomen show a well defined, poorly enhancing, soft tissue mass in the right suprarenal location with foci of calcifications (arrow). The mass is closely abutting the IVC and causing its displacement (outlined arrow). The mass was biopsied and diagnosed as Ganglioneuroblastoma

24.5.6 Carcinoid Tumor

On CT, these tumors appear as well-defined, rounded solid tumors with associated desmoplastic reactions in the mesentery manifesting as fibrotic strands emanating from the mass. They can also cause angulation, tethering, and fixation of adjacent bowel loops. They show avid enhancement after the administration of gadolinium, reflecting their hypervascular nature. Larger lesions tend to demonstrate necrosis. Characteristics suggesting malignancy include large primary tumor, central necrosis, vascular invasion, and calcification. These tumors have low signal intensity on T1-weighted images and high signal intensity on T2-weighted images. GRE sequences may show areas of calcifications as hypointense foci. A high index of clinical suspicion and appropriate diagnostic workup are important for early recognition because many carcinoid tumors are asymptomatic, and carcinoid syndrome is infrequent in children. Octreotide is a somatostatin analog commonly used in the treatment and diagnosis. Meta-iodobenzylguanidine (MIBG), a guanidine analog, is another radiotracer that concentrates in carcinoid tumors, including those not expressing somatostatin receptors. MIBG scan is helpful when pentetreotide imaging findings are negative. Because most carcinoid tumors are low-grade and well-differentiated, FDG PET/CT is not routinely used in the workup of these tumors.

24.5.7 Inflammatory Myofibroblastic Tumor

The inflammatory myofibroblastic tumor is a rare solid tumor of mesenchymal origin, which is most often found in the lung, mesentery, and omentum. Earlier, it was thought to be inflammatory in origin but is now considered a neoplasm of intermediate malignant potential because there is a propensity for local and regional recurrence and less than 5% risk of distant metastases. It commonly occurs in children and young adults, with a slight female preponderance. The symptoms depend on the site of the tumor, and the most common presenting symptom is pain in the abdomen. The imaging findings are nonspecific and variable. On USG, inflammatory myofibroblastic tumors typically appear as an ill- or well-defined, heterogeneous, solid, hypo, or hyperechoic mass. Calcifications or central hypoechoic regions correlating with necrosis may be seen, especially in large tumors. At CT, the mesenteric or omental inflammatory myofibroblastic tumor can be seen as a bulky, well-demarcated, homogeneous, or heterogeneous, spherical, or multilobulated mass. The CT attenuation can be hypo or iso-attenuating as compared to skeletal muscle, depending on the amount of myxoid or collagenous stroma. Contrast enhancement pattern includes early peripheral enhancement due to vascular tissue; and delayed central enhancement of fibrotic components (Figs. 24.14

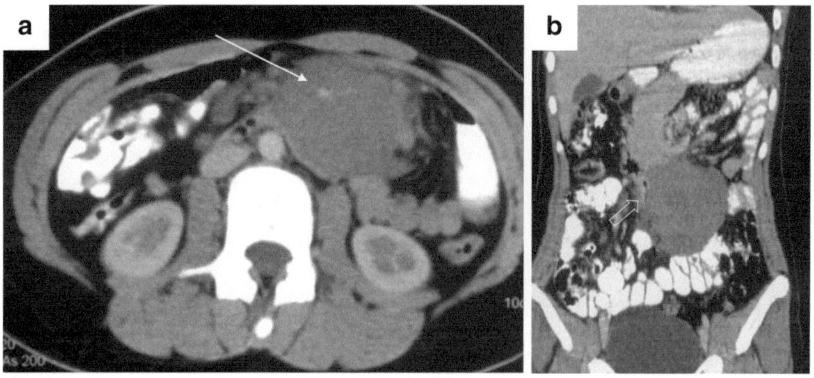

Fig. 24.14 (**a**, **b**): Axial and coronal CECT images of abdomen in a child show a well defined, homogeneously enhancing soft tissue mass with a foci of soft calcification within (arrow). The epicentre of the mass is in the mesentery and it is abutting bowel loops with maintained fat planes except for focal loss of fat plane with a jejunal loop (outlined arrow). Biopsy of the mass was performed and diagnosed as Inflammatory myofibroblastic tumor

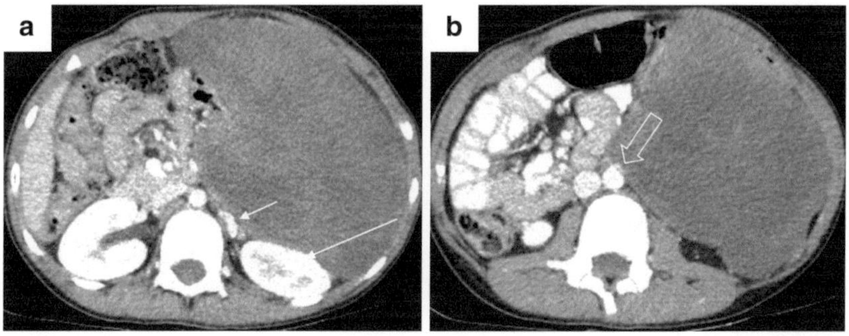

Fig. 24.15 (**a**, **b**): Axial CECT images showing a large, well defined, heterogeneously enhancing mass closely abutting the left kidney (arrow). The lesion also abuts abdominal aorta (outlined arrow) and left renal vessels (short arrow). The lesion is causing displacement of bowel loops and mesentery towards contralateral side. No calcification or fat noted within the mass. This lesion was proven to be an inflammatory myofibroblastic tumor

and 24.15). At MR imaging, inflammatory myofibroblastic tumors typically appear hypointense on T1-weighted images and hyperintense on T2-weighted images. Fibrotic stroma may appear dark on both T1- and T2-weighted images. The tumor commonly demonstrates heterogeneous enhancement and may exhibit delayed contrast enhancement of the fibrotic components.

24.5.8 Castleman Disease

Castleman disease, or angiofollicular lymphoid hyperplasia, is an idiopathic benign lymphoproliferative disorder that primarily affects young adults but can rarely occur in older children. It is broadly classified into two types: unicentric (local) and multicentric (disseminated) [32]. Unicentric disease is more common in children and follows a benign clinical course. The multicentric form has shown an association with human immunodeficiency virus, human herpesvirus 8 infection, and immune disorders [33, 34]. Unicentric Castleman disease appears as a well-defined, hypervascular, discrete mass or dominant mass with satellite nodules. The multicentric form of Castleman disease demonstrates hepatosplenomegaly, ascites, diffuse adenopathy, and thickening of retroperitoneal fascia [35]. USG imaging shows a well-defined, homogeneous, hypoechoic mass. Color Doppler interrogation may reveal large vessels at the periphery and

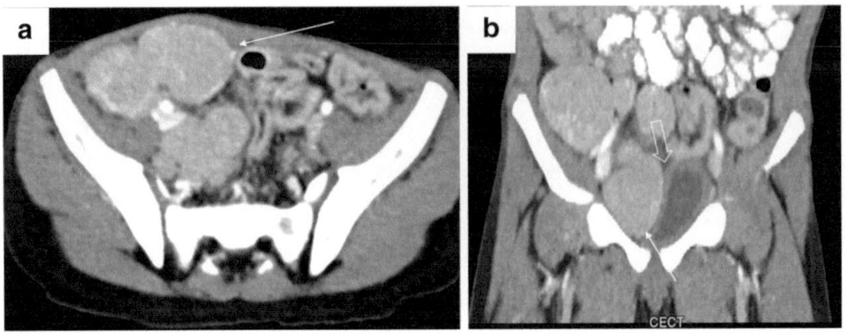

Fig. 24.16 (**a**, **b**): Axial and coronal CECT images show multiple variable sized, homogenous and intensely enhancing nodes (arrow) in the pelvis along the right iliac vessels. One of the mass is abutting the bladder with maintained fat planes and causing mass effect on bladder (outlined arrow). These masses were diagnosed as castleman disease on biopsy

extending centrally. Calcification is common and can be seen in 10%–31% of tumors. Enhancement is homogeneous in smaller masses but may be heterogeneous in larger masses (>5 cm) owing to areas of fibrosis or cystic necrosis (Fig. 24.16).

24.5.9 Mesenteric Fibromatosis

Mesenteric fibromatosis, also known as desmoid tumor, results from a benign proliferation of fibrous tissue. There is an association with familial adenomatous polyposis. Mesentery, particularly small bowel mesentery, is the most common location for desmoid tumors in Gardner syndrome. Previous trauma and surgery have also been implicated in its origin. Tumors may be solitary or multiple. These are locally aggressive tumors with a propensity to recur. A female preponderance has been reported as these tumors are associated with high estrogenic states. Mesenteric fibromatosis manifests as a focal well or ill-defined non-encapsulated mesenteric mass. The tumor may infiltrate adjacent structures like the bowel and lead to obstructive symptoms. At abdominal radiography, mass effect with displacement of bowel loops may be seen. In case it causes obstruction, signs of bowel obstruction may also be evident. At the ultrasound, they appear as well-defined solid masses with variable echogenicity. Rarely, they may present as ill-defined infiltrative, whorled soft-tissue thickening within the mesenteric fat usually causing angulation or spiculation of adjacent bowel loops. The imaging appearance of mesenteric fibromatosis depends on the histologic characteristics and vascularity of the lesion. They may be homogeneous with soft-tissue attenuation or heterogeneous due to collagenous/myxoid stroma in the tumor matrix. Poor enhancement after contrast administration is the rule, and they usually demonstrate progressive enhancement [36]. At MR, the majority of the lesions show low/intermediate signal intensity on T1-weighted sequences and appear heterogeneously hyperintense on T2-weighted images. When infiltrative, the tumor shows the characteristic "flame sign" feathery margins resembling a flame and can infiltrate local structures [37]. The mesenteric tumor often appears as a soft tissue mass with ill-defined margins and radiating spicules extending into the adjacent mesenteric fat ("whorled appearance") [37].

24.5.10 Desmoplastic Small Round Cell Tumor (DSRCT)

A desmoplastic small round cell tumor usually presents with a palpable abdominal mass. DSRCT is seen mostly in young patients and shows a marked male preponderance. It is most commonly seen to arise from the pelvic peritoneal cavity, the retrovesical or rectouterine space being the most frequent location. It can present as multifocal disease, nodular disease, diffuse omental and peritoneal disease, or a combination of these conditions. On ultrasound, the DSRCTs appear as lobulated, heterogeneous hypoechoic masses with increased vascularity. They might demonstrate interspersed cystic areas due to necrosis and hemorrhage [38]. These areas appear as hypoattenuating masses involving the peritoneal surfaces, omentum, and mesentery on unenhanced CT [38] (Fig. 24.17). Punctate or amorphous foci of calcification may be evident in 10–15% of patients. The largest mass is usually seen in the pelvic region (Fig. 24.18). On MRI, DSRCTs appear as heterogeneous isointense to hypointense masses on T1-weighted images. Patchy, mildly T1-hyperintense foci may represent intratumoral hemorrhage or calcification which can be differentiated on susceptibility-weighted imaging. On T2-weighted images, masses are usually heterogeneously hyperintense. T2 hypointense masses represent more fibrous stroma and densely packed cells within the tumor. Fluid-fluid levels are sometimes seen, suggesting hemorrhagic necrosis. On contrast-enhanced MRI, masses show heterogeneous enhancement. DWI sequence increases the conspicuity of peritoneal and visceral lesions in patients with DSRCT and aids in detecting subtle lesions [15, 38].

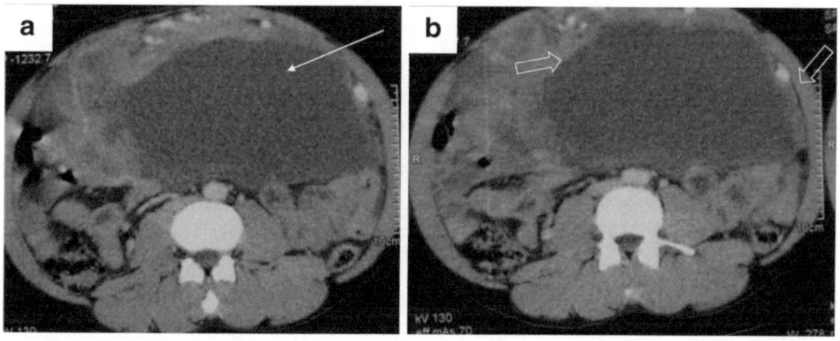

Fig. 24.17 (**a**, **b**): Axial CECT images of abdomen show a large, heterogeneously enhancing mass in the omentum with large central necrotic part and heterogeneous enhancement in the periphery of the mass (arrow). Multiple enlarged omental vessels are seen in the anterior surface of the mass (outlined arrow). The mass is displacing the bowel loops posterolaterally. No calcification was noted within the mass. Histopathological examination of the lesion showed desmoplastic small round cell tumor

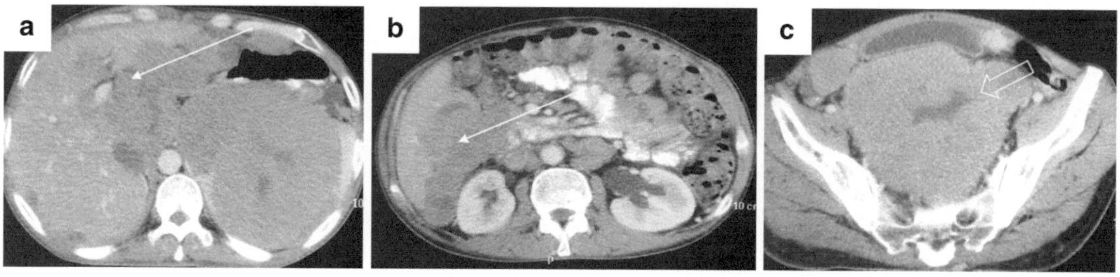

Fig. 24.18 (**a**–**c**): Axial CECT images reveal multiple, variable sized, enhancing soft tissue masses in the abdominopelvic cavity. The largest mass in the pelvis shows a central non enhancing necrotic area (outlined arrow). No calcification was noted within the lesions. Hypoenhancing ill defined lesions are also noted in the liver and in the gastro-splenic ligament location (arrow). Homogeneously enhancing lymph nodes are noted along the retroperitoneum. Biopsy of the lesion showed desmoplastic small round cell tumor

24.5.11 Nerve Sheath Tumor

Nerve sheath tumors occur in a younger age group and are usually benign. Schwannomas are the most common benign soft-tissue tumors occurring in the retroperitoneum accounting for 4% of retroperitoneal tumors. Neurofibromas can be solitary, diffuse, or plexiform types. Solitary neurofibromas (also known as localized, sporadic, or nodular) are most common (90%) and most often encountered in non-syndromic patients. Diffuse neurofibroma is uncommon and affects children and young adults. It most frequently involves the subcutaneous tissues of the head and neck. Plexiform neurofibromas may involve multiple fascicles, nerves, or even plexuses. They rarely can progress to malignant sarcomas. Diffuse and plexiform neurofibromas are more likely to be found in patients with NF1.

Various imaging features such as tail sign, split fat sign, target sign, and fascicular sign which are described for peripheral nerve sheath tumors are not so commonly seen in retroperitoneal nerve sheath tumors (Fig. 24.19). Plexiform neurofibromas on MR imaging appear as multinodular lesions that often feature the target sign and involve multiple nerve branches, creating a serpentine "bag-of-worms" configuration. They also show intense and homogeneous contrast enhancement. They appear bright on fluid-sensitive images and display homogeneous and moderate contrast enhancement closely mimicking a slow-flow vascular malformation. On diffusion-weighted Imaging, MPNSTs show low ADC values and restricted diffusion. On dynamic contrast-enhanced MR imaging, MPNSTs tend to display early arterial enhancement, a feature quite rare in benign nerve sheath tumors.

Most retroperitoneal schwannomas are benign. If associated with von Recklinghausen's disease, retroperitoneal schwannomas may undergo malignant transformation and exhibit irregular contours as well as distinct invasiveness into the adjacent tissue. Schwannomas are usually fusiform in shape, < 5 cm in size, and have intermediate (similar to muscle) signal intensity on T1-weighted images and high signal intensity on T2-weighted images. Rarely, a thin hypointense capsule (epineurium) can also be identified on T2, particularly if the tumor is surrounded by fat. Similar to retroperitoneal neurofibromas, retroperitoneal schwannomas also lack the typical split-fat sign and fascicular sign. The target sign is usually absent in large lesions or in schwannomas that have undergone cystic, hemorrhagic, or necrotic degeneration. The latter can mimic sarcomas on MR imaging. Calcification may be seen in approximately 23% of cases in retroperitoneal schwannomas. Cystic degeneration has been reported more in up to 66% of retroperitoneal schwannomas. Internal hemorrhagic areas in schwannomas show fallacious low ADC values, and these areas should be avoided when calculating the diffusion values by corroborating with T1-weighted images. Schwannomas also tend to display delayed enhancement on dynamic contrast-enhanced MR imaging.

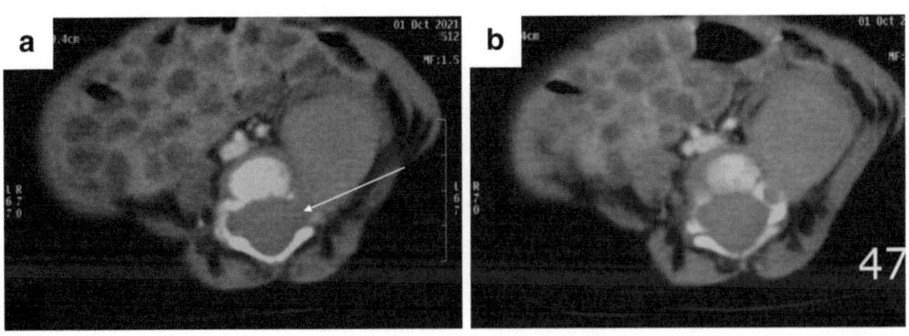

Fig. 24.19 (**a**, **b**): Axial CECT images of abdomen in a child show a homogeneously enhancing dumbbell shaped mass in the left paravertebral location which is causing widening of neural foramina (arrow) and is extending into the spinal canal. Biopsy of the lesion revealed neurofibroma

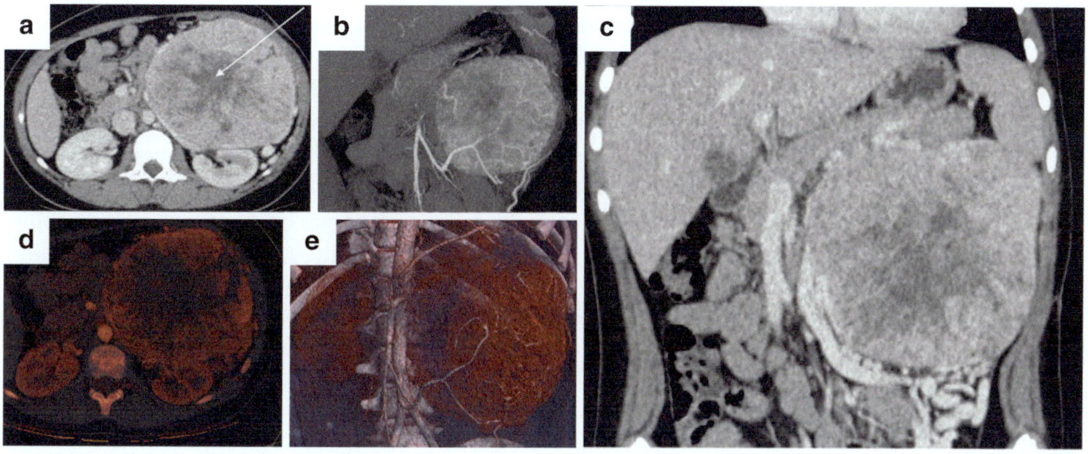

Fig. 24.20 (**a**–**e**): Axial (**a**) coronal MIP (**b**), coronal (**c**), axial Iodine map overlay (**d**) and volume rendered image (**e**) show a large heterogeneously intensely enhancing soft tissue mass with central hypoenhancing areas (arrow). The vascular supply to the mass is arising from multiple branches of abdominal aorta. Post-operative histopathology revealed solitary fibrous tumor

24.5.12 Solitary Fibrous Tumor

Solitary fibrous tumors (SFTs) are rare spindle-shaped cell tumors originating from dendritic mesenchymal cells. They mostly occur in the visceral pleura, but rarely in the retroperitoneum. These tumors appear as well-circumscribed, hypervascular masses with serpentine vessels along the periphery of the tumor (Fig. 24.20). Central hypoenhancing or non-enhancing areas may be seen in the tumor, which represent necrosis or cystic change. Calcification is rare and can be seen in large tumors.

At magnetic resonance (MR) imaging, SFTs appear as intermediate signal intensity mass on T1-weighted images and heterogeneous low signal intensity mass with flow voids on T2-weighted images and show intense enhancement. The imaging appearance, particularly the enhancement pattern on dynamic contrast-enhanced images varies depending on cellularity, vascularity, and the density of the collagenous or fibrous stroma. Hypervascular areas enhance intensely, the hypercellular areas show moderate enhancement, and areas of necrosis or cystic or myxoid degeneration do not enhance. Persistent or prolonged enhancement in the venous and delayed phases correlates with hypercellular areas, whereas mild enhancement in the arterial phase with increasing enhancement in the delayed phase correlates with the fibrous or collagenous stroma.

24.5.13 Primary Peritoneal Mesothelioma

Mesothelioma is a rare tumor involving the serosal cells of body cavities. Peritoneal mesothelioma specifically involves the serosa of the peritoneum and represents about 20% of these cases. Peritoneal epithelial malignant mesothelioma (PEMM) is seen in the pediatric population with a female preponderance. There is no association of PEMM with asbestos or radiation. Three variants of PEMM have been noted: diffuse malignant, localized malignant, and deciduoid peritoneal. The CT features of malignant peritoneal mesotheliomas can vary from a “dry” appearance, consisting of peritoneal masses to a “wet” appearance, consisting of ascites, irregular or nodular peritoneal thickening, and an omental mass. Calcified plaques are uncommon in malignant peritoneal mesotheliomas. Scalloping or direct invasion of adjacent abdominal organs may be seen. Differentials of a typical wet type of malignant peritoneal mesothelioma are peritoneal carcinomatosis, serous surface papillary carcinoma, lymphomatosis, and tuberculosis however, the amount of ascites is disproportionately small in relation to the degree of tumor dissemination in PEMM compared with peritoneal carcinomatosis. The incidence of liver metastasis and lymphadenopathy is also higher in peritoneal carcinomatosis.

24.5.14 Adrenal Adenoma

Adrenocortical adenoma is usually incidentally detected as most of these are nonfunctional and asymptomatic. The prevalence of adrenal adenoma increases with age. CT cannot differentiate between functioning adenomas and nonfunctioning adenomas, but the presence of ipsilateral or contralateral adrenocortical atrophy is strongly suggestive of a functioning adenoma. Noncontrast CT (NCCT) is a sufficient imaging modality for characterizing lipid-rich adenomas that measure 10 HU or less. However, washout CT is needed in case a lesion shows attenuation of >10 HU or has hyperdense foci (>10 HU), other than calcification or hemorrhage even when the other region of the lesion measures 10 HU or less on NCCT. Analyses of the NCCT histogram can provide a higher sensitivity than lesion attenuation measurement on NCCT and useful in patients with deranged renal function or hypersensitivity to iodinated contrast media. Adenoma-mimicking false-positive lesions that measure 10 HU or less on NCCT include adrenal hyperplasia, adenoma with coexisting non-adenoma, adrenal cyst, adrenocortical carcinoma, and pheochromocytoma. Most adenomas show early homogeneous enhancement and early washout in contrast to most malignant lesions. CECT is performed 60 seconds after the administration of the contrast material, and delayed contrast-enhanced CT (DCT) is performed 15 minutes after the administration of the contrast material. Absolute percentage washout (APW) and relative percentage washout (RPW) are calculated using lesion attenuation values on NCCT, CECT, and DCT as follows: APW = [CECT (HU) − DCT (HU)] × 100/[CECT (HU) − NCCT (HU)]. RPW = [CECT (HU) − DCT (HU)] × 100/CECT (HU). The thresholds of APW and RPW for an adenoma are 60% and 40%, respectively. Chemical-shift imaging (CSI) is an excellent MRI sequence for characterizing adenomas with abundant intracytoplasmic lipids, and these lesions show a signal drop in out-phase imaging (Fig. 24.21). Dual-energy CT can be used to characterize adrenal lesions with the help of virtual monochromatic images [39]. The lesion attenuation values decrease in 50% of adenomas on 80-kV, as compared to 140-kV, in contrast to Adrenocortical carcinomas (ACC) [40].

24.5.15 Myelolipoma

Adrenal myelolipomas are rare, benign incidentalomas of the adrenal gland characterized by the predominance of mature adipocytes. On imaging, they usually present as large masses with a variable amount of fat. Larger lesions (typically over 4 cm in size) can present with an acute retroperitoneal hemorrhage, or with vague mass-related symptoms. It has shown an association with

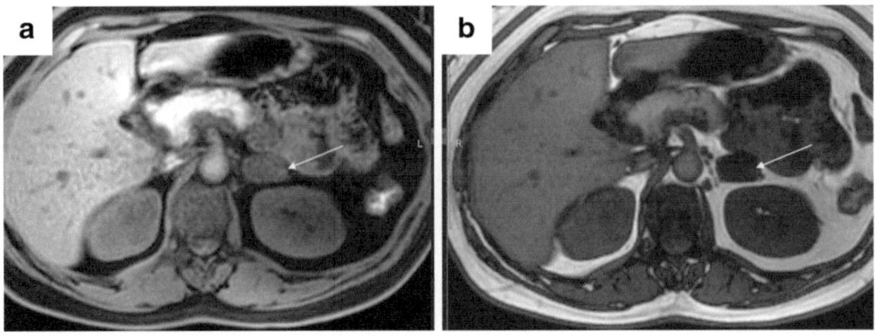

Fig. 24.21 (**a**, **b**): Chemical shift imaging (T1 in and opposed phase images **a**, **b**) showing a well defined focal lesion arising from the left adrenal gland with significant drop of signal in opposed phase (arrow) suggestive of adrenal adenoma

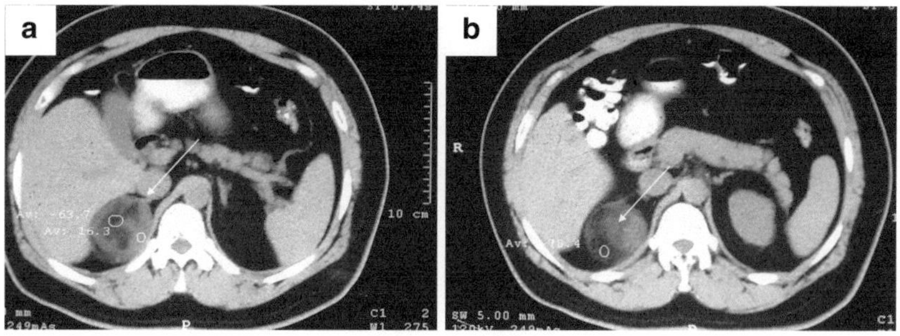

Fig. 24.22 (**a**, **b**): Axial CECT images of abdomen show a well defined, heterogeneous mass in right adrenal gland (arrow) with significant amount of macroscopic fat. The above features are diagnostic of adrenal myelolipoma

Cushing syndrome, congenital adrenal hyperplasia (21-hydroxylase deficiency), and Conn syndrome (primary hyperaldosteronism). On USG, they appear as a relatively well-defined heterogeneous mass of mixed hyper- and hypoechoic components. Areas of hemorrhage appear hypoechoic on ultrasonography. Fat within a myelolipoma can offer inertia to the ultrasound waves, resulting in the artifactual appearance of a discontinuous diaphragm. Small punctate calcifications may be seen in 25–30% of cases. On CT, they show a characteristic presence of macroscopic fat which usually occupies more than 50% of the tumor volume (Fig. 24.22). MRI shows a characteristic hyperintense mass on T1-weighted and T2-weighted sequences. Fat within the mass is suppressed on fat suppression imaging, but persistent high signal intensity areas may be seen in areas with myeloid tissue components or hemorrhage. In adrenal myelolipoma, fat saturation sequence leads to more signal loss than chemical shift imaging, because of the predominance of macroscopic fat.

24.5.16 Adrenal Pheochromocytoma

Pheochromocytomas are relatively rare catecholamine-secreting neuroendocrine tumors that arise from the chromaffin cells of the adrenal medulla. Less common extra-adrenal locations include the sympathetic chain in a cervical, thoracic, or pelvic location and rarely they may occur in the urinary bladder, spinal cord, and vagina. In children, 80% of pheochromocytomas occur in the adrenal gland, with bilateral adrenal involvement in 20%–40% of the cases. These tumors exhibit variability in symptoms and geographic distribution; therefore, biochemical markers and imaging are required to confirm the diagnosis. Pheochromocytomas are exceptionally rare in the pediatric population, but pediatric patients with pheochromocytoma, however, have a higher incidence of malignancy and genetic predisposition. Mutations of the protooncogene, RET; the tumor suppressor gene associated with von Hippel–Lindau disease, succinate dehydrogenase gene, Multiple endocrine neoplasia type 2, neurofibromatosis type 1, and familial paraganglioma syndromes. The tumor may be solid, mixed solid-cystic, or cystic. On NCCT, they can have low density to soft-tissue attenuation. Almost all pheochromocytomas have attenuation values of greater than 10 HU. Rarely, intracellular fat-containing pheochromocytomas may have attenuation less than 10 HU similar to adenomas resulting in signal loss on chemical-shift MRI. Hemorrhage can result in increased attenuation of pheochromocytoma. Calcifications are found in approximately 10% of pheochromocytomas. On contrast-enhanced CT (CECT), pheochromocytomas may show avid enhancement of the solid components, however, homogeneous or variable enhancement may also be seen. Contrast washout in pheochromocytomas is variable and may overlap with both benign and malignant lesions. Pheochromocytomas can have a classical "light-bulb" bright appearance on T2-weighted imaging with a signal intensity equivalent to cerebrospinal fluid (Fig. 24.23). In approximately 35% of cases, pheochromocytomas may have low signal intensity on T2-weighted imaging. Punctate signal voids representing tumor vessels create a salt-and-pepper pattern and are charac-

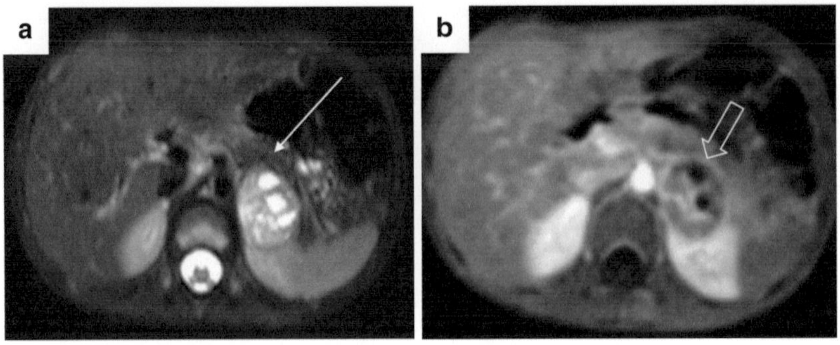

Fig. 24.23 (**a**, **b**): Axial T2 fat suppressed image (**a**), and axial post contrast images (**b**) reveal a well defined, heterogenous, solid cystic lesion (arrow) in the left adrenal gland which shows intense heterogeneous enhancement (outlined arrow). Plasma and urinary metanephrines were elevated in this child suggesting the diagnosis of pheochromocytoma

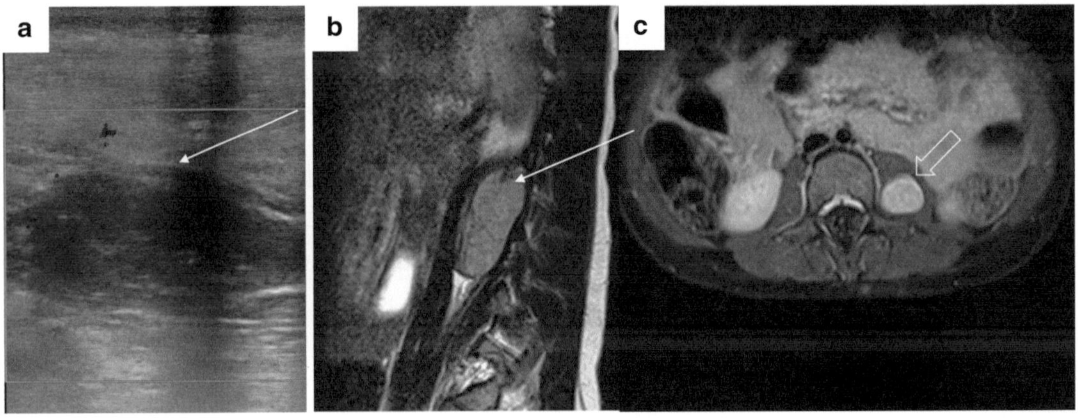

Fig. 24.24 (**a–c**): High resolution USG image of the left psoas muscle (**a**), sagittal T2W image (**b**), and axial post-contrast image (**c**) show a well defined, soft tissue mass (arrow) in the left psoas muscle demonstrating intense homogenous enhancement (outlined arrow). This lesion was diagnosed as paraganglioma based on the imaging and biochemical characteristics

teristically seen on T1- and T2-weighted images. 6-[18F] fluorodopamine PET and carbon-11 hydroxyephedrine PET are extremely useful in the detection and localization of pheochromocytoma. Iodine-131 or MIBG scintigraphy is often useful to localize, characterize, and exclude metastatic disease. Paragangliomas of sympathetic origin arising outside the adrenal gland show similar biochemical and imaging features that of pheochromocytomas except the fact that these tumors usually secrete normetanephrines rather than metanephrines unlike the latter (Fig. 24.24).

24.5.17 Adrenal Cortical Carcinoma

Adrenocortical carcinoma (ACC) is a rare, aggressive, malignant tumor arising from the adrenal cortex. It has a bimodal peak of incidence (less than 5 years old and between 30 and 50 years of age). Childhood ACC is clinically and biologically distinct from the adult tumor with affected pediatric patients typically presenting with signs and symptoms of endocrine excess, such as precocious puberty, Cushing syndrome, or virilization. Genetic syndromes

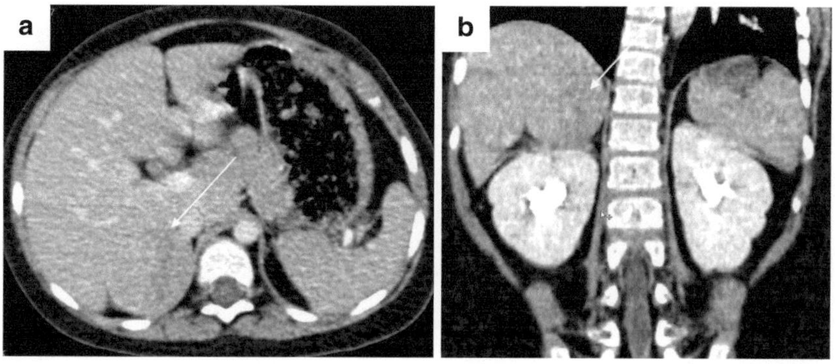

Fig. 24.25 (**a**, **b**): Axial and coronal CECT images of abdomen show a well defined, homogeneous, solid lesion arising from the right adrenal gland (arrow) which shows enhancement on post-contrast images. The child presented with cushing syndrome and hirsutism which led to the imaging diagnosis of adrenal cortical carcinoma which was proven later on post-operative histopathology

associated with ACC include Li-Fraumeni syndrome, Carney complex, Beckwith-Wiedemann syndrome, Familial Adenomatous Polyposis Coli, and MEN type 1. On ultrasound, a small ACC (<3 cm) typically is a homogeneous solid mass with internal vascularity. Larger masses often are heterogeneous and show areas of necrosis. CT characteristically shows a heterogeneously enhancing mass that displaces or invades adjacent organs (Fig. 24.25) About 25% of ACCs show central calcification. On MRI, ACC has an intermediate T1 signal, and T2 signal, and enhances heterogeneously on contrast-enhanced images. Imaging features suspicious for malignancy include size >4 cm, heterogeneous enhancement, venous invasion, indistinct margins, central necrosis, intratumoral calcifications, local invasion, and distant metastasis [39, 40].

24.5.18 Metastasis

It is one of the most common neoplasms affecting the peritoneum, mesentery, and omentum. It can be focal or diffuse. A pseudomyxoma peritonei-like appearance with scalloping of the solid organs has been described in rhabdomyosarcoma, Wilms tumor, Burkitt lymphoma, germ cell tumor, and dendritic cell sarcoma. Ascites is seen in most cases with peritoneal spread. On imaging, it can present as omental or peritoneal heterogeneously enhancing masses of variable size with hemorrhage, necrosis, and occasional calcifications depending on the characteristics of the primary tumor. Other imaging findings include enhancing nodules, masses, omental caking, and fibronodular stranding. Mesenteric thickening may produce pleated or stellate patterns on computed tomography (Fig. 24.26).

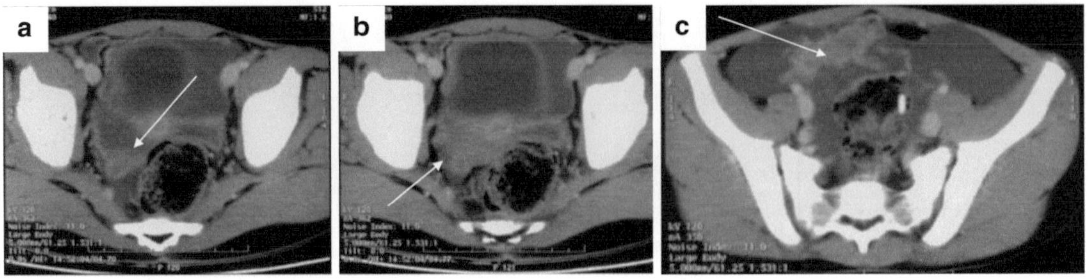

Fig. 24.26 (**a**–**c**): Axial CECT images of abdomen in a girl show diffuse, homogeneously enhancing nodular peritoneal thickening (arrow). There is minimal ascites with nodular thickening of peritoneal lining at places. These features are suggestive of peritoneal deposits in a case of ovarian germ cell tumor

24.6 Conclusion

There is a wide spectrum of tumors of retroperitoneum, mesentery, and omentum in the pediatric population. Knowledge of the spectrum of tumors and their distinctive clinical and imaging features is crucial to the diagnosis. The algorithmic approach may help in easier classification and narrow down the differential diagnosis.

24.7 Reporting Template

Size	[—x—x—] cm
Location	< retroperitoneum> <intraperitoneum>
Intraperitoneal	Right supramesocolic: <subphrenic> < anterior subhepatic> < posterior subhepatic> < lesser sac> Left supramesocolic: <left subhepatic> < anterior left subphrenic> < perisplenic space> Inframesocolic space: R/L > <paracolic gutter: R/L> Pelvic: <paravesical> < rectovesical space> <retrouterine> <omentum><mesentery>
Retroperitoneal	<lateral compartment: Anterior pararenal / posterior pararenal/ perirenal> < great vessel compartment> < posterior compartment>
Number	<single> <multiple>
Tumor type	<solid> <cystic> <mixed>
Cystic lesion	<unilocular / multilocular> < wall: Thin /thick> < Septation: Present/absent/thick/thin> < soft tissue nodule/ enhancing component/ focal mural thickening/ papillary projection >
Margins	< ill-defined> < well-defined> <infiltrative>
Content	<homogenous /heterogenous> <fat> <calcification> <necrosis> <hemorrhage> <mucin>
MRI signal	<T1:Hyper/iso/hypo> < T2:Hyper/iso/hypo> < DWI/ADC:Restriction/facilitation>
Enhancement	<mild> <moderate> <avid> < early/delayed>
Mass effect	<infiltration of adjacent structures> < vascular invasion>
Bowel involvement	< displaced> <infiltration> <obstruction>
Lymph nodes	<present/ absent>
Ascites	<present/ absent>
Metastasis	<present/ absent>
Other findings	
Syndromic association	
Impression	<provisional/differential diagnosis>

References

1. Whittington JM, Stevens SD, Evers BM. Diseases of the peritoneum, retroperitoneum, mesentery, and omentum. In: Wang TC, Camilleri M, Lebwohl B, Lok AS, Sandborn WJ, Wang KK, et al., editors. Yamada's atlas of gastroenterology [internet]. 1st ed. Wiley; 2022 [cited 2024 Jan 12]. pp. 556–63. Available from: https://onlinelibrary.wiley.com/doi/10.1002/9781119600527.ch64
2. Tirkes T, Sandrasegaran K, Patel AA, Hollar MA, Tejada JG, Tann M, et al. Peritoneal and retroperitoneal anatomy and its relevance for cross-sectional imaging—erratum. Radiographics. 2019;39(3):912.
3. ACS M, Dadras A, Blaj S, Leebmann H, Piso P. Selection criteria for Cytoreductive surgery and Hyperthermic intraperitoneal chemotherapy with special emphasis on laparoscopy as an efficient tool. In Vivo. 2022;36(3):1367–74.
4. Omentum a powerful biological source in regenerative surgery – PMC [Internet]. [cited 2024 Jun 25]. Available from: https://www.ncbi.nlm.nih.gov/pmc/articles/PMC6700267/
5. Sharma M, Rai P, Babu R, Senadhipan B. Imaging of peritoneal ligament by endoscopic ultrasound. Endosc Ultrasound. 2015;19(4):15–27.
6. Kose S. Role of computed tomography in the evaluation of peritoneal Carcinomatosis. J Belg Soc Radiol. 107(1):27.
7. Ruess L, Frazier AA, Sivit CJ. CT of the mesentery, omentum, and peritoneum in children. Radiographics. 1995;15(1):89–104.
8. Chung EM, Biko DM, Arzamendi AM, Meldrum JT, Stocker JT. Solid tumors of the peritoneum, omentum, and mesentery in children: radiologic-pathologic correlation: from the radiologic pathology archives. Radiogr Rev Publ Radiol Soc N Am Inc. 2015;35(2):521–46.
9. Gale HI, Gee MS, Westra SJ, Nimkin K. Abdominal ultrasonography of the pediatric gastrointestinal tract. World J Radiol. 2016;8(7):656–67.
10. Toprak H, Kiliç E, Serter A, Kocakoç E, Ozgocmen S. Ultrasound and Doppler US in evaluation of superficial soft-tissue lesions. J Clin Imaging Sci. 2014;27(4):12.
11. Anupindi SA, Halverson M, Khwaja A, Jeckovic M, Wang X, Bellah RD. Common and uncommon applications of bowel ultrasound with pathologic correlation in children. Am J Roentgenol. 2014;202(5):946–59.
12. Ballard DH, Mazaheri P, Oppenheimer DC, Lubner MG, Menias CO, Pickhardt PJ, et al. Imaging of Abdominal Wall masses, Masslike lesions, and diffuse processes. Radiographics. 2020;40(3):684–706.
13. Yu L, Liu X, Leng S, Kofler JM, Ramirez-Giraldo JC, Qu M, et al. Radiation dose reduction in computed tomography: techniques and future perspective. Imaging Med. 2009;1(1):65–84.
14. Layne KA, Dargan PI, Archer JRH, Wood DM. Gadolinium deposition and the potential for toxicological sequelae—a literature review of issues surrounding gadolinium-based contrast agents. Br J Clin Pharmacol. 2018;84(11):2522–34.
15. Patel CM, Sahdev A, Reznek RH. CT, MRI and PET imaging in peritoneal malignancy. Cancer Imaging. 2011;11(1):123–39.
16. Ramashankar PC, Shah NK, Giraddi G. Lymphatic malformations: a dilemma in diagnosis and management. Contemp Clin. Dent. 2014;5(1):119–22.
17. Ghritlaharey R, More S. Chylolymphatic cyst of mesentery of terminal ileum: a case report in 8 year-old boy. J Clin Diagn Res. 2014;8:ND-05.
18. Jahanvi V, Kelkar A. Chemical shift imaging: an indispensable tool in diagnosing musculoskeletal pathologies. SA J Radiol. 2021;25(1):2061.
19. Solanki S, Badwal S, Nundy S, Mehta NN. Cystic lesions of the adrenal gland. BMJ Case Rep. 2023;16(5):e254535.
20. Yacoub JH, Clark JA, Paal EE, Manning MA. Approach to cystic lesions in the abdomen and pelvis, with radiologic-pathologic correlation. Radiographics. 2021;41(5):1368–86.
21. de Boer HC, Musson R. Imaging features of myxoid soft-tissue tumours. Clin Radiol. 2023;78(9):635–43.
22. Subhawong TK, Fishman EK, Swart JE, Carrino JA, Attar S, Fayad LM. Soft-tissue masses and Masslike conditions: what does CT add to diagnosis and management? AJR Am J Roentgenol. 2010;194(6):1559–67.
23. Fat-containing Retroperitoneal Lesions: Imaging Characteristics, Localization, and Differential Diagnosis | RadioGraphics [Internet]. [cited 2024 Jun 26]. Available from: https://pubs.rsna.org/doi/10.1148/rg.2016150149
24. Al-Dasuqi K, Irshaid L, Mathur M. Radiologic-pathologic correlation of primary retroperitoneal neoplasms. Radiographics. 2020;40(6):1631–57.
25. Choyke PL, Hayes WS, Sesterhenn IA. Primary extragonadal germ cell tumors of the retroperitoneum: differentiation of primary and secondary tumors. Radiogr Rev Publ Radiol Soc N Am Inc. 1993;13(6):1365–75; quiz 1377–8.
26. Singh AP, Jangid MK, Morya DP, Arun G, Gupta P, Sharma M, et al. Retroperitoneal Teratoma in an Infant. J Case Rep. 2015;4(2):317–9.
27. Tiu A, Sovani V, Khan N, Hooda S. Primary retroperitoneal mature cystic teratoma (dermoid cyst) in a 51-year-old male:case report and historical literature review. SAGE Open Med Case Rep. 2017;23(5):2050313X17700745.
28. Hermann AL, L'Herminé-Coulomb A, Irtan S, Audry G, Cardoen L, Brisse HJ, et al. Imaging of pediatric testicular and Para-testicular tumors: a Pictural review. Cancers. 2022;14(13):3180.
29. Ganglioneuroma and Ganglioneuroblastoma Imaging: Practice Essentials, Radiography, Computed Tomography. 2024 Jan 29 [cited 2024 Jun 27]; Available from: https://emedicine.medscape.com/article/340723-overview?form=fpf

30. Guan YB, Zhang WD, Zeng QS, Chen GQ, He JX. CT and MRI findings of thoracic ganglioneuroma. Br J Radiol. 2012;85(1016):e365–72.
31. Abele N, Langner S, Felbor U, Lode H, Hosten N. Quantitative Diffusion-Weighted MRI of Neuroblastoma Cancers. 2023;15(7):1940.
32. Wojtyś M, Piekarska A, Kunc M, Ptaszyński K, Biernat W, Zaucha JM, et al. Clinicopathological comparison and therapeutic approach to Castleman disease—a case-based review. J Thorac Dis. 2019;11(11):4859–74.
33. Castleman Disease: The Great Mimic | RadioGraphics [Internet]. [cited 2024 Jun 27]. Available from: https://pubs.rsna.org/doi/10.1148/rg.316115502
34. Guayboon T, Chinthammitr Y, Sukpanichnant S, Horthongkham N, Angkasekwinai N. Human herpesvirus 8-associated multicentric Castleman disease in a patient with advanced HIV infection: a case report. Medicine (Baltimore). 2021;100(49):e28077.
35. Imaging Spectrum of Castleman's Disease | AJR [Internet]. [cited 2024 Jun 27]. Available from: https://ajronline.org/doi/full/10.2214/ajr.182.3.1820769
36. Koeller KK, Alamo L, Adair CF, Smirniotopoulos JG. From the archives of the AFIP: congenital cystic masses of the neck: radiologic-pathologic correlation. Radiographics. 1999;19(1):121–46.
37. Rosa F, Martinetti C, Piscopo F, Buccicardi D, Schettini D, Neumaier CE, et al. Multimodality imaging features of desmoid tumors: a head-to-toe spectrum. Insights Imaging. 2020;25(11):103.
38. Morani AC, Bathala TK, Surabhi VR, Yedururi S, Jensen CT, Huh WW, et al. Desmoplastic small round cell tumor: imaging pattern of disease at presentation. Am J Roentgenol. 2019;212(3):W45–54.
39. Park JJ, Park BK, Kim CK. Adrenal imaging for adenoma characterization: imaging features, diagnostic accuracies and differential diagnoses. Br J Radiol. 89(1062):20151018.
40. Gupta RT, Ho LM, Marin D, Boll DT, Barnhart HX, Nelson RC. Dual-energy CT for characterization of adrenal nodules: initial experience. Am J Roentgenol. 2010;194(6):1479–83.

25 Pancreatic and Biliary Neoplasms

Srishti Sharma and Adity Prakash

25.1 Introduction

All solid tumors are rare in childhood. Pancreatic neoplasms particularly are uncommon in children. Their prevalence has been estimated to be around 1–2 cases per ten million children in the United States [1]. The increasing use of abdominal imaging helps us to diagnose these tumors with confidence. This helps in saving time and resources and the patient is also not subjected to unnecessary procedures. Structured reporting of pancreatic imaging provides superior evaluation of pancreatic masses and facilitates surgical planning. It allows surgeons to take decisions about tumor resectability more confidently.

25.2 Imaging Protocol

25.2.1 Ultrasound

Pancreatic masses in children are often first identified on sonography. Ingestion of water may improve pancreatic visualization by displacing air within the stomach. Sometimes, prone imaging may be needed for better visualization [2]. The non-ionizing nature and easy availability are the biggest advantages of ultrasound. But it is of limited use in staging and surgical planning. Cross-sectional imaging is essential for these purposes.

25.2.2 Computed Tomography (CT)

Cross-sectional imaging techniques like computed tomography are often used for characterization of pediatric pancreatic tumors because of its excellent spatial resolution and multiplanar capabilities. It allows excellent evaluation of the extension of the lesion as well as vascular involvement. However, because of the risks of ionizing radiation in children, MRI is also increasingly being used for the assessment of pediatric masses.

The usual pancreatic protocol contains at least an arterial and a venous phase study as described in Table 25.1. Delayed phase at 3 min and precontrast imaging are optional. (Table 25.1).

25.2.3 Magnetic Resonance Imaging (MRI)

MRI is increasingly being used for tumor staging in pediatric age group. In addition to the multiplanar capabilities of CT, it also has the advantages of providing high spatial resolution in the

S. Sharma (✉)
Department of Radiodiagnosis, All India Institute of Medical sciences, Patna, India

A. Prakash
Department of Radiodiagnosis, Kalinga Institute of Medical Sciences, Bhubaneswar, Odisha, India

I. Kumar et al. (eds.), *Practical Approach to Imaging in Pediatric Oncology*,
https://doi.org/10.1007/978-981-96-8158-7_25

Table 25.1 CT protocol for pancreatico-biliary tumors

CT scanner	Multidetector CT (16 slice and above is preferred)
Tube potential	120 kVp
Tube current	Automated tube current modulation
Oral contrast	Neutral contrast (water)
Phases 1. Late arterial phase: 30–35 s 2. Portal venous phase: 65–70 s	
Acquisition/interslice gap	Submillimeter acquisition preferable/none

Table 25.2 MRI protocol for pancreatico-biliary tumors

Sequence	Useful for
T2-weighted axial and coronal	For anatomy
Axial STIR	Index mass and metastasis evaluation
T1 in phase and opposed phase	To rule out mimics of pancreatic neoplasm
3D MRCP	Pancreaticobiliary ductal system
Diffusion-weighted imaging	Improve primary and metastatic lesion detection and also assess response to chemotherapy
Axial T1 with and without fat suppression	
Triphasic 3D post-contrast imaging with fat suppression	To detect lymphadenopathy and metastasis

absence of ionizing radiation. A basic protocol is as described below. Table 25.2 provides a standard MRI protocol for pancreatico-biliary tumors.

25.3 CT vs MRI

CT has traditionally been used for evaluation, tagging, and presurgical planning of pediatric pancreatic tumors. But CT entails ionizing radiation which becomes more important when dealing with the pediatric age group. Though rare, the potential of adverse contrast media reaction also cannot be ruled out. So the use of other cross-sectional imaging techniques like MRI has increased. Several studies have shown similar performance of CT and MRI in the presurgical evaluation of pancreatic cancer [3]. MRI offers better lesion detection and lacks ionizing radiation, other than the fact that it provides excellent spatial resolution [4]. In the evaluation of pancreaticoblastomas, the European Cooperative Study Group for Pediatric Rare Tumors (EXPeRT) within the EU-funded PARTNER (Paediatric Rare Tumors Network—European Registry) project has recommended the use of any cross-sectional imaging for staging of pancreaticoblastoma [5]. If there is dilatation of the common bile duct or pancreatic ducts, contrast-enhanced MRI cholangiopancreatography may obviate the need for a dedicated endoscopic procedure [4]. MRI has become the cross-sectional modality of choice for the evaluation of pediatric liver masses, both primary and metastatic [6].

25.4 Image Evaluation

The stepwise interpretation approach outlined below is a practical guide to assess various pancreatic malignancies.

EXAM: Transabdominal ultrasound with color Doppler

Findings:

- Location: head, uncinate process, body, tail
- Solid/cystic nature based on Echogenicity: <Anechoic – cyst> <hypoechoic – mass/cyst with internal echoes> <hyperechoic-mass/fat containing mass/cyst with internal bleed>
- Measurements in orthogonal plane
- Doppler to look for intralesional vascularity in case of solid masses: <Flow present-solid> <Flow absent-Avascular mass/Complex cystic collection>
- Other findings

EXAM: Cross-sectional Imaging (CT/MRI)

Table 25.3 Standard reporting template for pancreatico-biliary neoplasms

Size of lesion	<Max diameter in 3 orthogonal planes>
Anatomical location	Pancreas: <Head> <Neck> <Body> <Tail> <Diffuse> Biliary: <common bile duct> <Common hepatic duct> <Primary confluence> <Intra-hepatic> <Length of involvement>
Composition of tumor	<Predominantly solid> <Mixed solid-cystic> <Predominantly cystic> <Completely cystic> <Intra-tumoral necrosis> <Intra-tumoral hemorrhage> <Septations> <Capsule>
Tumor margins	<circumscribed> <infiltrative>
Non-contrast phase morphology	<Hypodense> <Isodense> <Hyperdense> <Heterogeneous>
Calcifications	<Within tumor> <Outside tumor> <Clustered> <Punctate> < curvilinear> <chunky> <peripheral> <central>
Arterial phase enhancement	<Hyperenhancing> <Iso Enhancing> <Hypoenhancing> <Heterogeneous enhancement> <Rim enhancement
Portal venous phase enhancement	<Hyperenhancement> <Iso Enhancement> <Hypoenhancement> <Heterogeneous enhancement> <Peripheral enhancement> <Washout>
Relation with main pancreatic duct	<Dilated> <Non-Dilated> <Involved> <Abrupt cut-off>
Pancreatic duct side branches	<not visible> <ectatic> <dilated> <cystically dilated>
Relation with common bile duct	<Involved> <Uninvolved> <Dilated> <Non-Dilated> <Abrupt cut-off> <primary biliary confluence-involved/univolved>
Intra-hepatic biliary radicles	<Non-dilated> <Focal dilatation> <Diffuse dilatation-mild, moderate, severe> <secondary biliary confluence-involved/uninvolved>
Arterial involvement	<Celiac axis> <Common hepatic artery> <Right or left hepatic artery> <Superior mesenteric artery> <Gastroduodenal artery> <Splenic artery> <Aorta> <Arc of contact> <maintained fat plane> <abutment> <encasement> <displaced> <luminal stenosis> <occlusion>
Venous involvement	<Superior mesenteric vein> <Splenic vein> <Portal vein> <Inferior vena cava> <Arc of contact> <Maintained fat plane> <Abutment> <Encasement> <Displaced> <Contour irregularity> <Tear-drop deformity> <luminal stenosis> <Tumor thrombus>
Nodal involvement	<Local> Regional> <Distant> <Pancreatico-duodenal> <along splenic artery> <splenic hilar> <pre-aortic> <para-aortic> <precaval> <aorto-caval> <porto-caval> <laterocaval> <Periportal>
Metastasis	<no metastasis> <liver> <lungs> <bones> <Brain> <Omentum> <Peritoneum> <malignant ascites> <further study needed>
Resectability status	<Resectable> <Borderline resectable> <Unresectable>

Findings: A standard reporting template for pancreatico-biliary tumors has been detailed in Table 25.3.

25.5 How to Fill the Checklist

25.5.1 Age of Presentation

While some pancreatic tumors can be seen in both pediatric and adult population, there are some that are exclusively seen in the pediatric age group. Pancreatoblastoma is a tumor of younger children with a mean age of presentation of 4.5 years. These tumors also have a male predilection (M:F ratio: 1.3:1) [7–15]. Solid-pseudopapillary tumors are most commonly diagnosed in adolescent girls and the mean age at diagnosis is 21.9 years [16, 17]. Zhou et al. suggested that SPN is the most common pancreatic tumor of Asian children [18].

Pancreatic neuroendocrine tumors may be diagnosed in older aged children (more than 10 years of age). But in children with syndromes like multiple endocrine neoplasia type 1 (MEN 1), it presents at a younger age [19]. Persistent hyperinsulinemic hypoglycemia of infancy or nesidioblastosis can be diagnosed within the first days of life, although sometimes it presents later in infancy [20, 21]. Acinar cell carcinomas and ductal adenocarcinomas are tumors of adults, however may be seen in children with genetic or familial predisposition such as those with Puetz Jeghers syndrome, hereditary pancreatitis, hereditary non-polyposis colon cancer, familial atypical multiple mole melanoma, and BRCA2 gene carriers [22]. If they do occur, they generally affect older children. Figure 25.1 shows a flowchart to characterize pancreatic tum.

25.5.2 Size of Lesion

Most pediatric pancreatic tumors are quite large at presentation. Pancreatoblastomas present as large solitary masses with mean diameter up to 10.6 cm. Similarly, solid pseudopapillary tumors are also quite large and solitary. Neuroendocrine tumors vary widely in size. Functional neuroendocrine tumors like insulinomas are diagnosed earlier with the mean diameter of approximately 2–2.2 cm [23, 24]. Gastrinomas are also diagnosed earlier but usually are larger than insulinomas. Glucagonomas are also relatively large when diagnosed with a mean diameter of 7.6 cm at the time of presentation. The non-functional NET can be very large measuring more than 20 cm in diameter. The benign NETs have smaller size (<=2 cm diameter) whereas malignant ones have larger size (>3 cm diameter) but there is significant overlap.

Acinar cell carcinomas when present in pediatric population also present as a large mass with a mean size of 10 cm [25, 26]. Among the cystic tumors of pancreas, serous cystadenomas are <2 cm in size whereas mucinous cystadenomas are >2 cm in size but they are rare in children. Figure 25.2 shows a flowchart for classification of pancreatic tumors according to their size.

25.5.3 Location of Lesion

Different pancreatic masses have different propensity to involve different parts of the pancreas. The location of the tumor is also important because tumors at different locations present differently. A tumor at head of pancreas often has obstructive jaundice as the first presenting symp-

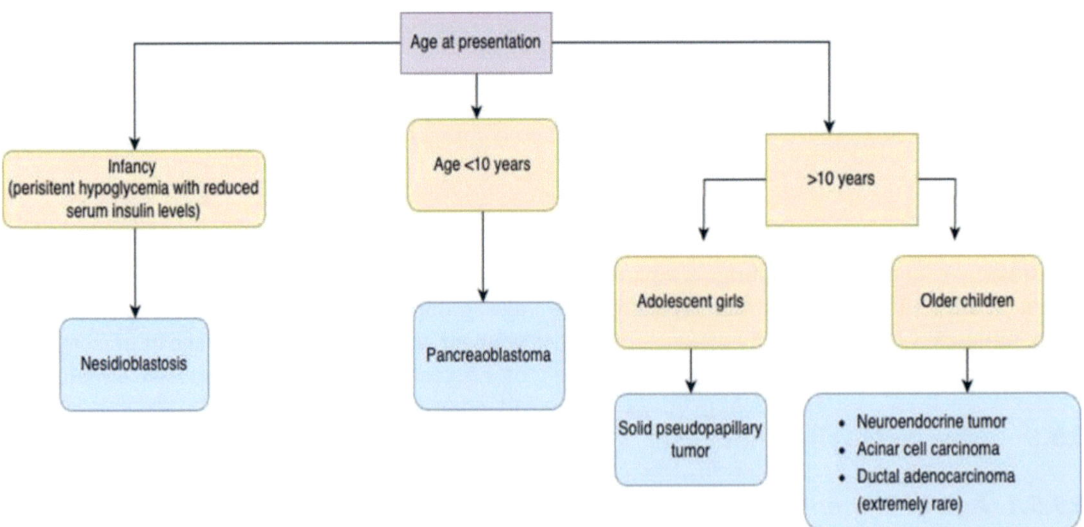

Fig. 25.1 Flowchart to characterize pancreatic tumors based on age of presentation

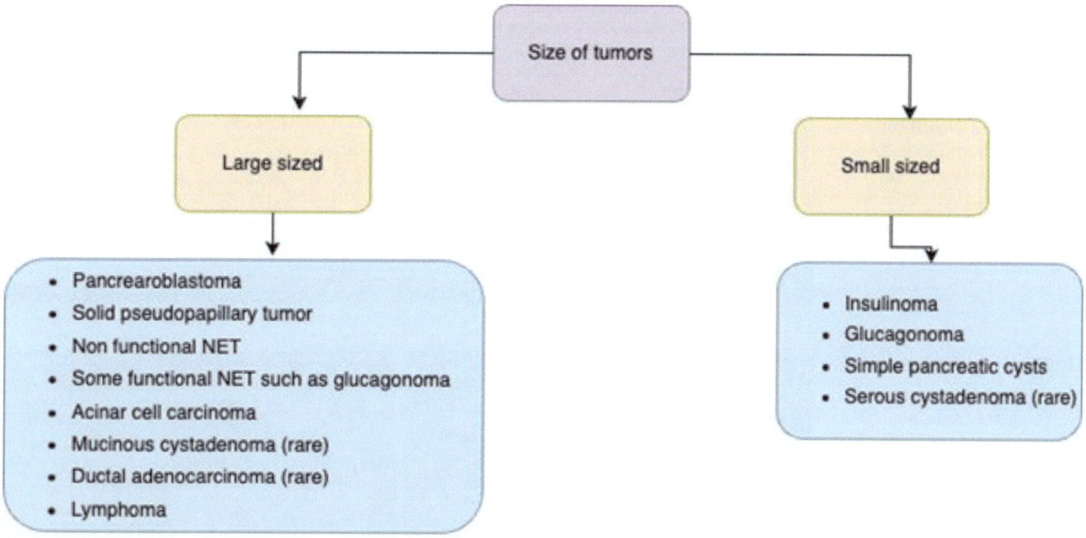

Fig. 25.2 Classification of pancreatic tumors according to their size

tom and they are detected early when their size is still small whereas a tumor at body or tail of pancreas often gets detected late and are quite large at presentation. Some pediatric tumors such as pancreatoblastoma may be so large that it is often difficult on imaging to identify the organ of origin. A study by Montemarano et al. suggested that pancreas is identified as the organ of origin on imaging in only 50% of pancreatoblastoma. These tumors even after involving the head of pancreas do not cause obstructive jaundice or dilatation of biliary tree due to their soft consistency [27].

Solid pseudopapillary tumors have been reported to occur throughout the pancreas, although some researchers have observed a propensity for the tail [28, 29]. Papavramidis reported that approximately 35.9% of these tumors arise in the pancreatic tail and 34% in the pancreatic head [30]. Like pancreaticoblastomas, obstructive jaundice is rare. While 65% of pancreatic insulinoma arise in the body and tail, gastrinomas have a predilection for the head of pancreas. Approximately 1% of insulinomas can be extra-pancreatic whereas 30% of gastrinomas can occur in extrapancreatic sites like stomach, duodenum, and proximal jejunum [19]. Gastrinomas often occur in the gastrinoma triangle which is formed by joining the points at junction of cystic duct and common bile duct, head and neck of pancreas, and second and third portions of the duodenum.

Non-functional pancreatic islet cell tumors generally involve the head of pancreas. Acinar cell carcinoma does not have any preferential location and can involve any part of the pancreas. Diffuse involvement of the pancreas may occur in lymphoma and diffuse adenomatosis (previously called diffuse nesidioblastosis) [31, 32].

25.5.4 Composition of Tumor

Pancreatic masses may be solid, cystic, or mixed solid-cystic. Solid tumors include pancreatoblastoma, NET, acinar cell, nesidioblastosis, lymphoma, and ductal carcinoma. Cystic tumors include simple pancreatic cysts, pancreatic pseudocyst, serous and mucinous cystadenomas. Solid pseudopapillary tumors are round to ovoid-shaped tumors and may be either completely solid or mixed solid-cystic [33]. Smaller SPN tend to be solid whereas larger ones are often cystic. Intra-tumoral hemorrhage is common in SPN and often fluid-debris levels are seen on imaging. SPN has a thick fibrous capsule that is well seen on imaging (Fig. 25.3).

The NETs are homogeneous solid mass but NETs also often develop a cystic core consisting

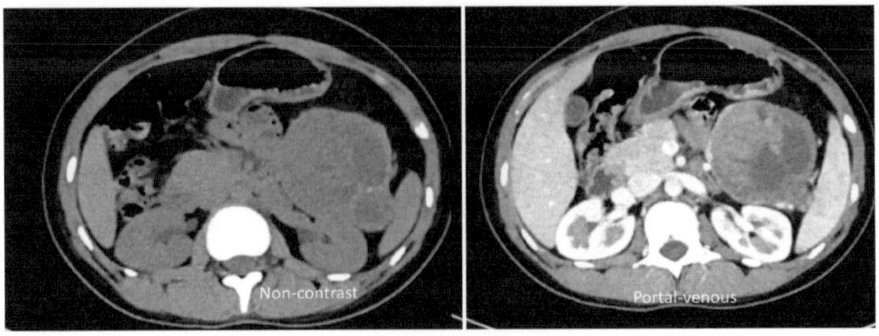

Fig. 25.3 Pre and post contrast axial CT scans of a case of Solid pseudopapillary epithelial neoplasm in the tail of the pancreas. Note the fibrous capsule and peripheral enhancing solid portion of the tumor

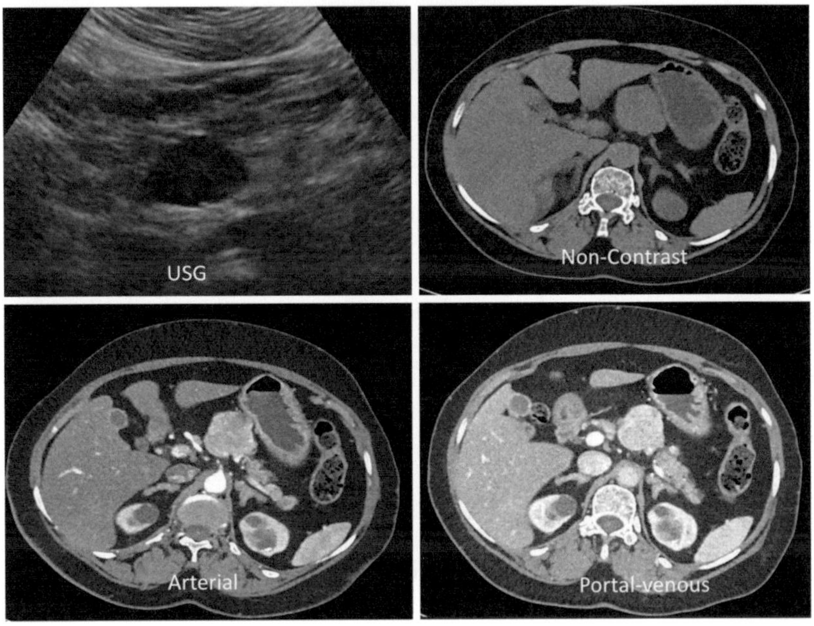

Fig. 25.4 Insulinoma of pancreas. USG and CT imaging findings. Enhancement characteristics in all three phases

of hemorrhage and necrosis if large in size. Gastrinomas are more heterogeneous than insulinomas on imaging (Fig. 25.4). Pancreatoblastomas are very heterogeneous in composition and often show internal hemorrhagic and necrotic areas on imaging. The tumor is frequently multiloculated and contains septations. Serous cystadenomas are microcystic tumors with multiple tiny cysts (>6 in number) and central scar. Mucinous cystadenomas are macrocystic with larger cysts (<6 in number). Figure 25.5 provides an algorithmic approach to diagnose pancreatic tumor based on tumor composition and clinical history.

25.5.5 Calcification

Many pancreatic tumors may show internal calcifications. These calcifications are best appreciated on CT but may also be seen on X-ray and ultrasound. Small punctate, curvilinear, or clustered calcifications may be present in pancreatoblastoma [34]. Calcifications are also seen in solid pseudopapillary tumors in one-third cases, commonly in its thick fibrous capsule [35]. Small calcifications may be present within larger neuroendocrine tumors and cast posterior acoustic shadow on ultrasound. Up to 50% cases of acinar cell carcinoma may show calcifications, which

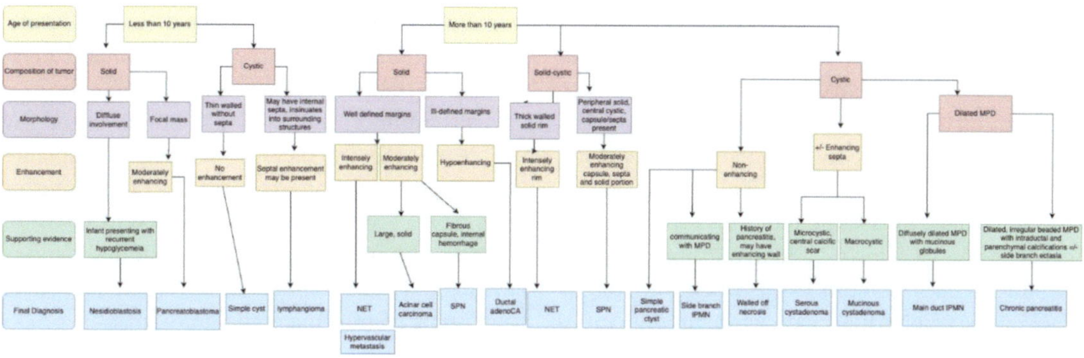

Fig. 25.5 Approach to pancreatic neoplasms

can be punctate or chunky and located either peripherally or centrally. Tooth-like calcification can be seen in intrapancreatic dermoid cyst.

25.5.6 Tumor Margins

Most pediatric pancreatic tumors have a well-demarcated margin. Pancreatoblastoma mostly has a well or partially circumscribed margin although there are few reports of infiltrative margin as well. The margins often show multiple lobulations in pancreatoblastoma [36]. Similarly, solid pseudopapillary tumor is often well-demarcated and shows a fibrous capsule. Neuroendocrine tumors are also discrete and have a well-defined margin. Acinar cell carcinoma is considered by some authors as the mature counterpart of pancreatoblastoma. Hence, they also have the well-demarcated margin as that of pancreatoblastoma. Few rare reports of ductal adenocarcinoma in children have described them as tumors with infiltrative margin.

25.5.7 Enhancement

Enhancement of a tumor is compared to the enhancement of pancreatic parenchyma. The tumors become more conspicuous after intravenous contrast and they may either be hypoenhancing, isoenhancing, or hyperenhancing to the pancreas. Pancreatoblastomas enhance heterogeneously and their enhancement is often greater than that of pancreatic parenchyma. In solid pseudopapillary tumor, enhancement is noted only in the solid component or fibrous capsule of the tumor, most often in the periphery with non-enhancing cystic components centrally.

Neuroendocrine tumors show avid enhancement and are best detected in the early arterial phase where they enhance more than the pancreatic parenchyma [37]. Even cystic NETs show avid ring enhancement. Acinar cell carcinoma demonstrated more enhancement than ductal adenocarcinoma but less than neuroendocrine tumors. Ductal adenocarcinomas show less enhancement than normal pancreas. The central scar of serous cystadenomas and the septations within mucinous cystadenoma may also show enhancement.

25.5.8 Relation with Pancreatic Duct

Most pancreatic tumors of children have a non-ductal origin. Hence, pancreatic duct dilatation is not generally a feature of pediatric pancreatic malignancies. However, if large, tumors may compress the main pancreatic duct. Advanced tumors may rarely also invade the pancreatic duct. Pancreatic duct dilatation is seen in tumors of ductal origin such as the rare ductal adenocarcinoma in hereditarily predisposed older children.

25.5.9 Relation with Bile Duct

As mentioned earlier, pancreatoblastomas do not cause biliary dilation even after involving the pancreatic head due to their soft consistency. However, few cases of pancreaticoblastomas causing biliary invasion have been reported previously [36]. Similarly, jaundice is rare in solid pseudopapillary tumors even when the tumor involves the head of the pancreas. Neuroendocrine tumors also do not cause biliary tree dilatation.

25.5.10 Arterial Involvement

Large tumors infiltrate surrounding structures and may lead to arterial encasement. An arc of contact more than 180° between the tumor and the artery makes the tumor unresectable. The most common arteries that may be involved by pancreatic cancer include celiac trunk, superior mesenteric artery, and common hepatic artery. In very advanced cases, aorta may also be involved.

If a tumor has no contact with either celiac trunk, common hepatic artery or superior mesenteric artery, it is considered resectable. If a tumor contacts the common hepatic artery only while all other vessels are free, it is considered borderline resectable. If more than 180° contact between tumor and either celiac axis or superior mesenteric artery is present, the tumor is unresectable [37]. Malignant pediatric pancreatic tumors such as pancreatoblastoma, acinar cell carcinoma, and malignant neuroendocrine tumors invade the adjacent arteries when advanced. Solid pseudopapillary tumors tend to displace vessels rather than encase them.

25.5.11 Venous Involvement

Large malignant tumors of pancreas may encase veins. They may also lead to venous thrombosis. A tumor vein contact less than or equal to 180° without any contour irregularity or tear drop deformity of the vein is still considered resectable. However, if the tumor vein contact is more than 180°, or there is vein contour irregularity or tear drop deformity or presence of tumor thrombus within the vein and reconstruction and anastomosis is not possible, it is unresectable [38].

The common veins which are involved by pancreatic tumors include portal vein, splenic vein, superior mesenteric vein, and rarely inferior vena cava. Portal and mesenteric vein invasion has been reported in pancreatoblastoma. Venous encasement and venous thrombosis have also been reported in acinar cell carcinoma.

25.5.12 Nodal Involvement

Malignant pancreatic tumors may show local, regional, and distant lymphadenopathy. In case of large tumors such as pancreatoblastoma, local lymphadenopathy cannot be adequately assessed with imaging. In cases of malignant neuroendocrine tumor, the presence of regional lymph nodes does not mean a worse prognosis but metastasis to the liver does. Acinar cell carcinoma may spread to regional and distant lymph nodes.

25.6 Peripancreatic Lymph Node Stations

Peripancreatic lymph nodes have been standardized according to the Japan Pancreas Society guidelines [39] which have mostly been given in relation to pancreatic adenocarcinomas. To summarize, malignancies involving head of pancreas spread to pancreaticoduodenal group of lymph nodes. Those involving the body and tail spread to nodes along splenic hilum and artery. From these locations, the tumor can spread to more proximal locations along the celiac and superior mesenteric arteries [40].

25.6.1 Metastasis

At presentation, metastasis is seen in up to 37% of pancreatoblastoma, most common site being the liver [41]. Less commonly metastasis may also occur in the lung and brain. There are case reports of metastasis of pancreatoblastoma to the omentum, colon, spleen, kidney, and adrenals. Metastasis may develop in cases of solid pseudo-papillary tumors occurring in adults, but such cases of metastasis are very rare in the pediatric age group. Patients of SPN will benefit from surgical tumor debulking even if complete resection is not possible.

More than 90% of insulinomas are benign, do not metastasize, and have a good prognosis. Gastrinomas, on the other hand, are malignant in more than 50% cases. Metastasizing gastrinomas that arise in extrapancreatic locations have better prognosis. Due to the slow-growing nature of these tumors, these patients have long survival rates even with liver metastasis. Acinar cell carcinomas have slightly better prognosis than ductal adenocarcinoma. The prevalence of metastasis is high in ductal adenocarcinomas of childhood. The rarity of this tumor in the pediatric age group leads to a low index of suspicion causing a delay in diagnosis.

25.7 Biliary Neoplasms

Benign biliary neoplasms are rare in children. These can be intrabiliary hepatic adenomas, biliary papillomatosis, cystadenomas, inflammatory fibroblastic tumors, and neuroendocrine tumors. All these tend to have non-specific imaging appearances and are often diagnosed on histopathology.

Roy et al. [42] have described a case of intrahepatic biliary adenoma which was misdiagnosed on imaging as hepatoblastoma. Biliary papillomatosis is another rare entity described with only 140 reported cases that too in adults [43]. Biliary cystadenoma should be suspected as a differential when a cystic mass is encountered in the liver [44]. Inflammatory fibroblastic tumor has a non-specific appearance however can be suspected on MRI. These tend to be hypo to isointense on T1-weighted images and markedly hypointense on T2-weighted images. They will show enhancement on delayed images [45]. Tonhoffer et al. have also reported a case of Intrabiliary neuroendocrine tumor in a 6-year-old child mimicking type 1 choledochal cyst on imaging studies.

Choldedochal cysts predispose to cholangiocarcinoma. Presence of enhancing nodular papillary projections along the walls of choledochal cyst is suggestive of development of cholangiocarcinomas (Fig. 25.6). Rhabdomyosarcomas of the biliary tract are rare botryoid groups of childhood tumors with very poor prognosis. On imaging, a heterogeneous or hypodense mass is seen distending the common bile duct with intrahepatic biliary radicles dilatation. If the mass becomes very large, it may invade surrounding structures such as vessels and liver parenchyma.

Primary neoplasms of the gallbladder consist of cholesterol polyps, adenomas, epithelial hyperplasia, and very rarely gastric heterotopia. [46, 47]. Some of these lesions may be incidentally detected. Surgery is advisable in these lesions if they are symptomatic or if the size exceeds 1 cm. Other cases can be kept under ultrasound surveillance. On imaging most of these conditions have a non-specific imaging

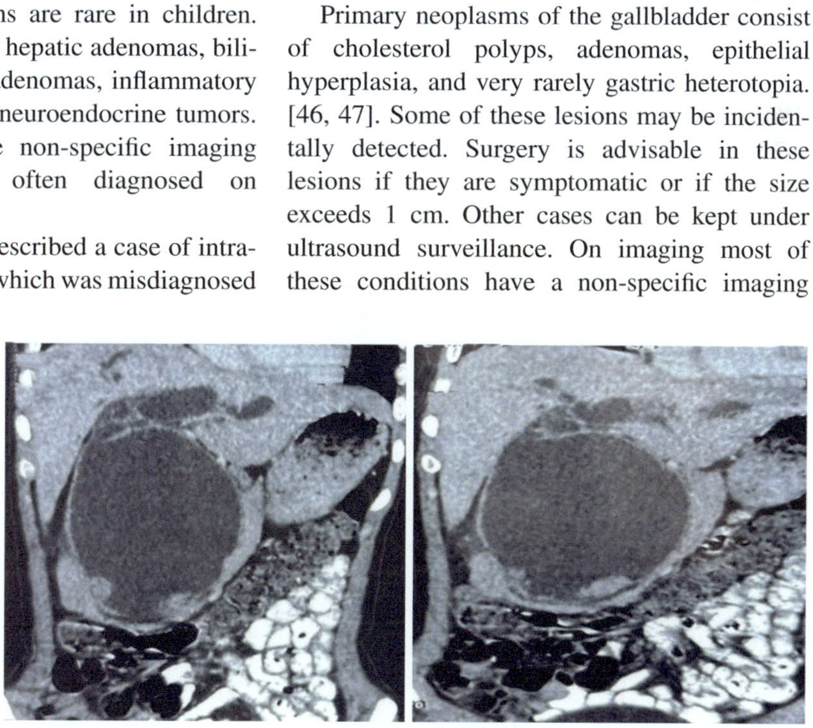

Fig. 25.6 In a 13-year-old girl, a known case of Type I choledochal cyst, coronal CT shows multiple enhancing solid mural nodules in a cystically dilated common bile duct. A diagnosis of cholangiocarcinoma was established on biopsy of the enhancing nodules

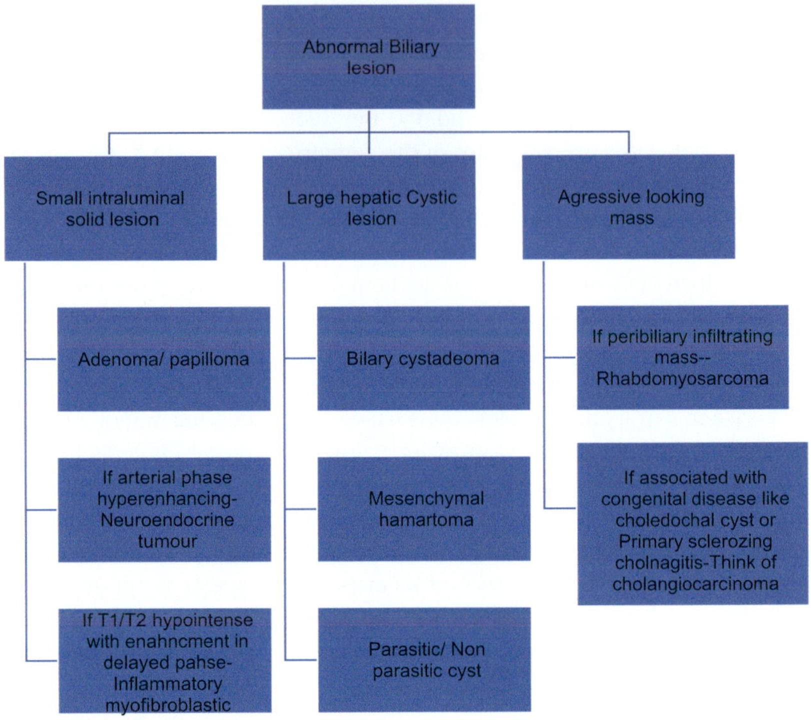

Fig. 25.7 Approach to diagnosis of pediatric biliary tumors

appearance. But imaging does play an important role in surgical planning. Figure 25.7 provides an algorithmic approach to diagnosis of Pediatric Biliary neoplasms.

25.8 Post-operative Imaging

It is essential that a radiologist be familiar with the normal expected findings of pancreatico-biliary surgery and post-surgical complications. The most common surgeries done for a pancreatic tumor include pancreatico-duodenectomy (Whipple's procedure), distal pancreatectomy with or without splenectomy, central quadrantectomy, and sometimes complete pancreatectomy. The common surgeries done for biliary neoplasms include Whipple's procedure, Kasai procedure, or partial hepatectomy depending on the location of the tumor.

Common expected imaging findings after surgery include mild fat stranding, surgical site edema, perivascular cuffing, pneumobilia, few locules of intraperitoneal free air (must be resolving), few prominent lymph nodes, pancreatic parenchymal atrophy, post-operative scarring, and transient post-surgical collections. Various complications of pancreatico-biliary surgeries include pancreatic leak, pancreatic fistula, recurrent pancreatitis, pancreatico-jejunal anastomosis stricture or dehiscence, hepatico-jejunal anastomosis stricture, hepatico-jejunal anastomosis leak, vascular erosion, pseudoaneurysm formation, vascular thrombosis, organ infarcts, gastrojejunostomy anastomosis leak or stricture, marginal ulcer formation, afferent limb syndrome, abscess formation and tumor recurrence.

Transient post-surgical collection can be differentiated from other complicated collections on imaging. Transient post-surgical seromas are homogeneous, do not have thick rim enhancement, do not communicate with main pancreatic duct, do not involve the anastomotic sites and regress on serial follow-ups. Collection from pancreatic leak is typically heterogeneous and may show internal fat foci. Peripheral enhancement can be seen in encapsulated pancreatic leak and abscess. Mild fat stranding is normal in the early post-operative period. A diagnosis of recurrent pancreatitis should be considered only when fat stranding is combined with other features of pancreatitis such as enlarged pancreas, peripancreatic collections with increased serum amylase and lipase levels. Post-operative scarring can mimic tumor recurrence. Both of these entities can show enhancement on post-contrast study. Diffusion-weighted imaging and perfusion imaging may help differentiate the two.

References

1. Qi X, Zhou B, Liang F, et al. Prognostic factors of pancreatic tumors in children and adolescents: a population study based on the surveillance, epidemiology, and end results database. BMC Gastroenterol. 2024;24:108.
2. Trout AT, Ayyala RS, Murati MA, Squires JH, Callahan MJ, Chavhan GB, Abu-El-Haija M, Anupindi SA. Current state of imaging of pediatric pancreatitis: AJR expert panel narrative review. AJR Am J Roentgenol. 2021;217(2):265.
3. Chen FM, Ni JM, Zhang ZY, Zhang L, Li B, Jiang CJ. Presurgical evaluation of pancreatic cancer: a comprehensive imaging comparison of CT versus MRI. Am J Roentgenol. 2016;206(3):526–35.
4. Shet NS, Cole BL, Iyer RS. Imaging of pediatric pancreatic neoplasms with radiologic-histopathologic correlation. Am J Roentgenol. 2014;202(6):1337–48.
5. Bien E, Roganovic J, Krawczyk MA, Godzinski J, Orbach D, Cecchetto G, Barthlen W, Defachelles AS, Ferrari A, Weldon CB, Brecht IB. Pancreatoblastoma in children: EXPeRT/PARTNER diagnostic and therapeutic recommendations. Pediatr Blood Cancer. 2021;68:e29112.
6. Schooler GR, Squires JH, Alazraki A, Chavhan GB, Chernyak V, Davis JT, Khanna G, Krishnamurthy R, Lungren MP, Masand PM, Podberesky DJ. Pediatric hepatoblastoma, hepatocellular carcinoma, and other hepatic neoplasms: consensus imaging recommendations from American College of Radiology Pediatric Liver Reporting and Data System (LI-RADS) Working Group. Radiology. 2020;296(3):493–7.
7. Qiu L, Trout AT, Ayyala RS, Szabo S, Nathan JD, Geller JI, Dillman JR. Pancreatic masses in children and young adults: multimodality review with pathologic correlation. Radiographics. 2021;41(6):1766–84.
8. Tsukimoto I, Watanabe K, Lin JB, Nakajima T. Pancreatic carcinoma in children in Japan. Cancer. 1973;31(5):1203–7.
9. Grosfeld JL, Vane DW, Rescorla FJ, McGuire W, West KW. Pancreatic tumors in childhood: analysis of 13 cases. J Pediatr Surg. 1990;25(10):1057–62.
10. Jaksic T, Yaman M, Thorner P, Wesson DK, Filler RM, Shandling B. A 20-year review of pediatric pancreatic tumors. J Pediatr Surg. 1992;27(10):1315–7.
11. Lack EE, Cassady JR, Levey R, Vawter GF. Tumors of the exocrine pancreas in children and adolescents: a clinical and pathologic study of eight cases. Am J Surg Pathol. 1983;7(4):319–27.
12. Shorter NA, Glick RD, Klimstra DS, Brennan MF, LaQuaglia MP. Malignant pancreatic tumors in childhood and adolescence: the Memorial Sloan-Kettering experience, 1967 to present. J Pediatr Surg. 2002;37(6):887–92.
13. Vane DW, Grosfeld JL, West KW, Rescorla FJ. Pancreatic disorders in infancy and childhood: experience with 92 cases. J Pediatr Surg. 1989;24(8):771–6.
14. Horie A, Yano Y, Kotoo Y, Miwa A. Morphogenesis of pancreatoblastoma, infantile carcinoma of the pancreas. Report of two cases. Cancer. 1977;39(1):247–54.
15. Roebuck DJ, Yuen MK, Wong YC, Shing MK, Lee CW, Li CK. Imaging features of pancreatoblastoma. Pediatr Radiol. 2001;31(7):501–6.
16. Todani T, Shimada K, Watanabe Y, Toki A, Fujii T, Urushihara N. Frantz's tumor: a papillary and cystic tumor of the pancreas in girls. J Pediatr Surg. 1988;23(2):116–21.
17. Buetow PC, Buck JL, Pantongrag-Brown L, Beck KG, Ros PR, Adair CF. Solid and papillary epithelial neoplasm of the pancreas: imaging pathologic correlation in 56 cases. Radiology. 1996;199(3):707–11.
18. Zhou H, Cheng W, Lam KY, Chan GC, Khong PL, Tam PK. Solid-cystic papillary tumor of the pancreas in children. Pediatr Surg Int. 2001;17(8):614–20.
19. Service FJ, McMahon MM, O'Brien PC, Ballard DJ. Functioning insulinoma: incidence, recurrence, and long-term survival of patients—a 60-year study. Mayo Clin Proc. 1991;66(7):711–9.
20. de Lonlay P, Fournet JC, Touati G, et al. Heterogeneity of persistent hyperinsulinaemic hypoglycaemia: a series of 175 cases. Eur J Pediatr. 2002;161(1):37–48.
21. Fekete CN, de Lonlay P, Jaubert F, Rahier J, Brunelle F, Saudubray JM. The surgical management of congenital hyperinsulinemic hypoglycemia in infancy. J Pediatr Surg. 2004;39(3):267–9.
22. Klimstra DS, Heffess CS, Oertel JE, Rosai J. Acinar cell carcinoma of the pancreas: a clinicopathologic study of 28 cases. Am J Surg Pathol. 1992;16(9):815–37.
23. Buetow PC, Parrino TV, Buck JL, et al. Islet cell tumors of the pancreas: pathologic-imaging correlation among size, necrosis and cysts, calcification, malignant behavior, and functional status. AJR Am J Roentgenol. 1995;165(5):1175–9.
24. Gouya H, Vignaux O, Augui J, et al. CT, endoscopic sonography, and a combined protocol for preoperative evaluation of pancreatic insulinomas. AJR Am J Roentgenol. 2003;181(4):987–92.
25. Grosfeld JL, Clatworthy HW Jr, Hamoudi AB. Pancreatic malignancy in children. Arch Surg. 1970;101(3):370–5.

26. Hoorens A, Lemoine NR, McLellan E, et al. Pancreatic acinar cell carcinoma: an analysis of cell lineage markers, p53 expression, and Ki-ras mutation. Am J Pathol. 1993;143(3):685–98.
27. Williams T, Babyn P. The pancreas. In: Stringer D, Babyn P, editors. Pediatric gastrointestinal imaging and intervention. 2nd ed. Hamilton: Decker; 2000.
28. Frantz V. Tumors of the pancreas. In: Atlas of tumor pathology. Section 7, fascicles 27 and 28. Washington, DC: Armed Forces Institute of Pathology; 1959. p. 32–3.
29. Mao C, Guvendi M, Domenico DR, Kim K, Thomford NR, Howard JM. Papillary cystic and solid tumors of the pancreas: a pancreatic embryonic tumor? Studies of three cases and cumulative review of the world's literature. Surgery. 1995;118(5):821–8.
30. Papavramidis T, Papavramidis S. Solid pseudopapillary tumors of the pancreas: review of 718 patients reported in English literature. J Am Coll Surg. 2005;200(6):965–72.
31. Berrocal T, Prieto C, Pastor I, Gutierrez J, al-Assir I. Sonography of pancreatic disease in infants and children. Radiographics. 1995;15(2):301–13.
32. de Lonlay-Debeney P, Poggi-Travert F, Fournet JC, et al. Clinical features of 52 neonates with hyperinsulinism. N Engl J Med. 1999;340(15):1169–75.
33. Balthazar EJ, Subramanyam BR, Lefleur RS, Barone CM. Solid and papillary epithelial neoplasm of the pancreas: radiographic, CT, sonographic, and angiographic features. Radiology. 1984;150(1):39–40.
34. Lee JY, Kim IO, Kim WS, Kim CW, Yeon KM. CT and US findings of pancreatoblastoma. Journal of computer assisted tomography. 1996 May 1;20(3):370–4.
35. Kosmahl M, Seada LS, Janig U, Harms D, Klöppel G. Solid-pseudopapillary tumor of the pancreas: its origin revisited. Virchows Arch. 2000;436(5):473–80.
36. Montemarano H, Lonergan GJ, Bulas DI, Selby DM. Pancreatoblastoma: imaging findings in 10 patients and review of the literature. Radiology. 2000;214(2):476–82.
37. Semelka RC, Ascher SM. MR imaging of the pancreas. Radiology. 1993;188(3):593–602.
38. Hong SB, Lee SS, Kim JH, Kim HJ, Byun JH, Hong SM, Song KB, Kim SC. Pancreatic cancer CT: prediction of resectability according to NCCN criteria. Radiology. 2018;289(3):710–8.
39. Dolay K, Malya F, Akbulut S. Management of pancreatic head adenocarcinoma: from where to where? World J Gastrointest Surg. 2019;11:143–54. https://doi.org/10.4240/wjgs.v11.i3.143.
40. Kumar I, Sharma S, Prakash A, Aggarwal P, Shukla RC, Verma A. CT-based definition and structured reporting of abdominal lymph node stations. Indian J Radiol Imaging. 2022;32(01):62–70.
41. Gupta AK, Mitra DK, Berry M, Dinda AK, Bhatnagar V. Sonography and CT of pancreatoblastoma in children. AJR Am J Roentgenol. 2000;174(6):1639–41.
42. Roy AK, Das NN. Pediatric intrahepatic bile duct adenoma – rare liver tumor: a case report. World J Gastrointest Surg. 2019;11(11):414–21.
43. Singh A, Sharma N, Panda SS, Bajpai M, Jana M. Benign papillomatosis of common bile duct in children: a rare case report. J Indian Assoc Pediatr Surg. 2014;19(1):44.
44. Wood JA, McLeary MS, Thomas RD, Zuppan CW. Biliary cystadenoma in a child: CT and MR appearances. Pediatr Radiol. 1998;28(12):922.
45. George V, Tammisetti VS, Surabhi VR, Shanbhogue AK. Chronic fibrosing conditions in abdominal imaging. Radiographics. 2013;33(4):1053–80.
46. Stringer MD, Ceylan H, Ward K, Wyatt JI. Gallbladder polyps in children—classification and management. J Pediatr Surg. 2003;38(11):1680–4.
47. Zhuang Y, Wu Z, Shi J, Wu Y, Lv F. Yolk sac tumor of biliary tract: a rare biliary space-occupying entity in children. J Pediatr Surg Case Rep. 2022;76:102102.

Imaging of Gonadal and Extragonadal Pelvic Tumors

26

Aishvarya Shri Rajasimman, Akshay D. Baheti, Vasundhara Rhushikesh Patil, Kunal Bharat Gala, Nitin Sudhakar Shetty, and Suyash Sureshchandra Kulkarni

26.1 Background

Pelvic neoplasms in children can be broadly divided into gonadal and extragonadal tumors. Gonadal tumors, namely ovarian and testicular neoplasms, are predominantly germ cell tumors or less commonly sex cord stromal tumors. Germ cell tumors are the commonest pelvic neoplasms, constituting of about 2–3% of all neoplasms in population under 15 years of age [1], with teratomas being the common benign neoplasm and dysgerminomas and yolk sac tumors comprising the common ovarian and testicular malignant neoplasms respectively [2]. Ovarian surface epithelial tumors are rare in children. Extragonadal pelvic neoplasms include neoplasms occurring in the uterus, urinary bladder, and prostate which are predominantly rhabdomyosarcomas (RMS). Sacrococcygeal teratomas and bone primary neoplasms are the other non-gonadal pelvic neoplasms. A detailed classification of the gonadal and extragonadal tumors is presented in Table 26.1 [3, 4].

All authors have reviewed and approved the final manuscript.

A. S. Rajasimman · A. D. Baheti (✉) · V. R. Patil · K. B. Gala · N. S. Shetty · S. S. Kulkarni
Department of Radiodiagnosis, Tata Memorial Centre & Homi Bhabha National Institute, Mumbai, Maharashtra, India
e-mail: patilvr@tmc.gov.in; galakb@tmc.gov.in; shettyns@tmc.gov.in; kulkarniss@tmc.gov.in

I. Kumar et al. (eds.), *Practical Approach to Imaging in Pediatric Oncology*,
https://doi.org/10.1007/978-981-96-8158-7_26

Table 26.1 Classification of gonadal and extragonadal pelvic neoplasms. Adapted from WHO classification 2022

Gonadal neoplasms	
Germ cell tumors	Gonadoblastoma seminoma embryonal carcinoma yolk sac tumor Choriocarcinoma Teratoma (immature and mature) mixed germ cell tumor dysgerminoma
Sex cord-stromal tumors of the testis	Leydig cell tumor Sertoli cell tumor Granulosa cell tumor Tumors in the fibroma-thecoma group Mixed and other sex cord-stromal tumors Fibroma/thecoma
Surface epithelial neoplasm (ovary)	Serous cystadenoma/carcinoma Mucinous cystadenoma/carcinoma Endometrioid cystadenoma/carcinoma Clear cell carcinoma Brenner tumor
Others	Gonadal lymphoma Leukemic infiltration Metastasis
Extragonadal neoplasms	
Pelvis	Germ cell tumors including sacrococcygeal teratoma Rhabdomyosarcoma (RMS) Desmoplastic small round cell tumor (DSRCT) Pelvic bone neoplasms—Ewing's sarcoma & chondrosarcoma Neuroblastoma
Uterus, cervix	Rhabdomyosarcoma
	Leiomyosarcoma
Vagina	Rhabdomyosarcoma
	Clear cell adenocarcinoma
	Endodermal sinus tumor
Bladder and prostate	Rhabdomyosarcoma
	Leiomyosarcoma
	Lymphoma/leukemia
	Inflammatory myofibroblastic tumor (IMT)

26.2 Clinical Presentation and Diagnostic Workup

Patients with ovarian tumors commonly present with abdominal swelling or pain [5]. Ovarian tumors may also have nausea and vomiting if associated with torsion or rupture. On the other hand, nearly 90% of testicular neoplasms in children present as a painless scrotal swelling [6]. Apart from swelling or pain, extragonadal tumors also present with complaints of urinary retention or constipation secondary to mass effect.

Gonadal tumors may also be associated with endocrine abnormalities. In tumors that secrete estrogen, symptoms like precocious puberty, breast enlargement, and abnormal vaginal bleeding/menstrual abnormalities can be seen in girls. Boys could present with gynecomastia, which is associated with sex cord stromal tumors [2, 7]. On the other hand, androgen-producing tumors like Sertoli-Leydig cell tumor present with features of virilization in girls, including hirsutism, enlarged clitoris, and voice change [8], and with precocious pubertal changes in boys [6]. Rarely, a gonadal neoplasm may be diagnosed in a prenatal ultrasound or asymptomatically picked up during childhood.

Sometimes, a pelvic swelling or abdominal distension might be the presenting complaint in cases of pelvic bony neoplasms or rare tumors like DSRCT (desmoplastic small round cell tumors). DSRCT are rare neoplasms that occur in adolescents between 18 and 21 years [9, 10].

Imaging plays a crucial role in the diagnostic work-up. A transabdominal ultrasound is usually the initial investigation of choice. It is inexpensive, readily available, and radiation-free. If a neoplasm is suspected on ultrasound, cross-sectional imaging in the form of CT/ PET-CT or MRI is performed. Further imaging recommendations/guidelines are detailed ahead. For adnexal and testicular masses, evaluation of tumor markers serves as an equally important tool to aid the

Table 26.2 List of commonly associated tumor markers and neoplasms

Tumor marker	Associated neoplasm
Alpha-feto protein (AFP)	Yolk sac tumor Mixed GCTs Immature teratoma (less common) Embryonal carcinoma (less common) Sertoli-Leydig cell tumor (rare)
Beta human chorionic gonadotropin (B-HCG)	Seminoma and NSGCT of testis Choriocarcinoma Mixed GCTs Embryonal carcinoma Dysgerminoma (rare)
Inhibin	Granulosa cell tumor
Lactose dehydrogenase (LDH)	Dysgerminoma

diagnosis. The tumor markers and the associated neoplasms have been briefed in Table 26.2 [8].

26.3 Consensus or Guidelines

The Children's Oncology Group (COG) and the Society of Pediatric Radiology oncology committee (SPR) under the guidance of International Society of Pediatric Oncology (SIOP) and The American Society of Pediatric Hematology/Oncology came up with a white paper on imaging recommendations in 2022 for testicular, ovarian, and extragonadal pelvic tumors. The important recommendations are discussed below with their grades of recommendation. Grades of the recommendations are based on the quality of the evidence. It ranges from Grade A which is a recommendation based on high-quality good evidence, to Grade D which is based on low-quality evidence that does not have proven research-based evidence or has very limited studies.

(i). **Preferred Modality of Imaging:**

- The initial modality of investigation as the patient presents is an ultrasound (USG) for all gonadal and extragonadal tumors (Grade A). An ultrasound in most of the cases could potentially rule out the non-neoplastic findings like a hemorrhagic ovarian cyst, hydrocele, epididymal cyst, appendicitis, torsion, etc., and picks up any suspected mass.
- Ultrasound is both highly sensitive and specific for testicular masses. In current practice, USG alone is considered adequate for scrotal evaluation (Grade B). The role of MRI to further characterize a testicular neoplasm is very limited.
- In all suspected testicular neoplasms the rest of the abdomen should be screened with CT or MRI for nodal and metastatic workup (Grade A).
- Although Ovarian Adnexal Reporting and Data System (ORADS) has not been validated in the pediatric population, the relevant lexicon may be used to describe complex cysts (Grade B) [2].
- Chest CT is indicated in malignant testicular and ovarian neoplasms since germ cell tumors (GCTs) have high predilection to metastasize to lungs (Grade C and D respectively). For the same reason, any suspected extragonadal teratoma should also be screened with a CT chest. For other extragonadal tumors, a chest screening to be planned on a case-by-case basis as some of them may be local in nature.
- For ovarian and extragonadal neoplasms detected on ultrasound, further evaluation needs to be performed with a CT, MRI, or FDG PET/CT as appropriate. The decision for the subsequent investigation of choice will vary based on the underlying pathology. For example, an adnexal mass on ultrasound with raised tumor markers (beta-HCG/AFP) is diagnostic of a germ cell tumor. This would require metastatic work-up with a CECT chest, abdomen, and pelvis (as performed in the author's institution) or with CE-MRI abdomen and pelvis and non-contrast CT chest. On the other hand, a paratesticular rhabdomyosarcoma or a bony Ewing's sarcoma would require an FDG PET/CT for staging. An MRI may

be performed for a pelvic rhabdomyosarcoma to identify the site of the primary (bladder, prostate, vaginal, etc.) and as a problem solving tool in clinically relevant situations. Any ovarian cyst more than 7.5 cm regardless of other features should be evaluated by an MRI (Grade C) [2, 11].

- Intravenous contrast is recommended for all ovarian and extragonadal neoplasms both during staging and in follow-up. A single-phase CT should suffice, and multiphasic studies are not required.
- Administration of oral contrast is recommended in females with ovarian or nongonadal pelvic masses (Grade D) [2].
- If the metastatic screening shows an indeterminate finding on CT/MRI, an FDG-PET scan may be considered for further evaluation.

(ii). **Staging:**

A dedicated staging for pediatric gonadal and extragonadal tumors was devised by COG (Table 26.3) [12, 13]. The COG staging incorporates both surgical and imaging features.

Following the COG staging, the Malignant Germ Cell International Consortium (MAGIC) was formed in 2009 to stratify the risk among the pediatric germ cell tumors (Table 26.4).

In testicular neoplasms, the COG system of staging is followed in pre-pubertal children whereas the use of National Comprehensive Cancer Network (NCCN) staging is used in post-pubertal children [7].

No dedicated staging is available for sacrococcygeal teratomas. Updated staging by COG and modified TNM for rhabdomyosarcoma was published in 2022 [14]. Respective TNM staging is presented below along with imaging features.

Table 26.3 Staging in testicular, ovarian, and extragonadal germ cell tumors. Adapted from the COG staging for GCTs

Stage	Testis	Ovary	Extragonadal
I	Limited to testis. No lymph node involvement	Limited to ovary. No lymph nodes	Complete resection with negative margins
II	Microscopic disease in scrotum or cord. Tumor markers fail to reach normal level	Microscopic residual disease. Peritoneal disease—Negative. Failure of tumor markers to normalize	Microscopic residual disease. Lymph nodes—Negative. Failure of tumor markers to normalize
III	Retroperitoneal lymph node involvement. No visceral or extra-abdominal involvement	Gross residual disease. Lymph node metastasis, contiguous visceral involvement (bladder, intestine, omentum)	Lymph node positive. Gross residual disease
IV	Distant metastases	Distant metastases	Distant metastases

Table 26.4 Risk stratification of gonadal and extragonadal tumors in children. Adapted from the MAGIC consortium [13]

Risk group	Age	Location	COG stage
Low	Any	Testis, ovary, extragonadal	I
Standard	< 11	Testis	II, III, IV
	< 11	Ovary	II, III, IV
	< 11	Extragonadal	II, III, IV
	≥ 11	Testis	II, III
	≥ 11	Ovary	II, III
	≥ 11	Extragonadal	II
Poor	≥ 11	Testis	IV
	≥ 11	Ovary	IV
	≥ 11	Extragonadal	III, IV

26.4 Overall Approach and Reporting Template

While evaluating a pediatric pelvic tumor, the origin of the tumor, size, and morphological features should be primarily assessed to create a differential diagnosis. A large ill-defined lesion with aggressive behavior would suggest an underlying malignant neoplasm. Diffusion restriction and enhancement parameters would supplement in the diagnosis. The presence of fat and calcification in an ovarian or extragonadal lesion would be suggestive for a teratoma. Based on the size and margin of the lesion, a mature and immature teratoma can often be differentiated [8]. Additional features like endometrial hyperplasia in a prepubertal girl can raise the suspicion for an estrogen-secreting tumor. Correlation with tumor markers is mandatory for any scrotal or adnexal/large pelvic lesion.

Involvement of adjacent structures and the presence of nodes are needed for staging any gonadal or extragonadal neoplasm. The report should also comment on the presence or absence of peritoneal disease and distal metastasis. Below is an example of a basic reporting template for gonadal or extragonadal tumor in Table 26.5. However, this needs to be tailored for individual tumors.

Table 26.5 Reporting template

Lesion epicenter	<Testis> <ovary> <extragonadal>
Size	[---x---x---]cm
T1 and T2 morphology	Hypo/iso/hyperintense
Diffusion restriction	Present/Absent
Enhancement	Homogeneous/heterogeneous
Margin	Well-defined/ill-defined/infiltrative
If testicular,	
Both testes in scrotal sac?	Yes/ undescended testis
Scrotal wall involvement	Present/Absent
Epididymis	Involved/Normal
Microlithiasis	Yes/No
Nodes involved	Retroperitoneal nodes <2 cm/ 2–5 cm/ > 5 cm
Non-regional nodes	Yes/No
Distal metastasis	Yes/No, if yes—Mention site
If ovarian,	
Appearance	Unilocular/multilocular cystic with/without solid component, solid (O-RADS morphologies)
Laterality	Unilateral/Bilateral
Fat	Present/absent
Hemorrhage	Present/Absent
Calcifications	Present/Absent
Tumor limited to ovary	Yes/No
Uterus or other pelvic structures involved	Yes/No
Endometrial hyperplasia	Yes/No
Retroperitoneal nodes	Suspicious/benign/indeterminate, <10 mm/> 10 mm
Peritoneal disease	Present/Absent
Non-regional lymph nodes	Yes/No
Distal metastasis	Yes/No, if yes mention site
If extragonadal,	
Epicenter appreciable from amongst the non-gonadal pelvic organs	Yes/No
	If yes mention—Prostate/seminal vesicles/urinary bladder/uterus/cervix/vagina
Calcification	Present/Absent
Other pelvic visceral involvement	Yes/No
Nodes	Present/Absent, if present—Mention sites
Peritoneal disease	Present/Absent
Distal metastasis	Present/Absent
Bone involvement	Present/Absent

26.5 Pathology

The pathogenesis of gonadal neoplasms has been attributed to intra-uterine and perinatal risk factors like cryptorchidism, gonadal dysgenesis, or sex chromosomal abnormalities [15]. For example, girls with Turner's syndrome are more predisposed to develop gonadoblastomas, ovarian germ cell tumors, and dysgerminomas. Similarly, Klinefelter's and Swyer (hypoplastic gonads with feminization in cytogenetic male) syndromes are also associated with increased risk of gonadal and extragonadal neoplasms.

Many theories exist for the pathology of GCTs, though the commonly accepted one is the holistic concept. This concept believes that the GCTs arise from pluripotent germ cells which are capable of differentiating into embryonic or extra-embryonic tissues. Tumorigenesis and development are also dependent on the tumor microenvironment, which is supported by the fact that certain histologies are predominant at certain sites compared to others. For example, teratomas and yolk sac tumors are common in the sacrococcygeal region whereas the GCTs in vagina are almost always pure yolk sac tumors. Genetic susceptibility and environmental factors have been postulated to have been associated with RMS. Syndromes like Li-fraumeni, Neurofibromatosis I, Beckwith-Wiedemann, etc., are among those that are seen frequently in children with RMS [16].

DSRCT is a multifocal primary peritoneal sarcoma that occurs secondary to chromosomal translocation between EWS and WT1 genes. The resultant chimeric protein results in the development of DSRCT [9].

26.6 Imaging Features

(a) **Testicular Neoplasms:**

USG is the primary tool in the evaluation of testicular neoplasms, with high sensitivity. Most of the testicular neoplasms appear as well-defined hypoechoic lesions with or without cystic/necrotic changes, calcifications, hemorrhage, etc. Doppler and elastography could add vital information regarding the vascularity and the hardness of the tumor.

No imaging modality is specific in identifying the subtype of GCT, but this is a moot point as tumor markers help identify most of them accurately. Teratomas compared to other tumors have certain specific findings like the presence of fat and calcifications. Mature teratomas are predominantly cystic and well-defined, whereas an immature teratoma is larger than mature [6] (Fig. 26.1). Juvenile granulosa cell tumor can sometimes present type, has more solid components, and shows more areas of necrosis and hemorrhage. These are poorly vascularized when compared to other GCTs. Juvenile granulosa cell tumor can sometimes present as a well-defined multi-loculated cyst with thick septa or as a solid mass with multiple cysts [6].

Rest of the tumors show non-specific imaging findings that make it difficult to predict the histological diagnosis solely on imaging (Fig. 26.2).

Other non-neoplastic differentials like hematoma or infarction may also appear hypoechoic. They however would have a different clinical presentation (history of trauma or acute pain respectively) and would not demonstrate vascularity. Focal orchitis could also mimic a neoplasm, but the clinical presentation is usually with fever, pain, and tenderness [15]. Presence of

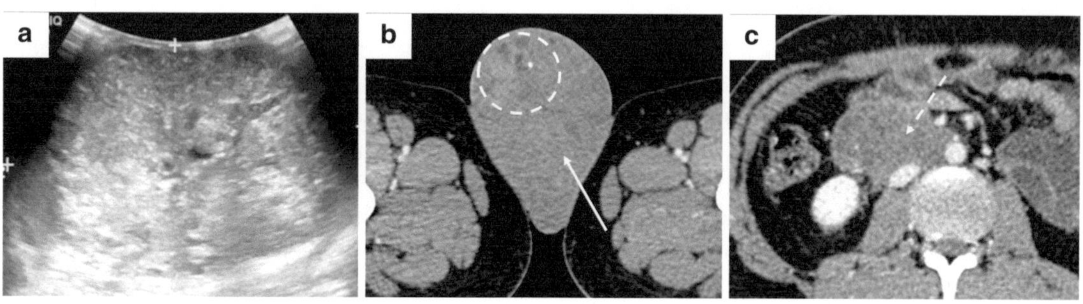

Fig. 26.1 A 15-year-old boy presented with scrotal mass. **a** Scrotal ultrasound shows enlarged testis replaced by a hyperechoic lesion. **b** Axial portal venous phase image shows a well-defined predominantly solid lesion (arrow) with focal area of fat and small specks of calcifications (dashed circle). **c** Note the metastatic retroperitoneal nodal mass (dashed arrow). HPR—Mature teratoma

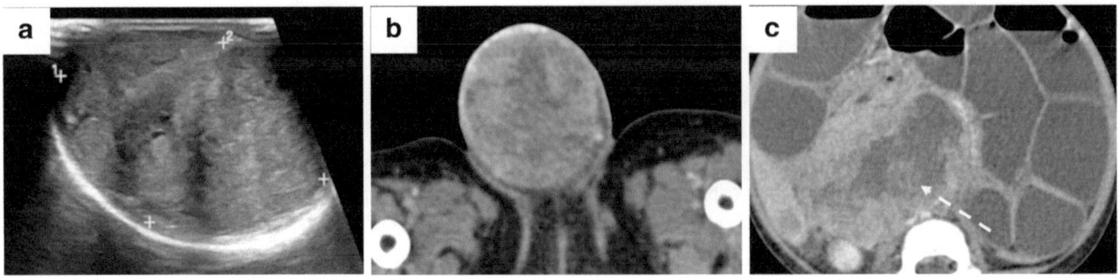

Fig. 26.2 A 2-year-old boy presented with scrotal swelling and abdominal pain. **a** Scrotal ultrasound showing an ill-defined heteroechoic lesion in the right testis. **b** CECT portal venous phase axial image showing a heterogeneously enhancing right testicular lesion. **c** Note the large necrotic retroperitoneal nodal mass (dashed arrow) and small bowel dilatation. HPR—Yolk sac tumor of testis

Table 26.6 TNM staging of testicular neoplasms [15]

Tumor	
Tx	Tumor cannot be assessed
T0	No evidence of primary tumor
T1	Tumor confined to testicle and epididymis
T2	Tumor breaches tunica vaginalis or spreads to adjacent lymphatics
T3	Tumor grows into spermatic cord
T4	Tumor reaches till scrotal skin
Node	
Nx	Regional lymph nodes cannot be assessed
No	No regional lymph nodes visible on imaging
N1	Lymph node—Greatest dimension <2 cm
N2	Lymph node—Greatest dimension 2–5 cm
N3	Lymph node—Greatest dimension >5 cm
Metastasis	
M0	No distal metastasis
M1a	Tumor in non-regional lymph node or in lungs
M1b	Metastasis in other organs

microlithiasis in the setting of an existing neoplasm warrants an annual screening USG [7].

Retroperitoneal nodes are the regional nodes for testis. A short axis diameter of 7–8 mm is used to distinguish between N0 and N1. However, for N1, N2, and N3 stages, the long axis diameter is used for staging [15]. Refer Table 26.6.

(b) **Ovarian neoplasms:** Ultrasound is the first-line investigation to confirm the ovarian origin and to rule out other etiologies. Though it is difficult to differentiate between the histological types, variable imaging findings help us predict between the benign versus malignant ovarian neoplasms and to some extent identify the tumor subtype, unlike testicular lesions where differentiation is almost impossible.

26.7 Germ Cell Tumors

Teratomas are the most common pediatric ovarian tumors, with mature teratomas constituting about 50% of benign pediatric ovarian neoplasms [8]. Mature teratomas are predominantly cystic with substantial macroscopic fat, along with variable amounts of calcification and other contents like hair, sebum, etc., On USG, they appear as unilocular cystic lesions with echogenic fat within, with a hyperechoic nodule, called Rokitansky nodule. Other features in USG include areas of coarse calcifications, fat-fluid level or ‘dermoid mesh’ sign, defined as the appearance of floating hair fibers/strands within the cyst. The Rokitansky nodule sometimes causes significant acoustic attenuation thus inhibiting proper/complete evaluation of the lesion, labeled as the ‘tip of the iceberg’ phenomenon [17]. They present as a well-defined cystic lesion with macroscopic fat and coarse calcification on CT and MRI (Fig. 26.3). Hounsfield (HU) values on CT and gradient echo opposed phase T1 could help identify doubtful fat components.

Immature teratomas are usually larger, multicystic with more solid components, and minimal (less than 5–10%) macroscopic fat. Specks of calcifications may be present along the walls or septae (Fig. 26.4). Immature teratoma may be

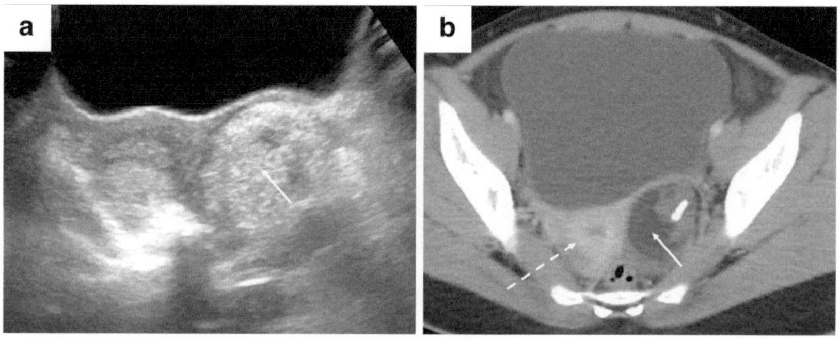

Fig. 26.3 A 13-year-old girl presented with intermittent abdominal pain. **a** Ultrasound pelvis shows a well-defined hyperechoic fat-echoic lesion in left adnexa. **b** Axial portal venous phase images showing a well-defined predominantly cystic lesion with fat-dense areas and a tooth (arrow). Note the normal uterus (dashed arrow). HPR—Mature teratoma

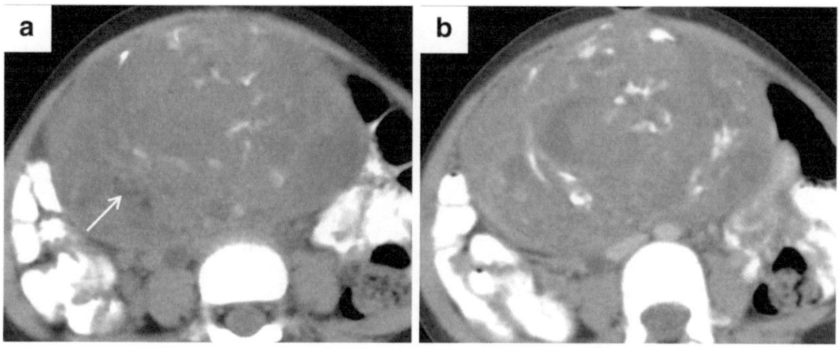

Fig. 26.4 An 8-year-old girl was brought with abdominal swelling that is inzcreasing in size since 2 weeks. **a** Axial non-contrast CT shows a large heterogenous lesion in the pelvis with small amounts of fat (arrow) and areas of calcification. **b** Axial portal venous phase image shows heterogeneous enhancement of the solid component. HPR—Immature teratoma

associated with elevated AFP levels and is more common in younger children.

Teratomas could be associated with torsion or rupture. An associated finding of tenderness, fluid in abdomen should raise the suspicion and careful evaluation should be done for timely intervention [18].

Dysgerminomas are the female counterpart tumor to seminomas. These are associated with gonadal dysgenesis and syndromes like Turner's syndrome and can arise from gonadoblastomas. On USG, these are solid or solid-cystic hypoechoic tumors with septa showing vascular flow on Doppler imaging. Calcifications and necrosis are less commonly seen. They present as a multi-lobulated heterogeneously enhancing solid/solid-cystic lesion on CT/MRI. The septa within the lesion show intense enhancement and appear T2 hypointense on MRI [17] (Fig. 26.5). Normal AFP and beta-HCG levels in the presence of an adnexal mass are an indicator of the diagnosis. Though non-specific, elevated LDH levels could help indicate the lesion.

Other germ cell tumors like yolk sac tumor, non-gestational choriocarcinoma, and embryonal carcinoma have non-specific imaging findings. They present as heterogeneously enhancing masses with variable amounts of cystic and solid components, hemorrhage, and necrosis. Yolk sac tumors are especially aggressive with increased incidence of hematogenous and peritoneal spread [8] (Fig. 26.6).

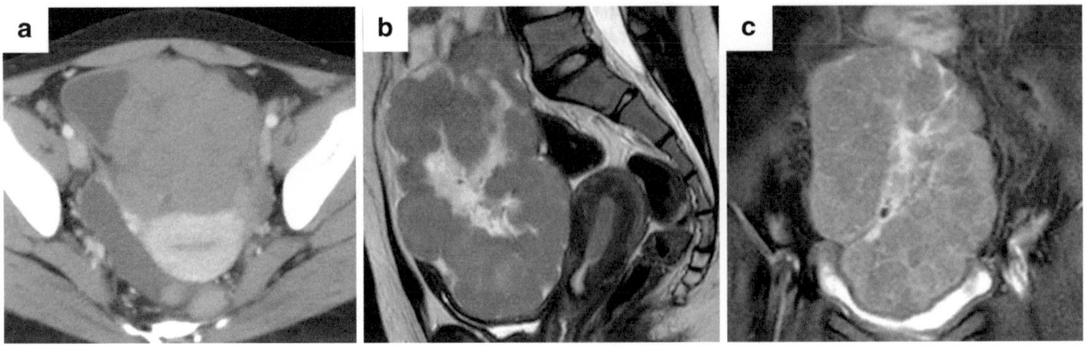

Fig. 26.5 A 15-year-old girl presented with abdominal pain. **a** Axial portal venous phase image shows a well-defined lobulated predominantly solid lesion without any necrosis. **b and c** Sagittal T2W image showing a well-encapsulated solid lesion with lobulations and homogeneous enhancement on post-contrast coronal images. HPR—Dysgerminoma

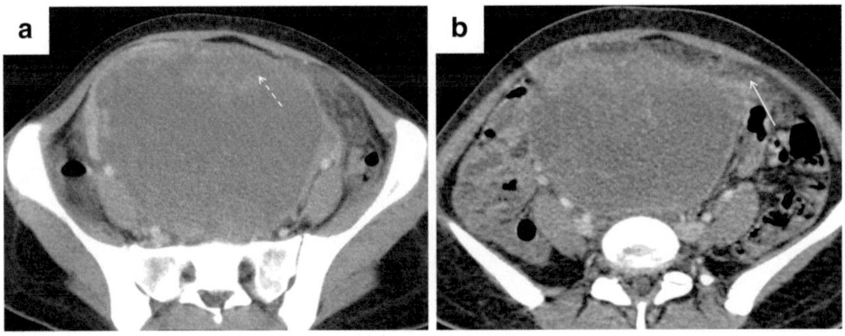

Fig. 26.6 A 17-year-old girl presented with abdominal pain and vomiting for 1 week with AFP of 75954.5 ng/ml. **a and b** Axial portal venous phase CT shows a cystic lesion with mild sheet-like enhancement in the periphery (dashed arrow). Note the omental caking (arrow). HPR—Yolk sac tumor of ovary

26.8 Other Ovarian Neoplasms

Among the non-germ cell tumors in ovary, granulosa cell tumors are the most common. It is divided into adult and juvenile types. Juvenile granulosa cell tumor is more common in the prepubertal age group and presents with precocious puberty. It could be associated with Ollier and Maffucci syndromes [8]. They could be either solid, solid-cystic, or completely cystic. A sponge-like pattern of solid with multiple cystic areas has been characteristically described for juvenile granulosa cell tumors, although not common. Since these are estradiol-secreting tumors, they can be associated with endometrial thickening (Fig. 26.7). Juvenile and adult types cannot be differentiated on imaging; the former has a better prognosis [17].

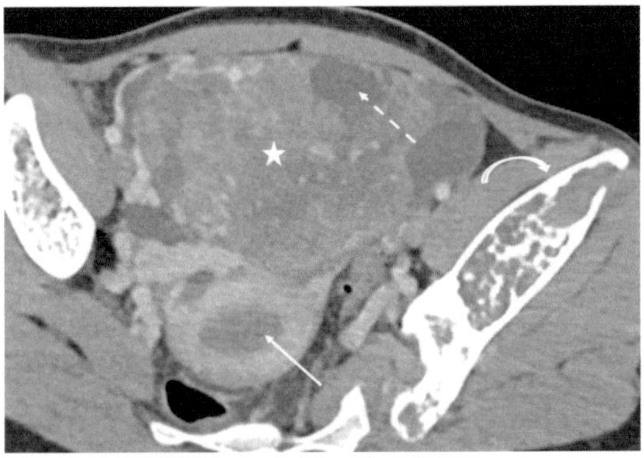

Fig. 26.7 A 16-year-old girl presented with abdominal pain and irregular menstrual cycles. The axial CECT image shows a large heterogeneous adnexal mass (star) with areas of cystic changes (dashed arrow). Note the endometrial hyperplasia (arrow) and bone metastasis (curved arrow). Inhibin was >8000 pg/ml and the lesion was proved as granulosa cell tumor (juvenile)

Sertoli-Leydig cell tumors are very rare in children and have non-specific imaging findings (Fig. 26.8). They are associated with androgen secretion and virilization symptoms.

The fibroma-thecoma group of tumors may sometimes be present in this patient group. These are solid tumors that appear hypointense on T2 owing to the collagen content and show mild homogeneous enhancement with a type I time-intensity curve on dynamic contrast-enhanced sequences. Sometimes, calcification and cystic changes can be seen [8, 18].

Epithelial tumors like cystadenoma and cystadenocarcinomas of serosal and mucosal origin are very rare in children and are not discussed here. Their imaging features are similar to that in adults. Borderline tumors are more common in this age group compared to frankly malignant tumors.

Ovarian metastases from rhabdomyosarcomas and neuroblastomas can also be seen rarely [17]. The staging of ovarian tumors is presented in Table 26.7 [19].

(a) **Non-gonadal Neoplasms:**

Uterus: Uterine neoplasms are rare in children. The rarely encountered ones are malignant neoplasms like leiomyosarcoma and rhabdomyosarcoma [20].

Vagina: The common vaginal neoplasms are rhabdomyosarcomas; these are more common than uterine RMS. The lesion usually presents with a polypoidal lesion projecting through the introitus or as vaginal bleeding. RMS may be embryonal, alveolar, and pleomorphic subtypes. These are locally aggressive lesions that occupy the vaginal canal and invade adjacent pelvic structures. They appear heterogenous with varying areas of necrosis or hemorrhage [20]. Botryoid RMS is a variant of embryonal RMS, typically seen in vagina and is characterized by grape-like appearance with multiple T2 hyperintense cystic areas that are peripherally enhancing [21, 22] (Fig. 26.9). Retroperitoneal lymph nodal involvement or distal metastases to liver, lung, and bone may be seen. FDG PET/CT is the investigation of choice for RMS.

Other rare neoplasms in vagina are endodermal sinus tumors and clear cell adenocarcinoma. These are indistinguishable from RMS on imaging [20].

Table 26.7 Revised International Federation of Gynecology and Obstetrics (FIGO) staging for ovarian tumors

Stage	Findings
Ia	Tumor limited to one ovary, no malignant cells in ascites or peritoneal washing
Ib	Similar to Ia, but involves both ovaries
Ic	Lesion involves one or two ovaries with capsule rupture or malignant cells in ascites
IIa	Tumor in ovary with involvement of uterus or fallopian tubes
IIb	Tumor in ovary with involvement of other intraperitoneal pelvic structures
IIIa	Positive retroperitoneal nodes or microscopic extra-pelvic involvement
IIIb	Positive macroscopic peritoneal metastases ≤2 cm with or without retroperitoneal nodes
IIIc	Positive macroscopic peritoneal metastases >2 cm with or without retroperitoneal nodes
IVa	Pleural effusion positive for malignant cells
IVb	Distal parenchymal metastasis

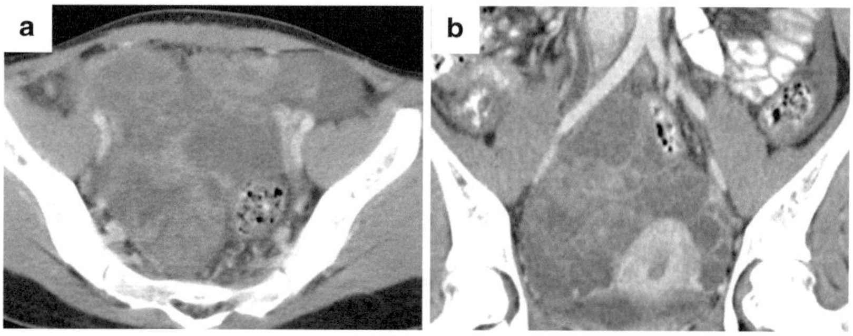

Fig. 26.8 An 18-year-old girl presented with mild abdominal pain. **a and b** Axial portal venous phase CT shows a solid-cystic lesion with heterogeneous enhancement. HPR—Sertoli Leydig cell tumor of ovary

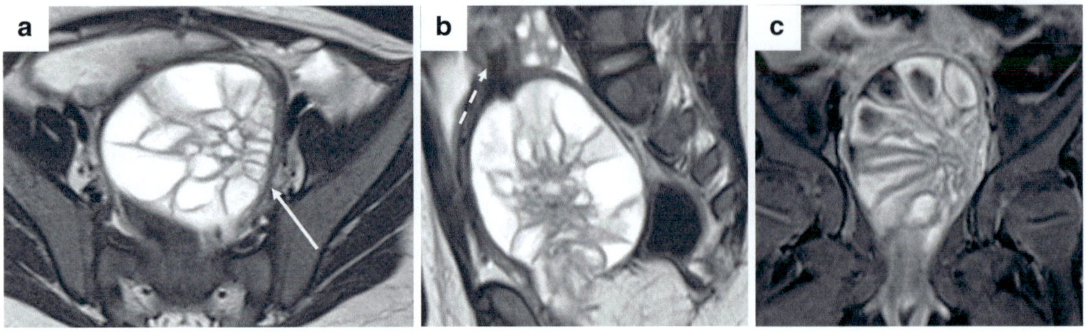

Fig. 26.9 A 19-month-old girl presented with whitish discharge per vagina. **a and b** The axial and sagittal T2 image shows a heterogeneous mass in the cervix and vagina with classic grape-like appearance (arrow) with normal uterus (dashed arrow). **c** Note the heterogenous enhancement on post contrast coronal image

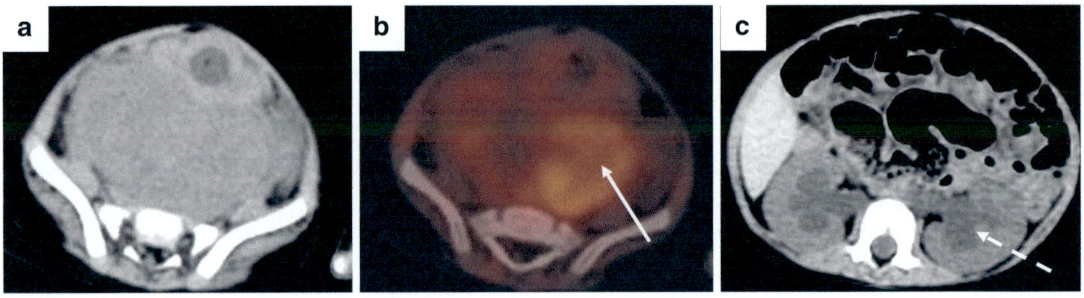

Fig. 26.10 An 11-month-old boy was brought with abdominal distension and poor urine flow. **a** Axial non-contrast PET-CT shows a large heterogenous lesion posterior to the urinary bladder displacing it anteriorly. **b** and **c** Note the FDG avidity within the lesion (arrow) in fused image and bilateral hydronephrosis secondary to ureteric compression (dashed arrow). HPR—Prostatic rhabdomyosarcoma

Bladder and prostate: Malignant tumors are more common in bladder and prostate than benign lesions. Rhabdomyosarcomas are the most frequently occurring bladder and prostatic neoplasm in this age group. Leiomyosarcomas, lymphoma, and leukemic involvement of the bladder are the other malignant neoplasms that can be rarely seen [20]. Though USG is used as the primary tool for detection, a CT/MRI is best for characterizing the lesion and pinpointing the organ of origin. The malignant lesions can be identified by their large size, heterogeneous enhancement and extravesical extension, and infiltration of adjacent structures (Figs. 26.10 and 26.11). Variable amounts of hemorrhage or necrosis can be seen. Both CT and MRI are used for local assessment and staging [21]. RMS commonly metastasizes to lungs, chest CT is done for screening. Though rare in children, inflammatory myofibroblastic tumors (IMT) can also occur. These are characterized by their classic location near the dome of the bladder.

Pelvis: The most common non-visceral pelvic neoplasms are seen in the presacral space. Most of these are germ cell neoplasms, sacrococcygeal teratomas, followed by rhabdomyosarcomas. Germ cell tumors of the pelvis are similar to gonadal GCTs in imaging appearance which has been discussed above, demonstrating both solid and cystic components. Other differentials like neuroblastomas and chordomas may also be seen. RMS and sacrococcygeal teratoma are discussed in more detail below.

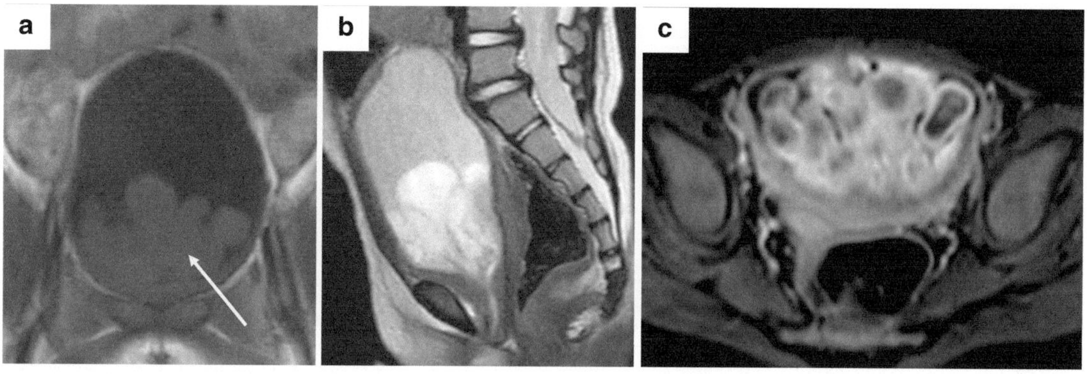

Fig. 26.11 A 2-year-old girl was brought with complaints of straining during micturition. **a** and **b** Coronal T1 and sagittal T2 images show a polypoidal lesion in the bladder (arrow). **c** Axial post-contrast imaging shows peripheral enhancement of the cystic spaces. HPR—Botryoid rhabdomyosarcoma of urinary bladder

Table 26.8 TNM staging of rhabdomyosarcomas [16]

TNM staging		
T stage	T1—Confined to the organ of origin	
	T2—Invades adjacent tissues T2a—≤ 5 cm T2b—> 5 cm	
N stage	N0—No metastatic nodes	
	N1—Regional nodes involved	
Site	**TNM**	**Stage**
Non-bladder, prostate	Any T, any N, M0	I
Bladder, prostate	T1, N0, M0 T2a, N0, M0	II
Bladder, prostate	T2b, N0, M0 Any T, N1, M0	III
Any site	Any T, any N, M1	IV

26.9 Rhabdomyosarcoma

RMS is the most common neoplasm of the genitourinary tract in both female and male children, with peak incidence in children under 5 years. It accounts for 4% of all malignant neoplasms in children. As discussed earlier, RMS has embryonal, alveolar, and pleomorphic subtypes of which embryonal is the common subtype in the genitourinary tract [16]. Botryoid RMS is a variant of embryonal type that occurs in vagina and bladder, with better prognosis. Alveolar RMS has the worst prognosis. On imaging, RMS presents as aggressive heterogeneously enhancing tumors with areas of necrosis and hemorrhage [21]. The staging as per the revised COG guidelines of RMS is tabulated in Table 26.8.

Table 26.9 Types of sacrococcygeal teratomas based on epicenter of the tumor

Types of sacrococcygeal teratomas	
I	Completely external
II	Partly external and partly internal
III	Predominantly internal (pelvic) with a small external component
IV	Intrapelvic

26.10 Sacrococcygeal Teratoma

These are the most common presacral neoplasms in children. They may be benign or malignant in etiology. They have been classified into different types based on location (Table 26.9) [23].

These appear as a heterogeneous lesion in the pelvic cavity with or without an external component showing cystic changes, fat, and calcifications (Fig. 26.12). They may be associated with anorectal malformations. If detected on prenatal USG, a fetal MRI has to be performed to assess other associated anomalies and to plan the management of the pregnancy [11].

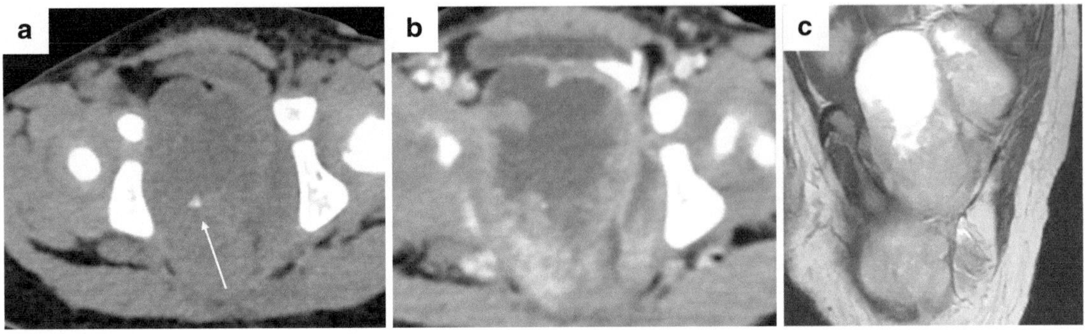

Fig. 26.12 A 12-month-old girl presented with lower back swelling. **a** Axial plain CT shows a large lesion with a focal calcification (arrow). **b** Axial portal venous phase image shows a heterogeneously enhancing solid-cystic lesion. It is a type III (predominantly pelvic and partly external). **c** Sagittal T2W image showing a large heterogenous lesion with cystic areas. HPR—Sacrococcygeal teratoma

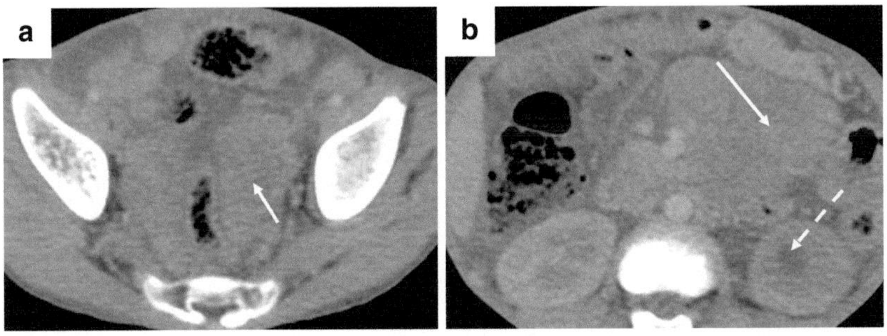

Fig. 26.13 A 12-year-old boy presented with abdominal distension and pain. **a** and **b** Axial portal venous phase images showing multiple peritoneal masses (arrows) with ascites. Note the large mass in retroperitoneal region causing upstream left hydronephrosis (dashed arrow). HPR - desmoplastic small cell round tumor

26.11 DSRCT

Desmoplastic small round cell tumors are aggressive peritoneal tumors presenting as multiple echogenic masses on ultrasound. On CT/MRI, DSRCT appears as multiple large well-defined enhancing diffuse peritoneal and omental masses with no obvious primary site of origin, often with the largest of these being in the pelvis (Fig. 26.13). It can sometimes present as a large solitary mass as well. When multiple masses are present, the largest mass would be considered as a dominant mass or epicenter of the disease [10]. Areas of cystic/necrosis, hemorrhage, or calcifications could also be seen within these lesions. Metastasis to organs like liver, lung, and spleen can also be picked up in cross-sectional imaging [9, 10]. Differentials include metastatic sarcoma and germ cell tumors.

26.12 Other Neoplasms

A low-lying neuroblastoma may present as a heterogeneous or homogenous lesion in the pelvis (Fig. 26.14). Chordoma is not common in children, but when present poses a close differential to sacrococcygeal teratoma. However, chordoma shows a very high signal on T2 [20, 24]. Pelvic Ewing's sarcomas and osteosarcomas of pelvic bones can also occur. Both are bony neoplasms that demonstrate a wide zone of transition and aggressive periosteal reaction with cortical destruction and associated soft tissue. Detailed description of these neoplasms is beyond the scope of this chapter.

While making a clinical diagnosis, imaging along with the knowledge of symptomatology and tumor markers plays a crucial role. An algorithmic approach for imaging evaluation of the gonadal and extragonadal neoplasms in children is presented below (Fig. 26.15).

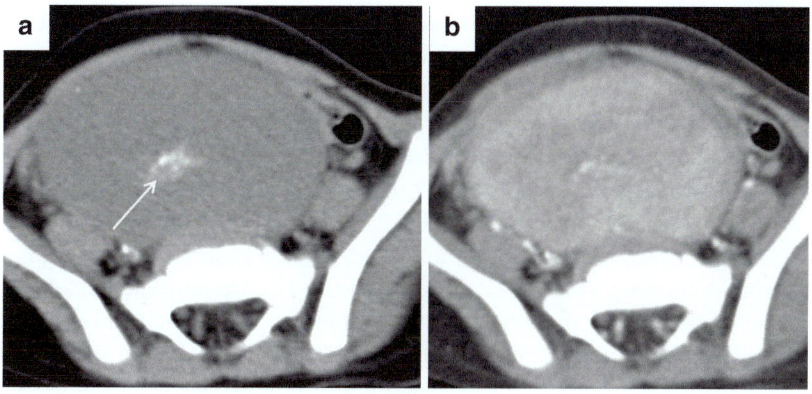

Fig. 26.14 A 1-year-old boy was brought with abdominal swelling. **a** Axial non-contrast CT shows a well-defined lesion in the pelvis with calcification (arrow). **b** Axial portal venous phase image shows heterogenous enhancement of the lesion. HPR—Neuroblastoma

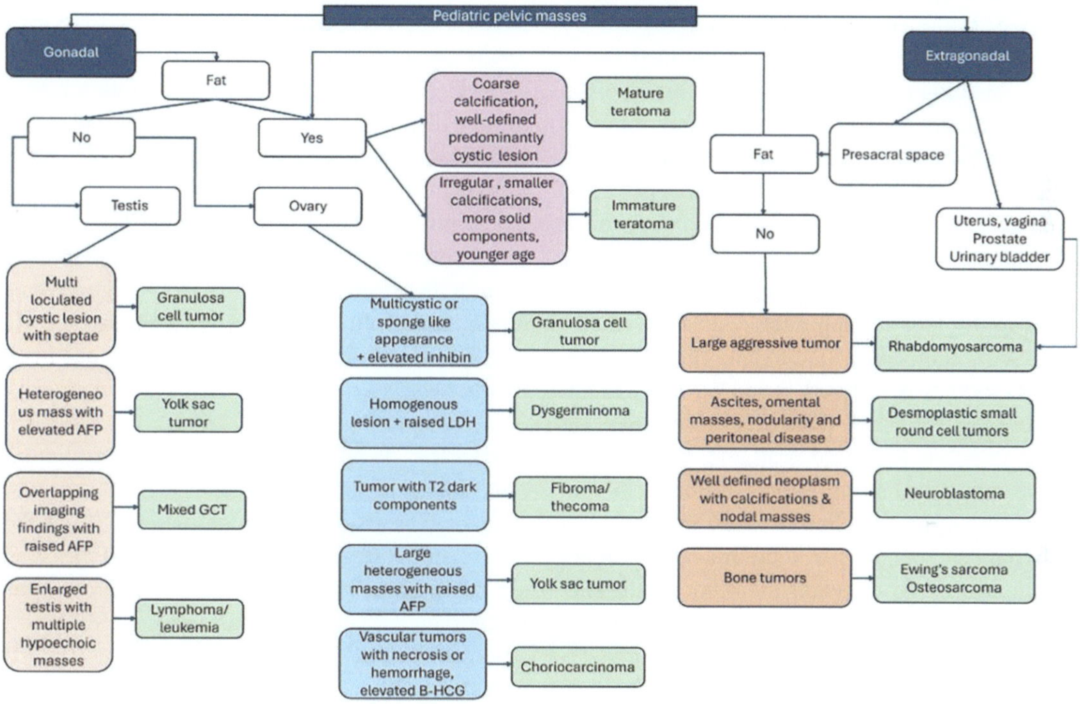

Fig. 26.15 Flowchart for algorithmic approach of gonadal and extragonadal lesions

26.13 Management

Ovarian and testicular neoplasms are not usually biopsied to avoid seeding. In testicular malignancies radical inguinal orchidectomy is the standard treatment. A testicular sparing surgery can be performed if the lesion is benign with some residual normal appearing salvageable testicular tissue. Testicular enucleation is recommended in benign tumors especially in cases of pre-pubertal boys. If malignancy is suspected during the microsurgical exploration, the surgery should be preferably converted to an inguinal orchidectomy [6].

Stage I patients with non-seminomatous tumors combined chemotherapy with bleomycin, etoposide, and cisplatin with active surveillance for a minimum of 5 years. Whereas in seminoma, the patients are subjected to adjuvant single-agent carboplatin chemotherapy or adjuvant radiation or surveillance for 5 years.

During surveillance, serum markers are monitored with USG and CT chest or radiographs in frequencies as discussed above. Stages II and III are treated with intense chemotherapy regimen followed by resection of the residual tumor if any. In the case of pulmonary or liver metastases, metastatectomy can be performed [15].

Benign ovarian tumors are managed with ovarian-preserving surgery to preserve fertility. Preservation of both ovaries is the goal in children as far as possible. Laparoscopy is preferred especially in the setting of a benign tumor. However, a laparotomy may be required based on the size of the tumor. Surgery is followed by adjuvant chemotherapy which is planned based on the histological diagnosis of the tumor [24]. The commonly followed chemotherapy regimen is BEP (bleomycin, etoposide, cisplatin) [18]. When the child presents with acute symptoms like pain a timely diagnosis and management of ovarian torsion should be made [25].

The gold standard treatment for RMS is usually a multimodality approach consisting of surgery with adjuvant/neoadjuvant chemotherapy and RT which is tailored based on the patient. However, no formal treatment guidelines for pediatric pelvic RMS are available. In sacrococcygeal teratomas, an upfront resection with coccygectomy is done in eligible cases. In the case of malignant sacrococcygeal teratomas, the surgery is followed by an adjuvant radiotherapy or chemotherapy. In unresectable cases, neoadjuvant chemotherapy with PEB (cisplatin, etoposide, and bleomycin) [26]. After chemotherapy, an attempt to resect the residual mass is suggested. Even in the presence of metastases, neoadjuvant platinum-based chemotherapy is given followed by a complete tumoral resection [27].

DSRCT does not have a standard chemotherapy regimen, and chemotherapy drugs like cyclophosphamide, doxorubicin, vincristine, ifosfamide, and etoposide are used. Cytoreductive surgery and hyperthermic peritoneal perfusion with chemotherapeutic drugs have also been tried to improve patient outcomes [10].

26.14 Surveillance Protocols

The primary aim of surveillance imaging is to detect local or distal recurrence before symptoms present. Surveillance includes clinical follow-up along with tumor markers and imaging.

Ovarian Neoplasms For ovarian neoplasms, the currently available surveillance is different based on the histology of the neoplasm. For most GCTs which secrete beta HCG or AFP, biochemical surveillance using tumor markers is the key as biochemical recurrence precedes imaging recurrence. In sex cord stromal tumors, the recurrence rate is rare after 3 years. Imaging plays a greater role in surveillance of non-secretory tumors like dysgerminomas. The society of gynecological oncologists recommends surveillance imaging every 2–4 months for the first 2 years in dysgerminoma [2]. Unlike in adults, routine follow-up with CT might not be appropriate in children with germ cell tumors. COG guidelines recommend follow-up imaging with either USG or MRI. However, no specific interval has been mentioned.

Testicular Neoplasms Most of the testicular neoplasms in children recur within the first 2 years. The guidelines recommend USG of the contralateral testis to be performed. For COG stage I disease, a chest radiograph at follow-up is recommended for metastasis surveillance, whereas chest CT is recommended for stage II and above [7].

Extragonadal GCTs Chest radiograph and abdominopelvic MRI or CT is recommended every 3 months, and every 6 months and then every yearly for 5 years from the time of diagnosis. After two years, MRI could be replaced with USG. Post-treatment assessment in sacrococcygeal teratomas should look for the change in the size of the tumor, changes in the enhancement, and necrosis. Surveillance imaging with CT/MRI at 3–6 months interval for first year is recommended. Chest radiograph would suffice for a non-metastatic presentation, whereas a CT is indicated for a metastatic sacrococcygeal teratoma for 2 years from diagnosis. Also, AFP and LDH are to be monitored every 2–6 months for the first year after resection.

Rhabdomyosarcoma Post-chemotherapy assessment with MRI and PET-CT is recommended. For patients with metastasis, a follow-up with chest CT is recommended. For surveillance of local disease, an abdominopelvic MRI is recommended every 3 months for the first year, every 4 months for next 2 years, and every 6 months for next one year [11].

Advances and Updates A recent study suggested that symptom-wise imaging picked up more relapses than following surveillance protocols in urologic neoplasms of childhood. Research regarding iterative reconstructions and detective technologies is ongoing with an aim to improve image quality and reduce radiation exposure in children undergoing CT. Though kid-friendly scanning rooms are already in practice, attempts are being made with MRI-compatible goggles to play videos for kids to distract them. Recently, novel mechanical devices or advanced imaging protocols are used to acquire motion-sensitive sequences [28].

Novel molecular targeting agents are being explored for translocation related to DSRCT [10].

In summary, radiologists play a vital role in diagnosing pelvic neoplasms and guiding in patient management. Pre-surgical planning and surveillance imaging for detecting relapses are other important roles of imaging. Strategies should be made to reduce scan time and radiation exposure.

Acknowledgments None.

Funding The authors did not receive funding from any organization for the submitted work.

Disclosures The authors have no conflict of interest to disclose.

Financial Interests The authors declare they have no financial interests.

References

1. Schneider DT, Terenziani M, Cecchetto G, Olson TA. Gonadal and Extragonadal germ cell tumors, sex cord stromal and rare gonadal tumors. In: Schneider D, Brecht I, Olson T, Ferrari A, editors. Rare tumors in children and adolescents. Pediatric oncology. Berlin/Heidelberg: Springer; 2012. https://doi.org/10.1007/978-3-642-04197-6_39.
2. Behr GG, Morani AC, Artunduaga M, et al. Imaging of pediatric ovarian tumors: a COG diagnostic imaging committee/SPR oncology committee white paper. Pediatr Blood Cancer. 2023;70(Suppl 4):e29995. https://doi.org/10.1002/pbc.29995.
3. Moch H, Amin MB, Berney DM, et al. The 2022 World Health Organization classification of Tumours of the urinary system and male genital organs—part a: renal, penile, and testicular Tumours. Eur Urol. 2022;82:458–68. https://doi.org/10.1016/j.eururo.2022.06.016.
4. Mehra P, Aditi S, Prasad KM, Bariar NK. Histomorphological analysis of ovarian neoplasms according to the 2020 WHO classification of ovarian tumors: a distribution pattern in a tertiary care center. Cureus. 2023;15(4):e38273. https://doi.org/10.7759/cureus.38273.
5. Schultz KAP, Sencer SF, Messinger Y, et al. Pediatric ovarian tumors: a review of 67 cases. Pediatr Blood Cancer. 2005;44:167–73. https://doi.org/10.1002/PBC.20233.
6. Sangüesa C, Veiga D, Llavador M, Serrano A. Testicular tumours in children: an approach to diagnosis and management with pathologic correlation. Insights Imaging. 2020;11:74. https://doi.org/10.1186/s13244-020-00867-6.
7. Behr GG, Morani AC, Artunduaga M, et al. Imaging of pediatric testicular tumors: a COG diagnostic imaging committee/SPR oncology committee white paper. Pediatr Blood Cancer. 2023;70(Suppl 4):e29988. https://doi.org/10.1002/pbc.29988.
8. Heo SH, Kim JW, Shin SS, et al. Review of ovarian tumors in children and adolescents: radiologic- pathologic correlation. Radiographics. 2014;34:2039–55. https://doi.org/10.1148/rg.347130144.
9. Morani AC, Bathala TK, Surabhi VR, et al. Desmoplastic small round cell tumor: imaging pat-

tern of disease at presentation. Am J Roentgenol. 2019;212:W45–54. https://doi.org/10.2214/AJR.18.20179.
10. Bent MA, Padilla BE, Goldsby RE, DuBois SG. Clinical characteristics and outcomes of pediatric patients with desmoplastic small round cell tumor. Rare Tumors. 2016;8:24–6. https://doi.org/10.4081/rt.2016.6145.
11. Pace E, Johnson TS, Kao SC, et al. Imaging of pediatric extragonadal pelvic soft tissue tumors: a COG diagnostic imaging committee/SPR oncology committee white paper. Pediatr Blood Cancer. 2023;70(Suppl 4):e29966. https://doi.org/10.1002/pbc.29966.
12. PDQ Pediatric Treatment Editorial Board. Childhood Extracranial germ cell tumors treatment (PDQ®): health professional version. In: PDQ cancer information summaries [internet]. Bethesda (MD): National Cancer Institute (US); 2002; 2024. https://pubmed.ncbi.nlm.nih.gov/26389316.
13. Weil BR, Billmire DF. Management of Germ Cell Tumors in pediatric patients. Surg Oncol Clin N Am. 2021;30:325–38. https://doi.org/10.1016/j.soc.2020.11.011.
14. Crane JN, Xue W, Qumseya A, et al. Clinical group and modified TNM stage for rhabdomyosarcoma: a review from the children's oncology group. Pediatr Blood Cancer. 2022;69(6):e29644. https://doi.org/10.1002/pbc.29644.
15. Moreno CC, Small WC, Camacho JC, et al. Testicular tumors: what radiologists need to know—differential diagnosis, staging, and management. Radiographics. 2015;35:400–15. https://doi.org/10.1148/rg.352140097.
16. Skapek SX, Ferrari A, Gupta AA, et al. Rhabdomyosarcoma. Nat Rev Dis Primers. 2019;5(1):1. https://doi.org/10.1038/s41572-018-0051-2.
17. Hanafy AK, Mujtaba B, Yedururi S, et al. Imaging in pediatric ovarian tumors. Abdominal Radiol. 2020;45:520–36. https://doi.org/10.1007/s00261-019-02316-5.
18. Mahadik K, Ghorpade K. Childhood ovarian malignancy. J Obst Gynecol India. 2014;64:91–4. https://doi.org/10.1007/s13224-014-0533-4.
19. Javadi S, Ganeshan DM, Qayyum A, et al. Ovarian cancer, the revised FIGO staging system, and the role of imaging. Am J Roentgenol. 2016;206:1351–60. https://doi.org/10.2214/AJR.15.15199.
20. Shah RU, Lawrence C, Fickenscher KA, et al. Imaging of pediatric pelvic neoplasms. Radiol Clin North Am. 2011;49:729–48. https://doi.org/10.1016/j.rcl.2011.05.007.
21. Pai DR, Ladino-Torres MF. Magnetic resonance imaging of pediatric pelvic masses. Magn Reson Imaging Clin N Am. 2013;21:751–72. https://doi.org/10.1016/j.mric.2013.07.002.
22. Houghton JP, McCluggage WG. Embryonal rhabdomyosarcoma of the cervix with focal pleomorphic areas. J Clin Pathol. 2007;60:88–9. https://doi.org/10.1136/jcp.2005.034769.
23. Groff DB. Pelvic neoplasms in children. J Surg Oncol. 2001;77(1):65–71. https://doi.org/10.1002/jso.1068.
24. Damle L. Diagnosis and Management of Pelvic Masses in children and adolescents. Postgraduate Obst Gynecol. 2011;31:1–6. https://doi.org/10.1097/01.PGO.0000394779.37584.41.
25. Khaja A, Frazier L, Weil BR, et al. Interdisciplinary Management of Malignant Ovarian Tumors in the pediatric and adolescent age group. J Pediatr Adolesc Gynecol. 2022;35:260–4. https://doi.org/10.1016/j.jpag.2021.10.006.
26. Kondagunta GV, Motzer RJ. Chemotherapy for advanced germ cell tumors. J Clin Oncol. 2006;24:5493–502. https://doi.org/10.1200/JCO.2006.08.7882.
27. Yadav D, Acharya S, Bagga D, et al. Sacrococcygeal teratoma: clinical characteristics, management, and long-term outcomes in a prospective study from a tertiary care center. J Indian Assoc Pediatr Surg. 2020;25:15. https://doi.org/10.4103/jiaps.JIAPS_219_18.
28. Davis JT, Wagner LM. Imaging of childhood urologic cancers: current approaches and new advances. Transl Androl Urol. 2020;9:2348–57. https://doi.org/10.21037/tau-19-839.

Part V

Interventional Radiology

27 Non-vascular Pediatric Interventional Oncology

Shikhar Garg and Shyamkumar N. Keshava

27.1 Introduction

Interventional oncology (IO) is a subspeciality of interventional radiology (IR) that has transformed the management of pediatric cancer by offering minimally invasive diagnostic and therapeutic procedures.

Pediatric patients present unique challenges, as children differ from adults in their anatomy, physiology, and disease patterns. IR procedures are less invasive than traditional surgical methods, making them particularly suitable for young patients who have limited tolerance for extensive procedures.

This chapter explores the various non-vascular IO techniques used in the management of pediatric cancer patients, focusing on their applications, benefits, and considerations unique to the pediatric population.

The indications for interventional radiology in pediatric cancer patients are broad and cover a range of applications—including diagnostic procedures, curative interventions, enhancement of therapeutic outcomes, management of complications, and palliative care.

S. Garg · S. N. Keshava (✉)
Department of Interventional Radiology, Division of Clinical Radiology, Christian Medical College, Vellore, Tamil Nadu, India

27.2 Special Considerations in the Pediatric Population

1. Case Selection: Before scheduling a case, the radiologist needs to assess the necessity of the procedure. It is vital to consider non-invasive or lower-risk choices that are accessible to the patient. Often, additional imaging reveals a safer alternative to the problem at hand. A basic blood work-up, including a coagulation profile, is mandatory before any procedure, and appropriate corrections to coagulopathy are required. The spectrum of IR is wide, It is crucial to take on cases where the necessary expertise is available and the hospital has sufficient resources to manage any potential complications, for example, endovascular embolization for a post-biopsy bleed.
2. Radiation Exposure: Children are more sensitive to radiation, so minimizing radiation is critical. This can be achieved by optimizing imaging techniques for the least radiation and using ultrasound guidance whenever possible. It is also important to monitor the cumulative radiation dose in children requiring multiple procedures.
3. Anatomical and Physiological Differences: As children have smaller anatomical structures, there is a lack of specialized hardware for this patient group. They also have a lower circulating blood volume and lower threshold for complications. The interventionist should

I. Kumar et al. (eds.), *Practical Approach to Imaging in Pediatric Oncology*,
https://doi.org/10.1007/978-981-96-8158-7_27

be cognizant of this fact while planning the procedures and employ techniques to account for the smaller size and more delicate structures. Anatomical structures change with growth, so interventions must be tailored to the child's age and size, with anticipation of future growth.

4. Sedation and Anesthesia: Children often will require sedation or anesthesia. It is important to address the anxiety of both the child and their family. Techniques such as distraction and the presence of parents during induction are helpful.
5. Parental Involvement: It is essential to obtain consent from parents or legal guardians, with clear explanations of risks, benefits, and alternatives. It is important to involve parents in the decision-making process.
6. Post-procedure Care: Close monitoring is essential in the post-procedure period. It is wise to have an ICU bed arranged before the procedure for post-procedure monitoring, in case of a complication.

27.3 Diagnostic Applications

27.3.1 Image-Guided FNAC & Biopsy

Commonly biopsied structures include lymph nodes, liver, abdominal masses, chest, and bone lesions. Even for larger lesions, image-guided biopsy is useful in localizing a better tract with less vascularity to plan the course of the needle and trajectory.

Image guidance (US, MRI, or CT) offers high accuracy with low complication rates.

It is essential to confirm the indication of biopsy and whether any additional imaging may reveal a safer target for biopsy. Functional imaging modalities such as PET-CT or contrast-enhanced CT, MRI, or ultrasound can be used to predict metabolically active parts of the tumor that can then be targeted for needle biopsy.

Due to the lack of body fat in a child, ultrasound visibility is usually very good, making it an attractive option but the margin of error is smaller, and the risk of collateral damage is substantially higher as critical structures are often very close. It is better to use a co-axial system for biopsy to avoid puncturing the organ multiple times to obtain an adequate sample [1]. The co-axial system also allows for plugging of the tract with gel foam to reduce bleeding risks (Fig. 27.1). The interventionist should be well-versed with the hardware and know about the throw length and cutting length of the needle [2]. An FNAC with better safety but inferior diagnostic yield should be considered for high-risk lesions.

Biopsy samples obtained with radiological guidance have been shown to reach a definitive diagnosis with high diagnostic yield and low complication rates [3–5].

Biopsy material should be correctly labeled and sent for appropriate analysis. It is a good practice to discuss with the referring team before the procedure what samples are required for analysis.

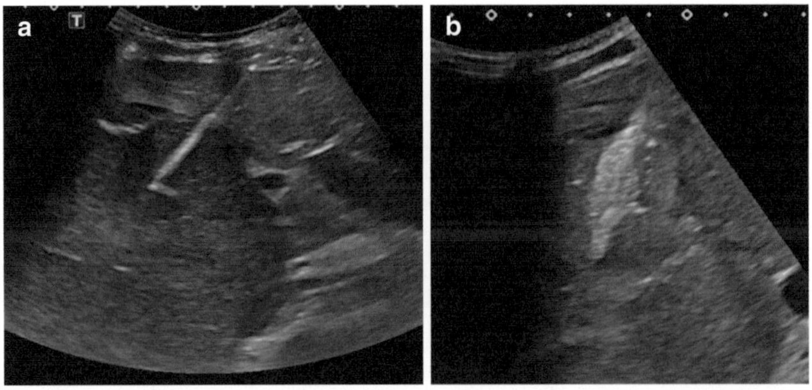

Fig. 27.1 (**a**) Ultrasound-guided liver biopsy using co-axial system in a 8-year-old boy. (**b**) Gelfoam plugging of the tract

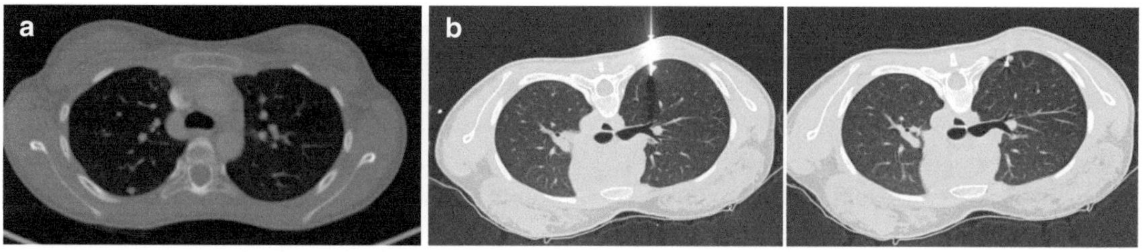

Fig. 27.2 (**a**) Sub-centimetric lung nodule in a 13-year-old girl with metastatic paraganglioma. (**b**) Needle placement followed by coil localization under CT guidance

27.3.2 Tumor Localization

In some specific situations, it is essential to mark a lesion preoperatively to be able to successfully identify it and avoid either insufficient excision or excessive removal of healthy tissue. Localization of the tumors intraoperatively can be challenging either due to deep location or non-solid presentation (e.g., ground glass opacity). IR-guided localization techniques can help these surgeries. Under image guidance, a needle is advanced into the lesion, quite similar to a biopsy. Localization then can be performed with injection of methylene blue or short coils placed through the needle (Fig. 27.2). Radio-opaque metallic markers (such as micro coils and fiducial markers) may also be placed to help localization of the tumor for SBRT (stereotactic body radiotherapy) [6].

27.4 Therapeutic Applications

27.4.1 Percutaneous Drainage

27.4.1.1 Image-Guided Drains

These are some of the most performed procedures in pediatric IR. Drainage can be performed on almost all organ systems. Indications for drainage include abscesses, hematomas, and post-surgical collections. Techniques of drainage are similar to adult drainage procedures other than the need for anesthesia, small catheters, conservative radiation exposure, and close monitoring of vital signs and fluid balance following the procedure. The choice of which type of imaging is used for guidance can be based on the highest likelihood of success and radiation exposure. It is important to avoid transgressing solid organs while placing a drain. In the absence of a direct window, transhepatic or transgastric access may be used.

Drainages are performed with Seldinger technique using an 18G needle for access followed by serial dilatation and drain insertion over an 035″ wire. In hard-to-access targets, a micropuncture needle (21G) with an 018″ wire can be used, which can be upsized for an 035″ wire to place the drain. Pigtail catheters are preferred for most drainage procedures.

Drains should be fixed with sutures and adequate dressing as children may tend to pull them out. Daily rounds for these patients are paramount to monitor drain output, infection, dislodgement, and pericatheter leak. The patient and relatives may have to be counseled for positional drainage to obtain adequate clearing up of the collection. The drain may be removed if the output is <10 mL/day and if the collection has resolved.

27.4.2 Percutaneous Nephrostomy

Percutaneous nephrostomy is performed to relieve urinary tract obstruction and decompression of an infected urinary tract. The kidneys have a higher risk of bleeding as compared to other solid organs. It is wise to make sure that patients' coagulation profile is within normal limits. The interventional procedure can be performed solely on ultrasound guidance in a grossly dilated system, and a combined US and fluoroscopic guidance for other procedures. The patient can be positioned prone or lateral decubitus position. Access to the system is always under ultrasound guidance. An attempt should be made to enter the renal capsule only once and to avoid inadvertent transgression of the colon on the way to the kidney. In a grossly dilated system, an 18G access may be taken, but for mildly dilated systems we use a Neff set (Neff Percutaneous Access Set, Cook Medical). Brodel's avascular line is a zone of relative avascularity at the junction of the anterior two-thirds and posterior one-third of the kidney. The ideal nephrostomy can be targeted at this avascular zone to minimize vascular complications. However, the operator may target other areas to successfully establish access. A direct tract to access the renal pelvis without transgressing the renal parenchyma should be avoided at all costs.

27.4.3 Percutaneous Biliary Interventions

Percutaneous biliary interventions are essential in managing biliary obstructions in pediatric oncology patients. Obstructions can arise due to primary hepatic tumors, metastatic disease, or because of complications from surgical or chemotherapy treatments. Indications to perform biliary interventions include providing relief of obstruction to reduce bilirubin levels and reduce symptoms of raised bilirubin. Careful review and assessment of the site of obstruction by cross-sectional imaging is crucial for planning the procedure. The drains should be planned to maximize the amount of drainage. Putting a drain in type 4 Bismuth-Corlette obstruction may not significantly reduce bilirubin levels due to non-communication of the dilated biliary segments. These procedures are done using combined ultrasound and fluoroscopic guidance with access to the biliary tree established preferably by ultrasound guidance. The initial puncture is performed using a 22G Chiba needle (Cook medical) which allows an 018″ wire. A co-axial dilator system (Neff Percutaneous Access Set, Cook Medical) is used to access the biliary system which allows upsizing to a 035″ system. An 8-12Fr drain is then placed making sure the holes of the drainage catheter are within the biliary system.

27.4.4 Ablation of Tumors

Generally, ablation is performed in well-localized tumors/metastasis. Advantages of ablation procedures include low morbidity and mortality of the procedures, relatively low cost, easily repeatable, and minimally invasive techniques. This technique involves the destruction of tumor tissue using extreme temperatures, electrical currents, or chemical agents and is usually performed using imaging guidance such as ultrasound or CT. Patient selection for ablation is best done after a multidisciplinary meeting. Usually, ablations are performed for lesions that are not amenable to surgery or those that recur after surgery. Ablations can be performed in nearly all organ systems, common indications for ablation are metastatic or primary hepatic lesions, lung metastasis, and musculoskeletal metastasis (Fig. 27.3). The most commonly performed ablative methods are RFA (radiofrequency ablation) and MWA (microwave ablation), newer modalities like

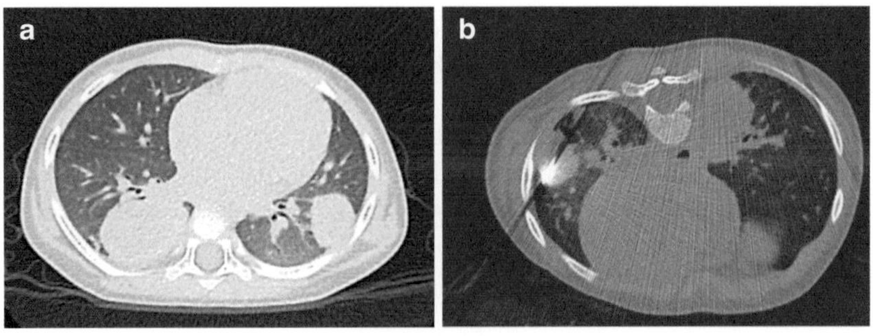

Fig. 27.3 (**a**) Lung metastasis from a Wilms tumor in a 2-year-old girl. (**b**) Microwave ablation probe placed under CT guidance

cryoablation and IRE (irreversible electroporation) have some specific applications but are not widely available [7, 8].

The procedure is performed under general anesthesia. Imaging guidance is crucial for the precise targeting of the tumor and avoiding damage to surrounding healthy tissues. A probe is inserted through the skin and guided to the tumor site, where the ablation energy is delivered to destroy the tissue. It is vital to calculate the ablation zone to keep in mind nearby vital structures. Planning of needle placement should be done in such a way as to maximize the amount of tumor ablation with minimal collateral damage.

27.4.5 Osteoid Osteoma Ablation

Osteoid osteoma is a benign bone tumor commonly affecting the long bones and infrequently the vertebrae. They are seen typically affecting males in the second decade. The typical radiographic appearance is a small lytic focus with a central sclerotic nidus and sclerosis of the surrounding bone. These have a classical clinical presentation of pain at night which is relieved by salicylates (oral medication). CT imaging is the modality of choice for the diagnosis of this lesion and helps in the planning of treatment. CT-guided thermal ablation is the treatment of choice for these lesions. Pre-procedure and post-procedure VAS (visual analog score) are recorded and are used as a marker of successful ablation. In case of complete resolution of pain, repeat post-procedure imaging may not be necessary.

Access to the lesion is obtained using a bone biopsy needle with manual screwing or with the help of an electric drill. Once inside the lesion, the biopsy needle is exchanged for an ablation probe using the back end of a short Amplatz wire and a peel-away sheath [9, 10]. It is ideal to place the needle in the center of the lesion to achieve complete ablation of the tumor (Fig. 27.4). Larger lesions may be divided into two and ablated twice with overlapping ablation zones. For ablation of osteoid osteomas in weight-bearing bones, the patients are advised to avoid weight-bearing on the treated limb with the help of crutches for 4–6 weeks. Complications are rare and include recurrence of lesions due to inadequate ablation, osteomyelitis, and nerve damage.

27.4.6 Pain Management

IR plays a crucial role in managing pain for pediatric oncology patients, offering minimally invasive techniques that provide relief when conventional pain management strategies are inadequate.

Peripheral nerve blocks are used when systemic analgesics (the first line of treatment) are ineffective due to significant side effects. Peripheral nerve blocks offer a focused approach by administering local anesthetic agents combined with corticosteroids, near the peripheral nerves to achieve targeted pain relief. This technique provides effective pain relief while minimizing the systemic side effects associated with other forms of analgesia.

Sympathetic nerve blocks are a type of interventional procedure used to manage pain when the pain is related to the sympathetic nervous system. Sympathetic blockade with local anesthetic

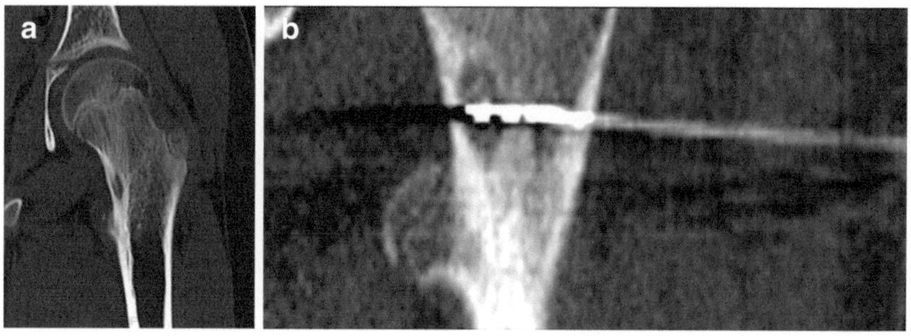

Fig. 27.4 (**a**) Typical osteoid osteoma in the femur of a 13-year-old boy. (**b**) Microwave ablation probe placed in the nidus under CT guidance

agents is used diagnostically to evaluate if the pain is sympathetically mediated. Once the block is proven effective, the use of chemical neurolysis with alcohol or thermal ablative modalities may provide a longer-lasting effect. If successful, these procedures may significantly reduce or in some cases eliminate the need for opioid therapy.

The celiac plexus innervates the foregut and midgut, and blocking this plexus can provide significant pain relief, particularly for malignancies affecting these organs. The superior hypogastric plexus, which innervates the hindgut structures and pelvic organs, can be targeted for blockade to treat persistent or intractable pelvic and rectal pain that has not responded to conservative treatments. Additionally, the ganglion impar, responsible for innervating the distal structures of the pelvis, can be blocked to alleviate pain associated with malignant conditions of the vulva, rectum, and anus, as well as intractable sacral and perineal pain caused by malignancy.

Vertebral compression fractures in some patients can be a source of intractable pain. Vertebroplasty is a technique in which medical-grade bone cement is injected into the collapsed vertebrae under fluoroscopic guidance. This cement hardens quickly, stabilizing the vertebra and providing immediate pain relief in many cases.

27.5 Conclusion

Interventional radiology has emerged as a pivotal field, offering innovative, minimally invasive treatments for a variety of malignancies. It provides effective alternatives to traditional surgery or systemic therapies. By directly targeting tumors and minimizing damage to surrounding healthy tissue, non-vascular interventions not only improve patient outcomes but also enhance quality of life by reducing recovery times, pain, and overall treatment burden. As technology advances, the role of interventional radiology is expected to grow in the management of pediatric oncology patients providing targeted and patient-centered care.

References

1. Roebuck DJ. Paediatric interventional oncology. Cancer Imaging. 2010;10(1A):S27–34.
2. Patra A, Keshava SN. Biopsy with side-cutting coaxial needle – knowing the "cutting length" and "throw length.". Indian J Radiol Imaging. 2021;31(04):933–8.
3. Bondera T, Schubert P, van Zyl A, Pitcher R, Bagadia A. Diagnostic yield and accuracy of paediatric image-guided fine needle aspiration biopsy of deep organ tumours. SA J Radiol. 2022;26(1):2485.
4. Serati L, Morosi C, Barretta F, Collini P, Calareso G, Chiaravalli S, et al. Diagnostic yield and accuracy of image-guided percutaneous core needle biopsy of paediatric solid tumours: an experience from Italy. Pediatr Hematol Oncol J. 2021;6(1):12–7.
5. Mitton B, Seeger LL, Eckardt MA, Motamedi K, Eilber FC, Nelson SD, et al. Image-guided percutaneous core needle biopsy of musculoskeletal tumors in children. J Pediatr Hematol Oncol. 2014;36(5):337–41.
6. Tsoumakidou G, Saltiel S, Villard N, Duran R, Meuwly JY, Denys A. Image-guided marking techniques in interventional radiology: a review of current evidence. Diagn Interv Imaging. 2021;102(12):699–707.
7. Koo KSH, Lungren MP, Aguado A. Interventional oncology for hepatic malignancy in children. Dig Dis Interv. 2019;03(03):193–202.
8. Gómez FM, Aguado A, Barnacle AM, Runge JH, Temple M. Opportunities for interventional radiology in paediatric oncology. EJC Paediatr Oncol. 2024;3:100139.
9. Ahmed M, Keshava SN, Moses V, Mammen S, Jacob KM, Madhuri V. Use of a vascular sheath for introduction of radiofrequency ablation probe during radiofrequency ablation of osteoid osteoma. Indian J Radiol Imaging. 2015;25(04):365–7.
10. Garge S, Keshava SN, Moses V, Chiramel GK, Ahmed M, Mammen S, et al. Radiofrequency ablation of osteoid osteoma in common and technically challenging locations in pediatric population. Indian J Radiol Imaging. 2017;27(01):88–91.

28 Vascular Interventional Oncoradiology

Shoban Haridass and Shyamkumar N. Keshava

28.1 Introduction

Pediatric interventional radiology (IR) is an emerging sub-specialty of IR, which warrants dedicated training to handle complex endovascular procedures. An image guidance is used to perform a myriad of minimally invasive procedures, ranging from simple vascular access to complex interventions in children. Interventions in the pediatric age group vastly differ from the adult population, as various factors like patient selection, radiation protection, vascular access, hardware selection, and drug dosing are to be taken into consideration for a safe outcome.

28.2 Special Considerations in Pediatric Interventions

28.2.1 Patient Selection

Certain pathologies are distinctive in pediatric patients. A pediatric interventional radiologist must be familiar to the spectrum of conditions that are unique to children. An out-patient department with child-friendly environment helps to reduce the anxiousness in children. A tumor in the children causes significant emotional burden to the family, hence an empathetic approach to assess and counsel for the procedure is important. Selection of an appropriate image guidance for the procedure is crucial to keep the radiation exposure at minimal.

28.2.2 Radiation Protection

Children are at higher risk of radiation-induced cancer than adults. This is attributed to the presence of rapidly dividing cells and the longer longevity of the pediatric population as compared to adults. Every essential step must be taken to keep the radiation exposure as minimal as possible. 'Image gently, step lightly' is an awareness campaign that emphasizes the importance of radiation safety and highlights considerate practice in minimizing radiation exposure in children undergoing IR procedures.

28.2.3 Anesthesia

Even for the simpler and shorter procedures, moderate sedation or general anesthesia is required in many instances for the control of anxiety, pain, and excessive motion. A dedicated anesthetist trained in handling children is essential.

S. Haridass · S. N. Keshava (✉)
Christian Medical College, Vellore, India

I. Kumar et al. (eds.), *Practical Approach to Imaging in Pediatric Oncology*,
https://doi.org/10.1007/978-981-96-8158-7_28

Nature of food	Fasting duration prior to GA A (hours)
Clear fluid	2 h
Breast milk	4 h
Formula feed	6 h
Solid	6 h

Hypothermia prevention is important, as children are prone to temperature dysregulation. Preheated blankets and nominal room temperature are used to avoid hypothermia.

28.2.4 Informed Consent

Informed consent is essential part of clinical practice, it helps the patient/parents to make decision in provision of health care. The age limit for providing consent is >18 years in India and this may vary according to the jurisdictions. Commonly, parents or the legal guardian provide consent for procedures in pediatric population.

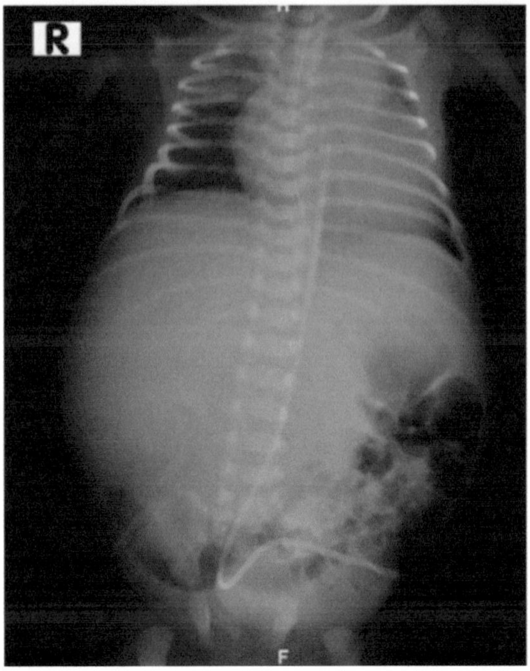

Fig. 28.1 Umbilical arterial access

28.2.5 Vascular Access and Hardware Selection

The common femoral artery is the most commonly used vascular access. Ultrasound guidance and the use of a micropuncture needle (21G) have minimized access-related complications in the pediatric population. In neonates in the first week of life, umbilical vascular access can be utilized for vascular interventions (Fig. 28.1). As dedicated pediatric hardware is not available in most cases, thorough knowledge about the details of the adult hardware is essential when used in children. 'Rule of 5': cranio-cervical vasculature attains almost the adult size by 5 years of age and thus most of the hardware meant for an adult population can be used.

28.2.6 Iodinated Contrast

Iodinated contrast is used in all vascular interventional procedures. The total volume of contrast must be limited to 2–3 mL/kg. For many vascular interventions, this might be a limiting factor. Utilization of small-volume syringes and bi-plane angio-suite allows minimizing the total volume of contrast used.

28.3 Arterial Interventions

28.3.1 Preoperative Embolization of Hypervascular Tumors

Excision of a hypervascular tumor is a nightmare for surgeons. Intraoperative bleeding can be life-threatening. The benefits of preoperative embolization of highly vascular tumors are manifold. Embolization de-vascularizes the tumor and helps in the reduction of blood loss during surgery, aids completion of excision of the tumor, and reduces the duration of surgery and complications [1]. Embolization can be performed via a trans-arterial route or through a percutaneous approach. Polyvinyl alcohol (PVA) particles, gel foam, and liquid embolic agent like glue are the commonly used embolic agents in the trans-arterial approach and glue is preferred in the percutaneous approach. The common hypervascular tumors which require preoperative embolization are juvenile nasopharyngeal angiofibroma (JNA), paraganglioma, hemangioma, hemangioendothelioma, and bone tumors like aneurysmal bone cyst and giant cell tumor. Embolization of intra-cranial tumors like choroid plexus papilloma and choroid plexus carcinoma is also less commonly performed.

JNA is a benign, highly vascular tumor of the nasopharynx seen in young adolescent males [2]. These lesions are epi-centered in sphenopalatine foramen. They can extend medially into the nasopharynx and laterally into the infratemporal fossa. Extension into the paranasal sinuses, orbit, and skull base is frequently encountered. Surgical excision of the tumor is the treatment of choice. These lesions are highly vascular and lack a capsule; hence surgery is associated with a higher risk of blood loss. Preoperative embolization is used to overcome the surgical difficulty. The internal maxillary artery and ascending pharyngeal artery are the common arterial feeders supplying JNA. On carotid angiogram, dense tumoral blush is noted in the corresponding location. Before embolization, it is essential to cautiously look for the aberrant origin of the ophthalmic artery from the middle meningeal artery and ECA—ICA anastomosis to avoid complications like blindness and stroke. Even if there are no obvious ECA-ICA anastomosis visible on angiogram, they always exist. Detailed knowledge about the expected locations of these dangerous anastomoses is important. The arterioles consisting of these anastomoses are frequently less than 100 μm, hence particle size larger than 150 μm should be used. (Fig. 28.2).

Direct puncture of the lesion can be performed through the nasopharynx or percutaneously via

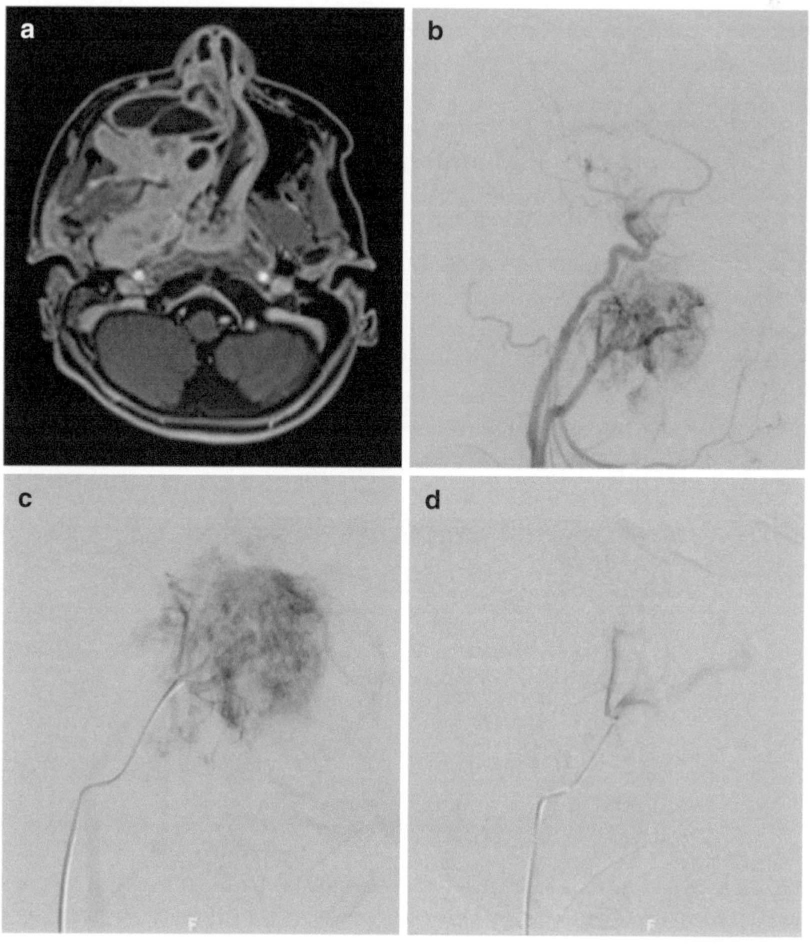

Fig. 28.2 (**a**) Post-contrast MRI—Intensely enhancing mass in left pterygopalatine fossa, (**b**) Tumoral blush with supply from left internal maxillary artery, (**c**) Selective angiogram of left internal maxillary artery, (**d**) Post-embolization angiogram shows stasis of contrast

the para-maxillary, supra, or infra-zygomatic approach. A 21/22G needle is used to access the lesion. Under fluoroscopic guidance, the needle is positioned based on the landmark technique and the location of the tip of the needle can be confirmed using dynaCT. Contrast is injected through the needle to confirm intra-tumoral location and assess the spread of the contrast. Embolization is performed using dilute glue. The percutaneous approach is preferred in tumors with a major supply from ICA branches, and when the trans-arterial approach is technically challenging due to tortuosity of the artery, or when the artery is small in caliber or complicated by spasm or dissection.

In a meta-analysis published by Diaz et al. there was a mean reduction in blood loss of 798 ml in the embolized group. Interestingly in the study, the direct tumor puncture group showed lower recurrence and complication rates as compared to the trans-arterial embolization group [3].

28.3.2 Embolization of Vascular Tumors with Hematological Disorder

The International Society for the Study of Vascular Anomalies categorizes vascular anomalies into vascular malformation and vascular tumors. Vascular malformation is non-neoplastic and arises due to abnormality in morphogenesis. On the other hand, vascular tumors are neoplastic, arising due to the proliferation of endothelial cells.

The most common vascular tumor is hemangioma. Many of these lesions demonstrate an expected growth pattern with an increase in size in the first year of life with involution by the next 5–7 years. Asymptomatic lesions do not require any treatment and can be followed up. Lesions that are symptomatic and those that are associated with hematological disorder mandate treatment. Tufted angioma and Kaposiform hemangioendothelioma can be associated with Kasabach-Merritt phenomenon (KMP) [4]. KMP is characterized by low platelet and fibrinogen levels, consumptive coagulopathy, and elevated D-dimer levels. Though KMP is less common, it can be life-threatening. An established treatment protocol for KMP is not available. KMP is traditionally treated by medical management with corticosteroids or chemotherapeutic drugs (e.g., cyclophosphamide), surgery, or embolization. Not all children show satisfactory results to medical management. Complete surgical excision can be curative, however it is not always possible due to reasons like larger size of the lesion, multi-compartmental extent, difficult anatomical location, and high risk of bleeding. In medically refractory KMP or when surgery is not feasible, endovascular treatment with trans-arterial embolization with PVA, gel foam, glue, or percutaneous glue injection can be performed (Fig. 28.3).

Trans-arterial embolization improved the hemoglobin and platelet count within 48 h and this effect was sustainable up to 6 months in a study published by Jimenez et al. [5]

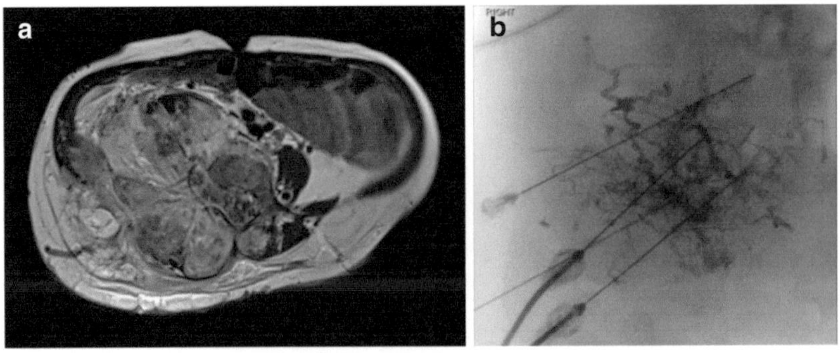

Fig. 28.3 Trans-arterial embolization in a 3-month-old child with biopsy-proven kaposiform hemangioendothelioma with Kasabach-Meritt phenomenon. (**a**) MRI abdomen—T2-weighted imaging shows a large multi-compartmental lesion in right lumbar region. (**b**) Direct tumoral puncture and glue injection

28.3.3 Hemostatic Arterial Embolization

The clinical presentation of a tumoral bleed ranges from mild, self-limiting event to a major catastrophic episode mandating a timely intervention. With the increasing incidence and prevalence of cancer, footfall in the casualty department owing to emergency indications among cancer patients has shown an uprising trend [6].

Various etiologies of the tumoral bleed include spontaneous rupture of the tumor, mostly owing to its rapid growth, neo-angiogenesis, and rupture of the fragile vessels, tumor-induced coagulopathy, and erosion of the adjacent vessels [7]. They can also be iatrogenic: anticoagulation or chemotherapy-induced, rupture of vessels following radiotherapy, and bleeding after biopsy or surgery. In such cases, a CT scan reveals active extravasation from the tumor or indirect signs like pseudo aneurysm, sentinel clot sign adjacent to the tumor, hemoperitoneum, or spasm of the feeding vessel can be seen. Hemostatic embolization is a minimally invasive endovascular technique to control bleeding which aims to occlude the bleeding vessel or devascularize the tumor at the expected site of rupture. Embolic agents like PVA particles, gel foam, coil, or glue can be used based on the location of the bleed and the nature of the vessel (Fig. 28.4). Covered stenting might be required in case of tumor-induced erosion of a vessel which cannot be sacrificed.

Biopsy of the tumor is essential to identity the nature of the lesion. They also play an important role in identification of the genetic background, staging, and assessment of response to therapies. Tumor with increased vascularity has a propensity to bleed following biopsy. Steps to prevent bleeding like correction if the coagulation profile is deranged, utilization of ultrasound guidance for real-time sampling, co-axial needle technique to avoid piercing of the tumoral capsule several times, and plugging the biopsy tract with gel foam must be adopted.

28.3.4 Trans-arterial Chemo-Embolization for Tumors

Systemic chemotherapy has multiple side effects due to widespread dissemination of chemotherapeutic agents into systemic circulation. Trans-arterial chemoembolization (TACE) delivers chemotherapeutic agents directly into the tumor via the feeding arteries, hence the systemic concentration of the drug is lower, maintaining high intra-tumoral drug concentration. Also, the dwell time of intra-tumoral chemotherapeutic agent increases up to 25% as a result of occlusion of feeding arteries [8]. TACE is well established in adult patients, however in children the data available is scarce.

Hepatocellular carcinoma (HCC) in pediatric population is less common as compared to adults and only one-third are associated with chronic liver disease in children. Risk factors for pediatric HCC include hereditary disorders like tyrosinemia, alpha 1 anti-trypsin deficiency,

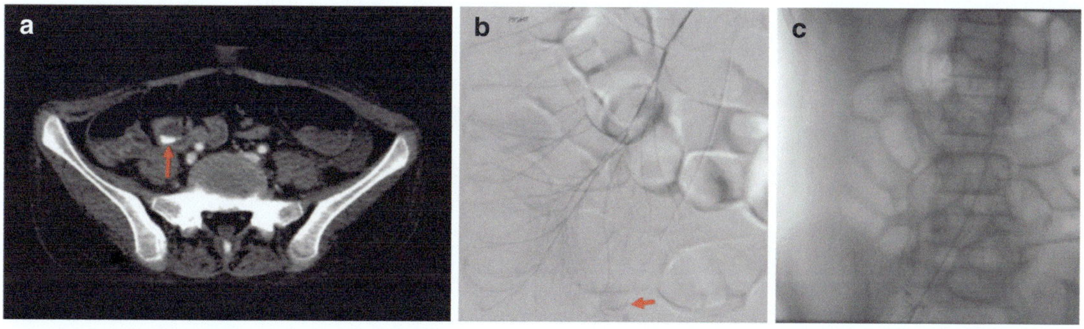

Fig. 28.4 Hemostatic arterial embolization of lower GI bleed in a child with extra nodal NK/T cell lymphoma with secondary hemophagocytic lymphohistiocytosis. (**a**) Active contrast extravasation in terminal ileum, (**b**) superior mesenteric angiogram confirms active extravasation (red arrow), (**c**) post-embolization glue cast noted

congenital biliary atresia, and primary biliary cirrhosis [9]. Resection of the tumor is the standard treatment option for pediatric HCC. TACE is indicated in unresectable tumors, which aids in down-staging the tumor and making them amenable for resection/bridging therapy prior to transplantation/palliative in case of extensive disease. Contraindications include decompensated chronic liver disease, invasion of main portal vein, severe cardiac disease, hepatic encephalopathy, renal failure, and uncorrectable coagulopathy. MRI is preferred over CT scan in children for pre-procedure evaluation of the disease extent. Doxorubicin (up to 50 mg) is one of the commonly used drugs for TACE in HCC. In a retrospective study performed by Weiss et al. TACE was performed in 8 patients with unresectable HCC. 6 out of 8 patients underwent transplantation with a mean interval of 141 days. Two patients died of progressive disease [10]. Similar to HCC, hepatoblastoma is also primarily supplied by hepatic arteries, TACE in unresectable hepatoblastoma is a safe and effective treatment option with similar intent [11].

Retinoblastoma (RB) is the most common intra-ocular malignancy in childhood. They are frequently diagnosed before 4 years of age. They can be sporadic or secondary to germline mutation involving the RB1 gene (chromosome 13). International Intraocular Retinoblastoma Classification categorizes RB into groups A-E. Cryotherapy, laser ablation, and intravenous chemotherapy are traditionally used treatment options for RB based on the staging. Trans-arterial chemo-embolization (TACE) is a well-established endovascular treatment option in the management of retinoblastoma [12]. TACE for retinoblastoma is indicated as a primary treatment option in patients with group B-D unilateral disease and group D-E bilateral disease (Fig. 28.5).

Mephalan (3–7.5 mg) is the most commonly used chemotherapeutic agent, and other less commonly used drugs are carboplatin and topotecan. The tip of the microcatheter is advanced preferably into the retinal branch of the ophthalmic artery, and the chemotherapeutic agent is delivered slowly. The retinal branch can be confirmed by the presence of a choroidal blush on the angiogram. If the ophthalmic artery is not visualized on an internal carotid angiogram, the internal maxillary artery must be evaluated for aberrant origin of the ophthalmic artery (Fig. 28.6). Peri-orbital edema and conjunctival chemosis are the commonly observed self-resolving complications after TACE. Major complications like stroke and blindness can occur rarely.

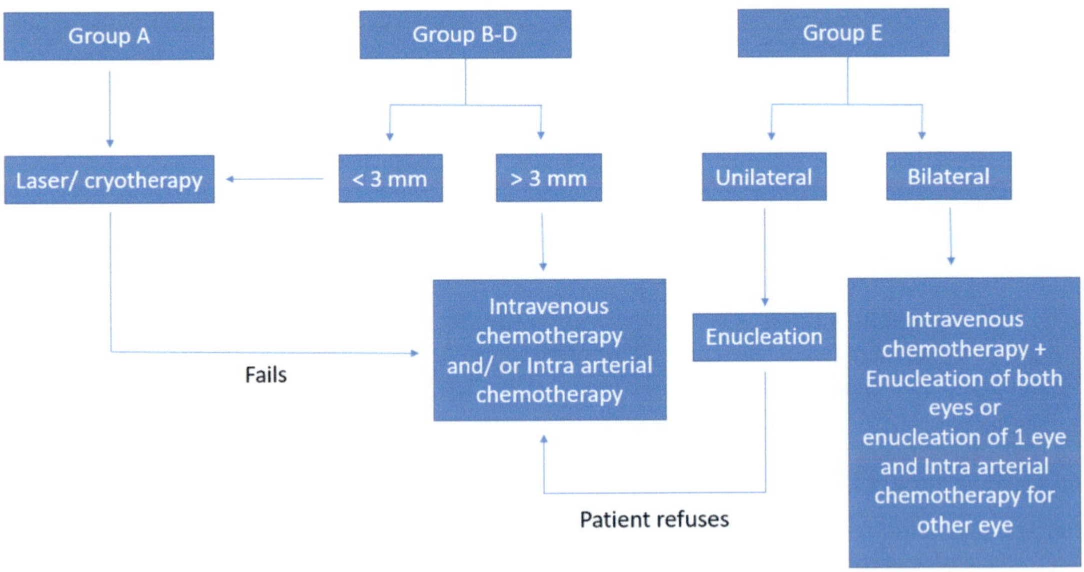

Fig. 28.5 Treatment algorithm in the management of intraocular retinoblastoma

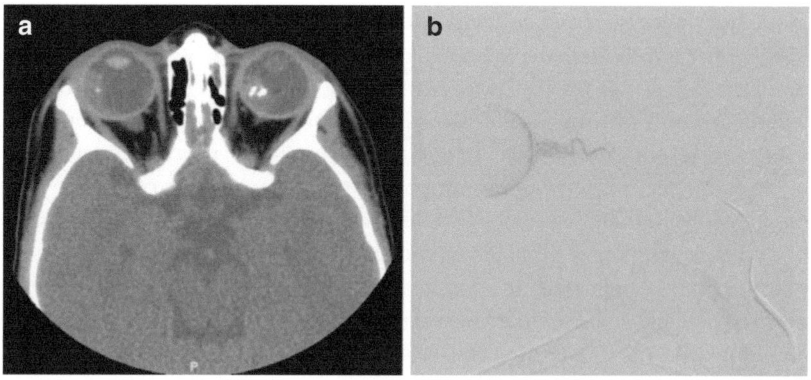

Fig. 28.6 (**a**) Bilateral retinoblastoma in a 3-year-old child, (**b**) selective cannulation of retinal branch of right ophthalmic artery for chemo-embolization (choroidal blush is noted)

Castela et al. in their study performed 130 intra-arterial chemotherapy procedures in 28 eyes. The mean survival without recurrence was 84.2% in the primary group vs 66.7% in the secondary group. Three patients had permanent adverse effects like cataract, vitreous hemorrhage, and choroidal ischemia [13].

28.4 Complications Specific to Arterial Interventions in Tumor and its Management

1. *Post-embolization syndrome*—It is a frequently encountered adverse event following trans-arterial embolization, characterized by fever, nausea, vomiting, and abdominal pain. It occurs as a result of inflammatory response to the necrotic tissue. They usually occur within first 3 days and are self-limiting. The management is conservative, mainly focusing on symptomatic management with analgesics, anti-emetic, and steroids.
2. *Tumor lysis syndrome (TLS)*—TLS is a rare but potentially lethal complication of trans-arterial embolization. They are frequently seen with hematological malignancies following initiation of chemotherapy. The diagnosis is mainly based on lab values, characterized by hyperuricemia, hyperkalemia, hyperphosphatemia, and hypocalcemia with or without acute renal failure. Early diagnosis and management can help to prevent untoward consequences.

28.5 Venous Interventions

28.5.1 Non-tunneled Vascular Catheter Placement

Vascular access is one of the most commonly performed IR procedures in the pediatric age group. Accessing the vessel in the pediatric age group is challenging due to the small caliber of the vessel and the less cooperative nature of the child. Examples of non-tunneled vascular catheters in children are the central line and PICC line (Peripherally Inserted Central Catheter). The central line catheter placement is indicated in children with difficult peripheral venous access, those requiring vasopressor support, and parenteral nutrition. The internal jugular vein is the most commonly accessed vein for central line placement. PICC line catheter placement is indicated in patients requiring long-term intravenous antibiotics. The right or left basilic vein is punctured with a micropuncture needle and a 3 or 4F catheter is placed.

28.5.2 Tunneled Vascular Catheter Placement

Hickman and chemo port are examples of tunneled vascular catheters. The main advantage of the currently available tunneled venous catheter is the presence of a dacron cuff that is placed in the subcutaneous tunnel. The cuff is placed 2–3 cm away from the skin exit point of the catheter. The cuff acts as a barrier in preventing ascending infection from the exit point. In similarity with non-tunneled catheters, the internal jugular vein is commonly accessed. From the technical point of view, under ultrasound guidance, the in-plane technique is utilized in tunneled catheter placement as opposed to an off-plane technique in non-tunneled catheter placements. Hickman catheter and chemo port placement are indicated in children requiring plasmapheresis or bone marrow transplantation and long-term chemotherapy, respectively.

The main advantage of chemo port insertion is the avoidance of frequent peripheral venous access which leads to thrombophlebitis and skin discoloration due to the toxic nature of the chemotherapeutic drugs. The Huber needle is a type of right-angled, non-coring needle that is used to access the silicon diaphragm of the chemo port. Chemo ports carry a lesser chance of infection as compared to other tunneled catheters due to the nature of absence of any external component. The tip of the catheter is placed at the junction of the superior vena cava and right atrium or upper one-third of the right atrium.

28.6 Complications Specific to Venous Interventions in Tumor and its Management

1. *Infection*—Catheter-related infections (CRI) are common in onco-patients as a result of immuno-suppression. CRI includes exit site infection, tunnel infection, and bacteremia. Strict sterility during procedure must be adhered to prevent such occurrence. Septicemia is associated with significant morbidity and mortality in these patients. There is no consensus regarding the prophylactic role of usage of pre- or intra-procedure antibiotics. Main stay of management includes antibiotics. Patients that are refractory to medical management require catheter removal.
2. *Catheter malfunction*—One of the most common adverse events after catheter placement is malfunction. This can be due to thrombus at the catheter tip or fibrin sheath. Linogram/venogram helps to identity the abnormity. Catheter tip thrombus requires anti-coagulation or intra-catheter thrombolytic infusion. Fibrin sheath at the tip of chemo-port catheter acting as a one-way valve does not commonly require any treatment as it doesn't affect infusion of chemotherapeutic agents into the vascular system.
3. *Pleural or vascular injury*—Inadvertent injury to adjacent structures like carotid or subclavian artery and pleura can result in hematoma formation/other forms of vascular injury or pneumo/hemothorax, respectively. Management of vascular injury varies based on its nature.

References

1. Ashour R, Aziz-Sultan A. Preoperative tumor embolization. Neurosurg Clin N Am. 2014;25(3):607–17.
2. Giorgianni A, Molinaro S, Agosti E, Terrana AV, Vizzari FA, Arosio AD, et al. Twenty years of experience in juvenile nasopharyngeal Angiofibroma (JNA) preoperative endovascular embolization: an effective procedure with a low complications rate. J Clin Med. 2021;10(17):3926.
3. Diaz A, Wang E, Bujnowski D, Arimoto R, Armstrong M, Cyberski T, et al. Embolization in juvenile nasopharyngeal Angiofibroma surgery: a systematic review and meta-analysis. Laryngoscope. 2023;133(7):1529–39.
4. Sun X, Xu M, Lv K, Ma X, Wu L, Ouyang T. Comprehensive therapy for infant vascular tumor associated with Kasabach–Merritt phenomenon—single-center primary experience. Front Pediatr. 2022;10:924422.
5. Celis-Jiménez A, Meza-López AS, Santana-Cárdenas CL, Cortés-Barrios DG, Requena-Torres BG, Tiznado-García HM. Management of Kasabach–Merritt phenomenon with transarterial embolization in patients with kaposiform hemangioendothelioma: case series. J Vasc Anom. 2021;2(3):e014.
6. Sung H, Ferlay J, Siegel RL, Laversanne M, Soerjomataram I, Jemal A, et al. Global cancer statistics 2020: GLOBOCAN estimates of incidence and mortality worldwide for 36 cancers in 185 countries. CA Cancer J Clin. 2021 May;71(3):209–49.
7. Revel-Mouroz P, Mokrane FZ, Collot S, Chabbert V, Rousseau H, Meyrignac O, et al. Hemostastic embolization in oncology. Diagn Interv Imaging. 2015;96(7–8):807–21.
8. West HJ, Jin JO. Transarterial chemoembolization. JAMA Oncologia. 2015;1(8):1178.

9. Varol Fİ. Pediatric hepatocellular carcinoma. J Gastrointest Cancer. 2020 Dec;51(4):1169–75.
10. Weiss KE, Sze DY, Rangaswami AA, Esquivel CO, Concepcion W, Lebowitz EA, et al. Transarterial chemoembolization in children to treat unresectable hepatocellular carcinoma. Pediatr Transplant. 2018;22(4):e13187.
11. Yang T, Yang J, Tan T, Pan J, Hu C, Li J, et al. Cure of hepatoblastoma through transcatheter arterial chemoembolization. Glob Pediatr Health. 2017;4:2333794X17742750.
12. Management of intraocular retinoblastoma: ICMR consensus guidelines | Indian J Pediatr [Internet]. [cited 2024 Nov 1]. Available from: https://link.springer.com/article/10.1007/s12098-024-05095-0
13. Castela G, Providência J, Monteiro M, Oliveiros B, Silva S, Brito M, et al. Effectiveness of intra-arterial chemotherapy for the treatment of intraocular retinoblastoma: relevance of a multidisciplinary setting. Clin Ophthalmol Auckl NZ. 2023;17:487.

MIX
Papier aus verantwortungsvollen Quellen
Paper from responsible sources
FSC® C105338

If you have any concerns about our products,
you can contact us on
ProductSafety@springernature.com

In case Publisher is established outside the EU,
the EU authorized representative is:
Springer Nature Customer Service Center GmbH
Europaplatz 3, 69115 Heidelberg, Germany

Printed by Libri Plureos GmbH
in Hamburg, Germany